Atlas of PREIMPLANTATION GENETIC DIAGNOSIS

Third Edition

Edited by

Anver Kuliev, MD, PhD

Svetlana Rechitsky, PhD

and

Oleg Verlinsky, MS

Reproductive Genetics Institute
Chicago, Illinois, USA

CRC Press
Taylor & Francis Group
Boca Raton London New York

CRC Press is an imprint of the
Taylor & Francis Group, an **informa** business

Acknowledgments

We are indebted to our colleagues in the DNA, FISH, and embryology laboratories – Z Zlatopolsky, S Lerner, Y Illkevitch, I Kirillova, T Pakhalchuk, A Goodman, V Kukharenko, and G Wolf – for their participation in acquisition of the data and technical assistance.

CRC Press
Taylor & Francis Group
6000 Broken Sound Parkway NW, Suite 300
Boca Raton, FL 33487-2742

Printed and bound in India by Replika Press Pvt. Ltd.

Printed on acid-free paper
Version Date: 20140124

International Standard Book Number-13: 978-1-4665-9839-3 (Hardback)

Library of Congress Cataloging-in-Publication Data

Kuliev, Anver, author.
Atlas of preimplantation genetic diagnosis / Anver Kuliev, Svetlana Rechitsky, Oleg Verlinsky. -- Third edition.
p. ; cm.
Preceded by: An atlas of preimplantation genetic diagnosis / Yury Verlinsky and Anver Kuliev. 2nd ed. 2005.
Includes bibliographical references and index.
Summary: "Based on one leading center's experience with over 100,000 cases, the new edition of this extensively illustrated atlas provides a detailed manual for procedures and techniques in preimplantation genetic diagnosis. New topics in this edition include mutations, diseases with genetic predisposition, and HLA typing. The book provides insight from authors who are pioneers in some of the procedures described"--Provided by publisher.
ISBN 978-1-4665-9839-3 (hardcover : alk. paper)
I. Rechitsky, Svetlana, author. II. Verlinsky, Oleg, author. III. Verlinsky, Yury. Atlas of preimplantation genetic diagnosis. Preceded by (work): IV. Title.
[DNLM: 1. Preimplantation Diagnosis--methods--Atlases. 2. Genetic Diseases, Inborn--prevention & control--Atlases. WQ 17]

RG628.3.P74
618.3042--dc23 2014001255

Visit the Taylor & Francis Web site at
http://www.taylorandfrancis.com

and the CRC Press Web site at
http://www.crcpress.com

Contents

SECTION II Preimplantation Genetic Diagnosis Illustrated

Preface

Preimplantation genetic diagnosis is currently an established option for couples at risk for producing offspring with genetic disorders. With this option, they no longer have to face prenatal diagnosis and potential termination of affected pregnancies, but may from the very onset plan having only unaffected pregnancies and births of healthy offspring free of genetic disease. PGD can now be performed with an extremely high reliability, safety, and accuracy, reaching over 99% in leading PGD centers. Moreover, because of social or religious reasons affecting pregnancy termination policy in some populations and ethnic groups, PGD may be the only approach in preventing genetic disease and having a healthy child in those social settings.

Since the Second Atlas Edition, there have been dramatic technological developments that have raised PGD to the next level in every aspect, making possible the application of new and more advanced methods. Fluorescent *in situ* hybridization (FISH)–based methods for testing chromosomal aneuploidies and translocations are steadily being replaced by microarray technology for testing all 24 chromosomes. Biopsy procedures are shifting from the cleavage to the blastocyst stage, which seems to have a much less detrimental effect on the viability of the embryo. PGD for monogenic disorders and HLA typing are performed together with 24-chromosome aneuploidy testing in an attempt to improve pregnancy outcome in couples of advanced reproductive age, while preimplantation HLA typing is becoming a realistic hope for couples with an affected child requiring HLA-compatible stem cell transplantation treatment. The number of PGD cycles performed annually is also steadily increasing to as many as dozens of thousands, evidence that PGD has now become an integral component of the current genetics and assisted reproduction practices, changing the traditional concept of prevention of congenital disorders based on prenatal diagnosis and pregnancy termination, and allowing genetically disadvantaged couples to reproduce normally, while diminishing the risk of producing an abnormal offspring.

The current edition presents the data of the world's largest PGD series, while updating the current PGD technologies and relevant information about its accuracy, reliability, and safety. The detailed description of over 23 years of PGD experience of the group that pioneered PGD by the introduction of polar body analysis in 1990, initiated preimplantation HLA typing for the stem cell transplantation treatment in 1999, and first applied PGD for common late-onset diseases with genetic predisposition in 2002 will be of a special value for those who still face the challenge of setting up PGD services in various areas of the world or of incorporating it within existing assisted reproductive practices with the forthcoming increase of requests from a highly sensitive group of at-risk couples. The presentation of one of the world's largest experiences of PGD for HLA typing will clearly promote a wider application of stem cell therapy, which is already a reality for the increasing number of genetic and acquired conditions for which there are still no available treatments. The description of the collection of embryonic stem cells established in ongoing PGD practice is also of specific interest, as it provides the unlimited source and unique *in vitro* model for analyzing the primary mechanisms of congenital disorders.

From PGD services for complicated cases obtained from more than 100 PGD centers from all over the world, the presented data contains the experience of performing PGD for the unique or rare conditions that might not be seen in a single center even during a lifetime. In addition, this edition presents the first systematic experience of PGD for *de novo* mutations that was not possible previously, summarizes the extensive practical observation of PGD for various cancers, reflecting growing public interest, and describes the novel experience on PGD for inherited cardiac diseases, allowing couples carrying genes predisposing for cardiac disease to reproduce without much fear of having offspring with these genes that create the risk of premature or sudden death.

Finally, the current edition describes the first systematic experience of PGD for monogenic disorders and preimplantation HLA typing combined with 24-chromosome aneuploidy testing, which demonstrates an improved reproductive outcome in couples of advanced maternal age. So this edition may be useful as a practical manual for the planning and organization of the relevant component of genetics services and the establishment and performance of PGD within assisted reproductive practices. It may be useful also for assisted reproductive laboratory specialists as well as for reproductive biologists and medical and biology students interested in advanced biomedical research.

Introduction

Preimplantation genetic diagnosis (PGD) is no longer just a research tool, but an established procedure for assisted reproductive technologies (ART) and genetics practices. Dramatic technological developments in the last few years have completely changed the procedures described in the Second Edition of the Atlas, so significant revisions and updates are presented in this Third Edition.

The present availability of the practical experience of over 100,000 PGD cases makes it necessary to completely revise the current relevant information provided to the medical profession and patients on its accuracy, reliability, and safety to support a wider clinical application and improved access to PGD for those who may benefit from this technology. Technological developments have made PGD for Mendelian disorders 99.8% accurate in leading PGD centers, including ours, which has now been applied to over 300 genetic conditions of dominant, recessive, and X-linked inheritance. Our experience is still the largest in the world for monogenic disorders, which provides PGD for any genetic condition when identified in one of the parents or only in the affected child for the first time, even when there are no available family data or relevant haplotypes.

New sections have been added in each chapter describing the new developments of the improved PGD accuracy that may now be achieved in PGD centers worldwide. One of the new sections in Chapter 6 describes the methods for direct and indirect testing for mutations as a universal approach for tracing their inheritance, with special emphasis on PGD for *de novo* mutations, which previously presented a real challenge. As we have the world's most extensive experience in this area, this section presents PGD strategies for a variety of genetic disorders determined by *de novo* mutations of maternal or paternal origin with dominant, recessive, or X-linked modes of inheritance.

The other new section is devoted to expanding PGD indications, with special emphasis on PGD for diseases with genetic predisposition, such as particular cancers and cardiovascular disorders. As this is still limited to leading centers, the description of the available experience of hundreds of cases of PGD for common disorders performed in our center could be useful for developing similar programs in other centers, which have to be prepared to respond to the increasing number of requests from patients with breast or colon cancer, or for inherited cardiac disorders for which there may not be any sign of the disease other than premature or sudden death induced by certain medications or by activities such as excessive exercise.

Since our first description of PGD for HLA typing more than a dozen years ago, hundreds of similar cases have demonstrated an almost 100% success rate of stem cell transplantation to siblings with congenital or acquired bone marrow failures or immunodeficiencies. This updated section draws on this experience to illustrate the possible limitations and failures that will definitely help in expanding this technology for a wider practical application.

Of course, the major breakthrough in PGD has been the development and application of microarray technology for aneuploidy testing, which has fundamentally changed the procedure of testing for chromosomal disorders. New sections in Chapters 4, 5, and 6 describing the methods, problems, limitations, and outcomes of preimplantation 24-chromosome aneuploidy testing by array-CGH and SNP array have been added. This method is compared with data from FISH, which is still a gold standard, despite its very well-known disadvantages. These sections also analyze the basis for the recent controversy in PGD for chromosomal disorders—that of possible damage caused by embryo biopsy at the cleavage stage. This novel experience of shifting from FISH to microarray, and from blastomere biopsy to blastocyst biopsy, is described in detail as a basis not only for improving the testing accuracy, but also for contributing significantly to a positive reproductive outcome.

Much improvement has been also achieved in PGD for translocations, involving not only the traditionally used FISH technique but also PCR-based technologies and the application of microarray analysis, requiring significant expansion and updating of the corresponding section. The current progress in the conversion of the interphase nucleus of blastomeres to metaphase by the chemical conversion method, developed in our center, is also added to the previously described procedures. However, the main emphasis is on the application of microarray technology to translocations detection. Because there is still room for improvement, each case is carefully addressed while highlighting the technical details to be devised to avoid misdiagnoses.

In conclusion, the above brief description of the contents of the Third Edition shows that required updates have been introduced in almost all sections, with substantial revisions in PGD for chromosomal disorders and some monogenic conditions, including those determined by *de novo* mutations and diseases of later life determined by genetic predisposition. Overall, almost all the sections have been significantly revised, with corresponding additional or revised figures and tables.

SECTION I REVIEW OF CURRENT METHODS AND EXPERIENCE IN PREIMPLANTATION GENETIC DIAGNOSIS

1 Normal and abnormal human preimplantation development in relation to preimplantation genetic diagnosis and establishment of embryonic stem cell lines

INTRODUCTION

Preselection of oocytes and embryos with the highest developmental potential, currently based on morphological criteria, is of obvious practical importance for improving the efficiency and standards of assisted reproductive technologies (ART). To date, the available evidence shows that despite morphological parameters being of certain value for suspecting aneuploidy, they are not sufficient for excluding embryos from transfer, although it is known that a significant proportion of chromosomally abnormal embryos fail to reach the blastocyst stage. Thus the aneuploidy testing of oocytes and embryos is required for preselection of oocytes and embryos with a higher chance of resulting in viable pregnancy, which unfortunately is limited to only a small proportion of IVF centers.

Different approaches have been tested for possible prediction of the developmental potential of oocytes, such as pronuclear morphology scoring,[1,2] microtubule and microfilament organization assessment,[3] and first polar body (PB1) grading.[4–6] It is known that over one-third of oocytes obtained from women of advanced reproductive age have PB1 aneuploidies,[7] but because chromosomal studies are not readily available and require specialized expertise, PB1 morphological grading as a potential means for preselection of viable oocytes and embryos for transfer has been studied, since it could be easier to adopt into IVF practice. However, preliminary reports on the utility of PB1 morphology have been controversial, suggesting a positive correlation between well-shaped, rounded PB1 within a cohort and fertilization rates, embryo quality, and implantation rates,[4,5] or no correlation with fertilization but a positive correlation between implantation rates and the presence of fragmented PB1 within a cohort.[6] Moreover, these were retrospective studies in which the chromosomal status of the oocytes and embryos was not actually tested. Thus, the observations on the prospective study of PB1 morphology in relation to fertilization, chromosomal status, developmental potential of the resulting embryos, and the outcome of embryo transfer may still be of interest, as described below.

OOCYTES AT DIFFERENT STAGES OF MEIOSIS I

Current superovulation procedures create a population of follicles that are not totally synchronous in development.[8] Although the preoperative injection of human chorionic gonadotropin (hCG) may induce germinal vesicle breakdown (GVBD), the cytoplasmic maturation of the oocyte may not be complete and appropriate for the initiation of normal embryonic development. A number of ovarian markers have been demonstrated to be useful for predicting the developmental potential of oocytes.[9,10] Immature oocytes are usually retrieved from small follicles and may not have undergone GVBD. Accordingly, the surrounding cumulus cells are well compacted around the oocyte and difficult to remove. Although maturation *in vitro* for a proportion of these immature oocytes in culture and full development to the blastocyst stage can be achieved, the fertilization rate of the *in vitro* matured oocytes and the competence of embryos derived from such oocytes to establish a pregnancy is reduced.[11,12]

The first set of photographs demonstrates the heterogeneity of the oocyte–cumulus complex, which may represent the degree of maturity of the oocytes and their competence for fertilization, as well as the viability of the resulting embryos (Figures 1.1–1.4). As seen from these oocyte–cumulus complexes, obtained in the course of a standard ovarian hyperstimulation procedure, not all of the oocytes may be selected for testing, since detailed examination of the preovulatory oocyte is obscured by the large cumulus mass. Although the stage of maturation can be deduced from the state of expansion of the cumulus mass, the exact stage of maturation cannot be determined without removal of the cumulus cells. In fact, it was recently suggested that the molecular genetic testing of cumulus cells may become useful as a non-invasive way of testing the genetic status of the oocytes (see Chapter 7). Removal of the cumulus cells prior to insemination is not detrimental to fertilization and is performed using hyaluronidase. Information about the exact stage of maturation is obligatory for PGD, since only oocytes with a mature nucleus can be the source of PB1 and subsequently PB2 for genetic testing.

The accurate assessment of oocyte maturity is based on the absence of a germinal vesicle and the presence of PB1. The germinal vesicle in prophase I oocytes is more or less spherical in shape and usually contains a single eccentrically placed nucleolus (Figures 1.5 and 1.6). The germinal vesicle is centrally located within the cytoplasm in early immature oocytes and becomes more eccentrically located prior to GVBD (Figure 1.6). The typical metaphase I (intermediate) oocyte displays neither germinal vesicle nor PB1 (Figure 1.7). The cytoplasm of these oocytes is round and even, and slightly colored or granular. The dynamics of the oocyte's transition from prophase I to metaphase I, revealed by immunochemical staining, is presented in Figure 1.8. These examples illustrate variations of oocyte maturation and possible abnormalities at each of these stages that may influence the selection and availability of material for PGD.

OOCYTES AT METAPHASE II AND VARIATIONS IN FIRST POLAR BODY FORMATION

Despite a small proportion of immature oocytes, the majority of retrieved oocytes have a mature nucleus and are suitable for PGD. The typical metaphase II (mature, preovulatory) oocyte displays PB1, extruded within 36–40 h of hCG injection, which is usually round and non-fragmented, with its morphology differing from oocyte to oocyte.

PB1 is the byproduct of the first meiotic division, providing the material for evaluation of the resulting genotype of the corresponding oocyte following maturation. Therefore, observation of the transition of oocytes from prophase I to metaphase II, as well as the outcome of the second meiotic division, is of special relevance for PGD. Together with analysis of PB2, which is the byproduct of the second meiotic division, the majority of maternally derived genetic defects may be detected, to avoid the transfer of the embryos resulting from the corresponding abnormal oocytes. Neither polar body has any biological significance in preimplantation and post-implantation development, and may be removed and analyzed to investigate the genetic normality of oocytes. It is, of course, possible to obtain the genotype of an oocyte by direct analysis, but this would destroy the oocyte. Therefore, removal and analysis of PB1 and PB2 is the only way for evaluating the genetic quality of oocytes.

Figures 1.9–1.15 show mature oocytes, based on PB1 extrusion, but clear abnormalities are seen. PB1 formation in some of them (Figures 1.12–1.14) suggests possible errors in the corresponding oocytes and their derivatives.[13] Although most of these abnormalities are rare (Figures 1.16–1.19), such oocytes should be rather detected and removed from genetic testing. Avoidance of inclusions of cumulus cells (Figures 1.20–1.26) in the process of PB1 removal is of great practical importance for preventing DNA contamination, which might lead to misdiagnosis in PGD of single-gene disorders.

FIRST POLAR BODY MORPHOLOGY IN RELATION TO CHROMOSOMAL ABNORMALITY IN OOCYTES

Comparison of PB1 morphology with its chromosomal contents was performed on oocytes obtained from 90 patients in 91 IVF cycles for different indications, using a standard IVF protocol.[14] PB1 morphology was assessed in 831 mature oocytes prior to intracytoplasmic sperm injection (ICSI) (day 0) and at fertilization assessment (day 1), and sorted into three main categories: grade 1—a round or oval shape that may sometimes be flattened; grade 2—a non-fragmented PB1 of irregular shape; and grade 3—a partially or totally fragmented PB1 (Figure 1.27). PB1 observation was performed using an inverted microscope (Diaphot, Nikon, Garden City, NY, USA) with Hoffman modulation contrast optics and a magnification of ×200. Prior to ICSI, oocytes were rotated so that both the side and top of the PB1 could be observed. Oocytes were then followed up after ICSI, from fertilization through preimplantation development and embryo transfer. Data on PB1 grading for each oocyte were correlated to fertilization rate, day-3 embryo quality as to the number of cells and the degree of fragmentation, development to the blastocyst stage, and embryo transfer outcome.

Based on differing patient responses to hormonal stimulation, patients were divided into two groups, consisting of 42 poor responders (50 cycles; group I) in which the number of retrieved oocytes did not exceed ten, and 48 good responders (50 cycles; group II) with more than ten available oocytes. The chromosomal status of the resulting embryos was available for 49 patients in 50 cycles in which 395 oocytes and embryos were tested on day 1 (polar body analysis), day 3 (blastomere analysis), or both, using micromanipulation techniques and fluorescent *in situ* hybridization (FISH) analysis as described in Chapter 3.

The overall distribution of oocytes according to PB1 grades on day 0 and day 1 in group I and group II was as follows. The number of oocytes with PB1 of different grades on day 0 was similar and distributed equally in both patient groups. PB1 grading on day 1 revealed the changes of PB1 morphology in both patient groups for each grade category except grade 3. Overall, the grade changes were observed in 331 (36.2%) of 831 PB1, and were similar in both groups I and II. Significant differences for such changes were observed only for the oocytes with grade 2 PB1, 79.1% and 66.3% of which, in groups I and II respectively, became grade 3 on day 1.

Lower fertilization rates were observed for oocytes with grade-1 PB1 (69.5% in group I and 73.6% in group II), compared to grade 2 (85.5%) in group I, and to grade 3 (83.6%) in group II. The cleavage rates of embryos deriving from oocytes with different PB1 grades were similar in each PB1 category for each patient group. The morphological quality of the embryos, with respect to the degree of fragmentation observed on day 3 in relation to the oocytes with different PB1 grading, showed no difference in the three PB1 grades or patient groups, as demonstrated by the proportion of grade 1–2 embryos (little or no fragmentation present), resulting from oocytes with PB1 grades 1, 2 and 3.

Similar results were observed in the potential of embryos to reach the blastocyst stage on days 5 and 6. Of 109 group I embryos, 35 (32%) reached the blastocyst stage of development with 24 (22%) at a gradable expanded stage according to Gardner's criteria,[15] with no significant difference in any of the PB1 grade groups. The same was true for 555 group II embryos, of which 249 (44.9%) reached the blastocyst stage with 148 (26.7%) at a gradable expanded stage, again with no significant difference in any of the PB1 grade groups.

Implantation rates of 317 embryos, grouped according to the oocytes' corresponding PB1 grade from which they were derived, showed no difference, also taking into consideration the embryo transfers consisting of a combination of embryos in which there were two different PB1 grades. The overall implantation rates for group I, group II, and the group of PGD patients were 20.2%, 32.8%, and 22.5%, respectively.

Results of aneuploidy testing in 395 embryos deriving from oocytes with different PB1 grades obtained from 49 patients (50 cycles) of mean age of 37 years showed no differences in aneuploidy rates in any PB1 grade category, which were 75.9%, 65.3%, and 66.4% for PB1 grades 1, 2, and 3, respectively. The data also failed to reveal any difference in the frequency of error for each chromosome tested in relation to the PB1 grade, as seen from examples of normal PB1 morphology and abnormal chromosome pattern, as well as abnormal PB1 morphology and normal FISH results (Figures 1.28–1.31). A higher prevalence of aneuploidy for chromosomes 21 and 22 for all PB1 grades was observed, which is in agreement with the previous findings for women of advanced reproductive age.[7]

The data show that PB1 morphology may not be a useful predictor of developmental potential or chromosomal normalcy of the resulting embryos, whether in good or poor responders. Because PB1 morphology was graded in sequence before and after fertilization, it was possible to detect the grading changes we observed in more than one-third of the oocytes in both patient groups. These changes were significant for the intact, irregular-shaped grade-2 PB1, in which the majority on day 0 became grade 3 by day 1. Although this may be representative of post-extrusion changes, it appears to have no practical relevance, since all the clinical parameters studied showed no correlation with any of the PB1 grades. The relevance of the higher fertilization rate observed in oocytes with the irregular PB1 shape, compared to those with the regular shape PB1 in poor responders, as well as to those with the fragmented PB1 in good responders, is not clear, since these findings conflict with other data. Previous retrospective studies suggested no correlation,[6] or even the possibility of a positive relationship of PB1 morphology with higher fertilization rate.[4,5] These conflicting data may be attributed to the timing of the ICSI procedure in relation to the cytoplasmic maturation of the oocytes.

On the other hand, in contrast to previous reports, there was no relationship of PB1 morphology to the embryo quality and cleavage rate, which makes PB1 grading questionable for reliable preselection of cleavage-stage embryos for transfer. Furthermore, in contrast to the earlier findings of a positive relationship of PB1 morphology with blastocyst formation potential,[4] the prospective data showed no relationship in either good or poor responders. In addition, no relationship was observed between PB1 grading based on PB1 morphology and the outcome of embryo transfer, which was similar across patient groups. This is not in agreement with previous data, some of which suggested higher implantation and pregnancy rates for embryos derived from oocytes with intact, round versus fragmented PB1,[4,5] nor does it agree with another report that describes an association between higher implantation and pregnancy rates and cohorts of oocytes in which a greater percentage of fragmented PB1 are present.[6]

Finally, aneuploidy testing of embryos resulting from oocytes with different PB1 grading failed to reveal any relationship between PB1 morphology and karyotype, suggesting that PB1 morphology is not useful for diagnosing or screening for chromosomal aneuploidies in preimplantation development.

Other approaches have also been tested for possible prediction of the developmental potentials of oocytes, such as a prolonged absence of meiotic spindle birefringence, pronuclear morphology, and microtubule and microfilament organization,[16,17] but they still cannot be used as isolated parameters for preselection of embryos for transfer.

In conclusion, the data provide no evidence for any direct relationship of PB1 morphology or any of the above morphological parameters with chromosomal normalcy, embryo quality and developmental potential, and outcome of embryo transfer, suggesting that they have no prognostic value for the developmental potential of embryos to be used in preselection of embryos for transfer.

OOCYTES FOLLOWING FERTILIZATION AND SECOND POLAR BODY EXTRUSION

The occurrence of normal fertilization is usually assumed from the presence of two pronuclei within the ooplasm observed approximately 12–18 h after insemination and PB2 in the perivitelline space (Figure 1.32). PB2 formation is an important sign of the fertilization process, following exposure of mature oocytes to sperm by conventional insemination or intracytoplasmic sperm injection (ICSI). However, the fertilization process can be delayed, interrupted at any point, or proceed in some peculiar way, as shown in Figure 1.33. In some instances the penetration of sperm leads to premature condensation of the oocyte, eventually leading to premature condensation of the sperm chromatin; with the PB2 maybe or maybe not having been extruded, the oocyte enters metaphase III stage (Figure 1.34). In other cases, one (Figure 1.35), three (Figure 1.36), or four pronuclei (Figure 1.37) are formed. Also, the number and morphology of polar bodies can vary from zygote to zygote. The time of the appearance (usually 6–8 h after ICSI) or disappearance (usually 20–24 h after insemination) of pronuclei and their size and location in the ooplasm can also differ from oocyte to oocyte.[8]

As mentioned, without testing the PB2, the genotype of the oocyte cannot be adequately assessed. PB2 is extruded within the first two hours after insemination or ICSI. Pronuclei may be formed as early as 4 h post-insemination; the zygote is not yet formed at this stage, and is defined as prezygotic (pronuclear stage). Usually male and female pronuclei are still present 20 h post-insemination, so genetic testing of PB1 and PB2 may be completed before syngamy.[18] Technically, this may represent preconception, or pre-embryonic, diagnosis, and thus can avoid the discarding of embryos, which is not acceptable in some populations and ethnic groups.[19]

Pronuclear morphology has been demonstrated to be an important predictive indicator for embryo potential and also may be correlated with chromosomal content of the oocyte and embryo.[1,2] This is in agreement with the fact that the nuclear and cytoplasmic maturation should be synchronized to ensure normal meiosis resumption, fertilization, and cleavage. Any abnormality in formation of the paternal or maternal pronucleus and asynchrony of nuclear and cytoplasmic maturation processes may lead to fertilization failure and irregular cleavage. For example, in couples with severe infertility undergoing ICSI, the poorer pronuclear morphology observed was associated with higher chromosomal abnormalities in the resulting preimplantation embryos.[1] Analysis of pronuclear morphology in relation to the resulting nuclear morphology, polar body alignment, chromosomal status, and the outcome of the transfer of the resulting embryos revealed the relationship between chromosomal abnormalities and embryo quality with only a few pronuclear types.[2] Thus, a possible correlation between pronuclear zygote morphology, chromosomal content, and embryo development may, in the future, provide at least some help in predicting the presence of chromosomal abnormalities based on morphological characteristics and thus in preselecting embryos with higher developmental potential.

NORMALLY AND ABNORMALLY CLEAVING EMBRYOS

Since testing of PB1 and PB2 may provide the PGD option for only maternally derived single-gene and chromosomal disorders, embryo biopsy with blastomere or trophectoderm analysis is the basic approach for PGD of paternally derived conditions, as well as for X-linked disorders by gender determination.[20] As mentioned, the first cleavage of the zygote is observed no earlier than 20 h post-insemination, and cleavage continues every 12–18 h (Figures 1.38–1.45). However, asymmetric or asynchronous divisions can occur, resulting in uneven distribution of zygote cytoplasm, anucleate blastomeres, and fragmentation, as well as slowly developing embryos (Figures 1.46–1.52). One blastomere is usually removed for PGD at the six- or eight-cell stage (Figures 1.53a–d), i.e., not earlier than two days after insemination. For slowly developing embryos, biopsy is delayed, or in some cases their development prohibits testing entirely.

It has also been proposed that two blastomeres can be removed as a means of avoiding the problem of mosaicism in the cleavage-stage PGD for chromosomal aneuploidy, but the deleterious impact of such a procedure seems to be obvious from the outcome of PGD, which has been misinterpreted as a lack of beneficial impact of aneuploidy testing.[21,22] Moreover, the removal of two blastomeres instead of one could definitely reduce the implantation potential of the biopsied embryos to an extent that could not be compensated for even by preselection of aneuploidy-free embryos.[23,24] The point is well supported by indirect evidence from the study that assessed the loss of two cells from 5–8-cell embryos after they were frozen and thawed. It was shown in this study that the loss of two cells impacted implantation potential of the embryos by more than 50%, whereas the loss of one cell decreased it by only 10%, so the loss of implantation potential proved not proportional to the number of cells lost. The embryo biopsy impact can be validated by such cryopreservation data, since these data reflect embryo damage caused by routine loss of one or more cells—a condition similar to removal of cells for PGD. Overall, the potential improvement in ART outcome by selecting against abnormal embryos through PGD should far outweigh the potential damage caused by the biopsy procedure (10%) when only one cell is removed.

As will be shown below, there are limitations to PGD by blastomere biopsy due to the high rate of mosaicism[25–27] and allele-specific amplification failure in cleaving embryos.[28] Complete failure of amplification may be also observed when anucleate blastomeres are removed for testing. As in polar body sampling, embryo biopsy has been suggested to have no deleterious effects on the viability of the embryo,[29,30] although this cannot be completely excluded until more data are collected on the clinical outcomes of PGD at the cleavage stage. Nevertheless, blastomere biopsy remains one of the options for PGD in many centers around the world.

NORMAL AND ABNORMAL BLASTOCYST FORMATION

With the present tendency of *in vitro* fertilization centers to shift from cleavage stage to blastocyst transfer, blastocyst biopsy has come to be of great value for PGD of single-gene and chromosomal disorders.[31–33] There has recently been a clear shift from blastomere to blastocyst biopsy, which appears to be a better choice for microarray-based testing (Chapters 5 and 6). Stages of blastocyst formation are presented in Figures 1.54–1.66, including possible abnormalities determined by morphological appearance and special staining (Figures 1.58, 1.63, 1.64). Without such staining, some normal contracted blastocysts (Figure 1.62) may look abnormal. One of the major advantages of PGD using blastocyst biopsy is based on the premise that trophectoderm cells rather than the inner cell mass could be biopsied to avoid reducing the number of cells forming the fetus.[33] In contrast to cleavage-stage embryo sampling, not one or two, but a dozen cells may be biopsied from the trophectoderm, providing more reliable and accurate analysis.

However, despite the advantage of the blastocyst-based PGD, culturing embryos to the blastocyst stage is a real challenge, the success of obtaining the blastocyst differing considerably in different laboratories. Standardization is clearly needed to ensure an acceptable blastocyst rate. The culture system we have used to improve the success rate of culturing embryos to the blastocyst stage to over 60% of embryos is described below.

ESTABLISHMENT OF HUMAN EMBRYONIC STEM CELL LINES

PGD provides a novel source for the establishment of embryonic stem (ES) cells.[34,35] Although ES cells are usually derived from the culture of the inner cell mass (ICM) of the preimplantation blastocyst (Figure 1.67d–f), morula-stage embryos may also be used (Figure 1.67a–b).[36] In brief, the zona pellucida is removed and the morula placed under a middle density feeder layer to allow cells to outgrow and spread into the feeder layer over the next few days. The passage 0 or primary cell disaggregation is performed with ethylenediamine tetraacetic acid (EDTA) or ethylene glycol bis-2-aminoethyl ether-N,N2,N22,N2-tetraacetic acid (EGTA), and the loose cells are transferred back to the feeder layer to proliferate. Rapidly proliferating colonies are isolated and propagated further. The typical human morula-derived stem cells are shown in Figure 1.67c.

In contrast to morula, the establishment of human ES cells from a blastocyst involves immunosurgery, requiring the isolation and placement of the ICM on a feeder layer (Figure 1.67d). The typical outgrowth of ICM is shown in Figure 1.67e. The passage 0 is performed with EDTA, and the rounded cells are transferred back to a fresh feeder. As seen in Figures 1.67d and 1.67f, no morphological differences between human ES cells originating from ICM and from morula were observed. Nor were differences observed in the pattern of marker expression, including alkaline phosphatase (AP), TRITC immunofluorescence of Oct-4 expression, immunofluorescence of TRA-2-39 (L-AP), TRA-2-60, and TRA-2-80, detected by monoclonal antibodies labeled by FITC antigens SSEA-3 and SSEA-4 (Figure 1.68). The fact that these markers are expressed in the same colony of morula-derived ES cells that are characterized by specific AP expression is shown in Figure 1.69. As can be seen in Figure 1.70, there was no difference in patterns of marker expression in morula-derived ES cells cultured in feeder-layer-free medium.

The established human ES cell lines were maintained *in vitro* from 10 to 15 passages before freezing in sufficient amounts with controlled thawout.[37] Tests for differentiation *in vitro* through embryonic bodies, with subsequent disaggregation and cell culture, showed a wide range of cell types belonging to ectoderm, endoderm, and mesoderm. The cells were also shown to spontaneously differentiate *in vitro* into a variety of cell types, including neuron-like cells with dendrites and contracting primitive cardiocyte-like cells (Figure 1.71).

The current institutional repository contains 87 human ES cell lines, obtained from embryos with single-gene and chromosomal disorders. Fourteen lines have various chromosomal abnormalities, including four with chromosomal rearrangements, one with trisomy 14, one with triploidy, one with trisomy 13, two with trisomy 12, one with trisomy 21, and four with aneuploidy of sex chromosomes (one with 45, X+mar, one with 47, XXX, and two with 47, XXY, one of which was derived from the same embryo that was the source of the hESC line with Emery–Dreifuss (carrier)-type muscular dystrophy). The lines with genetic disorders include 24 with autosomal recessive disorders (10 with beta-globin mutations, one with Fanconi anemia, complementation group A, eight with cystic fibrosis, two with spinal muscular atrophy, and three with Sandhoff disease), 14 with X-linked disorders (one with adrenoleukodystrophy, two with fragile site mental retardation, two with ocular albinism, one with Becker muscular dystrophy, four with Emery–Dreifuss muscular dystrophy, and four with Duchenne muscular dystrophy), and 35 with autosomal dominant conditions (seven with neurofibromatosis type 1, one with Marfan syndrome, three with torsion dystonia, two with tuberose sclerosis, one with popliteal pterygium syndrome, seven with Facioscapulohumeral muscular dystrophy 1A, two with muscular dystrophy, three with Treacher Collins–Franceschetti syndrome, one with familial breast cancer BRCA-2, one with familial breast cancer BRCA-2 together with type I multiple endocrine neoplasia, and seven with Huntington's disease). These cell lines are currently used for research purposes in many countries around the world (RGI, Chicago, IL).[35,37]

REFERENCES

1. Kahraman S, Kumpete Y, Sertyel S, et al. Pronuclear scoring and chromosomal status of embryos in severe male infertility. *Hum Reprod* 2002; 17:3193–200.
2. Gianaroli L, Magli MC, Ferraretti AP, Fortini D, Griego N. Pronuclear morphology and chromosomal abnormalities as scoring criteria for embryo selection. *Fertil Steril* 2003; 80:341–49.

3. Van Blercom J, Davis P, Alexander S. Differential mitochondrial distribution in human pronuclear embryos leads to disproportionate inheritance between blastomeres: relationship to microtubular organization, ATP content and competence. *Hum Reprod* 2000; 15:2621–633.
4. Ebner T, Yaman C, Mose M, Sommergruber M, Feichtinger O, Tews G. Prognostic value of first polar body morphology on fertilization rate and embryo quality in intracytoplasmic sperm injection. *Hum Reprod* 2000; 15:427–30.
5. Balaban B, Urman B, Isiklar A, Alatas C, Aksoy S, Mercan R. The effect of polar body morphology on embryo quality, implantation and pregnancy rates. *Fertil Steril* 2001; 76(Suppl 1):S8.
6. Miller KF, Sinoway CE, Fly KL, Falcone T. Fragmentation of the polar body at the time of ICSI does not predict fertilization or early embryo development but may be associated with improved pregnancy and implantation. *Fertil Steril* 2001; 76(Suppl 1):S201.
7. Kuliev A, Cieslak J, Ilkevitch Y, Verlinsky Y. Nuclear abnormalities in series of 6733 human oocytes. *Reprod Biomed Online* 2003; 6:54–59.
8. Veeck LL. *An Atlas of Human Gametes and Conceptuses.* London, UK: Parthenon Publishing Group, 1999.
9. Van Blerkom J. Epigenetic influences on oocyte developmental competence: perifollicular vascularity and intrafollicular oxygen. *J Assist Reprod Genet* 1998; 15:226–34.
10. Gregory L. Ovarian markers of implantation potential in assisted reproduction. *Hum Reprod* 1998; 3(Suppl 4):117–32.
11. Eppig JJ, O'Brien M, Wigglesworth K. Mammalian oocyte growth and development. *Mol Reprod Dev* 1996; 44:260–73.
12. Smitz J, Cortvrindt R. Oocyte in-vitro maturation and follicle culture: current clinical achievements and future directions. *Hum Reprod* 1999; 14(Suppl 1):145–61.
13. Rosenbusch B, Schneider M. Maturation of binuclear oocyte from the germinal vesicle stage to metaphase II: formation of two polar bodies and two haploid chromosome sets. *Hum Reprod* 1998; 13:1653–55.
14. Verlinsky Y, Lerner S, Illkevitch N, et al. Is there any predictive value of the first polar body morphology for embryo genotype or developmental potential? *Reprod Biomed Online* 2003; 7:336–41.
15. Schoolcraft W, Gardner D, Lane M, Schlenker T, Hamilton F, Meldrum D. Blastocyst culture and transfer results in high pregnancy and implantation rates while reducing high order multiple gestations. *Fertil Steril* 1999; 72:604–9.
16. Van Blercom J, Davis P, Alexander S. Differential mitochondrial distribution in human pronuclear embryos leads to disproportionate inheritance between blastomeres: relationship to microtubular organization, ATP content and competence. *Hum Reprod* 2000; 15:2621–33.
17. Magli C, Capoti A, Stanghellini I, Ferraretti AP, Gianaroli L. Prolonged absence of meiotic spindles by birefringence imaging negatively affects normal fertilization and embryo development. *Reprod Biomed Online* 2011; 23:747–54.
18. Larsen W. *Human Embryology.* New York: Churchill Livingstone, 1994:18.
19. Kuliev A, Rechitsky S, Laziuk K, Verlinsky O, Tur-Kaspa I, Verlinsky Y. Pre-embryonic diagnosis for Sandhoff disease. *Reprod Biomed Online* 2006; 12:328–33.
20. Handyside AH, Kontogiani EH, Hardy K, Winston RML. Pregnancies from biopsied human preimplantation embryos sexed by Y-specific DNA amplification. *Nature* 1990; 344:768.
21. Staessen C, Platteau P, Van Assche E, Michiels A, Tournaye H, Camus M, Devroey P, Liebaers I, Van Steirteghem A. Comparison of blastocyst transfer with or without preimplantation genetic diagnosis for aneuploidy screening in couples with advanced maternal age: a prospective randomized controlled trial. *Human Reprod* 2004; 19:2849–58.
22. Mastenbroek S, Twisk M, Van Echten-Arends J, Sikkema-Raddatz B, Korevaar JC, Verhoeve HR, Vogel NEA, Arts EGJM, De Vries JWA, Bossuyt PM, Buys CHCM, Heineman MJ, Repping S, Van der Veen F. Preimplantation genetic screening in women of advanced maternal age. *New England J Med* 2007; 357:9–17.
23. Cohen J, Wells D, Munné S. Removal of two cells from cleavage stage embryos is likely to reduce the efficacy of chromosomal tests employed to enhance implantation rates. *Fertil Steril* 2007; 87:496–503.
24. Edgar DH, Bourne H, Jericho H, McBain JC. The developmental potential of cryopreserved human embryos. *Mol Cell Endocrinol* 2000 Nov 27; 169:69–72.
25. Munné S, Weier HUG, Grifo J, Cohen J. Chromosome mosaicism in human embryos. *Biol Reprod* 1994; 51:373–79.
26. Munné S, Alicani M, Tomkin G, Grifo J, Cohen J. Embryo morphology, developmental rates and maternal age are correlated with chromosomal abnormalities. *Fertil Steril* 1995; 64:382–91.
27. Delhanty JDA. Chromosome analysis by FISH in human preimplantation genetics. *Hum Reprod* 1997; 12(Suppl):153–55.
28. Rechitsky S, Strom C, Verlinsky O, et al. Allele drop out polar bodies and blastomeres. *J Assist Reprod Genet* 1998; 15:253–57.
29. Hardy J, Martin KL, Leese HJ, Winston RM, Handyside AH. Human preimplantation development in vitro is not adversely affected by biopsy at the 8-cell stage. *Hum Reprod* 1990; 5:708–14.
30. Verlinsky Y, Munné S, Simpson JL, et al. Current status of preimplantation diagnosis. *J Assist Reprod Genet* 1997; 14:72–75.
31. Meldrum DR. Blastocyst transfer – a natural evolution. *Fertil Steril* 1999; 72:216–17.
32. McArthur S, Marshall J, Wright D, de Boer K. Successful pregnancies following blastocyst (day 5) biopsy and analysis for reciprocal and Robertsonial translocations. Fifth International Symposium on Preimplantation Genetics, 2003, 5–7 June, Antalya, Turkey:33.
33. Muggleton-Harris AL, Glazier AM, Pickering S, Wall M. Genetic diagnosis using PCR and FISH analysis of biopsied cells from both the cleavage and blastocyst stages of individual cultured human preimplantation embryos. *Hum Reprod* 1995; 10:183.
34. Pickering S, Braude P, Patel M, Burns J, Bolton V, Minger S. Preimplantation genetic diagnosis as a novel source of embryos for stem cell research. *Reprod Biomed Online* 2003; 7:353–64.
35. Verlinsky Y, Strelchenko N, Kukharenko V, Shkumatov A, Rechitsky S, Verlinsky O, Kuliev A. Repository of human embryonic stem cell lines and development of individual specific lines using stembrid technology. *Reprod Biomed Online* 2006; 13:547–50.
36. Strelchenko N, Verlinsky O, Kukharenko V, Verlinsky Y. Morula derived human embryonic stem cells. *Reprod Biomed Online* 2004; 9:623–29.
37. Verlinsky Y, Strelchenko N, Kukharenko V, Shkumatov A, Rechitsky S, Verlinsky O, Kuliev A. Isolation of human embryonic stem cells from various stages of the human embryo. In Lakshmipathy et al. *Emerging Technology Platforms for Stem Cells.* Hoboken, New Jersey: Wiley, 2009;19–27.

2 Micromanipulation and biopsy of polar bodies, blastomeres, and blastocysts

In addition to standard *in vitro* fertilization (IVF) techniques,[1] four major micromanipulation procedures are involved in preimplantation genetic diagnosis (PGD): intracytoplasmic sperm injection (ICSI),[2,3] polar body removal,[4,5] day-3 embryo biopsy,[6] and day-5–7 blastocyst/trophectoderm biopsy[7] (TEB). The micromanipulation setup and tool construction needed for performing each of these procedures are presented below, with the equipment, materials, and reagents listed in Tables 2.1 and 2.2.

To perform procedures involved in PGD, at least six basic microtools need to be constructed:

- Holding pipette to fix and position the oocyte or embryo during a procedure
- Microneedle to create an opening in the zona pellucida
- Blunt micropipette 15 μm in diameter for polar body removal (PBR)
- Blunt micropipette 35 μm in diameter for blastomere biopsy (BB)
- Blunt micropipette 25 μm in diameter for trophectoderm biopsy
- Finely pulled micropipette 7–8 μm in inner diameter beveled to a 30° angle with the tip pulled to form a spike for ICSI

Three instruments—pipette puller, microforge, and beveler—are used for microtool construction. The first step involves the creation of a microneedle by softening the capillary tube glass by heat and pulling it to form an attenuated tip. This can be done by hand (for the holding pipettes), or by utilizing a Flaming–Brown mechanical pipette puller (Model P-87, Sutter Instrument Co.). The program and heating filament of the mechanical pipette puller are adjusted to give the desired length of the attenuated portion of the microneedle. The attenuated portion of the holding pipette is approximately 2 cm, while the microneedle for partial zona dissection (PZD) and micropipettes for biopsy procedures are approximately 1 cm. ICSI microtools are pulled using a Narishige puller (Model PB-7) in two steps, because of the small diameter (7–8 μm) required and the need for a short attenuated tip of 0.7 cm.

The holding pipette, after being pulled by hand, is prepared by means of the de Fonbrune-type microforge (Model MF-1, TPI Instruments). Under the microforge stereomicroscope equipped with an eyepiece reticule, the tip of the needle is broken to create an opening. This is accomplished by placing the part of the needle 200 μm in diameter on top of the glass ball surrounding the heating filament and increasing the temperature of the filament until the needle is fused to the glass ball. The power is then switched off, to cause an abrupt decrease in temperature and shrinkage of the heating filament, leading to a break in the tip of the microneedle.

The pipette tip is then flame-polished by being placed approximately 0.5 mm away from the glass ball while the temperature of the filament is increased to achieve melting of the glass. The pipette tip is moved away from the heating filament when the opening is almost closed, leaving an inner diameter of 15–30 μm. The attenuated portion of the micropipette is bent by being placed above the glass ball. The filament is heated until the glass begins to soften, so that the pipette tip bends under its own weight (at an angle of approximately 35°). This is done to all microtools so that they are parallel to one another and to the microscope stage during micromanipulation.

A microneedle for PZD is the least complicated tool to create. After a capillary tube is pulled on the Flaming–Brown mechanical pipette puller, the microneedle is simply bent on the microforge, as for all other microtools. The PZD microneedle is not connected to the microsyringe system but is simply installed in a micropipette holder and mounted to the micromanipulator.

To prepare blunt micropipettes for polar body removal or embryo biopsy, the same procedure is followed, except for the diameter of the micropipette and the duration of the flame-polishing. A shorter period with less heat will only smooth any rough edges without decreasing the size of the opening. To construct a micropipette with a particular diameter, after the capillary tube is pulled the newly created microneedle is transferred to the microforge. The attenuated portion of the microneedle is broken with the same steps followed as for the holding pipette, except that it is broken where it has approximately the desired diameter (15–16 μm for polar body removal, 25–30 μm for blastomere biopsy). The tool is flame-polished and bent, as previously described.

To prepare the ICSI pipette, the first pull accomplishes the melting and stretching of the glass to give a tapered tube, while the second accomplishes the attenuation in

Table 2.1 Equipment required for micromanipulation and biopsy

Equipment	*Supplier/Model*	*Quantity*
Laminar flow hood	Holten LFM 24725	1
Inverted microscope	Nikon Diaphot or Olympus IX-70	1
Laser ZILOS-tk	Hamilton Thorne	1
Hydraulic joystick	Nikon-Narishige MO202	2
Coarse manipulator	Nikon-Narishige MN188	2
Mounting adapter	Nikon-Narishige or Olympus-Narishige	1
Microinjector	Narishige IM-6 or IM-16	2
Stereomicroscope	Nikon SMZ-U or Olympus SZH 10	1
deFonbrune-type microforge	TPI Instruments Model MF-1	1
Microforge	Narishige MF-9	1
Pipette puller	Narishige PB-7	1
Pipette puller	Sutter P-87	1
Pipette beveler with power supply	Research Instruments	1
Microtorch	Blazer	1
Micropipette tool holder	Research Instruments	1

which the walls are almost parallel, resulting in a break with a final inner diameter of 7–8 µm. The microneedle is then beveled with a Research Instruments MBI microbeveler at a 30° angle to create a beveled micropipette. The tip of the needle is viewed through a monocular microscope (×400) to ensure proper beveling. Since water is used to wet the grinding wheel, water will enter the micropipette, so the tool is then connected to a syringe to rinse the tip with HPLC H_2O followed by pure grain alcohol, and blown dry by having air forced through it.

The Narishige microforge (MF-9) with compound microscope is used to create a spike at the tip of the micropipette. The spike is necessary for easier breakage of the oolemma when the oocyte is entered. Under a compound microscope (magnification of ×300), the micropipette is positioned so that the bevel faces the operator as it is lowered towards the heating filament, which is turned on by a foot pedal. As soon as the tip of the micropipette fuses with the glass ball surrounding the heating filament, the tool is raised while simultaneously releasing the foot pedal to switch the filament off, resulting in a spiked tip of the micropipette. Finally, the tool is bent with the use of the de Fonbrune-type microforge, similar to other microtools, to obtain the angle necessary for micromanipulations. Microtools are stored in a Petri dish, with clay or foam rubber to hold the pipettes in place to avoid breakage.

Equipment is placed in a laminar flow hood with an immersion heater circulator and a stereomicroscope. An inverted microscope with a stage warmer for fertilization assessment and micromanipulation is also placed in the hood. Special measures are taken to maintain the pH of the culture medium even when working under oil. This can be better controlled by use of gas flow meters that control the passage of the tri-gas mixture (5% CO_2, 5% O_2, 90% N_2) through humidifiers to incubator chambers located on the working surface of the hood.

For manipulation of gametes and embryos, coarse manipulators are mounted to the inverted microscope. The Narishige MO202 fine manipulator (hanging joysticks) provides good control of both the holding and the ICSI pipettes, as well as of biopsy micropipettes. Hydraulic control for all tools is performed using the Narishige IM-6 or, more recently, the IM-16 microsyringe injector. A Stoelting microsyringe (no. 51222) can also be used for holding and aspirating pipettes with a slight modification: the micrometer is connected to the plunger of the 100-µl microsyringe with epoxy to obtain suction. The whole hydraulic system is filled with light paraffin oil, with special attention paid to elimination of any air bubbles. Microtools needed for holding, biopsy, or injection are filled with silicone oil (12,500 centistokes) prior to attachment to the micropipette holders.

Several solutions are required for culture and micromanipulation procedures (see also Tables 2.1 and 2.2):

- Global medium supplemented with Plasmanate (5% volume:volume) or 5% LGPS (Life Global) for oocyte retrieval
- Polyvinylpyrrolidone (PVP) (10%) for ICSI
- Global medium supplemented with Plasmanate (10% volume:volume) or 10% LGPS for embryo culture, "assisted hatching" prior to transfer, and BB or TEB
- Mineral (Cook, Sage, etc.) or paraffin (e.g. IVF Online) oil, sterile and equilibrated, for oocyte and embryo culture and all micromanipulation procedures

Approximately 35 h after human chorionic gonadotropin (hCG) administration, oocytes are aspirated and

Table 2.2 Materials and reagents required for micromanipulation and biopsy

Materials	*Supplier*	*Catalog Number*
35x10-mm Petri dishes (Falcon)	Fisher Scientific	08-757-100A
60x15-mm Petri dishes (Falcon)	Fisher Scientific	08-757-100B
150x15-mm Petri dishes (Fisher)	Fisher Scientific	08-757-14
4-well culture dishes (Nunc)	Scientific Supply	176740
50-ml culture flasks (Falcon)	Fisher Scientific	10-126-1B
0.2-micron filters (1 liter flask)	Fisher Scientific	09-740-26A
Receiver flasks (1 liter) (Nalgene)	Fisher Scientific	09-740-25F
0.2-micron filters (150 ml) (Nalgene)	Fisher Scientific	09-740-31F
Sterile pasteur pipettes (plugged 9 inch)	In Vitro Scientific Products	600-900P
Extra large gloves (powder free)	Scientific Products	2D7853
Platinum wire for microforge (6 in.)	Fisher Scientific	13-766-10A
Drummond capillary tubes (30 μl)	Fisher Scientific	21-170J
Chemicals & Reagents	*Company*	*Catalog Number*
Global culture medium	Life Global	Ref: LGGG-100
Protein Supplement (LGPS)	Life Global	Ref: LGPS-050
HPLC water (Mallinckrodt)	Scientific Products	6795-1
10% PVP for ICSI M.W. 360,000	Fertility Technologies, Inc.	
Paraffin oil	LifeGlobal	LGPO-100
Mineral oil	Sage	4009W
Silicone oil 12,500 centistokes	Sigma Chemical	DMPS-12M
Hyaluronidase	Sigma Chemical	H-3757

collected in HTF culture medium supplemented with plasmanate (5%). Two to three hours after retrieval, oocytes are removed from culture and transferred to a four-well dish with medium containing hyaluronidase (80 U/ml) for 30 s and transferred to the adjacent wells of culture medium for denuding. Usually, within these few seconds, the cumulus cells begin to disperse. After 20 min in culture, by means of an attenuated flame-polished pipette with an inner diameter of 150–180 μm, the remaining corona cells are mechanically removed by pipetting. The oocytes are cleaned thoroughly in order to allow the PB1 to be visualized during micromanipulations. It is also of special importance for PGD of single-gene disorders to eliminate the risk of corona cell contamination. Once oocytes have been cleaned, they are collected into one of the four wells, and their maturity is determined by the presence of PB1, assessed with an inverted microscope. If no PB1 has been extruded, the oocytes are further cultured for possible maturation *in vitro*, which may take an additional 24 h in culture for germinal vesicle oocytes.

To ensure easy maneuvering on and off the microscope stage without having to realign the microtools for each manipulation, micromanipulation dishes are prepared using Falcon 1008 35 × 10-mm Petri dish lids. The dishes are positioned so that the Falcon label is seen at the top. Microdrops of the required medium are placed in the center of the lid at the 3, 6, 9, and 12 o'clock positions and covered with sterile equilibrated mineral oil. Each dish is kept separately by being placed in a larger 60 × 15-mm Petri dish with lid, so that only one dish at a time is removed for a procedure.

FIRST POLAR BODY REMOVAL

To perform PB1 removal, an opening in the zona pellucida of sufficient size is needed. A device for the mechanical PZD, called the 3D-PZD, has been developed, which is a modification of a two-dimensional PZD and enables the creation of three types of openings.[7] A cross-shaped opening is created for "assisted hatching" and a V-shaped opening for embryo biopsy (routinely used). If necessary, a square hole can also be created by four intersecting cuts made in the zona pellucida.

For PGD of single-gene disorders, all microtools are constructed in advance and exposed to ultraviolet radiation for 20 min. The medium can be supplemented with 0.05 mol/l sucrose to cause ooplasm shrinkage, increasing the perivitelline space and decreasing the chances of plasma membrane damage during the procedure (optional). Three 15-μl drops of medium without sucrose are placed at the 12, 3, and 6 o'clock positions and one 15-μl drop of medium containing sucrose (optional) is placed at the 9 o'clock position. The drops are overlaid with the sterile equilibrated mineral oil. The number of prepared dishes is equivalent to the number of mature oocytes retrieved, as a separate micromanipulation dish is used for each oocyte to reduce the chance of DNA contamination.

To perform PB1 removal, a holding pipette with an inner diameter of 15–30 µm is filled with silicone oil and connected to the microsyringe hydraulic system with the micropipette holder. A micropipette of approximately 15–16 µm is filled with silicone oil, and a PZD microneedle is attached to the micropipette holder and the second microsyringe hydraulic system. The aspirating micropipette and the microneedle are mounted onto a modified Leica double tool holder (no. 520143) or Narishige HD-21, and the tools are aligned so that they are parallel not only to the microscope stage but also to one another within the same field.

An oocyte is removed from the four-well dish and transferred to a micromanipulation dish into the microdrop at 9 o'clock. The dish is placed on the microscope stage, the instruments are lowered initially into the 12 o'clock microdrop, and the excess oil is removed from the outer surface of the pipettes. A small amount of medium is aspirated into both the holding and the aspirating micropipettes, to ensure the hydraulic system is easily controlled. The stage is then moved so that the microdrop containing the oocyte is brought into view. Once the oocyte has been secured by the holding pipette with the use of gentle suction, the oocyte is oriented with the microneedle so that PB1 is visualized at the 6 o'clock position (Figure 2.1a). Using the microneedle, the oocyte is rotated horizontally until the polar body is slightly out of focus (Figure 2.1b and c). The slit is made in the zona pellucida at the 4–5 o'clock position, passing tangentially through the perivitelline space and out at the 7–8 o'clock position (Figure 2.1d). The oocyte is released from the holding pipette and held by the microneedle (Figure 2.1e), which is brought to the top of the holding pipette and pressed to it, pinching a portion of zona pellucida (Figure 2.1f). By gently rubbing the microneedle against the holding pipette with a sawing motion, the cut is accomplished and the oocyte is released.

The oocyte is then rotated so that the opening is at the 5 o'clock position and PB1 is in focus (Figure 2.2b); the aspirating micropipette is passed through the opening to PB1 (Figure 2.2c) with gentle suction applied to aspirate the polar body into the micropipette (Figure 2.2d and e). Pressure from the hydraulic system is equilibrated prior to withdrawal of the aspirating micropipette to avoid damage to the oocyte. The oocyte is released from the holding pipette and all microtools are raised slightly before the microscope stage is moved, so that the drop of medium at the 6 o'clock position is visualized (Figure 2.2f).

The micropipette containing the PB1 is lowered to the bottom of the dish and the PB1 is expelled, with careful attention not to scratch the bottom of the dish with the microtool, avoiding PB1 adherence to the dish and breakage during its transfer to the microcentrifuge tubes containing lysis buffer. Transfer is accomplished by a separate sterile, attenuated Pasteur pipette (its tip heated over a microtorch and hand pulled and its attenuated portion broken and flame-polished to a diameter of 40 µm in a de Fonbrune microforge). In a laminar flow hood, under control of the stereomicroscope, each PB1 is aspirated into the attenuated portion of a Pasteur pipette with 5 µl of medium and expelled into the microcentrifuge tube. To ensure that the PB1 was not retained in the pipette, the tip of the Pasteur pipette is repeatedly flushed and examined in the same drop in which PB1 was located, under the stereomicroscope. If fluorescence *in situ* hybridization (FISH) analysis is required, the PB1 is not transferred, but removed from the microdrop at the time of fixation.

INTRACYTOPLASMIC SPERM INJECTION

ICSI is required for PGD for single-gene disorders to avoid sperm cell contamination when performing polar body removal or embryo biopsy. The procedure is shown in Figures 2.3 and 2.4.

On the day of retrieval, after follicular aspiration, micromanipulation dishes are prepared, their number usually determined by the number of mature oocytes retrieved (one oocyte is placed in one micromanipulation dish for ICSI for cases requiring PB1 removal on day 0). The lid of a 35 × 10-mm Petri dish is oriented so that the Falcon label is at the top. Three 10-µl drops of culture medium are placed in the center of a lid at the 6, 9, and 12 o'clock positions and the fourth drop containing 10% PVP in culture medium at the 3 o'clock position. The drops are covered with sterile filtered and equilibrated mineral oil. Also, along with the 35 × 10-mm Petri dishes, individual culture dishes are prepared. Each of these dishes is filled with sterile equilibrated oil, under which a drop (50 µl) of HTF medium or Global medium supplemented with plasmanate (10%) is placed. All micromanipulation and culture dishes are kept at 37°C, under 5% CO_2 and air, until use.

After 4 h from oocyte retrieval the tools (one holding pipette and one ICSI micropipette) are back filled with silicone oil (12,500 centistokes) and connected to microinjectors via silicone tubing and micropipette holders. They are then installed onto the mounted micromanipulators, the left micromanipulator controlling the holding pipette, the right the ICSI micropipette. Under the inverted microscope, tools are aligned facing one another, parallel to the microscope stage, and then raised.

Under the stereomicroscope the washed sperm are added to the drop containing 10% PVP to slow down sperm movement, thus facilitating selection of a morphologically normal sperm for injection. This also minimizes sperm adherence to the glass surface once the sperm is inside the injection micropipette. The micromanipulation dish, containing both sperm and oocytes, is transferred to the inverted microscope stage, and the microtools are lowered into the drop of culture medium at the 9 o'clock position to ensure complete control of fluid in and out of the microtools. The microtools are raised slightly and the dish is moved by use of the mechanical stage to the location of the PVP drop with sperm. The ICSI micropipette is lowered and both sperm and micropipette are brought into focus. A sperm is immobilized by gently rubbing its tail on the bottom of the dish and aspirated into the micropipette tail first (Figure 2.3a and b) by being raised slightly and moved to the drop containing the oocyte. Once the oocyte is brought into focus, the ICSI micropipette containing the immobilized sperm is lowered and brought into focus; once again, the fluid control and sperm movement within the pipette are assessed. Should the sperm become stuck in the micropipette, it is expelled and another sperm is retrieved, or if necessary the microtool is changed.

The holding pipette is lowered, and using gentle suction the oocyte is held in a semi-fixed position (Figure 2.3c and d), so that it can still be rotated to the appropriate position using the ICSI micropipette. The ICSI micropipette is brought to the 3 o'clock position, the outer edge of the oocyte is brought into focus, and the sperm is brought to the tip of the micropipette. The micropipette is guided through the zona pellucida into the center of the oocyte (through the slit opening if PB1 removal has occurred prior to ICSI) and a small amount of ooplasm is aspirated into the micropipette to ensure breakage of the membrane by a slow turning of the micrometer of the microinjector (Figure 2.3e). Once the membrane has been broken, the contents of the micropipette, i.e., ooplasm and the immobilized sperm, are expelled slowly into the oocyte and the micropipette is slowly withdrawn (Figure 2.3f). Complete control over aspiration and expulsion is needed to minimize the amount of medium deposited along with the sperm. The entire injection procedure for each oocyte takes approximately 2–3 min. After injection, each oocyte is placed in its own dish, and fertilization is assessed 16–18 h after ICSI.

FIRST AND SECOND POLAR BODY REMOVAL

PB1 removal after ICSI is performed by the same procedure described above, except for some modifications to avoid the damage of the meiotic spindle during the procedure. Initially, the oocyte is oriented so that the PB1 is seen at the 12 o'clock position (Figure 2.5a). With the use of the microneedle, the oocyte is rotated horizontally until the polar body is visualized directly in the center of the oocyte, facing the operator (2.5b). The first slit is made by entering the zona pellucida at the 1–2 o'clock position and passing tangentially through the perivitelline space and out at the 10–11 o'clock position (Figure 2.5c), and is accomplished as previously described (Figure 2.5d). The oocyte is then rotated so that the opening is at the 2 o'clock position and the PB1 is in focus (Figure 2.5e). The aspirating pipette is passed through the opening to the PB1 (Figures 2.5f, 2.6a and 2.6b), which is removed by gentle suction (Figure 2.6c and d). The oocyte is released and the PB1 is expelled from the micropipette (Figure 2.6e).

The PB2 is removed in the same way as the PB1, except that there is no need for PZD, since the opening in the zona pellucida was created prior to PB1 removal. The zygote is rotated into position so that the opening is at the 4–5 o'clock position (Figure 2.7a). The opening should be in focus when the micropipette is passed into the perivitelline space (Figure 2.7b). Once in the perivitelline space, the PB2 is brought into focus by advancing the micropipette towards it (Figure 2.7c). Using gentle suction, the PB2 is aspirated into the micropipette, and the procedure further continues as for PB1 removal (Figure 2.7d–f). Oocytes are returned to their culture dishes and examined for cleavage after 48 h.

In contrast to PGD for single-gene disorders, in which both PB1 and PB2 are removed separately in sequence, PB1 and PB2 are removed simultaneously for the purpose of PGD for chromosomal abnormalities. The procedure of simultaneous PB1 and PB2 biopsy, demonstrated in Figures 2.8–2.10, is similar to that performed for PB1 removal, except that it does not require the strict precautions for DNA contamination that are necessary when testing for single-gene disorders.

Although PB1 and PB2 are not expected to have any biological role in the development of the embryo, the subject has been explored by following up and evaluating the resulting micromanipulated oocytes at different stages of development.[8,9] No significant decrease in fertilization rate for oocytes after ICSI or in cleavage of the resulting embryos following PB1 removal was observed. The percentage of embryos entering cleavage was similar in biopsied and non-biopsied oocytes. There was also no increase in the percentage of polyspermic embryos. Data on the long-term effect of the procedure, from culturing the embryos to the blastocyst stage, demonstrate that the proportion of embryos reaching the blastocyst stage is similar to that known for non-micromanipulated oocytes. A follow-up study of the viability of the sampled oocytes through implantation and post-implantation development of the resulting embryos also suggested no detrimental effect. As will be described below, the procedure of PB1 removal has already been applied to tens of thousands of oocytes in the process of PGD for age-related aneuploidies and single-gene disorders, and showed no effect on fertilization, preimplantation or, possibly, post-implantation development. Furthermore, no deleterious effect was observed in the follow-up study of children born following PB1 and PB2 sampling.[10]

BLASTOMERE BIOPSY

Embryo biopsy is performed as soon as the embryo reaches a minimum of six cells, so as not to cause a considerable decrease in cell number at later stages of development.

As in PB1 removal, a mechanical approach to open the zona pellucida has been developed, called 3D-PZD, allowing the creation of a V-shaped triangular or square flap opening sufficient in size for a micropipette to pass through in order to remove the blastomere(s).

Micromanipulation dishes are prepared in the same way as for PB1 removal, in that all solutions are sterile filtered and equilibrated prior to use. The micromanipulation setup is the same as for PB1 removal, with two exceptions: the biopsy micropipette has a larger diameter of 25–30 μm, and biopsy may be performed using a calcium- and magnesium-free medium with HEPES buffer supplemented with plasmanate (5%) (optional) to temporarily disassociate tight cell gap junctions in compacting embryos for ease of cell removal. During aspiration the cell membrane may break, so a blastomere with a clearly visible nucleus is chosen so that its aspiration into the pipette can be controlled and the chance of losing genetic material is reduced.

Once a blastomere is chosen, the embryo is rotated so that the blastomere is at the 12 o'clock position (Figure 2.11a). The embryo is rotated slightly, horizontally, and the first slit is made (Figure 2.11b). The microneedle is passed from the 1–2 o'clock position tangentially through the perivitelline space and out at the 10–11 o'clock position (Figure 2.11b). The embryo is released and the first cut accomplished by rubbing the microneedle against the holding pipette (Figure 2.11c). The second cut is completed by entry into the first slit, advancing tangentially through the perivitelline space and ending at the 10–11 o'clock position (Figure 2.11d and e). The embryo is released from the holding pipette and held by the microneedle, and the cut is accomplished as previously described. This results in the creation of a V-shaped opening (see below) sufficient for passage of a 35-μm micropipette to remove a blastomere. If a larger opening is desired, two additional intersecting slits are made, creating a square opening. After the second cut, the embryo is rotated until the new slit is visible at the 12 o'clock position and then backward until the slit is slightly out of focus. The microneedle is passed through the slit opening and perivitelline space and out at the 10–11 o'clock position to make the third intersecting cut (Figure 2.11e). To complete the square and create a hole in the zona pellucida, the final cut is made by entering the first slit and passing through the perivitelline space (2.11f). The procedure results in an opening in the shape of a square, as seen in Figure 2.12a, after removal of the cut-out portion by microneedle. To complete the embryo biopsy procedure, the embryo is rotated until the opening is at 3 o'clock and then held firmly by suction from the holding pipette (Figure 2.12b). The micropipette is inserted (Figure 2.12c) and gentle suction is applied, to aspirate the blastomere slowly into the pipette to avoid breakage and disruption of the surrounding blastomeres (Figure 2.12d). Once the blastomere is aspirated, pressure within the pipette is equilibrated and the micropipette is withdrawn (Figure 2.12e). The blastomere is slowly expelled into the 6 o'clock microdrop (Figure 2.12f) and transferred to the microcentrifuge tube as in PB1 removal for single-gene disorders.

The same procedure is applied for embryo biopsy using a triangular opening in the zona pellucida as shown in Figure 2.13. Slight upward pressure is applied with the micropipette to the triangular flap, followed by insertion of the micropipette to remove a blastomere (Figure 2.13).

As for PB1 and PB2 removal, the follow-up studies of embryos after blastomere biopsy did not show any detrimental effect.[11] No increase in congenital malformation has been reported among more than 1000 children born following polar body or blastomere biopsy,[12,13] although further systematic study will be needed to monitor the clinical outcomes of PGD using PB1 and PB2 sampling or embryo biopsy and to collect further data on the safety of the procedures used in PGD for single-gene and chromosomal disorders.

BLASTOCYST BIOPSY

With the current tendency for blastocyst transfer, a robust method for blastocyst biopsy has been developed,[14,15] which has become a method of choice, particularly coupled with microarray-based 24-chromosome aneuploidy testing.[16–19] As an average blastocyst contains more than 100 cells, removal of 2–10 cells from the trophectoderm is very unlikely to have a detrimental effect on the blastocyst's development and particularly on the development of the fetus originating from the inner cell mass. The major advantage of this method is that a large amount of genetic material is available for testing. Having many cells to work with prevents hybridization and amplification failures. It also prevents misdiagnosis in mosaic embryos that may have both normal and abnormal cells, thereby increasing the reliability and accuracy of the diagnosis.

The procedure of blastocyst biopsy is demonstrated in Figure 2.14 (materials and equipment for blastocyst biopsy are presented in Tables 2.1 and 2.2). As seen in Figure 2.14, trophectoderm biopsy is performed at day 5 of development, when the trophectoderm is beginning to herniate through the zona pellucida. Several trophectoderm cells herniating through the zona pellucida at the opposite side of the inner cell mass are removed by smooth aspiration into the biopsy pipette with an internal diameter of 30 μm. Currently, to break down the tight junctions between trophectoderm cells, three laser shots are applied (with a duration of 0.7 msec pulse with each) (Figure 2.15). In the selection of embryos for blastocyst biopsy, poor-quality blastocysts and those with an early stage of herniation are avoided. While blastocyst biopsy is becoming the major method of choice for PGD, its potential use is also obvious for additional testing required to confirm the polar body or blastomere diagnosis. Detailed description of laser-assisted hatching and blastocyst biopsy is presented below.

The time for the analysis is limited by the implantation window of the blastocyst, which is less than 24 hours. Another limitation is the need for an optimum laboratory setup with culture conditions providing an acceptable rate of blastocyst development. Several culture systems and media have been developed for culturing embryos to the blastocyst stage *in vitro*, involving defined sequential culture media.[20] Sequential media pairs consist of one medium for culture from day 1 to day 3, and a second for culture from day 3 to blastocyst formation. The two media are purported to mimic the *in vivo* environment (oviduct and uterus, respectively) and also to reflect changes in the metabolic patterns of the embryo. However, a special single medium has since been designed (Global medium, which is a modified KSOMaa medium for human embryos) capable of supporting the development of human embryos from zygote to the blastocyst stage.[21]

There are currently three general approaches to the culture of human embryos from zygote to the blastocyst stage: (1) sequential culture with a change from medium 1 to medium 2 at day 3; (2) single medium with 2-step (interrupted) culture with a change to a fresh drop of the same medium at day 3; and (3) single medium, 1-step (uninterrupted) culture in which the embryos remain in the same drop from day 1 to day 5.[22] We used the last approach, with the average success rate of culturing embryos to blastocyst stage of over 60%.

To overcome the time-frame limitation available for blastocyst-sample shipment and genetic analysis, the technique of vitrification of biopsied blastocysts was introduced, allowing sufficient time for transfer of the diagnosed embryos in a subsequent frozen–thawed cycle. It appeared that this approach has also improved implantation and pregnancy rates, which could be also explained by the better receptivity of the uterus in unstimulated cycles. The major advantage of this method is that the embryo has already passed the natural self-correction mechanisms, overcoming the natural errors of the cleavage stage, and thus only persistent abnormalities are diagnosed.

In contrast to the traditional slow-freezing protocols, vitrification is a very quick freeze utilizing a high concentration of cryoprotectants that solidify without ice crystal formation. To perform vitrification, the embryos are placed in a loading device surrounded by a vitrification medium, which is then placed into liquid nitrogen, where it is stored. There are a variety of loading devices available, including the Cryotop, Cryoloop, Cryotip, Cryo-leaf, High Security Straws, and Rapid-i, but success of vitrification, measured by survival, implantation, and pregnancy rates, depends not only on the loading devices used, but also on the appropriate blastocyst selection, media protocol, freezing rate, warming rate, and operator-dependent factors.[23] Our protocol of freezing, which is based on standard Irvine Scientific Protocol with the use of Rapid-i™ Kit (Vitrolife Inc.) as a carrier, is presented below:

Reagents and Equipment

Vitrification Freeze Solutions, Irvine Scientific, Cat# 90133-DSO
Rapid-i Kit (Vitrolife)
Global medium (IVF Online Cat #LGGG-100)
LGPS (IVF Online, Cat #LGPS-050)
Paraffin oil (IVF Online Cat #LGPO-100)
or Washed oil (SAGE, Cat #ART-4009-5W)

The Stripper

140-µm, 200-µm, and 275-µm stripper tips
Micropipette 10–50 µl
Pipette aid (Sarstedt)
Falcon serological pipettes (1 ml, 5 ml)
Hamilton 710 Series 100-µl syringe
SmartBox™ (Vitrolife)
Rapid-i Sealer (Vitrolife)
Cryocane with goblet
Nitrogen storage tank
Brady labeler

(1) Fill the SmartBox with liquid nitrogen up to 1 cm from the Box's rim and place the lid on top of the box.
(2) Check each RapidStraw for possible damage. It is important that the RapidStraws are not bent. Place the label with patient's identification below the black mark at the top of the RapidStraw. Label the exact number of RapidStraws needed with the patient's identification.
(3) Place labeled RapidStraws in SmartBox filled with liquid nitrogen and make sure that the straws are securely attached to the magnet in the SmartBox.
(4) Prepare a suitable pipette of minimal volume depending on the size of blastocyst to transfer it between drops. The best time for blastocyst vitrification is when the diameter of the embryo reaches 140–180 µm (on day 5). But often we have more-expanded blastocysts on day 5 (especially from PGD cases), and it is important to prepare a transfer pipette not bigger than 200 µm (external diameter) to allow blastocyst with a small volume of medium to fill the hole of a RapidStraw. For PGD cases it is important to freeze blastocysts as soon as possible after biopsy, before re-expansion after collapse. For regular cases it is possible to prepare a transfer pipette for expanded blastocysts of 200 µm, to collapse them during pipetting in the medium before placing them in vitrification solution.
(5) Aseptically dispense one 20-µl drop of equilibration solution (ES) on a 90-mm Petri dish.
(6) Transfer embryo(s) (two maximum) to the ES drop and expose undisturbed for 6–10 min. Blastocysts

will shrink and then gradually return to original size, indicating that equilibration is complete.

Note: Observe the blastocysts during equilibration in the ES and wait for the disappearance of the perivitelline space to be sure that equilibration is completed. Time for equilibration depends on the size and quality of the embryo. For high-quality or small embryos equilibration does not take long: approximately 8 min. If the recovery of the volume of the blastocyst cannot be confirmed, stop equilibration after 15 min (maximum!), as this is long enough for equilibration.

(7) Two minutes prior to completion of above equilibration in ES, aseptically dispense four 20-μl drops of vitrification solution (VS) in a row.

(8) After the completion of equilibration, aspirate the embryo in the ES at the tip of pipette and transfer to VS1 with minimal volume. Blow the solution two times out of pipette to the outside of the drop before transferring embryo to the next VS. Keep the embryo in VS1 for 5 seconds.

(9) Transfer embryo to VS2 for 5 seconds.

(10) Transfer embryo to VS3 for 10 seconds.

(11) Transfer embryo to VS4 and keep for at least 30–40 seconds.

(12) Place the RapidStraw on the microscope stage with the flat side down. Locate the correct plane of focus, so that the hole of the RapidStraw is in view for easy loading.

(13) Collect the blastocyst with the transfer pipette, and keep it close to the end of the pipette. Slide the hole of RapidStraw into view on the microscope stage. Move the tip of the pipette close to the wall of the hole in RapidStraw and expel the blastocyst into the hole (it is important to avoid overfilling the hole to keep the embryo from floating out).

(14) Remove the stainless steel rod from RapidStraw and quickly place RapidStraw with the embryo inside vertically into the precooled straw sitting in the Smartbox. Cover the hole of straw immediately after insertion for few seconds to prevent the RapidStraw from accidentally popping out. Complete steps 8–14 within 60–90 seconds!

(15) Immediately seal the top of the RapidStraw using the Rapid-i Sealer. Inspect the seal to ensure that sealing was correctly performed. Incorrect handling and sealing can cause a pressure buildup inside that may result in damage or even explosion of the straw during the thawing.

(16) Move the sealed RapidStraw into the goblet in such a way that the RapidStraw with the embryo does not leave the liquid nitrogen, and add more nitrogen to the SmartBox up to 1 cm from the Box's rim.

(17) Transfer the cryocane with goblet to long-term storage.

Laser-assisted hatching

The goal of laser-assisted hatching is to create a hole or trench in the embryo's zona pellucida by laser zona drilling. Laser-assisted hatching (laser zona drilling) is performed on day 3 of embryo development (6–10-cell stage) inside the lid of a 35 × 10-mm Petri dish (Falcon 35-1008) in 5-μl drops of 10% Global medium covered with 2 ml of paraffin oil (LifeGlobal). The laser is set for creating a ~10–25 μm hole (laser pulse width is 300–500 μs). The hole should be wide enough to breach the zona pellucida (as seen at the focal plane when the embryo is observed at its largest diameter). The optimal diameter of a hole is determined by the thickness of the zona pellucida. Holes of wide diameter are necessary to accommodate a thick zona (one or more laser pulses). Holes of smaller diameter are preferred for thin zona. To minimize the risk of damage to blastomeres, as few laser pulses as possible should be administered at the lowest power levels possible to achieve safe zona drilling or thinning effects.

Trophectoderm biopsy

(1) Laser-assisted hatching is performed at the EBF, EB1, or EB2 stage of embryo development on day 4 or 5. The embryo's zona pellucida is drilled with one or more ZILOS-tk pulses at the high setting. The diameter of the drilled hole is 25–30 μm.[15]

(2) On day 5, 6, or 7 of normal embryo development (expanded blastocyst stage) the trophectoderm begins herniating through the hole. The embryo is transferred to the lid of a 35 × 10-mm Petri dish into 5 μl drops of 10% Global medium covered with 2 ml of oil. Each blastocyst is separated—one per biopsy dish—and placed into the appropriately numbered (from the bottom) drop in the Petri dish.

(3) The blastocyst is supported on a holding pipette and held at the floor of the Petri dish. Using a polished thin-walled biopsy pipette with an internal diameter of 15–25 μm, ~5 cells are drawn into the pipette and pulled away from the embryo. Separation from the rest of the trophectoderm is achieved by 2–5 pulses of the laser at the medium setting (laser pulse width 350–500 μs) aimed at the junction of the cells near the biopsy pipette. Biopsy time is not to exceed 2–3 min (Figure 2.15).

(4) The biopsied cells are transferred into the empty 5-μl drop of 10% Global medium in the same Petri dish at the 3 o'clock position.

(5) When the blastocyst has been biopsied, the dish is taken back to the dissecting scope and, observed by a witness, the blastocyst is placed into the appropriately numbered culture drop in the separate growth dish, which had been equilibrated at least 2 hours.

(6) Trophectoderm samples are transferred into properly labeled microcentrifuge tubes containing 2 μl of microarray buffer using individual attenuated pipettes (inner diameter 100 μm). Samples are transferred in a minimum possible volume of media, which should not exceed 2.5 μl (the transfer pipettes are changed between every sample). The box with microcentrifuge tubes containing microarray buffer working solution (2 μl per tube) is provided by the DNA lab. Microcentrifuge tubes are handled the same way as for PCR testing.

REFERENCES

1. Cohen J, Malter H, Talansky B, Grifo L. *Micromanipulation of Gametes and Embryos*. New York: Raven Press, 1992.
2. Palermo G, Joris H, Devroey P, Van Steirteghem AC. Pregnancies after intracytoplasmic injection of single spermatozoon into an oocyte. *Lancet* 1992; 340:17.
3. Palermo G. Assisted fertilization by intracytoplasmic sperm injection (ICSI). In Veeck LL, ed. *An Atlas of Human Gametes and Conceptuses*. Carnforth, UK: Parthenon Publishing Group, 1999:76–85.
4. Verlinsky Y, Cieslak J, Evsikov S. Techniques for micromanipulation and biopsy of human gametes and preembryos. In Verlinsky Y, Kuliev A, eds. *Preimplantation Genetics*. New York: Plenum Press, 1991:273–78.
5. Verlinsky Y, Cieslak J. Embryological and technical aspects of preimplantation genetic diagnosis. In Verlinsky Y, Kuliev A, eds. *Preimplantation Diagnosis of Genetic Disorders: A New Technique for Assisted Reproduction*. New York: Wiley-Liss, 1993:49–67.
6. Handyside A. Biopsy of human cleavage stage embryos and sexing by DNA amplification. In Verlinsky Y, Kuliev A, eds. *Preimplantation Genetics*. New York: Plenum Press, 1991: 75–83.
7. Cieslak J, Ivakhnenko V, Wolf G, Sheleg S, Verlinsky Y. Three-dimensional partial zona dissection for preimplantation genetic diagnosis and assisted hatching. *Fertil Steril* 1999; 71:308–13.
8. Verlinsky Y, Milayeva S, Evsikov S, et al. Preconception and preimplantation diagnosis for cystic fibrosis. *Prenat Diagn* 1992; 12:103–10.
9. Kaplan B, Wolf G, Kovalinskaya L, Verlinsky Y. Viability of embryos following second polar body removal in a mouse model. *J Assist Reprod Genet* 1995; 12:747–49.
10. Strom C, Levin R, Strom S, et al. Neonatal outcome of preimplantation genetic diagnosis by polar body removal: the first 109 infants. *Pediatrics* 2000; 106:650–53.
11. Hardy J, Martin KL, Leese HJ, Winston RM, Handyside AH. Human preimplantation development in vitro is not adversely affected by biopsy at the 8-cell stage. *Hum Reprod* 1990; 5:708–14.
12. Kuliev A, Verlinsky Y. Current features of preimplantation genetic diagnosis. *Reprod Biomed Online* 2002; 5:296–301.
13. Verlinsky Y, Cohen J, Munné S, et al. Over a decade of preimplantation genetic diagnosis experience – a multi-center report. *Fertil Steril* 2004; 82:292–94.
14. Muggleton-Harris AL, Glazier AM, Pickering S, Wall M. Genetic diagnosis using PCR and FISH analysis of biopsied cells from both the cleavage and blastocyst stages of individual cultured human preimplantation embryos. *Hum Reprod* 1995; 10:183.
15. McArthur S, Leigh D, Marshall J, de Boer K, Jansen R. Pregnancies and live births after trophectoderm biopsy and preimplantation genetic testing of human blastocysts. *Fertil Steril* 2005; 84:1628–36.
16. Schoolcraft WB, Fragouli E, Stevens J, Munné S, Katz-Jaffe MG, Wells D. Clinical application of comprehensive chromosomal screening in the blastocyst stage. *Fertil Steril* 2010; 94:1700–706.
17. Fragouli E, Alfarawati S, Daphnis DD, et al. Cytogenetic analysis of human blastocyst with the use of FISH, CGH, and aCGH: scientific data and technical evaluation. *Hum Reprod* 2011; 26:480–490.
18. Schoolcraft WB, Treff NR, Stevens JM, Ferry K, Katz-Jaffe M, Scott RT. Live birth outcome with trophectoderm biopsy, blastocyst vitrification, and single-nucleotide polymorphism microarray-based comprehensive chromosome screening in infertile patients. *Fertil Steril* 2011; 96:638–40.
19. Scott RT Jr., Ferry K, Su J, Tao X, Scott K, Treff NRT. Comprehensive chromosome screening is highly predictive of the reproductive potential of human embryos: a prospective, blinded, nonselection study. *Fertil Steril* 2012; 97:870–75.
20. Gardner DK, Lane M. Culture of viable human blastocysts in defined sequential serum-free media. *Hum Reprod* 1998; 13(Suppl.3):148–59.
21. Bigger JD, Racowsky C. The development of fertilized human ova to the blastocyst stage in KSOM (AA) medium: is a two-step protocol necessary? *Reprod Biomed Online* 2002; 5:133–40.
22. Rieger D. The use of global for 1-step (uninterrupted) culture from zygote to blastocyst. *Fertil Mag* 2012; 14:5–11.
23. Kader A, Choi A, Orief Y, Agrawal A. Factors affecting the outcome of human blastocyst vitrification. *Reprod Biol Endocrinol* 2009; 7:99.

3 Nuclear transfer techniques for preimplantation diagnosis and prospect for artificial gamete formation

VISUALIZATION OF POLAR BODY AND BLASTOMERE CHROMOSOMES

The possibility of reprogramming the donor cell nucleus by the recipient oocyte makes current developments in nuclear transfer (NT) techniques useful for improvement of the methods for preimplantation genetic diagnosis (PGD). For example, it has become possible to convert interphase nuclei of single blastomeres and the second polar body (PB2) into metaphase for performing PGD by full karyotyping (Figure 3.1; see description below). This is an essential improvement, because the current fluorescence *in situ* hybridization (FISH) technique allows chromosomes to be enumerated on interphase cell nuclei, though with the number of chromosomes studied being limited to the number of chromosome-specific probes available. Even with the applicaiton of the methods for re-hybridization of interphase nuclei for the second and the third time, such karyotyping cannot be practical.

In contrast to PB1, which consists of metaphase chromosomes and may be analyzed using whole-chromosome-specific fluorescence probes, PB2 forms a nucleus and never transforms into metaphase. We have developed various techniques for converting the PB2 into the metaphase stage. One of these approaches involved electrofusion of the mouse PB2 with intact or enucleated mouse zygotes, which resulted in PB2 nucleus transformation into the metaphase plate in 34% of cases. The same results were obtained by electrofusion of the PB2 with a foreign one-cell mouse embryo, with the proportion of metaphase plates reaching 65% when the recipient one-cell stage mouse embryo was enucleated.[1] The other approach involved the treatment of the one-cell-stage mouse embryos with okadaic acid (a specific inhibitor of phosphatases 1 and 2A), leading to visualization of PB2 chromosomes in up to 80% of cases.[2] The visualized PB2 chromosomes were unichromatid G1 premature condensed chromosomes of good quality, suitable for differential staining. However, in contrast to the mouse data, okadaic acid treatment of human PB2 led to further condensation of already pyknotic PB2 nuclei, so we developed a special technique to convert PB2 into metaphase chromosomes.

The technique for removal of PB2 was described in a previous chapter, with the only modification here being that the biopsy is performed in a medium without sucrose. The PB2 is introduced into oocyte cytoplasts (see Figure 3.2), which are usually obtained by the enucleation of metaphase II oocytes that remained unfertilized after *in vitro* fertilization (IVF) or intracytoplasmic sperm injection (ICSI), or of the metaphase II oocytes that were matured for 24–48 h *in vitro* from immature oocytes. Prior to enucleation, these ooplast recipients were incubated for 10–15 min in medium with 1 μg/ml cytochalasin D, 0.3 μg/ml nocodazole, and 0.5 μg/ml Hoechst 33342. As shown in the procedure steps for oocyte enucleation (Figure 3.3), PB1 is removed together with the nucleus of the oocyte. Because oocytes with failure of fertilization are used, special attention is paid to removing both the meiotic metaphase II spindle and the sperm chromosomes. The enucleated oocytes are then washed and transferred into culture medium for at least 1 h to recover before PB2 injection, which is essentially the same as ICSI. The pipette for intracytoplasmic PB2 injection is prepared in the same way as for biopsy tools, except for modification of the very tip of the needle, which is broken using a microforge. The resulting pipette has a tip broken perpendicularly, without any irregularities and with an inner diameter of 7–10 μm. Unlike the biopsy tools, these pipettes are not flame-polished. The same microforge is used to bend the tool to the desired angle. Prior to use, the micropipettes are treated with non-ionic detergent (NP10).

The procedure of intracytoplasmic PB2 injection is shown in Figures 3.4 and 3.5. PB2 is aspirated into an injection pipette, with care taken that the PB2 plasma membrane is broken, and the pipette is brought into the perivitelline space of the recipient cytoplast through the partial zona dissection (PZD) slit made during oocyte enucleation, and moved into the center of the cytoplast. Cytoplasm is aspirated into the pipette until the plasma membrane is broken, and the PB2 nucleus is expelled into the cytoplast (Figures 3.4 and 3.5). The reconstructed haploid embryos are cultured in standard medium for at least 1 h.

Oocyte activation is performed by electrofusion, with the use of a custom-made electrostimulation apparatus (XRONOS, Chicago, IL; Figure 3.6) in a fusion chamber consisting of two platinum wire electrodes glued to the bottom of a glass dish with a gap of 0.33 mm (Figures 3.4e and 3.5d). Electrofusion medium consists of 0.3 mol/l mannitol, 0.1 mmol/l $MgSO_4$, 0.05 mmol/l $CaCl_2$, and 0.5% polyvinylpyrrolidone, dissolved in

HPLC-grade water. The pH of the medium is adjusted to 7.4 by titration with 0.1 mol/l NaOH.

The reconstructed embryos are checked every 30 min starting at 24 h after activation, and fixed 45 min after the disappearance of PB2 pronuclei (Figure 3.7). Alternatively, premature chromosome condensation of the resulting PB2 pronuclei in the reconstructed embryos is induced by 1-h exposure to okadaic acid (5–10 μg/ml). To prevent embryo cytoplasm fragmentation, okadaic acid is diluted to the working concentration with phosphate-buffered saline containing 3 mg/ml bovine serum albumin and 0.5 μg/ml cytochalasin D. Hypotonic treatment of the embryos is avoided to prevent overspreading of chromosomes. Because there is also no need to improve the spreading of chromosomes during fixation, the embryos transferred from the fixative to the slide are simply left to dry out.

The sequence of PB2 nuclear transformation in foreign cytoplasm from the very beginning of its injection to the first mitotic division of the reconstructed embryo and premature chromosome condensation by okadaic acid is presented in Figures 3.7 and 3.8. As can be seen from immunocytochemical study, as early as 2 h after injection, tubulin microfilaments, initially present only around the PB2 nucleus, start to elongate into the cytoplasm, eventually forming the metaphase spindle of PB2 (Figure 3.8).

The whole procedure is usually completed within two days of PB2 removal, and so can be realized well before the embryo transfer. The procedure is started by PB2 removal a few hours after oocyte exposure to sperm or ICSI, followed by its injection into enucleated oocytes and electrofusion. The following day the embryos without pronuclei are fixed or exposed to okadaic acid prior to fixation, should the PB2 pronucleus still be present. Initially, 18 of 34 reconstructed embryos were able to be activated,[3] demonstrating the efficiency of the method for karyotyping of the PB2, which has also been applied for the PGD of translocations. (The karyotype of a PB2 obtained through the above procedure is presented in Figure 3.9.)

The same principle is used for visualization of individual blastomeres (Figures 3.1 and 3.10). Initially individual blastomere nuclei were transformed into metaphase chromosomes through blastomere fusion with enucleated human oocytes (Figure 3.11).[4] Although metaphases were obtained from 23 of 38 blastomeres treated by this method, its efficiency was not high enough to be applicable for PGD. This was due to the inability of a replicating nucleus to form metaphase chromosomes after induction of premature chromosome condensation (PCC). However, because biopsied blastomeres may be at any stage of the cell cycle at the time of biopsy, the timing of mitosis of the blastomere nucleus should be controlled; this can be achieved by the introduction of the blastomere into the cytoplasm of a cell at a known cell cycle. To achieve such reprogramming, the individual blastomeres are fused with intact or enucleated mouse zygotes at the pronuclear stage and known to be in the S phase of the cell cycle (Figure 3.12).

Frozen mouse zygotes (Charles River Laboratories, Wilmington, MA) may be used as recipient cytoplasts to induce conversion of the blastomere nucleus into metaphase. Although initially mouse zygotes were enucleated, there is no need for this step for most of the cases, as mouse and human chromosomes may be clearly distinguished.

Blastomere biopsy is performed in the same way as described in Chapter 2, except that only intact blastomeres with a clearly visible nucleus are chosen. Also, several precautions have to be taken to ensure the integrity of the blastomere plasma membrane during the biopsy procedure. Although intact blastomeres may be inserted microsurgically into the perivitelline space, this has appeared to be traumatic and so has been replaced by blastomere–zygote agglutination with phytohemagglutinin (Irvine Scientific, Santa Ana, CA). Before the procedure, the thawed mouse zygotes are freed of zonae pellucidae with acidic Tyrode's solution and pipetted through the flame-polished Pasteur pipettes with an internal diameter of 80 μm to separate the PB2. Using the flame-polished Pasteur pipettes with internal diameter of 100 μm, blastomere–zygote pairs are brought together and agglutinated in 300 μg/ml of phytohemagglutinin in protein-free human tubal fluid buffered with 20 mmol/l of HEPES in a four-well plastic dish (Nunc) (Figure 3.12a).

Electrofusion is induced in the same way as mentioned in the above section, except for substitution of 0.5% polyvinylpyrrolidone in the electrofusion medium by 0.1% with molecular weight 360,000 (kDa). Blastomere–zygote pairs are oriented between electrodes by hand, with the final orientation achieved with alternating current (500 kHz; 0.2 kV/cm for 2 s). Cell fusion is induced with a single direct-current pulse (1 kV/cm for 500 μs), and the results are assessed in 20 min (Figure 3.12b).

When human blastomeres are fused with intact mouse zygotes, the heterokaryons entering mitosis are identified under the dissecting microscope (Figure 3.12c–e). Because of the transparency of mouse cytoplasm, the disappearance of pronuclei and the formation of the joint metaphase plate are clearly visible. The heterokaryons with a persisting pronucleus are exposed for 1 h to 5 μmol/l of okadaic acid in phosphate-buffered saline containing 3 mg/ml of bovine serum albumin and 0.5 μg/ml of cytochalasin D (Figure 3.12f). After 10–15 min of incubation in a hypotonic solution (0.1% sodium citrate and 0.6% bovine serum albumin) the resulting mitotic heterokaryons are fixed in a cold 3:1 solution of methanol and acetic acid in a four-well plastic dish. When the cytoplasm clears, the heterokaryons are transferred onto slides and air-dried. Chromosome plates are assessed by phase contrast (Figure 3.13) and then used for standard chromosome analysis. For FISH analysis the slides are pretreated with formaldehyde and pepsin (Abbott Inc., Downers Grove, IL) (Figure 3.14).

Although the overall success rate of the procedure is as high as 83% (Figure 3.15), its efficiency can be further improved with experience.[5] Similar results were obtained by using bovine ooplasts for fusion with human blastomeres.[6] Our data show that some of the failures were due simply to the absence of the nucleus in biopsied blastomeres, or because the heterokaryons were fixed after they had already cleaved. It is also useful to perform blastomere biopsy no earlier than day 3 or day 4 to avoid the biopsy of two- and four-cell embryos, which would lead to accelerated heterokaryon cleavage. However, the success rate did not depend on whether mouse zygotes were enucleated before fusion with blastomeres, thus allowing simplification of the procedure by using intact mouse zygotes.

The procedure is quite simple and includes the following components. Mouse zygotes are thawed and freed of zonae pellucidae and PB2 1–2 h before electrofusion with human blastomeres. Four hours after fusion, heterokaryons are monitored for signs of the disappearance of pronuclei, and fixed at mitosis following hypotonic treatment. To avoid possible missing of mitosis, the heterokaryons may be cultured in the presence of microtubuli inhibitor, vinblastine or podophyllotoxin. All the embryos still left in the culture by the 9th hour after fusion are fixed following 1 h of pretreatment with okadaic acid.

This method has been applied for PGD of paternally derived reciprocal translocations and for confirmation of the PGD of chromosomal abnormalities performed by PB1 and PB2 FISH analysis, with a success rate of 83% (Figure 3.15). With the current success rate of blastomere nucleus conversion into metaphase, the method was applied to 89 clinical cycles for translocation carriers, resulting in the transfer of balanced or normal embryos in 68 of them, which yielded 22 unaffected pregnancies (see Chapter 5).

It was also reported that the blastomere metaphase can be obtained without the application of a specific conversion method.[7] To obtain analyzable chromosomes, the embryos were monitored closely from the second day after ICSI in order to identify the blastomere with nuclear breakdown, which was then biopsied and fixed within 1 h. This method was then modified by employing a 1-h culture of the biopsied blastomere in medium containing vinblastine, which resulted in a harvest of metaphase chromosomes of good quality (see Figure 3.16).

However, the method is still labor intensive and requires a considerable time for observation of the embryos under the microscope, so to simplify the process a chemical conversion method was introduced, which is quite simple and may be routinely used for "in house" PGD cases. To perform the procedure, the largest blastomere with one or two large nucleoli within the cell nucleus is selected for biopsy. Upon embryo biopsy, each blastomere is contained in microdrops of Global culture medium (LifeGlobal, USA) supplemented with Plasmanate (Bayer Biological, USA) 10% vol, caffeine (Sigma) (1 mmol/l), and a low dose of colcemid (Sigma) (<0.1 μg/ml) under mineral oil.[7,8] Blastomeres are incubated at 37°C in an atmosphere of 6% CO_2 and air for approximately 2–3 hours or until nuclear membrane breakdown is observed. Then the blastomeres are treated in a hypotonic solution, followed by fixation using a cold solution of methanol and glacial acetic acid, 3:1. Careful attention is paid so as not to overspread the chromosomes in order to avoid chromosome loss during fixation. Consequently not all metaphases are suitable for cytogenetic investigation by G-banding; however, they are suitable for FISH analysis to identify structural rearrangements (Figure 3.17).[9]

SPERM DUPLICATION

As seen above, the genetic composition of oocytes may reliably be tested through removal and examination of PB1 and PB2. However, no method is as yet available for testing the outcome of male meiosis, because genetic analysis destroys the sperm, making it useless for fertilization. To overcome this problem, the technique has been adopted, allowing duplication of a sperm prior to genetic analysis, so that one of the duplicated sperms can be used for testing and the other for fertilization and consequent transfer of the resulting embryo, provided that the genetic analysis of the corresponding duplicate shows a normal genotype.[10] To demonstrate the reliability of the technique, over 100 human sperm from chromosomally normal donors, as well as from translocation carriers, were injected into enucleated mouse oocytes, and the duplicated cells resulting from an overnight culture were tested by FISH to compare the chromosomal status of both daughter cells. All but 3% of the haploid cell pairs derived from the normal donors were identical for the chromosomes tested, while, as expected, a high proportion of the paired nuclei derived from the sperm of translocation carriers were chromosomally unbalanced, suggesting that ooplasm from mature mouse eggs can support the faithful replication of any human sperm genome, irrespective of the genotype.

A similar technique has been developed to duplicate human sperm using human oocytes (Figure 3.18), where the duplication of sperm may be performed (Figure 3.19) faithfully in only one-half of cases (Figures 3.20 and 3.21), in contrast to when using murine oocytes; the technique thus requires further testing before being applied clinically. This technique is expected to have important practical implications for PGD of paternally derived conditions, such as translocations, which are known to produce as much as 70% abnormal sperm on average.

The technique also has potential for research purposes, as shown in preliminary work devoted to the study of mosaicism.[11] Following duplication of human sperm in cow oocytes, a series of 31 resulting embryos were cultured up to the eight-cell stage, and tested by probes specific to chromosomes 13, 16, 18, 21, and 22. In all, 16% of the resulting sperm duplicates appeared not to be identical, which may further be related to the genetic differences between the donors involved. In fact, one of the three sperm donors for the above experiment produced mostly mosaic embryos in two PGD cycles. However, the rate of mosaicism in sperm duplicates of the three donors involved in this small series was similar, indicating that the generation of mosaic embryos, at least in the patients previously tested by PGD, may not be related to sperm genotype, but to the sperm centrosome.[12]

DEVELOPMENT OF ARTIFICIAL HUMAN GAMETES *IN VITRO*

One of the developments in micromanipulation and nuclear transfer has been the progress in the construction of artificial human gametes. Attempts were undertaken to create female and male gametes, with both demonstrating strong morphological evidence for haploidization.[13–15] However, insufficient cytogenetic evidence for haploidization has been presented, which would also be required to ensure the normalcy of the resulting gametes derived from the somatic cell nuclear transfer into the matured oocytes.

The technique is based on inducing nuclei of mitotic somatic cells to skip the S-phase of the cell cycle and undergo haploidization when introduced into oocytes, thus allowing artificial gametes to be obtained from somatic cells through the process of haploidization. We have shown that the efficiency of haploidization of donor cumulus cell nuclei differs depending on the stage of development of the enucleated recipient oocyte. This may be tested using the extruded polar bodies (PB), or generated pronulei, which also allow investigation of the correctness of chromosomal segregation. As seen from the flow chart (Figures 3.22a, b) the first step involves enucleation of *in vitro* matured metaphase II oocytes under the control of UV luminescence (Figures 3.23a, b), which is important to ensure the accuracy of chromosomal analysis of the resulting haploid nuclei. Then the cumulus cell nuclei, which are at G0 of the cell cycle, are introduced into ooplasts by injection (Figures 3.22c, d and 3.23c, d) and the oocytes are activated by electrostimulation delivered by the electrofusion device (XRONOS, Chicago, IL) (Figure 3.22e, f). Following oocyte activation, the chromosomes of the transferred nuclei segregate with the extrusion of polar bodies (Figure 3.22f), or form two pronuclei (Figures 3.22e, 3.23e, f and 3.24), both evidencing the formation of artificial gametes through somatic cell haploidization. Although the resulting pronuclei have similar morphology to pronuclei resulting from natural fertilization (Figures 3.24 and 3.25b), spatial differences are observed, with the pronuclei derived from natural fertilization migrating from the periphery to the center of the oocyte (Figure 3.25a), in contrast to the artificial pronuclei, which are closely positioned to each other from the very beginning, and remain in the same position, despite growing in volume (Figures 3.24 and 3.25b). FISH analysis (Figure 3.26) and DNA fingerprinting (Figure 3.27) of PB1 and pronuclei resulting from the haploidization procedure showed the haploid chromosomal set with the resulting DNA originating from the donor nuclei, with up to 90% of these haploid nuclei appearing to have chromosomal aneuploidies (Figure 3.28). This suggests that the use of the resulting haploid nuclei in gamete reconstruction procedures may still not be acceptable.

To determine whether incubation of nuclei in ooplast improves chromosomal segregation, two groups of a total of 122 reconstructed metaphase II oocytes were studied, one activated 5–7 h after nuclear transfer, and the other after 12–21 h. A higher activation rate in response to parthenogenetic stimulation was observed in the latter group, suggesting the need for a longer incubation period. An aneuploidy rate as high as approximately 90% was observed irrespective of incubation time, with the majority being of a complex nature, suggesting that prolonged incubation would not improve the accuracy of chromosomal segregation. Preliminary results suggest more accurate chromosomal segregation when PB1 and pronucleus were formed. The data show that although haploidization of somatic cells may be achieved using metaphase II oocyte cytoplasm, the aneuploidy rate is much higher than in normal meiosis.

Our preliminary data show that the aneuploidy rate in haploidization may be reduced by substituting recipient metaphase II oocytes with immature oocytes of metaphase I stage. This experiment was performed by the electrofusion of the G2 human fibroblast nuclei with metaphase I oocytes (Figure 3.29). Twelve hours following maturation two PB1s were extruded (Figure 3.30), one originating from the recipient nucleus, and the other from the donor fibroblast, with the overall efficiency of human metaphase I oocytes to haploidize the chromosome set of the G2 somatic cells as high as 80%. According to preliminary FISH results, the aneuploidy rate in the oocytes producing two metaphase II metaphases and two PB1s was comparable to control.

The available data, therefore, show that despite previous hopes of using nuclear transfer technology to produce female and male gametes through haploidization of somatic cells, the majority of the resulting haploid cells are chromosomally abnormal. Therefore, despite the feasibility of somatic cell haploidization by the use of the metaphase II oocyte cytoplasm, its clinical use cannot be considered at the present time.

As mentioned above, there is also a prospect of obtaining the male and female gametes using the stem cell technology based on the progress of differentiation of totipotent cells into different type of cells, including oocytes and sperm.[16] For example, male gametes originate from a small population of spermatogonial stem cells, which divide infinitely, supporting spermatogenesis throughout life in the male. It was demonstrated that these cells are able to undergo meiosis and generate haploid gametes *in vitro* and are functional, as shown by fertilization of mouse oocytes that resulted in viable embryos and birth of live mice.[17]

REFERENCES

1. Verlinsky Y, Dozortzev D, Evsikov S. Visualization and cytogenetic analysis of second polar body chromosomes following its fusion with one-cell mouse embryo. *J Assist Reprod Genet* 1996; 11:123–31.
2. Dyban A, De Sutter P, Verlinsky Y. Okadaic acid induces premature chromosome condensation reflecting the cell cycle progression in one-cell stage mouse embryos. *Mol Reprod Dev* 1993; 34:403–15.
3. Verlinsky Y, Evsikov S. Karyotyping of human oocytes by chromosomal analysis of the second polar body. *Mol Hum Reprod* 1999; 5:89–95.
4. Evsikov S, Verlinsky Y. Visualization of chromosomes in single human blastomeres. *J Assist Reprod Genet* 1999; 16:133–7.
5. Verlinsky Y, Evsikov S. A simplified and efficient method for obtaining metaphase chromosomes from individual human blastomeres. *Fertil Steril* 1999; 72:1–6.
6. Willadsen S, Levron J, Munné S, et al. Rapid visualization of metaphase chromosomes in single human blastomeres after fusion with in-vitro matured bovine eggs. *Hum Reprod* 1999; 14:470–74.
7. Tanaka A, Nagayoshi M, Awata S, et al. Preimplantation diagnosis of repeated miscarriage due to chromosomal translocations using metaphase chromosomes of a blastomere biopsied from 4-6 cell stage embryo. *Fertil Steril* 2004; 81:30–34.
8. Shkumatov A, Kuznyetsov V, Cieslak J, Ilkevitch, Verlinsky Y. Obtaining metaphase spreads from single blastomeres for PGD of chromosomal rearrangements. *Reprod Biomed Online* 2007; 14:498–503.
9. Kuliev A, Cieslak-Jansen J, Zlatopolsky Z, Kirillova I, Ilkevitch Y, Verlinsky Y. Conversion and non-conversion approach to preimplantation diagnosis for chromosomal rearrangements in 475 cycles. *Reprod Biomed Online* 2010; 21:93–99.
10. Willadsen S, Munné S, Schmmel T, Cohen J. Applications of nuclear sperm duplication. Fifth International Symposium on Preimplantation Genetics, 5–7 June 2003, Antalya, Turkey:35.
11. Munné S, Willadsen S, Schmmel T, Cohen J. Nuclear sperm duplication as a tool to study mosaicism. Fifth International Symposium on Preimplantation Genetics, 5–7 June 2003, Antalya, Turkey:55–6.
12. Silber S, Sadowy S, Lehahan K, et al. High rate of chromosome mosaicism but not aneuploidy in embryos from karyotypically normal men requiring TESE. *Reprod Biomed Online* 2002; 4(Suppl 2):20.
13. Lacham-Kaplan O, Daniels R, Trounson A. Fertilization of mouse oocytes using somatic cells as male germ cells. *Reprod Biomed Online* 2001; 3:205–11.
14. Tesarik J, Mendoza C. Somatic cell haploidization: an update. *Reprod Biomed Online* 2003; 6:60–65.
15. Galat V, Ozen S, Rechitsky L, Verlinsky Y. Is haploidization by human mature oocytes real? Fifth International Symposium on Preimplantation Genetics, 5–7 June 2003, Antalya, Turkey: 36–37.
16. Hayashi Y, Saitou M, Yamanaka S. Germline development from human pluripotent stem cells towards disease modeling of infertility. *Fertil Steril* 2012; 97:1250–59.
17. Nayernia K, Nolte J, Michelmann HW, et al. In vitro differentiation of embryonic stem cells give rise to male gametes that can generate offspring of mice. *Develop Cell* 2006; 11:1–8.

4 Preimplantation diagnosis for aneuploidies

INTRODUCTION

Although preimplantation genetic diagnosis (PGD) was initially introduced for pre-existing genetic conditions, its application appears to be of particular relevance for sporadic conditions, such as chromosomal abnormalities, that contribute significantly to pregnancy loss and infertility. At least three-quarters of all PGDs have been performed for age-related aneuploidies, resulting in the birth of thousands of healthy children. PGD is currently performed by three main approaches—the testing of biopsied trophectoderm cells at the blastocyst stage (day 5), blastomeres biopsied from the cleaving embryos (day 3), or polar bodies removed from matured and fertilized oocytes (day 0)—combined with fluorescent *in situ* hybridization (FISH) or microarray analysis.

As described in Chapter 2, embryo biopsy can be performed at day 3 (6–8-cell stage) or day 5 (over 100 cells), and enables testing for both maternally and paternally derived genetic abnormalities. First and second polar body (PB1 and PB2) removal (see Chapter 2), on the other hand, allows testing exclusively for maternally derived abnormalities, as can be seen from the schematic presentation of the possible errors in meiosis I and meiosis II shown in Figure 4.1. Each of these two approaches has advantages and disadvantages, and which one is applied depends on the clinical circumstances. For example, despite a reduction in embryo cell number, which may have an influence on embryo viability, embryo biopsy is performed for paternally derived chromosomal abnormalities, as well as for gender determination. In contrast, removal of PB1 and PB2, naturally extruded from oocytes in the process of maturation and fertilization, respectively, should not have any effect on embryo viability, although this provides no information on gender and paternal meiotic errors. The particular value of PB testing for PGD of aneuploidies is obvious from the fact that over 90% of chromosomal errors originate from maternal meiosis. This approach is also of importance owing to a relatively high rate of mosaicism at the cleavage stage, which is recognized as the major limitation of blastomere-based PGD for chromosomal disorders (see below).

PGD for aneuploidies is currently performed by FISH analysis using commercially available chromosome-specific probes (Abbott, Downers Groves, IL, USA; Rainbow Scientific, Inc., Windsor, CT, USA; BlueGnome Ltd, Cambridge, UK), or by microarray analysis, which is in the process of validation. FISH analysis was first applied in 1991 for gender determination using DNA probes specific for either the X or Y chromosome.[1] Since testing for only one of the sex chromosomes could lead to misdiagnosis of gender due to a possible failure of hybridization, a dual FISH was done involving the simultaneous detection of X and Y, each with a different color.[2] Additionally, the dual FISH analysis was combined with a ploidy assessment to improve the accuracy, by adding a centromeric probe specific for chromosome 18.[3,4] Testing was then extended to up to five autosomes, including chromosomes 13, 16, 18, 21, and 22 (Figures 4.2 and 4.3), and then to seven, eight, or even a dozen chromosomes, using additional rounds of rehybridization (Figures 4.4–4.6).[5–7] An additional round of re-hybridization is also used for testing the same chromosome by different probes when one of the probes provides controversial results, or when the fluorescent signal is too weak to make a determination (Figures 4.7).

The overall experience of preimplantation FISH analysis may at present be close to 100,000 clinical cycles, resulting, overall, in an improved pregnancy rate in poor-prognosis *in vitro* fertilization (IVF) patients,[8–11] although a few randomized controlled studies failed to confirm this. The majority of these cycles were performed by FISH analysis of blastomeres, while only a small proportion of cases were done by PB1 and PB2 analysis. A few dozens of thousands of unaffected pregnancies and healthy children have resulted, with the follow-up confirmation of the preselected abnormal embryos and babies born following the procedure indicating an acceptable accuracy of the FISH analysis, which is described below. Examples of normal FISH patterns in PB1, PB2, and blastomeres are presented in Figures 4.2 and 4.3 for five chromosomes, and Figures 4.4 and 4.5 for seven or nine chromosomes.

The reliability of the FISH technique for aneuploidy detection in blastomeres has been extensively studied.[12–15] By comparing the FISH results in the cleaving embryos to morphological abnormalities and maternal age, it was established that the observed chromosomal abnormalities were not related to the limitations of the FISH technique, but were due to the embryo variables. A high rate of mosaicism was observed at the cleavage stage, which was initially suggested to be particularly high in slow embryos exhibiting an arrested development. Furthermore, the accumulated experience showed that up to half of all cleaving embryos are mosaic (Figures 4.6, 4.8, and 4.9), representing a common feature of preimplantation embryo development at the cleavage stage.[13–17] Mosaicism currently represents a major limitation of the FISH analysis of aneuploidies performed at the cleavage stage, and it may obviously affect the diagnostic accuracy of PGD, resulting in the possible transfer of an affected embryo because one or a few cells were found to be normal as a result of mosaicism. Conversely, when the embryo is erroneously diagnosed as abnormal, while it is actually normal, the perfectly normal embryo may be untransferred, compromising the chances of the patient to become pregnant. It has recently been shown that mosaicism also presents diagnostic problems at the blastocyst stage[18] (Figures 4.6 and 4.8), involving also inner mass cells, despite the initial prediction that the abnormal cells are deviated mainly to the trophectoderm. As shown in Figures 4.6, 4.8, and 4.10–4.13, even embryos with monosomies, including those with double monosomies, are able to reach the blastocyst stage, comparable to trisomies (Figure 4.14).

The first attempt to use FISH analysis for testing PB1 was undertaken in 1994.[19–21] In this work, 130 unfertilized metaphase II oocytes were tested simultaneously with their PB1, using X-chromosome- and chromosome-18-specific probes. It was demonstrated that PB1 FISH data allow an exact prediction of the chromosome set in the corresponding oocytes. Each chromosome in PB1 was represented by double dots (signals), corresponding to two chromatids in each univalent (Figure 4.2). The data suggested that the number of signals (chromatids) in PB1 reliably predicts the corresponding number of signals (chromatids) in the metaphase II oocytes, therefore providing an excellent tool for the genetic preselection of oocytes. It was also of interest that, in addition to a normal distribution of signals in PB1 and the corresponding metaphase II oocytes, meiotic errors were also detected, confirming the accuracy of PB1 diagnosis for predicting the genotype of the corresponding oocyte. For example, in one PB1 four signals for chromosome 18 were detected, perfectly in accordance with the lack of the chromosome 18 signals in the corresponding metaphase II oocyte (chromosome 18 non-disjunction). This suggested that the chromosomal complements of the oocyte could be inferred from the testing of PB1, which can be removed following its extrusion from the mature oocyte with no potential influence on the embryo viability. Another interesting phenomenon was the observation of chromatid malsegregation as a possible cause of chromosomal aneuploidy in the resulting mature oocytes (see schematic presentation of possible errors in meiosis in Figure 4.1). In four oocytes, instead of the expected two signals, three were found in the metaphase II oocytes, which perfectly corresponded to a single signal in the corresponding PB1 (examples of the error leading to trisomy or monosomy 21 detected by PB1 testing are shown in Figures 4.15 and 4.16). Similar results have been reported by another group, confirming the diagnostic significance of PB1 FISH analysis for predicting the genotype of the preimplantation embryo.[22]

However, it became clear from the very beginning of the application of PB1 testing that the resulting genotype of the oocyte cannot be predicted without testing the outcome of the second meiotic division, by testing the PB2, extruded following fertilization of the oocyte.[23] It was shown that in contrast to the paired dots in PB1, each chromosome in PB2 was represented by a single dot (Figure 4.2), so the lack or addition of a signal for a particular chromosome provided evidence of a second meiotic division error. Although only 19 of 55 oocytes in this first study were tested by both PB1 and PB2, evidence for a possible error in both PB1 and PB2 was presented. These data suggested that some oocytes selected as normal, based on the PB1 FISH analysis, could still appear to be abnormal following non-disjunction in the second meiotic division (Figures 4.17 and 4.18). Therefore, FISH analysis of both PB1 and PB2, which allows detection of errors in both the first and second meiotic divisions, has become the basic requirement for PGD of aneuploidies (Figures 4.19–4.25).

Currently, more than 20,000 oocytes have been tested by FISH analysis, demonstrating the accuracy and reliability of PB1 and PB2 testing for predicting the karyotype of the corresponding oocyte and resulting embryo. The data demonstrated a greater than 50% aneuploidy rate in oocytes from IVF patients of advanced maternal age,[24–29] resulting from the errors in both the first and second meiotic divisions, in contrast to the previously accepted concept that aneuploidies mainly originate from meiosis I. These data were confirmed by microarray-based 24-chromosome testing, which will be described below.

PREPARATION OF POLAR BODIES, BLASTOMERES, AND TROPHECTODERM SAMPLES FOR FLUORESCENCE *IN SITU* HYBRIDIZATION ANALYSIS (FISH)

Preparation of PB1 and PB2

Equipment, materials, and reagents for preparation of PB1 and PB2 are listed in Tables 4.1–4.3, and presented in brief below:

Glacial acetic acid	Sigma #A-6283
Methanol	Sigma #M-3641
HPLC H_2O	Scientific Prod #6795-1
Microscope slides	Fisher #12-550-41
Micropipettes	Fisher #21-176-2A
50-ml culture flask	Fisher #10-126-1B
5-3/4 inch Pasteur pipettes	Fisher #13-678-20A
PGD stripper (MidAtlantic Diagnostics) or mouthpiece with tubing to hold micropipette	
Hanging drop slide (engrave a circle in the bottom center)	Fisher #12-560
Carbide marker for engraving glass	Fisher #13-378
Lead pencil and permanent marker	

Table 4.1 Equipment for fluorescence *in situ* hybridization (FISH) analysis of polar body, blastomere, and trophectoderm biopsy

Microscope (Nikon Microphot FXA) with epifluorescence attachment, 100-W mercury lamp, phase-contrast optics with ×10 objective, oil immersion objectives x63 and ×100
Single-bandpass filters (Chroma Technologies) for all fluorophores: DAPI (blue), FITC (green), TRITC (red), AQUA (aqua), FI5 (yellow), and F6 (blue)
Dual bandpass filters – FITC/TRITC (red and green) and aqua/blue
CCD camera, filter wheel, and computer with imaging software (Quips Imaging Workstation, Applied Imaging, Santa Clara, CA)
Inverted microscope with phase-contrast optics, ×10 and x20 objectives (Olympus CK 40, Olympus America)
Stereomicroscope
Air incubator (set at 37°C)
Water bath (capable of maintaining temperatures up to 100°C)
Microcentrifuge
Vortex
Calibrated thermometers (for incubator and water bath)
pH meter and standards
Micropipettes (0.5–10 µl, 2–20 µl, 20–200 µl) and appropriate sterile tips
Microtorch (Blazer Corporation GB 2001) or ThermoBrite 07J9-010 (Abbott)

Table 4.2 Materials for fluorescence *in situ* hybridization (FISH) analysis of polar body, blastomere, and trophectoderm biopsy

Materials and reagents	*Supplier*	*Catalog number*
Microscope (25 x 75 x 1-mm) frosted precleaned slides	Fisher	12-550-14
Drummond 1–5 µl pipettes	Fisher	21-176-2A
Drummond 25–50 µl pipettes	Fisher	21-176-2D
5 3/4-inch Pasteur pipettes	Fisher	13-678-20A
35 x 10-mm Petri dishes (Falcon 1008)	Fisher	08-757-100A
50-ml culture flask (Falcon 353014)	Fisher	10-126-1B
Coplin jars (12)	Fisher	08-817
4 glass dishes with removable tray	Fisher	08-812
Hanging drop slides	Fisher	12-560
Carbide marker for engraving glass	Fisher	13-378
22 x 30-mm coverslips (Corning)	Fisher	12-531A
Microcentrifuge tubes	Midwest Scientific	TT05B
Forceps (fine tip)	Fisher	08-953E
Parafilm	Fisher	13-374-10
Graduated cylinders and serological pipettes		
Mouthpiece with tubing to hold micropipette	Sigma	A-51 77
Lead pencil and fine point permanent marker		
Rubber bulb for blow-drying	Fisher	14-085

The procedure for preparation of polar bodies is as follows:

(1) Fixative (methanol and glacial acetic acid, 3:1) is prepared in a 50-ml culture flask on the day of fixation, and stored at ambient temperature.

(2) Micropipettes are pulled using the microtorch to obtain an attenuated tip with an inner diameter approximately 50 µm. If the diameter is too large, there is a greater potential for PB loss.

(3) Glass slides, although precleaned, may be cleaned again to remove any grease or dirt by applying a few drops of fixative and wiping with a lint-free tissue (Kimwipe).

(4) Fill the hanging drop slide or regular slide with HPLC H_2O using a pasteur pipette.

(5) After oocytes/zygotes have been manipulated and PB removal has been accomplished, the PB(s) can be

Table 4.3 Reagents for fluorescence *in situ* hybridization (FISH) analysis of polar bodies, blastomeres, and trophectoderm

Materials and reagents	*Supplier*	*Catalog number*
MultiVysion PB Panel (chromosomes 13, 16, 18, 21, and 22)	Vysis	32-131085
MultiVysion PGT (chromosomes X,Y, 13, 18, and 21)	Vysis	32-131080
MultiVysion 4 Color Custom (chromosomes X,Y, 17, and 15)	Vysis	32-131086
CEP X (DXZ1, alpha satellite) spectrum green	Vysis	32-132023
CEPY (DYZ1, satellite) spectrum aqua	Vysis	32-131024
CEP 17 (D1721) spectrum aqua	Vysis	32-131017
CEP 15 (D15Z1) spectrum green	Vysis	32-182015
Sub-telomeric 13q spectrum orange	Vysis	33-260013
Sub-telomeric 13q (green)	Cytocell	LPT13qg
Sub-telomeric 16q spectrum orange	Vysis	33-260016
Sub-telomeric 16p spectrum green	Vysis	33-252016
Sub-telomeric 18q spectrum orange	Vysis	33-260018
Sub-telomeric 21q spectrum orange	Vysis	33-260021
Sub-telomeric 22q spectrum orange	Vysis	33-260022
Sub-telomeric Xp/Yp spectrum green	Vysis	33-252023
Vectashield antifade	Vector Labs	H-1000
DAPI counterstain	Sigma	D-1388
Glacial acetic acid	Sigma	A-6283
Methanol	Sigma	M-3641
HPLC H_2O (Mallinckrodt Baker Inc.)	Scientific Products	6795-1
Bovine serum albumin	Sigma	A-3311
Sodium citrate	Fisher	S279-500
25-mg vials of pepsin	Vysis	30-806001
Magnesium chloride	Sigma	M-2393
Phosphate-buffered saline	Irvine Scientific	9235
Neutral buffered formalin (10%)	VWR	3239-4
20 x SSC	Vysis	32-804850
Ethanol series (70, 85, and 100%)	Fisher	A 407-4
NP-40	Vysis	32-804818
Immersion oil (fluorescence)	Fisher	12-371-IB
Sodium hydroxide solution (1 mol/l)	Vysis	930-65
Hydrochloric acid (2 mol/l)	Vysis	251-2

found in the micromanipulation dish in the 3 o'clock drop. Once PB is located using a micropipette, a small amount of water is aspirated to ensure proper control of fluid in and out of the pipette.

(6) After aspiration of a small amount of water, the PB is aspirated into the pipette and brought to the hanging drop slide containing water. The PB is released from the pipette by blowing gently until it is visualized in the center circle of the hanging drop slide.

(7) Once rinsed in the water, the PB is aspirated again into the pipette. Any oil surrounding the pipette is usually removed by going through the water. The PB is transferred to a clean slide. The resulting drop of water containing the PBs is encircled using the carbide marker.

(8) Prior to complete drying of the water, a drop of fixative is placed on top of the PB from the other PB-sized micropipette to obtain spreading of the chromatin.

(9) Another drop of fixative is placed on the PB and repeated if necessary until the cytoplasm dissolves. Careful attention is paid to observe this process to thoroughly remove all cytoplasm. The location of the chromatin is further defined by encircling it using the carbide marker, care being taken to only lightly engrave the glass to avoid interference from any glass fragments possibly created. Encircling is done to easily locate the chromatin when analyzing slides.

(10) A heavier circle is engraved on the bottom of the slide to locate the smaller circles and thus the chromatin at

the time of analysis. The oocyte number is engraved just below the circle.

(11) The slide is marked with the patient's name and the oocyte number, along with the number of PB(s) and/or pieces of chromatin by small circles. Polar bodies from two oocytes can be fixed in separate areas on one slide (the distance between two rough circles must be not less than 10 and not more than 20 mm).

(12) Slides can be stored at room temperature overnight before hybridization, or hybridized immediately. Results are obtained well within a reasonable time frame for embryo transfer.

Preparation of blastomeres

Equipment, materials, and reagents are mainly the same as above (Tables 4.1–4.3) with small modifications, which are presented in brief below:

Microscope slides	Fisher #12-544-2
Drummond 1–5 and 10-µl pipettes	Fisher #21-176-2B
35 × 10 mm Petri dishes	Fisher #08-757-100A
PGD stripper (MidAtlantic Diagnostics) or mouthpiece and tubing to hold pipette	
Carbide marker for engraving	Fisher #13-378
Glacial acetic acid	Sigma #A-6283
Methanol	Sigma #M-3641
HPLC H_2O (Mallinckrodt)	Scientific Prod #6795-1
Bovine serum albumin (BSA)	Sigma #A- 3311
Sodium citrate	Fisher #S279-500

The procedure for preparation of blastomeres is as follows:

(1) Prepare a hypotonic solution containing 6 mg/ml of BSA and 1% sodium citrate dissolved in HPLC H_2O. Filter through a 0.2-µm filter and store at 5°C.

(2) Prepare fixative solution by combining 3 parts methanol and 1 part glacial acetic acid. Shake well and store at ambient temperature. This solution should be prepared fresh each day.

(3) Engrave a circle in the bottom of a 35 × 10-mm Petri dish and add 3 ml of hypotonic solution.

(4) Using a microtorch, 1–5 and 10-µl pipettes are pulled to obtain an attenuated tip of approximately 80–100 µm in diameter.

(5) Aspirate a small amount of hypotonic solution into the pipette.

(6) The blastomere in a microdrop of culture medium may be located using a stereo- or inverted microscope. The size of the pipette opening (80–100 µm) is checked prior to picking up the blastomere to ensure that it is larger than the blastomere. Gently aspirate the blastomere into the pipette and transfer it to the Petri dish containing hypotonic solution, placing it within the engraved circle.

(7) After 1–5 min, the blastomere is aspirated into the pipette and transferred to a microscope slide with a small amount of hypotonic solution. The resulting drop of solution containing blastomere is gently encircled using a carbide marker.

(8) Under an inverted microscope, the blastomere is constantly observed until drying is almost complete. Just prior to crystallization of the hypotonic solution, the fixative is aspirated into the pipette (ID 50 µm) and dropped onto the blastomere. While constantly observing the cell, just before drying occurs, fixative is dropped again. This is done several times until the cytoplasm has dissolved, with only the nucleus remaining. A complete removal of the cytoplasm is essential to hybridization.

(9) The location of the nucleus is further defined by encircling with the carbide marker, with care taken to only lightly engrave the glass to avoid creating glass fragments. The heavier circle is engraved on the bottom of the slide to locate the smaller circles and thus the nucleus at the time of analysis.

(10) Below the circle, the embryo number is engraved. The exact location of the nucleus on the bottom of the slide is needed for the accuracy of probe application.

(11) The slide is marked with the patient's name and the embryo number, along with the nucleus quality (N+, N–, fragmented). Nuclei from two embryos can be fixed in separate areas on one slide (the distance between two rough circles must be not less than 10 and not more than 20 mm).

(12) Slides can be stored at room temperature overnight before hybridization, or hybridized immediately. Results are obtained well within a reasonable time frame for embryo transfer.

Preparation of biopsied trophectoderm cells

The materials required are similar to those presented in Tables 4.1–4.3, and include the following:

Microscope slides	Fisher #12-544-2
Drummond 1–5 and 10-µl pipettes	Fisher #21-176-2B
35 × 10-mm Petri dishes	Fisher #08-757-100A
Tween 20 (detergent)	Sigma #P-1379
PGD stripper (MidAtlantic Diagnostics) or mouthpiece and tubing to hold pipette	
Carbide marker for engraving	Fisher #13-378
Glacial acetic acid	Sigma #A-6283
Methanol	Sigma #M-3641
Hydrochloric acid (HCl)	Fisher #A144-212
HPLC H_2O (Mallinckrodt)	Scientific Prod #6795-1
Bovine serum albumin (BSA)	Sigma #A-3311
Sodium citrate	Fisher #S279-500

The procedure of trophectoderm biopsy preparation includes the following steps:

(1) Prepare a hypotonic solution containing 6 mg/ml of BSA and 1% sodium citrate dissolved in HPLC H_2O. Filter through a 0.2-μm filter and store at 5°C.

(2) Prepare a detergent solution containing 1% Tween 20 in 0.01 N HCl.

(3) Prepare fixative solution by combining 3 parts methanol and 1 part glacial acetic acid. This solution should be prepared fresh each day.

(4) Using a microtorch, 1–5 and 10-μl pipettes are pulled to obtain an attenuated tip approximately 80–100 μm in diameter.

(5) Aspirate a small amount of hypotonic solution into the pipette.

(6) The trophectoderm sample contained in a microdrop of culture medium may be located using a stereo- or inverted microscope. Gently aspirate the trophectoderm sample into the pipette and transfer it to the Petri dish containing hypotonic solution, placing it within the engraved circle.

(7) After 1 min, the trophectoderm sample is aspirated into the pipette and transferred to a microscope slide with a small amount of hypotonic solution. The resulting drop of solution containing trophectoderm sample is gently encircled using the carbide marker.

(8) Under an inverted microscope, the trophectoderm sample is constantly observed until drying is complete. Just after crystallization of the hypotonic solution, the Tween 20 solution is aspirated into the pipette (ID 50 μm) and is dropped onto the trophectoderm sample several times. In 1–2 min the cytoplasm starts dissolving and isolated nuclei come out of trophectoderm sample. After complete drying of the Tween 20 solution, fixative is dropped continuously to wash out any residual Tween 20. This is done until the detergent is completely removed, with only the nucleus remaining.

(9) The location of the nuclei is further defined by encircling them using the carbide marker, with care taken to only lightly engrave the glass to avoid creating glass fragments. The embryo number is engraved just below the circle.

(10) Prior to probe application, the whole area containing nuclei may be indicated on the bottom of the slide using a carbide marker. This defines the area in which to apply the probe.

(11) The slide is marked with the patient's name and the embryo number, along with the nucleus quality (N+, N–, fragmented). Nuclei from two embryos can be fixed in separate areas on the same slide (the distance between two rough circles must be not less than 10 and not more than 20 mm).

PRETREATMENT, PROBE APPLICATION, HYBRIDIZATION, AND WASHING

According to the classical method, slides are incubated in 2 × SSC (pH 7–7.5) for 10 min at 37°C, before being fixed for 5 min in 1% formaldehyde at ambient temperature. They are then washed for 5 min in 1 × PBS (pH 7–7.5) at ambient temperature, before being incubated for 5 min in 0.5 mg/ml pepsin in 0.01 mol/l HCl at 37°C. The slides are then washed for 5 min in 1 × PBS at ambient temperature and the back of the slide is drained and wiped to remove excess PBS before being sequentially immersed in 70%, 85%, and 100% ethanol at ambient temperature for 1 min each, and then air-dried and hybridized. Many steps may be omitted if chromatin is thoroughly isolated. Nevertheless, for fixed polar bodies and biopsied trophectoderm cells a 5-min incubation in pepsin at 37°C is important, followed by a 1-min wash in PBS and sequential immersing in 70%, 85%, and 100% ethanol at room temperature. Blastomere samples are exposed to pepsin for 1 min to remove residual cytoplasm. For the purpose of re-hybridization, prior to pretreatment, coverslips are removed from the slides and the slides are placed in methanol for 5 min to ensure fixation of the chromatin to the slide, and then placed in PBS, followed by sequential immersing in 70%, 85%, and 100% ethanol, 1 min in each.

Probe mixtures are prepared according to the manufacturer specifications. A three-color probe mixture is prepared by first centrifuging and then vortexing each of the probes of interest along with a vial of locus-specific identifier (LSI) hybridization buffer for 10 s. For 10 μl of working probe, 1 μl of each probe is added to 7 μl of LSI hybridization buffer in a small microcentrifuge tube, which is then vortexed prior to probe application. For a single chromosome probe mixture, 1 μl of probe and 2 μl of HPLC grade H_2O are added to 7 μl of hybridization buffer, which is then vortexed and centrifuged for 10 s.

MultiVysion five-color and four-color custom probe mixtures as well as some microdeletion probes are ready to use, so that after being brought to room temperature, they are centrifuged and vortexed prior to probe application. Prior to case use all working probe mixtures are validated on peripheral blood lymphocyte control slides and can be stored at 20°C for several months according to the manufacturer's expiration date.

Hybridization procedure

The hybridization procedure is as follows:

(1) Prior to probe application, 22 × 30-mm coverslips are cut into 8 × 8-mm smaller squares (dimensions depend on the size of the fixation area) using a carbide marker and stored in a glass Petri dish with lid.

(2) Parafilm is cut into approximately 22 × 22-mm squares and stored in a Petri dish.

(3) A humidification chamber for hybridization is prepared by placing a paper towel moistened with sterile filtered water into a glass (staining) dish, and the slide rack is placed inside and covered. The humidification chamber is warmed in an air incubator at 37°C prior to the application of the working probe. HYBrite or ThermoBrite (Abbot) eliminates manual steps and reduces hands-on time during FISH procedures.

(4) The working probe is removed from the freezer, centrifuged for 10 s, and mixed by vortexing.

(5) Using a micropipette, 1–3 µl of working probe, depending on the size of the marked fixation area, is applied to the marked area where the chromatin is located. Immediately after application of the probe, an 8-mm coverslip is placed on top using forceps. Air bubbles should be avoided, as they interfere with hybridization. If any air bubbles should appear, the coverslip is depressed lightly using forceps.

(6) Coverslips can be sealed using rubber cement or parafilm. When applying parafilm, adhesion to the slide may be ensured by applying pressure down around the coverslip with fingertips.

The StatSpin ThermoBrite System holds up to 12 slides. The lid seals tightly when closed, providing optimal chamber humidity. The system maintains uniform temperature across all slide positions. Slides can be easily added or removed with one hand.

The slides are placed on a slide warmer at 69°C for 8 min for simultaneous denaturation of both probe and specimen nucleic acids. Afterwards, they are removed from the slide warmer and quickly transferred to the humidification chamber, which is placed in a 37°C air incubator for hybridization to occur. HYBrite or ThermoBrite (Vysis) (Abbott) can be used instead of a slide warmer and humidification chamber for the simultaneous denaturation of probe and specimen nucleic acids. Water is added to each for humidity, which is especially important for overnight hybridizations. The HYBrite or ThermoBrite system holds up to 12 slides. The numeric keypad allows for easy programming of the settings in three modes of operation: denaturation/hybridization, hybridization, and fixed temperature.

Hybridization times vary with the first hybridization of the MultiVysion PB or PGT panel five-color probe mixture at 1–3 h followed by rehybridization with mixtures that may include sub-telomeric probes requiring a longer minimum hybridization of 4–5 h. Whole chromosome paints are hybridized for a minimum of 8 h.

Washing procedures

The following two wash protocols may be used, which do not require formamide.

Rapid wash I

This wash is used for 1–3-color probe mixtures including whole chromosome paints and MultiVysion PGT for chromosomes 13, 18, 21, X, and Y.

(1) A coplin jar is filled with approximately 50 ml of 0.4 × SSC/0.3% NP-40, pH 7.4 and is placed in a 73°C water bath. Using a calibrated thermometer, the temperature of the solution inside the jar is checked before adding slides for the wash procedure. The solution temperature should be 73 ± 1°C.

(2) A second coplin jar is filled with 50 ml of 2 × SSC/0.1% NP-40, pH 7.4 and placed at room temperature.

(3) Slide(s) are placed in the 0.4 × SSC/0.3% NP-40 immediately after removing the coverslip, and incubated for 5 min, no more than four slides at a time so as not to decrease dramatically the temperature of the wash solution.

(4) After 5 min the slide(s) are removed from the wash solution and placed in the coplin jar containing 2 × SSC/0.1% NP-40 at room temperature and incubated for 1 min.

(5) The slide(s) are removed from the wash solution, dipped in a coplin jar containing HPLC-grade water and placed vertically to drain on a paper towel in a dark area (such as a drawer).

This wash may be used also for MultiVysion PB panel probe, although Abbott recommends for this purpose Rapid wash II.

Rapid wash II

This wash is used for MultiVysion PB panel probe for chromosomes 13, 16, 18, 21, and 22, and the four-color custom probe for chromosomes X, Y, 15, and 17.

(1) A coplin jar is filled with 50 ml of 0.7 × SSC/0.3% NP-40, pH 7.4 and placed in a 73°C water bath. Using a calibrated thermometer, the temperature of the solution inside the jar is checked before adding slides for the wash procedure. The solution temperature should be 73 ± 1°C.

(2) A second coplin jar is filled with 50 ml of 2 × SSC/0.1% NP-40, pH 7.4 and placed at room temperature.

(3) Slides are placed in the 0.7 × SSC/0.3% NP-40 immediately after removing the coverslips, not to exceed more than four slides, and incubated for 7 min.

(4) After 7 min of incubation the slide(s) are removed from the wash solution and placed in the coplin jar containing 2 × SSC/0.1% NP-40 at room temperature and incubated for 1 min.

(5) The slide(s) are removed from the wash solution, dipped in a coplin jar containing HPLC-grade water and placed vertically to drain on a paper towel in a dark area (such as a drawer).

DAPI counterstain

Approximately 10 µl of DAPI counterstain is applied to each slide and covered with a 22 × 30-mm coverslip for three-color probe testing. The slides are blotted using a paper towel or paper blotter to spread evenly and remove excess medium from the slide. For hybridizations using MultiVysion five-color and four-color custom probe mixtures, Vectashield anti-fade mounting medium is applied without DAPI.

FLUORESCENT SIGNAL EVALUATION

Signals are determined under ×630 magnification using fluorescence immersion oil.

Fluorophores are readily photobleached by exposure to light. To limit this degradation, handle all solutions containing fluorophores in reduced light. This includes all steps involved in handling the hybridized slide. All steps that do not require light for manipulation (incubation and washes) are carried out in the dark.

Fluorescence microscopy is accomplished using a 100-W mercury lamp. The manufacturer's recommendations for the length of time the lamp may be used should be followed since prolonged use may result in dim signals, creating the potential for misdiagnosis. An adequate supply of replacement bulbs should be on hand.

For the MultiVysion PGT probe, chromosome X (alpha satellite DXZ1) is seen in blue, the Y chromosome (alpha satellite DYZ3) is seen in gold, chromosome 13 (13q14) is seen in red, chromosome 18 (alpha satellite D18Z1) is seen in aqua, and chromosome 21 (LSI 21q22.13–21q22.2) is seen in green. For the MultiVysion PB Panel probe, chromosome 13 (13q14) is seen in red, chromosome 16 (satellite II D16Z3) is seen in aqua, chromosome 18 (alpha satellite D18Z1) is seen in violet blue, chromosome 21 (LSI 21q22.13–21q22.2) is seen in green, and chromosome 22 (22q11.2) is seen in gold (Figures 4.2 and 4.3). Abbott manufactures sub-telomeric probes for chromosome p-arms in green and q-arms in gold (seen with red and yellow filters). Rainbow sub-telomeric probes are produced in red and green for both p- and q-arms. Some microdeletion probes contain two areas labeled in green and gold (Abbot) or green and red (Rainbow). All BlueGnome LSI and telomeric probes can be ordered in green or orange (better seen with a yellow filter).

Visualization of signals is performed using the appropriate single-bandpass filters for the probe fluorophores (red, green, blue, gold, aqua, and DAPI). Dual-bandpass filters are useful in distinguishing signals from non-specific fluorescence or bleed-through, which is sometimes seen with centromeric enumeration probes that hybridize to alphoid repeat sequences resulting in large bright signals.

When determining the number of signals present, the size and intensity of each signal is considered especially when in close proximity to another one. Chromosomes 13, 21, and 22 are identified using locus-specific identifier DNA probes that contain specific sequences homologous to the chromosomes of interest as well as unlabeled blocking DNA to suppress common sequences. This results in smaller round signals when compared to signals from centromeric enumeration probes, which hybridize to a greater number of alpha repeat sequences identifying chromosomes 15, 16, 17, 18, X, and Y. To improve the accuracy of diagnosis, especially in cases of split or missing signals, repeat hybridization with a probe that targets a different locus (e.g., with a sub-telomeric probe) for the same chromosomes is required, as shown in Figures 4.26–4.29.

Signals for different chromosomes that are within close proximity to one another to the point of overlapping, especially in cases of highly condensed chromatin, are distinguished from non-specific hybridization by close examination using both single- and dual-bandpass filters, or re-hybridization with telomeric probes (Figure 4.26). Upon imaging, the overlapping portion of the signals may appear yellow or even white because of the fluorophore combination. Use of an imaging system is highly recommended when using probe mixtures containing more than three colors.

The PB1 contains two chromatids for each chromosome, so the signals for each chromosome are paired, at least one domain apart, and of equal size (Figure 4.2). However, if the chromatids are in close proximity to one another, the signals may appear as one fluorescent strip, representative of two chromatids (Figures 4.16, 4.23, and 4.26). The PB2 contains single chromatids for each chromosome, therefore resulting in one fluorescent signal for each chromosome tested (Figure 4.2).

Two single-dot signals for each chromosome studied are normally observed in each blastomere nucleus (Figure 4.3). However, signals can appear as double dots depending upon the stage of the cell cycle and the degree of chromatin condensation and overspreading (Figures 4.27 and 4.28). After replication, a signal may appear as paired dots less than one domain apart or as a strip consisting of two interconnected dots. These signals are counted as one signal according to standard criteria.

If signals are of equal size and intensity and are two domains apart, they are counted as two separate signals. However, proximity of two separate signals may be even closer than two domains in highly condensed nuclei and must be considered in order to avoid a misdiagnosis. Size and intensity of the signals of the individual nuclei as well as additional nuclei on the same slide must be taken into consideration when distinguishing non-specific fluorescence from actual signals. Hybridization spots of lower intensity, smaller in size or with a flat, non-fluorescing appearance are not counted.

As with all cytogenetic testing, for quality assurance, two independent readers are required for each case.

ARRAY-BASED 24-CHROMOSOME ANEUPLOIDY TESTING

The development and application of microarray technology for PGD of chromosomal disorders allows a highly improved detection of chromosomally abnormal oocytes and embryos. A number of platforms for 24-chromosome testing are now available, but the most widespread for the purpose of PGD at this time is 24sure technology, developed by BlueGnome Ltd, Cambridge, UK. This technique can be applied to all biopsy materials, including PB1, PB2, blastomeres, and blastocysts and allows the completion of the test within 12 h. The protocol consists of at least five steps, including amplification (2 h), labeling (2.5 h), hybridization (3.5 h), washing (30 min), scanning (30 min), and data analysis (1 h). The technique tests all 24 chromosomes for any gain or loss with the BAC pooling strategy, which coupled with the uniquely designed software enables obtaining straightforward results on aneuploidy in a single cell. Currently two 24sure array formats are used for two applications. BACs spotted on the 24sure array are selected on the basis of having little variations in over 5000 hybridizations, so deliver the highest level of reproducibility and sensitivity in aneuploidy testing.

For additional analysis of chromosomal rearrangements, the 24sure+ array format is used, which has greater coverage of genome, including sub-telomeric and peri-centromeric regions, and also enables accurate characterization of arm level aneuploidy and other large-scale structural abnormalities. Each of these formats is used with Sure Ref reference DNA as a hybridization reference, which is well matched for quality to an amplified single cell. To provide a useful reference in interpreting the results, a sex-mismatched design is used, such as the use of male reference in the hybridization, which mismatches with the X chromosome in analysis of polar bodies.

The critical step of the procedure is whole-genome amplification with the Super Plex Single Cell Whole Genome Amplification Kit (Rubicon Technology Inc.), which is performed according to manufacturer's instructions. Specific quality control criteria for sample quality and quantity are used to ensure that only specific amplifications are labeled. The fluorescent labeling system (BlueGnome Ltd) is used for the labeling of the amplified samples of biopsy materials, as well as for the labeling of a commercially available reference DNA. Test and reference DNA co-precipitation, their denaturation, array hybridization, and the post-hybridization washes are done according to the manufacturer's instructions.

A laser scanner is used to excite the hybridized fluorophores and to read and store the resulting images of hybridization, using the special software provided by BlueGnome. Chromosome profiles are examined for gain or loss, or for structural rearrangement. The examples of array-CGH results are presented in Figures 4.30 and 4.31.

This approach has opened the possibility of combining aneuploidy testing for 24 chromosomes with PGD for single-gene disorders and preimplantation HLA typing. The list of conditions for which this combined approach has been used in our center includes gangliosidosis GM1, isolated hypertrophic cardiomyopathy, cystic fibrosis, fragile X, neurofibromatosis type 1, Niemann–Pick disease, congenital gangliosidosis, Huntington, and chronic granulomatous disease, to mention only a few (see Chapter 6 for the list of 55 conditions tested). The data show that 24-chromosome aneuploidy testing together with PGD for Mendelian disorders and HLA typing is feasible in a single comprehensive test, thus avoiding the need for additional biopsy procedures. The technique may presently be applied for a combined PGD of single-gene disorders, aneuploidies, and translocations (see Chapter 6).

CHROMOSOMAL ABNORMALITIES IN POLAR BODIES

Thus far, chromosomal abnormalities in polar bodies have been studied in more than 20,000 oocytes obtained from 3953 clinical cycles for IVF patients of advanced reproductive age (average age 39 years).[23–29] Based on the results of PB1 and PB2 testing, aneuploidy-free zygotes were preselected for transfer back to patients. The embryos resulting from abnormal oocytes, when available, were tested further to confirm the PB1- and PB2-based diagnosis (see examples in Figures 4.21–4.25). As shown in Figure 4.32, results were not obtained either because of failure of hybridization or because the polar bodies were lost in process of preparation. The results for both PB1 and PB2 were obtained in 73.5% of oocytes. The remaining oocytes had either PB1 (13.1%) or PB2 results (13.4%) (Figure 4.33).

A total of 9812 (46.81%) of these oocytes were with aneuploidies, of which 2921 (29.8%) had errors in both PB1 and PB2, 2983 (30.4%) in only PB1, and 3908 (39.8%) in only PB2. As expected, the aneuploidy rates rose with increasing maternal age, from 20% in patients 35 years of age to over 40% in patients of 40 years of age.

Comparable proportions of aneuploidies were detected in PB1 (31.1%) and PB2 (33.7%), suggesting that the observed aneuploidies originate equally from both meiosis I and II, which is contrary to the well-established concept of female meiosis I origin of chromosomal abnormalities. Almost one-third of the chromosomally abnormal oocytes were outcomes of sequential meiosis I and meiosis II errors, so almost one-third of meiosis II errors were associated with the preceding meiosis I errors. However, half of meiosis II errors are still observed to be independent from meiosis I errors, so the genotype of the resulting zygote cannot be predicted without testing the outcomes of both meiotic divisions. The biological significance of both meiotic errors may also be obvious from the age dependence of isolated errors of meiosis I and meiosis II, as well as of sequential meiosis I and meiosis II errors.[28]

The schematic representations of the types of errors observed in PB1 and PB2 are presented in Figures 4.34 and 4.35, showing at least two times higher frequency for missing signals (nullisomy) compared to extra signals (disomy) in PB1 (approximately 2:1 ratio), in contrast to a comparable distribution of missing and extra signals in PB2 (Figure 4.36). The majority of abnormalities in meiosis I are represented by chromatid errors, in contrast to the expected chromosomal non-disjunction suggested by previous traditional studies mentioned.[30] However, chromosomal errors are still observed in 6.3% of oocytes. Although both chromatid and chromosomal errors are involved in producing MII abnormalities, the frequency of chromatid errors is much higher than chromosomal ones (chromatid/chromosome error ratio 10:1) (Figure 4.37). Both of these meiosis I errors lead to aneuploidy in the resulting embryos, as demonstrated by the follow-up study of the embryos resulting from these oocytes, the transfer of which was avoided. Although the observed excess of missing signals in PB1 may be also attributable to technical errors, such as hybridization failure, it is also possible that a certain meiosis I mechanism exists for preventing an extra chromosome material extrusion into PB1 if meiotic errors occur during the oocyte maturation process.

A significant proportion of abnormalities in PB1 and PB2 were of complex origin, represented by errors in both meiotic divisions and/or involving more than one chromosome (Figure 4.38). Overall, 78.5% of complex abnormalities involved two or more chromosomes simultaneously, and 21.5% the same chromosome(s) in both PB1 and PB2.

Chromosome-specific patterns of meiotic errors are shown in Figure 4.39. The most frequent chromosomes involved in meiotic error were chromosomes 21 and 22, with the error of chromosome 21 deriving comparably from meiosis I and meiosis II, and the error of chromosome 22 deriving predominantly from meiosis II. Meiotic error involving chromosomes 13, 16, and 18 was much less frequent, and their error patterns were not similar. Chromosome 16 errors originated predominantly in meiosis II, in contrast to chromosome 13 and 18 errors, which derived more frequently from meiosis I.

Despite the need for testing of both PB1 and PB2, testing of meiosis I errors alone should reduce the aneuploidy rate in the resulting embryos at least by two-thirds. In addition, over one-third of these oocytes will be still aneuploid following the second meiotic division, so PB1 testing could still sufficiently improve the implantation and pregnancy rates in poor prognosis IVF patients, or ICSI patients, by applying ICSI selectively to the oocytes with aneuploidy-free PB1. On the other hand, only close to a half of the abnormalities deriving from second meiotic division may be detected by PB1 analysis as complex errors; therefore, to avoid the transfer of all the embryos resulting from aneuploid oocytes, testing of both PB1 and PB2 is still required. Overall, the direct testing of meiosis I and meiosis II errors allows avoiding the transfer of at least 50% of embryos resulting from aneuploid oocytes, which clearly contributes to the pregnancy outcome of the IVF patients. As PB1 and PB2 are extruded in a normal process of oocyte maturation and fertilization and thus have no biological significance in pre- and post-implantation development, their removal and testing may become a useful tool in assisted reproduction practices to identify the oocytes without nuclear abnormalities, which should help in the preselection of oocytes with the highest potential for establishing a viable pregnancy, significantly improving IVF efficiency.

As expected, microarray-based testing for 24 chromosomes detects higher than FISH (70%) aneuploidy rate in human oocytes through the application of array-CGH analysis in PB1 and PB2, confirming the above observations by FISH analysis (examples of normal and abnormal oocytes resulting from meiosis errors detected by array-CGH analysis of PB1 and PB2 are presented in Figures 4.40 and 4.41). The relevance of array-CGH for testing PB1 and PB2 has also been confirmed by other recent reports.[31–33]

CHROMOSOMAL ABNORMALITIES IN CLEAVING EMBRYOS AND BLASTOCYSTS

As shown above, approximately half of meiosis II errors are observed in the oocytes with prior errors in meiosis I. As a result of such sequential errors, almost one-third of the resulting zygotes may have been considered normal (euploid) (Figure 4.35), provided that the preceding errors in meiosis I and meiosis II have no effect on the further preimplantation development of the corresponding embryos. However, the follow-up testing of these embryos at the cleavage stage demonstrated subsequent errors in mitotic divisions in the resulting zygotes, leading to the development of chromosomally abnormal embryos that were unacceptable for embryo transfer. In all, only 18% of embryos deriving from the apparently balanced zygotes were euploid for the five chromosomes analyzed (Figure 4.42), while the remaining majority had chromosomal abnormalities (Figures 4.43 and 4.44).[34,35]

All of the chromosomally normal embryos appeared to result from zygotes with only one chromosomal error rescue, with none resulting from the zygotes balanced for two chromosomes. The fact that only a few resulting embryos (11%) were abnormal for the same chromosome for which sequential meiosis I and meiosis II led to the balanced set may suggest that the observed sequential errors in female meiosis may be attributable to a meiotic apparatus abnormality overall, rather than to a single-chromosome segregation defect, and further may lead to a general defect in the mitotic apparatus of the resulting embryos. This seems to be also in agreement with the observed types of aneuploidies detected in the resulting embryos, which in 79.3% of cases were represented by complex errors (Figures 4.45–4.47), including mosaicism, known to be highly prevalent at the cleavage stage.

According to the data on PGD for aneuploidies performed at the cleavage stage, at least 60% of embryos tested had chromosomal abnormalities.[10,36,37] Although the reported types of aneuploidies may differ in different studies, approximately half of these abnormalities are represented by mosaicism. As there was no information about the initial chromosome complement of the zygotes from which the mosaic embryos originated in any of these studies, the nature of mosaicism in preimplantation embryos is not known, despite its high prevalence and the potential clinical relevance. There were, however, some indirect observations, suggesting that the observed mosaicism at the cleavage stage may be of a different nature, with some mosaic types increasing with maternal age,[38] therefore probably stemming from female meiosis errors, while others are possibly attributable to immaturity of centrosome structures in sperm and are expected to be active from the first mitotic divisions of the zygote, as suggested for cases involving testicular sperm extraction (TESE) patients.[39] It may also be suggested that a significant proportion of mosaic embryos originate from oocytes that are aneuploid from the outset, through a process of trisomy "rescue." A possible high rate of further mitotic errors in cleaving embryos deriving from oocytes with complex aneuploidies may also explain the phenomenon of chaotic embryos, which make up almost half of the embryos with mosaicism. A comparable prevalence of aneuploidies in oocytes and embryos, with the differences in the types of chromosomal anomalies mainly attributable to a high frequency of mosaicism in cleavage-stage embryos, may also support a prezygotic origin of the majority of embryo chromosome abnormalities, including mosaicism.

The problem of mosaicism also remains in the application of array-CGH-based 24-chromosome aneuploidy testing to the cleavage stage biopsy material. It is expected that this problem may be overcome by the application of this technique to blastocyst biopsy samples, which may detect 10% or higher rates of mosaicism. Examples of aneuploidies detected by array-CGH 24-chromosome analyses in embryos confirmed by FISH analysis are shown in Figures 4.48–4.50.

Comparison of the chromosome-specific aneuploidy rates in oocytes and embryos may also be of relevance in understanding the relationship between oocyte and embryo abnormalities. The data show a higher rate for each chromosome error in oocytes compared to that in embryos, which may indicate a possible correction of some of the aneuploidies through the mechanism of "trisomy rescue," probably resulting in a certain proportion of mosaic embryos following the first three cleavage divisions. In fact, the exact data on the mosaicism rate in preimplantation development are not known, because only a limited number of the preimplantation embryos were fully studied, with the majority available from PGD for aneuploidies performed on a single biopsied blastomere, which may not be representative of the whole embryo. Although the possibility of postzygotic mitotic errors in cleavage-stage embryos euploid from the outset cannot be excluded, the proportion of the aneuploidy and mosaicism stemming from these errors and the impact of these postzygotic errors on the pre- and post-implantation embryo development are not known.

Based on the above data, it may be suggested that the most accurate preselection of embryos for transfer in PGD for aneuploidies may be performed by array-CGH analysis for 24 chromosomes couples with blastocyst biopsy. It may also be useful to perform a sequential testing of meiosis I, meiosis II, and mitotic errors, through sequential PBI, PB2, and embryo biopsy. This may enable the transfer of embryos with prezygotic chromosomal errors to be avoided, which seems to be the major source of chromosomal abnormalities in the embryo, and may also enable the detection of possible mitotic errors in embryos resulting from the euploid zygotes, the proportion of which cannot be evaluated at the present time. The accumulating data on such sequential sampling will help to evaluate possible differences in the viability of embryos with chromosomal abnormalities of meiotic and mitotic origin.

REFERENCES

1. Griffin DK, Handyside AH, Penketh RJA, et al. Fluorescent in-situ hybridization to interphase nuclei of human preimplantation embryos with X and Y chromosome specific probes. *Hum Reprod* 1991; 6:101–105.
2. Griffin DK, Wilton LJ, Handyside AH, et al. Dual fluorescent in-situ hybridization for the simultaneous detection of X and Y chromosome specific probes for the sexing of human preimplantation embryonic nuclei. *Hum Genet* 1992; 89:18–22.
3. Schrurs BM, Winston RML, Handyside AH. Preimplantation diagnosis of aneuploidy using fluorescent in-situ hybridization: evaluation using a chromosome 18-specific probe. *Hum Reprod* 1993; 8:296–301.
4. Munné S, Weier HUG, Stein J, et al. A fast and efficient method for simultaneous X and Y in-situ hybridization of human blastomeres. *J Assist Reprod Genet* 1993; 10:82–90.
5. Munné S, Lee A, Rozenwaks Z, et al. Diagnosis of major chromosome aneuploidies in human preimplantation embryos. *Hum Reprod* 1993; 8:2185–91.
6. Munné S, Magli MC, Bahçe M, et al. Preimplantation diagnosis of the aneuploidies most commonly found in spontaneous abortions and live births: XY, 13, 14, 15, 16, 18, 21, 22. *Prenat Diagn* 1998; 18:1459–66.
7. Bahçe M, Cohen J, Munné S. Preimplantation genetic diagnosis of aneuploidy: were we looking at the wrong chromosomes? *J Assist Reprod Genet* 1999; 16:154–59.
8. Kuliev A, Verlinsky Y. Thirteen-years experience of preimplantation genetic diagnosis. *Reprod Biomed Online* 2004; 8:229–35.
9. Gianaroli L, Magli MC, Ferraretti AP, Munné S. Preimplantation diagnosis for aneuploidies in patients undergoing in vitro fertilization with poor prognosis: identification of the categories for which it should be proposed. *Fertil Steril* 1999; 72:837–44.

10. Munné S. Preimplantation genetic diagnosis of numerical and structural chromosome abnormalities. *Reprod Biomed Online* 2002; 4:183–96.
11. Munné S, Sandalinas M, Escudero T, et al. Improved implantation after preimplantation genetic diagnosis of aneuploidy. *Reprod Biomed Online* 2003; 7:91–97.
12. Munné S, Alikani M, Tomkin G, et al. Embryo morphology, developmental rates and maternal age are correlated with chromosome abnormalities. *Fertil Steril* 1995; 64:382–91.
13. Munné S, Weier HUG, Grifo J, Cohen J. Chromosome mosaicism in human embryos. *Biol Reprod* 1994; 51:373–79.
14. Delhanty JDA, Griffin DK, Handyside AH. Detection of aneuploidy and chromosomal mosaicism in human embryos during preimplantation sex determination by fluorescent in situ hybridisation (FISH). *Hum Mol Genet* 1993; 2:1183–85.
15. Harper JC, Coonen E, Handyside AH, et al. Mosaicism of autosomes and sex chromosomes in morphologically normal monospermic preimplantation human embryos. *Prenat Diagn* 1994; 15:41–49.
16. International Working Group on Preimplantation Genetics. Current status of preimplantation diagnosis. *J Assist Reprod Genet* 1997; 14:72–75.
17. International Working Group on Preimplantation Genetics. 10th anniversary of preimplantation genetic diagnosis. *J Assist Reprod Genet* 2001; 18:66–72.
18. Evsikov S, Verlinsky Y. Mosaicism in inner cell mass of human blastocysts. *Hum Reprod* 1998; 13:3151–55.
19. Dyban A, Fredine M, Severova E, et al. Detection of aneuploidy in human oocytes and corresponding first polar bodies using FISH. Presented at the 7th International Conference on Early Prenatal Diagnosis, Jerusalem, Israel, 22–27 May, 1994: abstract 97.
20. Verlinsky Y, Cieslak J, Freidine M, et al. Pregnancies following pre-conception diagnosis of common aneuploidies by fluorescent in-situ hybridization. *Hum Reprod* 1995; 10:1923–27.
21. Dyban A, Fredine M, Severova E, et al. Detection of aneuploidy in human oocytes and corresponding first polar bodies by FISH. *J Assist Reprod Genet* 1996; 13:72–77.
22. Munné S, Daily T, Sultan KM, et al. The use of first polar bodies for preimplantation diagnosis of aneuploidy. *Hum Reprod* 1995; 10:1014–20.
23. Verlinsky Y, Cieslak J, Ivakhnenko V, et al. Birth of healthy children after preimplantation diagnosis of common aneuploidies by polar body FISH analysis. *Fertil Steril* 1996; 66:126–29.
24. Verlinsky Y, Cieslak J, Ivakhnenko V, et al. Pre-pregnancy genetic testing for age-related aneuploidies by polar body analysis. *Genet Test* 1998; 1:231–35.
25. Verlinsky Y, Cieslak J, Ivakhnenko V, et al. Polar body preimplantation diagnosis in aging IVF patients. *Ref Gynecol Obstet* 2000; 7:191–94.
26. Verlinsky Y, Cieslak J, Ivakhnenko V, et al. Chromosomal abnormalities in the first and second polar body. *Mol Cell Endocrinol* 2001; 183:S47–49.
27. Kuliev A, Cieslak J, Ilkevitch Y, et al. Chromosomal abnormalities in a series of 6733 human oocytes in preimplantation diagnosis for age-related aneuploidies. *Reprod Biomed Online* 2003; 6:54–59.
28. Kuliev A, Cieslak J, Verlinsky Y. Frequency and distribution of chromosomal abnormalities in human oocytes. *Cytogenet Genome Res* 2005; 111:193–98.
29. Kuliev A, Zlatopolsky Z, Kirillova I, Spivakova J, Cieslak-Jansen J. Meiosis errors in over 20,000 oocytes studied in practice of preimplantation aneuploidy testing. *Reprod Biomed Online* 2011; 22:2–8.
30. Angel R. First meiotic division nondisjunction in human oocytes. *Am J Hum Genet* 1997; 65:23–32.
31. Geraedts J, Montag M, Magli C et al. Polar body array CGH for prediction of the status of the corresponding oocyte. Part I: clinical results. *Hum Reprod* 2011; 26:3172-3180.
32. Magli C, Montag M, Koster M, et al. Polar body array CGH for prediction of the status of the corresponding oocyte. Part II: technical aspects. *Hum Reprod* 2011; doi:10.1093/humrep/der295.
33. Gabriel AS, Thornhill AR, Ottolini CS, et al. Array comparative genomic hybridization on first polar bodies suggests that non-disjunction is not the predominant mechanism leading to aneuploidy in humans. *J Med Genet* 2011; 48:433–437.
34. Kuliev A, Cieslak J, Zlatopolsky Z, et al. Origin of aneuploidies in preimplantation embryos. 2003 Fifth International Symposium on Preimplantation Genetics, 5–7 June 2003, Antalya, Turkey: 16–17.
35. Kuliev A, Cieslak J, Zlatopolsky Z, et al. Aneuploidy rescue after female meiosis I and follow up analysis of its outcome in resulting preimplantation embryos. *Am J Hum Genet* 2003; 73(Suppl):189.
36. Gianaroli L, Magli MC, Ferraretti AP. The in vivo and in vitro efficiency and efficacy of PGD for aneuploidy. *Mol Cell Endocrinol* 2001; 183:S13–18.
37. Munné S, Bahçe M, Sandalinas M. Differences in chromosome susceptibility to aneuploidy and survival to first trimester. *Reprod Biomed Online* 2003: webpaper 1058.
38. Munné S, Sandalinas M, Escudero T, et al. Some mosaic types increase with maternal age. *Reprod Biomed Online* 2002: webpaper 382.
39. Silber S, Sadowy S, Lehahan K, et al. High rate of chromosome mosaicism but not aneuploidy in embryos from karyotypically normal men requiring TESE. *Reprod Biomed Online* 2002; 4 (Suppl 2):20.

5 Preimplantation diagnosis for translocations

As described in the previous chapter, cytogenetic testing of single cells obtained from preimplantation embryos has previously been performed by interphase fluorescent *in situ* hybridization (FISH) analysis, which allows chromosome enumeration and detection of translocations on interphase cell nuclei.[1] However, the number of chromosomes studied by FISH is limited to the number of chromosome-specific probes available, which is presently surpassed by microarray analysis. Even with the currently available methods for re-hybridization of interphase nuclei for a second and third time, a complete karyotyping, even if possible, is not practical. The technique also had clear limitations for the detection of some rearrangements, such as chromosome insertions and inversions, so new approaches have now been developed, including methods for visualization of chromosomes in single cells (polar bodies (PB) and individual blastomeres), haplotyping by the use of a multiplex fluorescent PCR of highly polymorphic markers, and microarray-based technology, which will clearly improve the accuracy of preimplantation genetic diagnosis (PGD) for chromosomal disorders.[2–7]

One of the approaches for PGD of maternally derived translocations is first polar body (PB1) testing, based on the fact that PB1 never forms an interphase nucleus and so consists of metaphase chromosomes. It has been shown that PB1 chromosomes are recognizable when isolated 2–3 h after *in vitro* culture, with degeneration beginning 6–7 h after extrusion,[8] thus whole-chromosome painting or locus-specific probes may be applied for testing.[9] As shown in Figures 5.1–5.6, which demonstrate segregation during meiosis I, by testing PB1 using specific probes for chromosomes involved in translocation, unbalanced chromosome complements may be detected and avoided. Although the method resulted in a significant reduction in the rate of spontaneous abortions in the patients carrying translocations, yielding unaffected pregnancies and the birth of healthy children, it has been shown to be sensitive to malsegregation and/or recombination between chromatids (Figures 5.7–5.9), requiring a further follow-up analysis of the second polar body (PB2) in order to accurately predict the meiotic outcome following the second meiotic division. However, despite the progress in transforming PB2 into metaphase chromosomes via electrofusion of the PB2 nucleus with a foreign one-cell human embryo (see Chapter 3), the proportion of metaphase plates obtained did not exceed 65%, and a higher percentage would be necessary to be useful in clinical practice.[1] Therefore, alternative methods were developed to convert single blastomere nuclei into metaphase chromosomes following the fusion of single blastomeres with murine[3] (see Chapter 3) or bovine zygotes.[4] These methods appeared to be useful for PGD for both maternally and paternally derived translocation.

Initially individual blastomere nuclei were transformed into metaphase chromosomes through blastomere fusion with enucleated human oocytes,[3] but currently this is accomplished by the fusion of individual blastomeres with intact mouse zygotes at the pronuclear stage,[10] as described in Chapter 3. To date, the method has been applied for PGD of paternally derived reciprocal translocations, for chromosome inversions, and for confirmation of PGD for chromosomal abnormalities identified by PB1 and PB2 FISH analysis (Figures 5.10–5.14). In our experience of the 609 PGD cycles for balanced translocations, 133 were offered using the nuclear conversion method, 94 by chemical conversion, 90 using PB1 and PB2 testing, and the remaining by embryo biopsy and interphase analysis using FISH (Table 5.1) or, currently, array-CGH analysis.[10,11]

Examples of PGD cycles for translocations performed utilizing the nuclear conversion method are presented in Figures 5.10–5.14. Overall, the technique was applied to 767 blastomeres, which included 582 for reciprocal and 185 for Robertsonian translocations, resulting in successful nuclear metaphase conversion in as many as 635 (83%). This made possible the preselection of normal embryos or those with a balanced chromosomal complement for transfer in 73% of the cycles, resulting in a 32% pregnancy rate per transfer, with only 20% spontaneous abortions, compared to a nearly 90% spontaneous abortion rate before PGD in the same patients.

Examples of PGD for maternally derived translocations performed using PB1 and PB2 FISH analysis are shown in Figures 5.7–5.9, 5.13, and 5.14. In these cycles, the FISH results were obtained from 79% of the oocytes, allowing preselection of normal or balanced embryos for transfer in 63% of cycles, resulting in clinical pregnancies and the delivery of unaffected children. The proportion of abnormal oocytes and embryos detected varied depending on the types of translocations and their origin. The meiotic outcomes of female reciprocal translocations based on PB and blastomere analysis are presented in Figure 5.15, showing the most frequent segregation patterns, which are mainly in agreement irrespective of the method of analysis,

Table 5.1 List of translocations for which PGD was performed, FISH probes used, and the clinical outcome

Patients	*Cycles*	*Karyotype*	*FISH Probes*	*Embryo Transfers / Pregnancies / Deliveries (# of children born) (# of miscarriages*)*
28	35	45,XX,der(13;14)(q10;q10)	WCP 13, WCP 14, LSI 13 (13q14), tel 13q, tel 14q	32 / 13 / 9 (11) (4*)
1	1	45,XX,der(13;15)(q10;q10)	tel 13q, tel 15q	0 / 0
1	1	45,XX,der(13;21)(q10;q10)	tel 13q, tel 21q	1 / 1 / 1 (1)
1	1	45,XX,der(13;22)(q10;q10)	WCP 13, WCP 22, PB panel (chromosomes 13,16,18,21,22)	1 / 0
3	5	45,XX,der(14;21)(q10;q10)	WCP 14, WCP 21, LSI 21(21q22.13-q22.2), tel 14q, tel 21q	5 / 3 / 3 (3)
1	5	45,XX,der(14;22)(q10;q10)	WCP 14, WCP 22, tel 14 q, LSI 22 (22q11.2)	3 / 1 / 1 (1)
37	44	45,XY,der(13;14)(q10;q10)	WCP 13, WCP 14, LSI 13 (13q14), tel 14q	39 / 17 / 14 (15) (3*)
3	5	45,XY,der(13;15)(q10;q10)	WCP 13, WCP 15, LSI 13 (13q14), tel 15q	5 / 2 / 2 (2)
1	2	45,XY,der(14;15)(q10;q10)	tel 14q, tel 15q	0 / 0
6	13	45,XY,der(14;21)(q10;q10)	WCP 14, WCP 21, LSI 21	11 / 4 /3 (3) (1*)
1	2	45,XX,der(4),t(4;13)(q35;q12),-13	WCP 4, WCP 13, CEP 4, tel 4q, tel 13q	1 / 0
1	1	46,XX,t(1;3)(q32;q12)	CEP 3, tel 1q, tel 3q	0 / 0
1	1	46,XX,t(1;4)(q23;q31.1)	WCP 1, WCP 4, (CEP 18 as control)	1 / 0
1	1	46,XX,t(1;7)(p10;p10)	CEP 7, tel 1p, tel 7p	0 / 0
1	1	46,XX,t(1;7)(q23;p11)	WCP 1, WCP 7, CEP 1	1 / 1 / 1 (1)
1	1	46,XX,t(1;7)(p42.3;q32)	WCP 1, WCP 7, CEP 7, tel 1p, tel 7q	2 / 0
1	3	46,XX,t(1;8)(q42;p11.2)	WCP 1, WCP 8, CEP 1, CEP 8, tel 1q, tel 8p	3 / 2 / 1 (1) (1*)
1	1	46,XX,t(1;8)(q25;p11.2)	WCP 1, WCP 8, CEP 1, CEP 8, tel 1q, tel 8p	0 / 0
1	1	46,XX,t(1;9)(p36.3;p13)	CEP 9, tel 1p, tel 9p	0 / 0
1	2	46,XX,t(1;10)(q32.3;q24.3)	CEP 1, CEP 10, tel 1q, tel 10q	2 / 1 / 1 (1)
1	2	46,XX,t(1;10)(q42.1;q26.1)	WCP 1, WCP 10, CEP 10, tel 1q, tel 10q, PB panel	0 / 0
1	1	46,XX,t(1;11)(q32.1;p15.5)	CEP 11, tel 1q, tel 11p	1 / 1/ 1 (1)
1	1	46,XX,t(1;13)(q12;q32)	WCP 1, WCP 13, CEP 1, tel 1q, tel 13q	1 / 0
1	1	46,XX,t(1;14)(p34.3;q22.1)	WCP 1, WCP 14, CEP 1, tel 1p, tel 14q	1 / 0
1	2	46,XX,t(1;15)(q32;q26)	WCP 1, WCP 15, CEP 15, CEP 1, tel 15 q, tel 1q	2 / 1 / 1 (1)
1	3	46,XX,t(1;21)(q32;q22.1)	CEP 1, tel 1q, tel 21q	2 / 0
1	1	46,XX,t(1;22)(q25;q11.1)	CEP 1, tel 1q, tel 22q	1 / 0
1	1	46,XX,inv(1)	WCP 1, tel 1p, tel 1q	1 / 1 / 1 (2)
1	1	46,XX,t(2;3)(p13;q29)	WCP 2, CEP 3, tel 2p, tel 3q	1 / 0
1	1	46,XX,(2;4)(p11.1;q31.3)	CEP 4, tel 2p, tel4q	2 / 1 / 1 (2)
1	2	46,XX,t(2;5)(q13;q13)	WCP 2, WCP 5, CEP 2, tel 2q, tel 5q	1 / 0
1	1	46,XX,t(2;5)(q31.1;q31.1)	CEP 2, tel 2q, tel 5q	1 / 1/ 1 (1)
1	1	46,XX,t(2;5)(q33;p14)	WCP 2, WCP 5, tel 2q, tel 5p	1 / 0
1	1	46,XX,t(2;6)(q33;p23)	CEP 6, tel 2q, tel 6p	0 / 0
1	1	46,XX,t(2;8)(q11.2;q24.22)	CEP 2, CEP 8tel 2q	1 / 1 /1 (1)
1	2	46,XX,t(2;9)(q35;q34.3)	WCP 2, WCP 9, CEP 2, CEP 9, tel 2q, tel 9q	2 / 0
1	2	46,XX,t(2;10)(q31;q11.2)	WCP 2, WCP 10, CEP 2, tel 2q	1 / 0

Table 5.1 (*Continued*) List of translocations for which PGD was performed, FISH probes used, and the clinical outcome

Patients	*Cycles*	*Karyotype*	*FISH Probes*	*Embryo Transfers / Pregnancies / Deliveries (# of children born) (# of miscarriages*)*
1	1	46,XX,t(2;13)(q22;q33)	WCP 2, WCP 13, CEP 2, tel 13 q, LSI 13 (13q14)	1 / 1 / 1 (1)
1	1	46,XX,t(2;13)(q37;q21)	CEP 2, tel 2q, tel 13q	1/ 1/ 1 (1)
1	2	46,XX,t(2;14)(q33;q24.1)	CEP 2, tel 2q, tel 14q	0 / 0
1	1	46,XX,t(2;16)9q35;q24)	CEP 16, tel 2q, tel 16q	1 / 1 / 1 (2)
1	1	46,XX,t(2;16)(q37;p13.1)	WCP 2, WCP 16, CEP 16, tel 2q, tel 16p	0 / 0
1	2	46,XX,t(2;18)(q31.1;q21.3)	CEP 18, tel 2q, tel 18q	2 / 0
1	1	46,XX,t(2;20)(q37;q11.2)	WCP 2, WCP 20, CEP 2, tel 20q	0 / 0
1	1	46,XX,t(3;4)(p13;p35)	CEP 4, tel 3p, tel 4q	0 / 0
1	1	46,XX,t(3;5)(p25;q35.2)	WCP 3, WCP 5, tel 3p, tel 5q	1 / 0
1	1	46,XX,t(3;6)(p13;p15)	CEP 6, tel 3p, tel 6q	0 / 0
1	1	46,XX,t(3;6)(p26.2;q21)	WCP 3, WCP 6, CEP 6, tel 3p, tel 6q	1 / 1 / 1 (1)
1	1	46,XX,t(3;7)(p21;q22)	WCP 3, WCP 7, tel 7q, tel 3p	1 / 1 / 1 (1)
1	1	46,XX,t(3;8)(q21;q24.1)	CEP 3, CEP 8, tel 3q, tel 8q	1 / 1 / 1 (1)
1	1	46,XX,t(3;8)(q26.3;q24.3)	CEP 8, tel 3q, tel 8q	1 / 1 / 1 (2)
1	1	46,XX,t(3;8)(q27;q22)	WCP 3, WCP 8, tel 8q, CEP 8, CEP 3	1 / 0
1	1	46,XX,t(3;9)(p21;q22.33)	CEP 3, CEP 9, tel 3p, tel 9q	1 / 1 / 0 (1*)
1	3	46,XX,t(3;9)(q28;q33)	CEP 3, CEP 9, tel 3q, tel 9q	3 / 1 / 0 (1*)
1	1	46,XX,t(3;10)(p25;q15.1)	WCP 3, WCP 10, tel 3p, tel 10q, CEP 3, CEP 10	0 / 0
1	1	46,XX,t(3;12)(p13;q23)	CEP 3, CEP 12, tel 3p, tel 12q	1 / 0
1	4	46,XX,t(3;12)(q21;q24.33)	WCP 3, WCP 12, CEP 3, CEP 12, tel 3q	4 / 0
1	1	46,XX,t(3;12)(q25;q15)	CEP 3, CEP 12, tel 3q	1 / 0
2	2	46,XX,t(3;15)(q13.2;q22.3)	CEP 15, tel 3q, tel 15q	2 / 1 / 1 (2)
1	1	46,XX,t(3;19)(p25;p13.3)	WCP 3, WCP 19	1 / 0
1	1	46,XX,t(3;22)(q13.2;q11.2)	WCP 3, WCP 22, CEP 3, tel 3q, tel 22q	1 / 1 / 1 (1)
1	1	46,XX,t(4;5)(p15.2;q31.3)	WCP 4, WCP 5, CEP 4, tel 4p, tel 5q	1 / 0
1	3	46,XX,t(4;6)(p14;q21)	WCP 4, WCP 6, CEP 4, CEP 6, tel 4p, tel 6q	3 / 0
1	4	46,XX,t(4;8)(p16;p23.1)	WCP 4, WCP 8, CEP 4, tel 4p, tel 8p	4 / 0
1	1	46,XX,t(4;8)(p16;q24)	CEP 4, tel 4p, tel 8q	0 / 0
1	3	46,XX,t(4;8)(q27;q24)	WCP 4, WCP 8, CEP 4, tel 4q, tel 8q	1 / 0
1	1	46,XX,t(4;9)(p16.6;p13)	CEP 4, CEP 9, tel 4p, tel 9p	1 / 0
1	1	46,XX,t(4;10)(q21.3;q11.2)	WCP 4, WCP 10, CEP 10, tel 4q, tel 10q	0 / 0
1	1	46,XX,t(4;13)(p11;p12)	CEP 4, tel 4p, tel 4q, LSI 13	1 / 0
1	2	46,XX,t(4;13)(p14;q31)	WCP 4, WCP 13, tel 13q	0 / 0
1	2	46,XX,t(4;13)(q23;q21)	WCP 4, WCP 13, LSI 13(13q14), CEP 4, tel 4q	1 / 0
1	2	46,XX,t(4;16)(q33;p13.1)	WCP 4, WCP 16, CEP 4, tel 4q, tel 16p	2 / 0
1	2	46,XX,t(4;22)(q32;q13.1)	CEP 4, tel 4q, tel 22q	2 / 0
1	2	46,XX,t(4;14)(q21.3;q24.3)	WCP 4, WCP 14, tel 14 q, CEP 4	2 / 0
1	1	46,XX,t(5;7)(p14;p21)	WCP 5, WCP 7, tel 7p	1 / 0
1	1	46,XX,t(5;9)(q33.1;p13)	CEP 9, tel 5q, tel 9p	1 / 1 / 1 (2)

(*Continued*)

Table 5.1 (*Continued*) List of translocations for which PGD was performed, FISH probes used, and the clinical outcome

Patients	*Cycles*	*Karyotype*	*FISH Probes*	*Embryo Transfers / Pregnancies / Deliveries (# of children born) (# of miscarriages*)*
1	2	46,XX,t(5;10)(q11;q22.1)	WCP 5, WCP 10, CEP 10	2 / 0
1	4	46,XX,t(5;10)(q35;p11.2)	CEP 10, tel 5q, tel 10p	4 / 2 / 2 (2)
1	1	46,XX,t(5;11)(q13;p15)	WCP 5, WCP 11, CEP 11, tel 5q, tel 11p	0 / 0
1	1	46,XX,t(5;11)(p15.1;p15.1)	CEP 11, tel 5p, tel 11p	0 / 0
1	2	46,XX,t(5;13)(q23.1;q14.1)	WCP 5, WCP 13, tel 5q, tel 13q	0 / 0
1	2	46,XX,t(5;13)(p14;q22)	Cri-du-Chat, tel 13q	1 / 0
1	2	46,XX,t(5;13)(p15.3;q32.1)	WCP 5, WCP 13, rel 5p, tel 5q, tel 13q	1 / 0
1	1	46,XX,t(5;14)(p16.3;q22)	tel 5p, tel 5q, tel 14q	2 / 0
1	1	46,XX,t(5;14)(q35;q32.2)	WCP 5, WCP 14, tel 5q	0 / 0
1	1	46,XX,t(5;16)(p15.3;q24)	WCP 5, WCP 16, CEP 16, tel 5p, tel 16q	0 / 0
1	1	46,XX,t(5;18)(q12;p11.2)	WCP 5, WCP 18, CEP 18, tel 15q, tel 18p	1 / 1 / 1 (1)
1	1	46,XX,t(5;18)(q22;q12.2)	WCP 5, WCP 18, CEP 18, tel 15q, tel 18q	0 / 0
1	3	46,XX,t(5;20)(q33;q13.1)	tel 5q, CEP 20, tel 201	2 / 1 / 1(1)
1	2	46,XX,t(5;21)(q11.2;q22)	WCP 5, WCP 21, LSI 21 (21q22.13-q22.2), tel 21q, tel 5p, tel 5q	1 / 0
2	3	46,XX,t(5;21)(q31;q22.1)	WCP 5, WCP 21, LSI 5 (5q33-q34), LSI 21 (21q22.13-q22.2)	1 / 0
1	2	46,XX,t(6;7)(p11.2;q11.2)	CEP 6, tel 6p, tel 7q	0 / 0
1	1	46,XX,t(6;8)(q25;p21.1)	CEP 6, CEP 8, tel 6q, tel 8p	1 / 1 / 1 (2)
1	1	46,XX,t(6;9)(p25;q31)	CEP 6, tel 6p, tel 9q	0 / 0
1	1	46,XX,t(6;12)(q16.3;p12.2)	CEP 6, CEP 12, tel 12q	1 / 1 / 0 (0) (1*)
2	3	46,XX,t(6;13)(q21;q22)	WCP 6, WCP 13, LSI 13, tel 6q, tel 13q	1 / 1 / 1 (1)
1	1	46,XX,t(6;14)(q15;q13.1)	WCP 6, WCP 14, CEP 6, tel 6q, tel 14q	0 / 0
1	1	46,XX,t(6;15)(p21.3;q26.1)	WCP 6, WCP 15, CEP 15, tel 15q	1 / 1 / 1 (1)
1	2	46,XX,t(6;15)(q23;q26)	CEP 6, tel 6q, tel 15q	2 / 0
1	1	46,XX,t(6;19)(q;p)	CEP 6, tel 6q, tel 19p	1 / 0
1	1	46,XX,t(7;11)(p11.2;q24.2)	WCP 7, WCP 11, CEP 11, tel 11q	1 / 1 / 1 (1)
1	1	46,XX,t(7;13)(q36;q12)	WCP 7, WCP 13, LSI 13 (13q14), CEP 7, tel 7q	0 / 0
1	1	46,XX,t(7;14)(q33;q32.3)	WCP 7, WCP 14, CEP 7, tel7q, tel14q	1 / 0
1	1	46,XX,t(7;18)(q32;q23)	WCP 7, WCP 18, CEP 18	1 / 0
1	3	46,XX,t(7;19)(q22.3;p13.3)	WCP 7, CEP 7, tel 7q, tel 19p	3 / 2 / 2 (2)
1	1	46,XX,t(7;19)(q32;p13.2)	WCP 7, WCP 19, CEP 7, tel 7q, tel 19p	1 / 1 / 0 (0) (1*)
1	1	46,XX,t(7;19)(q34;p13.1)	CEP 7, tel 7q, tel 19p)	1 / 0
1	3	46,XX,t(7;22)(p22.3;p11.2)	CEP 7, tel 22q, tel 7p	1 / 1 / 1 (1)
1	1	46,XX,t(8;9)(q11.2;q32)	WCP 8, WCP 9, CEP 8, CEP 9, tel 8q, tel 9q	1 / 1/ 1 (1)
2	2	46,XX,t(8;10)(q22.1;q22.1)	WCP 8, WCP 10, CEP 10, tel 8q, tel 10q	1 / 0
1	3	46,XX,t(8;10)(q24.3;q24.1)	WCP 8, WCP 10, CEP 10, tel 10q, tel 8p, tel 8q	1 / 0
1	1	46,XX,t(8;10)(p10;p10)	WCP 8, WCP 10, CEP 10, tel 10p, tel 8p	1 / 0
1	1	46,XX,t(8;12)(q21.2;p13.3)	WCP 8, WCP 12, tel 12 p, CEP 12	0 / 0
1	1	46,XX,t(8;13)(q22.3;q12)	WCP 8, WCP 13, CEP 8, tel 8q, tel 13q	1 / 1 /1 (3)
1	1	46,XX,t(8;18)(q22.1;q12.3)	WCP 18, CEP 18, tel 81, tel 18q)	0/0

Table 5.1 (*Continued*) List of translocations for which PGD was performed, FISH probes used, and the clinical outcome

Patients	*Cycles*	*Karyotype*	*FISH Probes*	*Embryo Transfers / Pregnancies / Deliveries (# of children born) (# of miscarriages*)*
1	1	46,XX,t(8;18)(q24.13;q21.2)	CEP 18, tel 8q, tel 18q	0 / 0
1	2	46,XX,t(8;22)(q24.1;q11.2)	WCP 8, WCP 22, CEP 8	1 / 0
1	1	46,XX,t(9;10)(q32;p13)	WCP 9, WCP 10, CEP 10, tel 9q, tel 10p	1 / 1 / 1 (1)
1	1	46,XX,t(9;11)(q13;q13.5)	WCP 9, WCP 11, CEP 11, tel 11q	1 / 1 / 0 (0) (1*)
1	1	46,XX,t(9;11)(p24;q23.1)	WCP 9, WCP 11, CEP 11, tel 9p, tel 11q	1 / 1 / 1 (1)
1	1	46,XX,t(9;13)(q22.3;q12.3)	WCP 9, WCP 13, CEP 9, LSI 13 (13q14), tel 9q	0 / 0
1	1	46,XX,t(9;13)(p21;q21)	WCP 9, WCP 13, CEP 9, tel 9p, tel 13q	0 / 0
1	2	46,XX,t(9;13)(q22;q14)	WCP 9, WCP 13, CEP 9, LSI 13 (13q14), tel 9q	0 / 0
1	1	46,XX,t(9;15)(q21;q11)	CEP 9, CEP 15, tel 9q, tel 15q	1 / 0
1	1	46,XX,t(9;15)(q22.3;q14)	CEP 9, tel 9q, tel 15q	1/ 1/ 1 (1)
1	4	46,XX,t(9;16)(q34.3)(p13.1)	WCP 9, WCP 16, CEP 9, tel 9q, tel 16p	4 / 2 / 1 / (1) (1*)
1	1	46,XX,t(9;20)(q21.2;q11.2)	WCP 9, WCP 20, CEP 9, tel 9q, tel 20q	0 / 0
1	1	46,XX,t(9;20)(q32;q13.1)	CEP 9, tel 9q, tel 20q	1 / 0
1	1	46,XX,t(10;11)(p15;q23)	WCP 10, WCP 11, CEP 10, tel 10 p, tel 11q	1 / 1 / 1 (3)
1	1	46,XX,t(10;12)(p11.2;p13.3)	CEP 10, tel 10p, tel 12p	1 / 1 / 1 (1)
1	1	46,XX,t(10;12)(q26;q24.1)	CEP 10, tel 10q, tel 12q	1 / 1 / 1 (1*)
1	1	46,XX,t(10;13)(q24.3;q14.3)	CEP 10, tel 13q, tel 10q	1 / 0
1	1	46,XX,t(10;15)(q23;q21)	WCP 10, WCP 15, CEP 15	0 / 0
1	1	46,XX,t(11;13)(q13.1;q33.2)	CEP 11, tel 11q, tel13q	1 / 0
1	1	46,XX,t(11;14)(p15;q24)	WCP 11, WCP 14, CEP 11, tel 11p	0 / 0
1	1	46,XX,t(11;14)(p15;q32.1)	WCP 11, WCP 14, CEP 11, tel 11p	1 / 1 / 1 (1)
1	1	46,XX,t(11;14)(q22;q32)	CEP 11, tel 11q, tel 14q	1 / 0
1	1	46,XX,t(11;14)(q22;q23)	CEP 11, tel 11q, tel 14q	1 / 0
1	1	46,XX,t(11;15)(p15.5;q22.3)	CEP 11, tel 11p, tel 15q	1 / 1 / 1 (2)
1	1	46,XX,t(11;16)(q23;q22)	WCP 11, WCP 16, CEP 11, tel 11q, tel 16q	1 / 1 / 1 (1)
1	1	46,XX,t(11;17)(q13;q21)	CEP 11, tel 11q, tel 17q	0 / 0
1	1	46,XX,t(11;18)(p14.2;p11.2)	CEP 18, tel 11p, tel 18q	0 / 0
1	1	46,XX,t(11;18)(q22.3;q12.21)	CEP 11, tel 11q, tel 18q	0 / 0
1	1	46,XX,t(11;20)(p13;q11.2)	CEP 11, CEP 20, tel 11p, tel 20q	1 / 0
2	5	46,XX,t(11;22)(q23;q11.2)	WCP 11, WCP 22, CEP 11, tel 11q, LSI 22 (22q11.2)	4 / 1 / 1 (1)
1	1	46,XX/46,XX,t(11;22)(q23.3;q11.2)	CEP 11, tel 11q, tel 22q	1 / 1 / 1 (1)
1	6	46,XX,t(11;22)(q23;q11)	CEP 11, tel11q, tel22q	5 / 2 / 1 / (1) (1*)
1	1	46,XX,t(12;15)(p13.3;q13.3)	WCP 12, WCP 15, tel 12p, tel 15q, CEP 15	1 / 0
1	3	46,XX,t(12;18)(p11.2;p11.2)	CEP 18, tel 12p, tel 18p	2 / 0
1	4	46,XX,t(12;18)(p13.31;q21.32)	WCP 12, WCP 18, CEP 18, tel 12p, tel 18q	2 / 1/ 0 (0) (1*)
1	4	46,XX,t(12;18)(q15;q12.2)	CEP 12, CEP 18, tel 12q, tel 18q	4 / 0
1	2	46,XX,t(13;15)(q12.3;q13.3)	WCP 13, WCP 15, CEP 15, tel 13q, tel 15q	0 / 0
1	2	46,XX,t(13;15)(q14;q13)	WCP 13, WCP 15, CEP 15, tel 13q, tel 15q	1 / 1 / 1(2)

(*Continued*)

Table 5.1 *(Continued)* List of translocations for which PGD was performed, FISH probes used, and the clinical outcome

Patients	*Cycles*	*Karyotype*	*FISH Probes*	*Embryo Transfers / Pregnancies / Deliveries (# of children born) (# of miscarriages*)*
1	2	46,XX,t(13;19)(q14;p13.3)	WCP 13, WCP 19, tel 13q, tel 19p	2 / 1 / 1
1	2	46,XX,t(13;21)(q32;q22)	WCP 13, WCP 21, tel 13q, tel 21q	1 / 0
1	2	46,XX,t(14;18)(q24.3 ;p11.31)	WCP 14, WCP 18, CEP 18, tel 14q, tel 18p	1 / 0
1	1	46,XX,t(14;20)(q24.1;q11.2)	CEP 20, tel 14q, tel 20q	0 / 0
1	1	46,XX,t(14;20)(q31;q13.2)	CEP 20, tel 14q, tel 20q	1 / 1 / 1 (1)
1	2	46,XX,t(14;21)(q24.1;q22.1)	WCP 14, WCP 21, tel 14q	1 / 1 / 1 (1)
1	2	46,XX,t(16;17)(p13.3;q11.2)	WCP 16, WCP 17, CEP 17, tel 16p, tel 17q	2 / 2 / 2 (3)
1	1	46,XX,t(16;17)(p13.3;p13.1)	CEP 16, CEP 17, tel 16p, tel 17p	0 / 0
1	2	46,XX,t(16;18)(p13.1;p11.2)	CEP 16, tel 16p, tel 18p	2 / 0
1	2	46,XX,t(16;19)(q13;p13.3)	WCP 16, WCP 19, CEP 16, tel 16q, tel 19p	0 / 0
1	2	46,XX,t(17;18)(p13;pter)	WCP 17, WCP 18, CEP 17, tel17p, tel18p	2 / 1 / 1 (2)
1	1	46,XX,t(17;20)(p13.1;q11.21)	CEP 17, tel 17q, tel 20q	1 / 1 / 1 (1)
2	2	46,XX,t(19;22)(q13.3;q11.2)	tel 19p, tel 19q, tel 22q	1 / 0
1	4	46,XX,inv(X)(p22.3;q13)	CEP X, tel Xp/Yp, tel Xq/Yq	3 / 2 / 2 (2)
1	1	46,X,t(X;2)(p11.2;q23)	WCP 2, WCP X, CEP 2, CEP X, tel 2q	1 / 0
1	1	46,X,t(X;17)(p22.1;q21)	WCP 17, WCP X, CEP x, tel 17q	1 / 0
1	1	47,XX,+fis(19)(p10),+fis(19)(q10)	tel 19p, tel 19q	1 / 0
1	1	46,XX/46,XX,+21,der(21;21)(q10;q10)	PB panel, tel21	0 / 0
1	3	46,XY,t(1;2)(q42.3;q37.3)	WCP 1, WCP 2, tel1q, tel 2q, PB panel	1 / 0
1	1	46,XY,t(1;3)(p34.3;q26.2)	WCP 1, WCP 3, CEP 3, tel1p, tel3q, CEP X<CEP Y, tel21	1 / 1 / 1 (1)
1	1	46,XY,t(1;3)(p36.1;q27)	WCP 1, WCP 3, CEP 1, tel 1p, tel 3q	1 / 1 / 1 (1)
1	1	46,XY,t(1;3)(q42.3;q29)	WCP 1, WCP 3, CEP 3, tel 1q, tel 3q	1 / 0
1	1	46,XY,t(1;4)(q41;p22)	CEP 4, tel 1q, tel 4p	0 / 0
1	1	46,XY,t(1;4)(p32;q21)	WCP 1, WCP 4, CEP 4, tel 1p, tel 4q	1 / 1 / 1 (2)
1	1	46,XY,t(1;7)(q11;p13)	WCP 1, WCP 7, CEP 7, tel 1q, tel 7p	0 / 0
1	8	46,XY,t(1;8)(p13;q23)	WCP 1, WCP 8, CEP 8, CEP 1, tel 1q	5 / 0
1	1	46,XY,t(1;8)(q42.1;q24.1)	WCP 1, WCP 8, tel 1q, tel 8q	1 / 1 / 1 (2)
1	1	46,XY,t(1;9)(p36.3;q32)	CEP 1, CEP 9, tel 1p, tel 9q	1 / 1 / 0 (1*)
1	1	46,XY,t(1;10)(p13;p11.2)	CEP 10, tel 1p, tel 10p, tel 1q	1 / 0
1	2	46,XY,t(1;15)(p13;q21.2)	CEP 15, tel 1p, tel 15q	0 / 0
1	2	46,XY,t(1;16)(q32.1;q12.1)	CEP 16, tel 1q, tel 16q	2 / 1 / 1 (1)
1	2	46,XY,t(1;21)(p13;q11.2)	WCP 1, WCP 21, CEP 1	2 / 0
1	1	46,XX,t(1;22)(q25;q11.1)	CEP 1, tel 1q, tel 22q	1 / 0
1	1	46,XY,t(2;3)(q21;p13)	WCP 2, WCP 3, CEP 2, tel 2q, tel 3p	0 / 0
1	3	46,XY,t(2;3)(p25;q13)	CEP 2, tel 2p, tel 3q	3 / 1 / 1 (1)
1	3	46,XY,t(2;4)(q21.1;q31.1)	WCP 2, WCP 4, CEP 4, tel 2q, tel 4q	2 / 1 / 1 (1)
1	2	46,XY,t(2;5)(q11.2;q33.3)	CEP 2, tel 2q, tel 5q	2 / 0
1	1	46,XY,t(2;6)(p13;p25)	CEP 2, CEP 6, tel 2p, tel 6p	1 / 0
1	1	46,XY,t(2;7)(p13;q36)	CEP 7, tel 2p, tel 7q	1 / 1 / 1 (1)

Table 5.1 (*Continued*) List of translocations for which PGD was performed, FISH probes used, and the clinical outcome

Patients	*Cycles*	*Karyotype*	*FISH Probes*	*Embryo Transfers / Pregnancies / Deliveries (# of children born) (# of miscarriages*)*
1	1	46,XY,t(2;7)(q32.1;q33)	CEP 7, tel 2q, tel 7q	1 / 1/ 1 (1)
1	1	46,XY,t(2;8)(q37.3;p11.2)	CEP 2, CEP 8, tel 2q, tel 8p	1 / 1 / 1(2)
1	1	46,XY,t(2;8)(p15;p11.2) inv(10) (p11.2;q21.2)	WCP 2, WCP 8, tel 8p, CEP 2, CEP 8, PB panel	1 / 0
1	1	46,XY,t(2;9)(q36;p22)	CEP 9, tel 2q, tel 9p	0 / 0
1	1	46,XY,t(2;11)(p13.3;p15.1)	WCP 2, WCP 11, CEP 2, CEP 11, tel 2p	1 / 0
1	1	46,XY,t(2;11)(q33;q23.3)	CEP 11, tel 2q, tel 11q	1 / 0
1	1	46,XY,t(2;12)(q32.3;q24.33)	CEP 2, tel 2q, tel 12q	1 / 0
1	1	46,XY,t(2;14)(q32.2.;q32.3)	CEP 2, tel 2p, tel 2q, tel14q	1 / 0
1	1	46,XY,t(2;17)(p21;q23)	CEP 17, tel 2p, tel 17q	0 / 0
1	1	46,XY,t(2;17)(p23;p25)	WCP 2, WCP 17, CEP 17, tel 2p, tel 17q	2 / 1 / 1 (1)
1	3	46,XY,t(2;18)(p13;q11)	WCP 2, WCP 18, CEP 18	2 / 1 / 1 (1)
1	1	46,XY,t(2;18)(p25;q23)	CEP 2, CEP 18, tel 2p, tel 18q	1 / 1 / 1 (2)
1	1	46,XY,t(2;19)(p25.1;p13.11)	WCP 2, WCP 19, tel 2p, tel 19p, CEP 4	1 / 1 / 0 (0) (1*)
1	1	46,XY,t(2;21)(q31.1;q11.2)	WCP 2, WCP 21, CEP 2, tel 2q, tel 21q	1 / 1 / 0 (0) (1*ect)
1	6	46,XY,t(3;5)(p26;q35.1)	WCP 3, WCP 5,CEP 3, tel 3p, tel 5q	5 / 1 / 1 (1)
1	4	46,XY,t(3;6)(q27.1;p21.1)	WCP 3, WCP 6, CEP 6 tel 3q, tel 6p	4 / 2 / 2 (2)
1	1	46,XY,t(3;7)(p24;p21)	WCP 3, WCP 7, tel 3p	1 / 0
1	1	46,XY,t(3;9)(q25.3;q22.3)	CEP 3, CEP 9, tel 3q, tel 9q	1 / 0
1	2	46,XY,t(3;10)(q21;p14)	WCP 3, WCP 10, CEP 10	0 / 0
1	1	46,XY,t(3;10)(q21;q24.1)	WCP 3, WCP 10, CEP 10, tel 3q, tel 10q	1 / 0
1	4	46,XY,t(3;10)(p26;q24.1)	WCP 3, WCP 10, CEP 3, CEP 10, tel 3p, tel 10q	2 / 0
1	3	46,XY, t(3;10)(q27;q25.2)	CEP 10, tel 3q, tel 10q	2 /2 / 2 (2)
1	1	46,XY,t(3;12)(p23;p13.3)	CEP 3, tel 3p, tel 12p	1 / 1 / 1(2)
1	1	46,XY,t(3;14)(q13.3;q24.1)	CEP 3, tel 3q, tel14q	1 / 0
1	1	46,XY,t(3;15)(q23;q13)	CEP 15, tel 3q, tel 15q	1 / 0
1	4	46,XY,t(3;21)(p21;q22.3)	WCP 3, WCP 21, tel 3p, tel 21q	2 / 0
1	1	46,XY, t(3;21)(q12;q11.2)	tel 3p, tel 3q, tel 21q	1 / 1 / 0 (0) (1*)
1	5	46,XY,t(4;5)(q33;q22)	WCP 4, WCP 5, CEP 4, tel 4q, tel 5q	5 / 1 / 0 (0) (1*)
1	1	46,XY,t(4;6)(p16;q25.3)	WCP 4, WCP 6, CEP 6, tel 4p, tel 6q, PB panel	2 / 1 / 1 (2)
1	1	46,XY,t(4;6)(q25;q21)	WCP 4, WCP 6, CEP 6, tel 6q	0 / 0
1	1	46,XY,t(4;8)(p16.1;p23.1)	CEP 4, tel 4p, tel 8p	1 / 0
1	2	46,XY,t(4;8)(q25;p23.1)	WCP 4, WCP 8, CEP 4, tel 4q, tel 8p	1 / 0
1	2	46,XY,t(4;10)(q21.3;q24.1)	WCP 4, WCP 10, CEP 4, tel 4q, tel 10q	1 / 0
1	5	46,XY,t(4;11)(q35.2;p14.3)	WCP 4, WCP 11, CEP 4, tel 4q, tel 11p	4 / 2 / 2 (2)
1	1	46,XY,t(4;13)(q35;q22.1)	WCP 4, WCP 13, tel 4q, tel 13q	0 / 0
1	1	46,XY,t(4;14)(p16;q23)	CEP 4, tel 4p, tel 14q	0 / 0
1	2	46,XY,t(4;15)(q21.3;q11.2)	WCP 4, WCP 15, CEP 4, tel 4q, tel 15q	2 / 0
1	1	46,XY,t(4;17)(q31.1;p13)	WCP 4, WCP 17, CEP 4, tel 4q, tel 17p	1 / 0
1	2	46,XY,t(4;22)(p15.3;q13.3)	CEP 4, tel 4p, tel 22q	1 / 1 / 1(2)

(*Continued*)

Table 5.1 (*Continued*) List of translocations for which PGD was performed, FISH probes used, and the clinical outcome

Patients	*Cycles*	*Karyotype*	*FISH Probes*	*Embryo Transfers / Pregnancies / Deliveries (# of children born) (# of miscarriages*)*
1	2	46,XY,t(4;22)(q31.1;q11.2)	WCP 4, WCP 22, tel 4q, tel 22q	2 / 1 / 1 (2)
1	1	46,XY,t(5;6)(q22;q22.2)	WCP 5, WCP 6, tel 5q, tel 6q	1 / 0
1	1	46,XY,t(5;7)(q21.2;q36)	WCP 5, WCP 7, tel 7q, CEP 7, tel 5p	1 / 1 / 1 (1)
1	2	46,XY,t(5;8)(p15.3;p21.1)	CEP 8, tel 5p, tel 8p	2 / 1 / 1 (1)
1	1	46,XY,t(5;9)(q35;q34)	CEP 9, tel 5q, tel 9q	1 / 1 / 1 (2)
1	8	46,XY,t(5;10)(q35.2)(q26.13)	WCP 5, WCP 10, CEP 10, tel 5q, tel 10q	6 / 1 / 1 (1)
1	1	46,XY,t(5;11)(q23.2;q24.2)	CEP 11, tel 5p, tel 5q, tel 11q	1 / 0
1	1	46,XY,(5;12)(p14;p13.33)	CEP 12, tel 5p, tel 12p	0 / 0
1	1	46,XY,t(5;14)(p10;q10)	WCP 5, WCP 14, tel 5p, tel 14q, Cri-du-Chat	1 / 1 / 1 (2)
1	2	46,XY,t(5;15)(q31;q22)	CEP 15, tel 5q, tel 15q	1 / 0
1	1	46,XY,t(5;18)(q13.1;q21.1)	WCP 5, WCP 18, CEP 18, tel 5q, tel 18q	1 / 0
1	1	46,XY,t(6;7)(q23;q36)	WCP 6, WCP 7, CEP 7	1 / 1 / 1 (1)
1	1	46,XY,t(6;8)(q21;q13)	WCP 6, WCP 8, CEP 6, CEP 8, tel 6q, tel 8q	1 / 0
1	2	46,XY,t(6;8)(q21;q32.1)	WCP 6, WCP 8	1 / 0
1	1	46,XY,t(6;8)(q23.3;q21.1)	WCP 6, WCP 8, CEP 6, tel 6q, tel 8q	2 / 0
1	1	46,XY,t(6;9)(p12;q34.1)	CEP 6, CEP 9, tel 6p	0 / 0
1	1	46,XY,t(6;10)	CEP 6, CEP 10, tel 6q, tel 10q	1 / 1 / 0 (0) (1*)
1	4	46,XY,t(6;13)(q23.1;q14.3)	CEP 6, WCP 13, WCP 6, tel 13q, tel 6q	3 / 2 / 2 (3)
1	2	46,XY,t(6;13)(q23;q32)	CEP 6, tel 6q, tel 13q	2 / 1 / 1 (1)
1	1	46,XY,t(6;14)(p23;q24.3)	WCP 6, ECP 14, CEP 6, tel 6p, tel 14q	1 / 1 / 1 (1)
1	1	46,XY,t(6;16)(q21;q13)	CEP 6, tel 6q, tel 16q	1 / 1 / 1 (1)
1	1	46,XY,(6;16)(p24;p13.2)	CEP 6, CEP 16, WCP 6, WCP 16, tel 6p, tel 16p	1 / 1 / 0 (0) (1*ect)
1	4	46,XY,t(6;17)(p25;p13)	CEP 6, tel 6p, tel 17p	4 / 1 / 1 (1)
1	2	46,XY,t(6;18)(qter;qtr)	WCP 6, WCP 18, CEP 6, tel 6q, tel 18q	2 / 1 / 1 (1)
1	2	46,XY,t(6;21)(p12.2;q22.2)	CEP 6, tel 6q, tel 21q	2 / 1 / 1 (1)
1	1	46,XY,t(6;21)(q22.2;q22.2)	CEP 6, tel 6q, tel 21q	1 / 1 / 1 (1)
1	1	46,XY,t(7;8)(q21.3;q23.3)	CEP 8, tel 7q, tel 8q	1 / 1 / 1 (1)
1	1	46,XY,t(7;10)(q36;p11.2)	WCP 7, WCP 10, CEP 10, tel 7q, tel 10p	1 / 0
1	1	46,XY,t(7;12)(p15.1;p13)	CEP 7, tel 7p, tel 12q	0 / 0
1	1	46,XY,t(7;19)(q36;q31.1)	WCP 7, WCP 19, CEP 7, tel 7q, tel 19q	0 / 0
1	1	46,XY,t(7;21)(p11.2;q22.2)	WCP 7, WCP 21, CEP 7, tel 7p, tel 21q	1 / 0
1	1	46,XY,t(8;10)(q22.1;q22.1)	WCP 8, WCP 10, CEP 10, tel 8q	1 / 1 / 1 (2)
1	1	46,XY,t(8;11)(p23;p13)	WCP 8, WCP 11, CEP 11, tel 8p, tel 11p	1 / 1 / 1 (1)
1	2	46,XY,t(8;19)(p23.1;q13.3)	WCP 8, WCP 19, CEP 8, tel 8p, tel 19q	2 / 1 / 1 (1)
1	1	46,XY,t(9;11)(p22;q23)	WCP 9, WCP 11, CEP 11, tel 9p, tel 11q	1 / 0
1	1	46,XY,t(9;15)(q13;q11)	CEP 9, CEP 15, tel 9q, tel 15q	1 / 1 / 1 (1)
1	2	46,XY,t(10;11)(p11.1;q25)	CEP 10, tel 10p, tel11q	2 / 1 / 1 (1)
1	1	46,XY,t(10;11)(q23;q23) / 46,XY	CEP 11, tel 10q, tel 11q	1 / 1 / 1 (1)
1	1	46,XY,t(10;13)(p12;p11.2)	WCP 10, WCP 13, CEP 10	1 / 0
1	1	46,XY,t(10;16)(p10;q10)	CEP 10, tel 10p, tel 16q	1 / 0

Table 5.1 (Continued) List of translocations for which PGD was performed, FISH probes used, and the clinical outcome

Patients	*Cycles*	*Karyotype*	*FISH Probes*	*Embryo Transfers / Pregnancies / Deliveries (# of children born) (# of miscarriages*)*
1	1	46,XY,t(10;22)(q24.1;p12)	WCP 10,WCP 22, LSI 22 (22q11.2), tel 10q, CEP 10	1 / 1 / 1 (1)
1	2	46,XY,t(10;22)(q25;q13.3)	WCP 10,WCP 22, LSI 22 (22q11.2), tel 10q, CEP 10	2 / 0
1	2	46,XY,t(11;14)(q23;q32)	WCP 11,WCP 14, CEP 11, tel 11q, tel 14q	2 / 0
1	1	46,XY,t(11;20)(p15;q13.12)	WCP 11,WCP 20, tel 11p	1 / 1 / 1 (1)
1	1	46,XY,t(11;22)(q13.1;q13.3)	CEP 11, tel 11q, tel 22q	0 / 0
1	1	46,XY,t(11;22)(q23.3;q11.2)	CEP 11, tel 11q, LSI 22 (22q11.2)	0 / 0
1	2	46,XY,t(11;22)(q23.3;11.23)	CEP 11, tel 11q, tel22q	1 / 0
3	5	46,XY,t(11;22)(q23;q11.2)	WCP 11,WCP 22, CEP 11 tel 11q, tel 22q	4 / 2 / 1 (1) (1*)
1	2	46,XY,t(11;22)(q25;q12)	WCP 11,WCP 22, CEP 11, tel 11q	1 / 0
1	2	46,XY,t(12;13)(q24.1;q12.2)	CEP 12, tel 12q, tel 13q	2 / 0
1	2	46,XY,t(12;15)(p13.3;q24)	WCP 12,WCP 15, CEP 12, CEP 15, tel 15q	1 / 1 / 1 (2)
1	1	46,XY,t(12;19)(p13.3;q13.4)	CEP 12, tel 12p, tel 19q	1 / 0
1	2	46,XY,t(12;20)(q23;p13)	WCP 12,WCP 20, CEP 12, tel 12q, tel 20p	2 / 2 / 2 (2)
1	1	46,XY,t(13;20)(q12.11;q11.23)	tel 13q, tel 20p, tel 20q	0 / 0
2	3	46,XY,t(13;20)(q22;q11.2)	WCP 13,WCP 20	0 / 0
1	1	46,XY,t(13;21)(q14;q11.2)	WCP 13,WCP 21, tel 13q, tel 21q	1 / 1 / 0 (0) (1*)
1	4	46,XY,t(13;21)(q32;q22)	WCP 13,WCP 21, LSI13, tel 13q, tel 21q	1 / 1 / 1 (1)
1	1	46,XY,t(14;15)(q32.2;q26.1)	CEP 15, tel 14q, tel 15q	1 / 1 / 0 (0) (1*)
1	2	46,XY,t(14;20)(q24.1;q11.2)	WCP 14,WCP 20, tel 14q, tel 20q	0 / 0
1	1	46,XY,t(14;20)(q32.1;q13.1)	tel 14q, tel 20p, tel 20q	0 / 0
1	1	46,XY,t(15;16)(q13;q13)	WCP 15,WCP 16, CEP 15	1 / 0
1	3	46,XY,t(15;17)(q24;q21.3)	WCP 15,WCP 17, tel 15q, tel 17q, CEP 15, CEP 17	3 / 1 / 1 (2)
1	1	46,XY,t(16;20)(q12.3;q13.1)	WCP 16,WCP 20, CEP 16, CEP 20, tel 16q, tel 20q	1 / 0
1	3	46,XY,t(18;20)(p11.2;q13.3)	WCP 18,WCP 20, CEP 18, tel 18p, tel 20q	3 / 2 / 1 (1) (1*)
1	1	46,XX,ins(10;13)(q22.3;q14.1q21)	CEP 10, tel 10q, LSI 13, tel 13q	1 / 0
1	1	46,XY,ins(18;11)(q23;p14.1p13)	CEP 11, LSI 11p, tel 18q	1 / 0
1	1	46,XY, inv(2)(p16;q23)	tel 2p, tel 2q, LSI 2p14, LSI 2q21.2	1 / 0
1	2	46,XY,inv(5)(p13;q13)	Xcyte 5 (Metasystems), tel 5p, tel 5q	2 / 0
1	2	46,XX,inv(5)(p15.1;q13.1)	Cri-du-Chat (Vysis), Cri-du-Chat / Sotos (Cytocell)	2 / 1 / 1 (1)
1	3	46,XY,inv(5)(p15.3;q33.1)	LSI 5p, tel 5p, tel 5q, Cri-du-Chat	3 / 1 / 1 (1)
0	1	46,XY,inv(5)(p15.3;q33.1)	LSI 5p, tel 5p, tel 5q,Cri-du-Chat	1 / 1 / 1 (0) (1*)
1	1	46,XY,inv(5)(p31.1;q33.1)	LSI 5p, tel 5p, tel 5q, Cri-du-Chat	1 / 1 / 1 (1)
1	1	46,XY,inv(8)(p22;q22)	CEP 8, tel 8p, tel 8q	1 / 0
1	1	46,XY, inv(9)	Conversion failed / no result	0 / 0
1	1	46,XY,inv(12)(p13.3;q14.1)	LSI ETV breakapart probe, CEP 12, tel 12q	1 / 0

(Continued)

Table 5.1 (*Continued*) List of translocations for which PGD was performed, FISH probes used, and the clinical outcome

Patients	*Cycles*	*Karyotype*	*FISH Probes*	*Embryo Transfers / Pregnancies / Deliveries (# of children born) (# of miscarriages*)*
1	1	46,XY,inv(22)(q11.2;q12.2)	LSI 22q11.22, LSI 22q12.1	1 / 1 / 0 (1*ect)
1	1	48,XY,idic(15)(q11.1)	CEP 15, tel 15q, 15q22, 15p11.2	1 / 0
1	1	Del17p13.1	CEP 17, tel 17p, p53	1 / 1 / 0 (0) (1*)
1	4	46,XX,del(22)(q21.2;q11.2)	DiGeorgie / VCFS TUPLE 1 region probe & 22 q13.3	4 / 1 / 1 (2)
1	3	46,XX,r(15)	CEP 15, tel 15q, PWP	2 / 0
1	1	46,XY,t(9;6)(q22;q15q23.1)	G-Banding, WCP 6, WCP 9, CEP 6	0 / 0
1	1	46,XX,t(2;3;21)(q11.2;p11.2;q11.2)	WCP 2, WCP 21, CEP 3, tel 2q, tel 21q	0 / 0
1	3	46,XX,t(8;10)(p23.3;q14.1) & 45,XY,der(13;14)(q10;q10)	WCP 8, WCP 10, CEP 8, pel 8p, tel 10q & WCP 13, WCP 14, tel 13q, tel 14q	3 / 0
1	1	44,XY,der(13;14)(q10;q10) × 2 & 45,XX,der(13;14)(q10;q10)	tel 13q, tel 14q	1 / 0
395	**609**			**456 / 177 / 145 (176) (32*)**

\# of miscarriages includes 3 cases of ectopic pregnancies (ect)
WCP – whole chromosome paint
LSI – locus specific identifier
tel – sub-telomeric
CEP – centromeric enumeration probe
G-Banding – Giemsa Stain

except for chromatid exchange, which can be detected only by sequential PB1 and PB2 analysis (Figures 5.7–5.9, 5.13). Complex errors were identified with PB analysis using a combination of centromeric and sub-telomeric probes, which detects non-disjunction events occurring in meiosis I and II involving single chromatids (Figure 5.14). This may also explain the higher rate of 3:1 segregation observed with blastomere analysis, since these may have been the product of a different segregation pattern in conjunction with anaphase II non-disjunction. The segregation patterns for paternally derived translocations, when compared to patterns observed from blastomere analysis of maternally derived translocations, showed similar tendencies, predominantly represented by alternate and adjacent I segregation, with a lower adjacent II pattern observed (Figures 5.16–5.20). In embryos tested for maternally derived reciprocal translocations, 76.1% unbalanced embryos were predicted, leaving only 23.9% suitable for transfer, of which 12.6% were balanced and 11.3% normal. The testing of embryos for paternally derived reciprocal translocations resulted in the prediction of 69% unbalanced embryos, leaving 31.0% of embryos suitable for transfer, 16.1% being balanced and 14.9% normal.

Testing of embryos for maternally derived Robertsonian translocations (Figures 5.15, 5.21–5.23) resulted in the prediction of 69.7% unbalanced embryos, with the remaining 30.3% embryos suitable for transfer, 16.8% of them balanced and 13.5% normal. Similarly, the testing of embryos for paternally derived Robertsonian translocations allowed identification of 52.1% unbalanced embryos, with the remaining 47.9% being suitable for transfer, 28.6% balanced and 19.3% normal.

Our overall experience shows normal/balanced embryos were available for transfer in 72% of the cases. Clinical pregnancies were obtained in 38% of transfer cycles in which the mean number transferred was 1.6 embryos, resulting in a 38% pregnancy rate, and a 33% live-birth rate. In those couples with known pregnancy history prior to undertaking PGD, there was a spontaneous abortion rate of 85%, not to mention the birth of affected children. This is in contrast to the spontaneous abortion rate of approximately 20% and only healthy children born after PGD, demonstrating the tremendous positive impact that PGD has on the clinical outcome of pregnancies in couples carrying balanced chromosome translocations (Figure 5.24).

As previously mentioned, the detection rates of embryos suitable for transfer depended on the types of the translocations tested. For example, the clinical outcome is poorer in reciprocal than Robertsonian translocations, with the pregnancy rates of 23% and 28%, respectively. As may be expected, there was also a relationship between the poorer clinical outcome and the proportion of unbalanced embryos in these PGD cycles. In PGD cycles with the proportion of unbalanced complements under 75%, the pregnancy rate was 30% per cycle, compared to 11% in PGD cycles with an unbalanced rate of over 75%.

Although the application of the conversion technique to visualize chromosomes in single blastomeres improves the accuracy of the diagnosis by analysis of metaphase chromosomes using a combination of commercially available probes, a high frequency of mosaicism in the cleavage-stage embryos, arising from anaphase lag or nuclear fragmentation, still presents problems for diagnosis (Figures 5.25, 5.26). Follow-up analysis of unbalanced embryos, including those in which chromatid malsegregation or recombination was identified by the analysis of PB1 and in which subsequent testing of PB2 indicated a balanced or normal embryo, revealed a mosaicism rate of 40%. Different cell lines, including normal and balanced, were present that if investigated only by embryo biopsy may have led to misdiagnosis. Therefore, our PGD strategy for maternally derived translocations may still be based on PB1 and PB2 testing, applying the blastomere nucleus conversion technique if further testing is required. To avoid transferring the embryos with aneuploidy, which may be prevalent in preimplantation embryos resulting from carriers of balanced translocations, re-hybridization with a five-color probe for chromosomes 13, 16, 18, 21, and 22 may be useful, as shown in Figure 5.25. This may presently be done by array-CGH, applicable to PGD for both 24-chromosome aneuploidy testing and rearrangements.

It was also demonstrated that embryos with unbalanced chromosome complements have the potential to reach the blastocyst stage of embryo development in extended culture. Of 420 unbalanced embryos cultured for a further period, 151 (36%) reached the blastocyst stage, confirming that some of the detected chromosomal rearrangements may not be lethal in preimplantation development, and may be eliminated either during implantation or post-implantation development,[12] explaining an extremely high spontaneous abortion rate in couples carrying translocations. As mentioned, our data suggest close to five-fold reduction of spontaneous abortions following PGD cycles for translocations, in agreement with previous data.[13–15]

In addition to avoiding of expensive and time-consuming customized breakpoint-spanning probes applied at the initial stages of PGD for translocations,[12] the conversion technique used was highly accurate based on the follow-up testing of embryos predicted to be abnormal and on confirmatory prenatal diagnosis of the ongoing pregnancies or testing of the newborn babies. The method also allows balanced and normal embryos to be distinguished, which cannot be achieved by currently available interphase FISH analysis (Figures 5.10–5.12).

However, as mentioned, the conversion method is still labor intensive, so to simplify the process of conversion a chemical method was introduced (see above), which is quite simple and may be routinely used for "in house" PGD cases. At present, more than 100 cycles were performed by the chemical conversion method, applied to over 1000 blastomeres.[11] Metaphases were obtained in 71%, with the examples of chemical conversion presented in Chapter 3 (Figure 3.17) and Figure 5.27.

Because PGD is almost the only hope for couples with translocations to be able to have an unaffected child without fear of repeated spontaneous abortions, increasing numbers of PGD cycles for this indication have been performed. As seen from Table 5.1, more than 600 clinical cycles have been performed, resulting in 177 clinical pregnancies and births of unaffected children.

Of special importance is the current shift of testing for translocations from FISH to microarray technology, which despite some limitations allows accurate detection of the majority of chromosomal rearrangements (Figures 5.28 and 5.29). Although no prior work-up seems necessary for performing the array-based testing, at least a 650-band level on parental karyotypes is required for consideration on the choice of FISH or array-CGH approach, as its accuracy is adversely affected even by slightest imprecision of the break points, being unable to detect translocated fragments smaller than 4–5 Mbp. The testing strategy also depends on the position of the fragments, as some of the 3:1 segregation patterns in translocation involving acrocentric chromosomes are not detectable by array-CGH. According to our preliminary data, at least one-quarter of cycles originally considered for array-CGH were performed by FISH analysis as the more reliable approach. The advantage of performing array-CGH, combined with blastocyst biopsy, is the possibility of concomitant 24-chromosome aneuploidy testing in patients of advanced reproductive age. However, the microarray-based approach, although expected to be universal, may not yet be sufficiently accurate for smaller rearrangements at the particular position of smaller segments.

Overall, we performed PGD cycles for 609 carriers of chromosomal rearrangements, including those done by FISH and array-CGH, which resulted in 177 (39%) pregnancies of known outcomes, and birth of 176 unaffected children. The data on the meiotic outcome may explain the observed 85% spontaneous abortion rate in patients prior to undergoing PGD, which was reduced to 18% after PGD, demonstrating the tremendous positive impact of PGD on the clinical outcome of pregnancies in translocation carriers. The data suggest that PGD is the only option for patients with translocations, who are at an extremely high risk for spontaneous abortions and birth of an affected child.

REFERENCES

1. Scriven PN, Handyside AH, Mackie Ogilvie C. Chromosome translocations: segregation modes and strategies for preimplantation genetic diagnosis. *Prenat Diagn* 1998; 18:1437–49.
2. Verlinsky Y, Evsikov S. Karyotyping of human oocytes by chromosomal analysis of the second polar body. *Mol Hum Reprod* 1999; 5:89–95.

3. Verlinsky Y, Evsikov S. A simplified and efficient method for obtaining metaphase chromosomes from individual human blastomeres. *Fertil Steril* 1999; 72:1–6.
4. Willadsen S, Levron J, Munne S, et al. Rapid visualization of metaphase chromosomes in single human blastomeres after fusion with in-vitro matured bovine eggs. *Hum Reprod* 1999; 14:470–74.
5. Traversa MV, Carey L, Leigh D. A molecular strategy for routine preimplantation genetic diagnosis in both reciprocal and Robertsonian translocation carriers. *Hum Reprod* 2010; 16:329–337.
6. Treff NR, Northrop LE, Kasabwala K, Su J, Levy B, Scott RT. Single nucleotide polymorphism microarray-based concurrent screening of 24-chromosome aneuploidy and unbalanced translocations in preimplantation human embryos. *Fertil Steril* 2011; 95:1606–612.
7. Colls P, Escudero T, Fischer J, et al. Validation of array comparative genome hybridization for diagnosis of translocations in preimplantation human embryos. *Reprod Biomed Online* 2012; 24:621–29.
8. Verlinsky Y, Kuliev A. *Preimplantation Diagnosis of Genetic Diseases: A New Technique for Assisted Reproduction*. New York: Wiley-Liss, 1993.
9. Munne S, Morrison L, Fung J, et al. Spontaneous abortions are significantly reduced after preconception genetic diagnosis of translocations. *J Assist Reprod Genet* 1998; 15:290–96.
10. Verlinsky Y, Cieslak J, Evsikov S, et al. Nuclear transfer for full karyotyping and preimplantation diagnosis of translocations. *Reprod Biomed Online* 2002; 5:302–07.
11. Kuliev A, Cieslak-Jansen J, Zlatopolsky Z, Kirillova I, Ilkevitch Y, Verlinsky Y. Conversion and non-conversion approach to preimplantation diagnosis for chromosomal rearrangements in 475 cycles. *Reprod Biomed Online* 2010; 21:93–99.
12. Evsikov S, Cieslak J, Verlinsky Y. Survival of unbalanced translocations to blastocyst stage. *Fertil Steril* 2000; 74:672–76.
13. Munné S, Sandalinas M, Escudero T, et al. Outcome of preimplantation genetic diagnosis of translocations. *Fertil Steril* 2000; 73:1209–18.
14. Munné S. Preimplantation genetic diagnosis of numerical and structural chromosome abnormalities. *Reprod Biomed Online* 2002; 4:183–96.
15. Gianaroli L, Magli MC, Ferraretti AP, et al. The beneficial effects of PGD for aneuploidies support extensive clinical application. *Reprod Biomed Online* 2005; 10:633–40.

6 Preimplantation diagnosis for single-gene disorders

Preimplantation genetic diagnosis (PGD) for single-gene disorders is based on the testing of oocytes or embryos to preselect and transfer only normal embryos back to the patient to achieve an unaffected pregnancy and the birth of a healthy child. As in PGD for chromosomal disorders, it is performed by testing either single blastomeres removed from eight-cell preimplantation embryos or a number of cells from blastocysts, or by testing female gametes by the removal and genetic analysis of the first and second polar bodies (PB1 and PB2). However, the latter approach cannot be applied for testing paternally derived abnormalities or for gender determination, which can be detected only by genetic analysis of single cells removed from the cleaving- or blastocyst-stage embryo. Therefore, the two methods are complementary, and their application is dependent upon the PGD objectives in the individual patient.

Overall, the experience of using PGD for single-gene disorders is now more than 12,000 cases, showing that it is an established alternative to traditional prenatal diagnosis and can be reliably applied as an integral part of genetic practice.[1–3] Our experience, which is the world's most extensive in one center, is presented in Table 6.1.

UPDATED PROCEDURE OF SINGLE-CELL DNA ANALYSIS FOR PGD OF SINGLE-GENE DISORDERS

Principles of PGD using first and second polar bodies

The principle of PGD of single-gene disorders using PB1 and PB2 analysis is presented in Figure 6.1. As seen from this figure, there are three genetic possibilities for the PB1 genotype from a heterozygous woman. If no crossover occurs, the PB1 will be homozygous (either normal or affected), but in the event of a crossover, the PB1 will be heterozygous. If a crossover does not occur and the PB1 is homozygous for the mutant gene, the oocyte must contain two copies of the normal gene and any embryo from this oocyte can be transferred. If the PB1 is homozygous for the normal gene, the maternal contribution to the embryo must be the mutant gene.

In the event that a crossover occurs, the PB1 will be heterozygous and analysis of the PB2 is required to predict which maternal allele will be present in the fertilized oocyte (Figure 6.1). If the PB2 contains the normal gene, the oocyte will be affected, and if the PB2 contains the mutant gene the oocyte will have the unaffected gene. The crossover rate varies with the distance of the locus being studied from the centromere and perhaps with other, as yet, undelineated mechanisms. Our experience has shown a high rate of crossover, limiting the number of embryos available for transfer based on PB1 analysis, thus sequential two-step analysis of the PB1 and PB2 in genetic analysis of oocytes is required.[4] As will be demonstrated below, the highest accuracy of diagnosis can be achieved if a crossover occurs, as in this case both mutant and normal alleles are detected, so that the finding of the mutant allele in the PB2 indicates that the resulting oocyte is free of the mutation.

DNA analysis using conventional PCR analysis in single cells

Genetic analysis in single cells, allowing performance of PGD for single-gene disorders, became possible after the introduction of the polymerase chain reaction (PCR) technique,[5] which is an *in vitro* technique for the amplification of specific DNA sequences. PCR is a cycling process in which the number of DNA targets doubles in each cycle (a flow chart for single-cell genotyping is shown in Figure 6.2). The basic PCR components include a DNA template (10 pg–500 ng), DNA polymerase (0.5–2.5 units), primers (0.1–1.0 µmol/l), dNTPs (50–200 µmol/l of each), buffer (pH 8.3–9.5), and $MgCl_2$ (1.5–3.0 µmol/l). PCR allows a single gene to be copied more than a billion times in a matter of hours. It consists of three basic steps: denaturation, annealing, and extension.

(1) Denaturation is carried out at 94–96°C for 0.5–2.0 min during regular cycles and leads to melting of the template into single strands, eliminating the secondary structure.

(2) The annealing temperature allows primers to hybridize to the template, varying with the strand-melting temperature of the primers, with standard reactions using 45–60°C for 1–2 min.

(3) Extension is carried out at 72°C, which is optimal for Taq polymerase, completing the synthesis of the new DNA strand. PCR can be efficiently carried out using only two temperatures: one for denaturation and the other for annealing and extension (also called two-step PCR or turbo PCR).

Table 6.1 Overall current experience of PGD for single-gene disorders

DISEASE	*GENE*	*Type of Inheritance*	*No. of Patients*	*No. of Cycles*	*No. of ET*	*No. of Embryos*	*Pregnancy*	*Birth*	*ONGOING*
HLA genotyping			46	109	70	105	22	18	1
Ichthyosis congenita, harlequin fetus type	ABCA12	AR	1	1	0	0	0	0	0
Surfactant metabolism dysfunction, pulmonary 3 (SMDP3)	ABCA3	AR	1	1	1	2	1	1	0
Cholestasis, progressive familial intrahepatic 2	ABCB11	AR	1	1	1	2	0	0	0
Hyperinsulinemic hypoglycemia, familial 1 (HHF1)	ABCC8	AR	1	10	6	15	2	1	0
Adrenoleukodystrophy (ALD)	ABCD1	XL	10	22	14	23	5	4	0
HLA + adrenoleukodystrophy	ABCD1	XL	2	5	1	1	0	0	0
ACYL-CoA dehydrogenase medium-chain deficiency	ACADM	AR	1	5	5	12	1	1	0
ACYL-CoA dehydrogenase very long-chain deficiency	ACADVL	AR	4	5	5	10	1	1	0
Telangiectasia, hereditary hemorrhagic, of Rendu, Osler, and Weber; HHT	ACVRL1	AD	1	2	2	4	1	0	1
HLA + thrombotic thrombocytopenic purpura, congenital; TTP	ADAMTS13	AR	1	2	2	4	1	1	0
Joubert syndrome 3; JBTS3 Joubert syndrome 6; JBTS6	AHI1 TMEM67	AR	2	2	1	2	0	0	0
Succinic semialdehyde dehydrogenase deficiency	ALDH5A1	AR	2	3	3	8	1	1	0
Hypophosphatasia, infantile	ALPL	AR	5	5	4	7	3	4	0
Alport syndrome, X-linked; ATS	AMMECR1	XL	3	7	7	11	3	3	0
Hyalinosis, infantile systemic	ANTXR2	AR	1	1	1	2	1	1	0
Adenomatous polyposis of the colon	APC	AD	10	23	21	38	5	3	1
Androgen insensitivity syndrome; AIS	AR	XL	1	1	0	0	0	0	0
Kennedy disease	AR	XL	1	2	2	2	0	0	0
Metachromatic leukodystrophy	ARSA	AR	1	2	2	2	0	0	0
Chondrodysplasia punctata 1, X-linked recessive; CDPX1	ARSE	XL	1	2	2	3	0	0	0

Argininosuccinic aciduria (ASA)	ASL	AR	1	2	2	3	0	0	0
Canavan disease	ASPA	AR	1	2	2	4	2	2	0
Citrullinemia, classic	ASS1	AR	1	1	1	3	0	0	0
Ataxia–telangiectasia; AT	ATM	AR	1	3	2	3	1	1	0
Darier–White disease; DAR	ATP2A2	AD	1	1	1	1	1	1	0
Spinocerebellar ataxia 1; SCA1	ATXN1	AD	1	2	2	4	1	1	0
Spinocerebellar ataxia 2; SCA2	ATXN2	AD	6	13	13	26	5	7	0
Machado–Joseph disease; MJD	ATXN3	AD	1	3	2	3	2	3	0
Spinocerebellar ataxia 7; SCA7	ATXN7	AD	2	3	3	7	2	1	0
Breast cancer 1; BRCA1	BRCA1	AD	25	40	31	54	18	23	0
Breast cancer 2; BRCA2	BRCA2	AD	14	36	23	39	10	13	0
Agammaglobulinemia, X-linked, type I	BTK	XL	3	5	5	11	2	3	0
Mosaic variegated aneuploidy syndrome 1; MVA1	BUB1B	AR	1	1	1	2	1	0	0
Migraine, familial hemiplegic, 1; FHM1	CACNA1A	AD	1	1	1	2	1	2	0
Spinocerebellar ataxia 6; SCA6	CACNA1A	AD	1	2	1	1	0	0	0
HLA + immunodeficiency with hyper-IgM, type 1; HIGM1	CD40LG	XL	6	11	7	11	4	3	0
Immunodeficiency with hyper-IgM, type 1; HIGM1	CD40LG	XL	4	9	9	13	3	3	0
Epileptic encephalopathy, early infantile, 2	CDKL5	XL	1	1	1	2	1	1	0
Epileptic encephalopathy, early infantile, 2 CDKL5	CDKL5	XL	1	1	1	2	1	1	0
Cystic fibrosis; CF	CFTR	AR	278	423	359	703	182	192	8
Choroideremia; CHM	CHM	XL	2	4	4	7	3	4	0
Myotonia congenita, autosomal dominant	CLCN1	AD	1	1	1	2	1	1	0
Myotonic dystrophy 2; DM2	CNBP	AD	1	1	1	2	1	1	0
Metaphyseal chondrodysplasia, Schmid type; MCDS	COL10A1	AD	1	1	1	2	1	1	0
Stickler syndrome, type I; STL1	Col11A1 Col2A1	AD	3	8	6	17	0	0	0

(Continued)

Table 6.1 (*Continued*) Overall current experience of PGD for single-gene disorders

DISEASE	*GENE*	*Type of Inheritance*	*No. of Patients*	*No. of Cycles*	*No. of ET*	*No. of Embryos*	*Pregnancy*	*Birth*	*ONGOING*
Osteogenesis imperfecta congenita; OIC	COL1A1 PPIB	AD	17	44	35	59	12	13	2
Ehlers–Danlos syndrome, type iv, autosomal dominant	COL3A1 COL5A1 PLOD1	AD	4	5	4	6	4	5	0
Epidermolysis bullosa dystrophica	COL7A1 LAMB3 PLEC1 LAMA3		11	15	11	19	5	6	0
Epiphyseal dysplasia, multiple, 1; EDM1	COMP	AD	2	2	1	3	0	0	0
Carbamoyl phosphate synthetase I deficiency	CPS1	AR	1	1	1	2	0	0	0
Carnitine palmitoyltransferase II deficiency	CPT2	AR	1	1	1	1	1	1	0
Cystinosis, nephropathic; CTNS	CTNS	AR	1	1	1	1	0	0	0
HLA + granulomatous disease, chronic, X-linked; CGD	CYBB	XY	4	10	7	10	3	2	0
Congenital adrenal hyperplasia (CAH)	CYP21A2	AR	7	12	11	21	7	8	0
Myopathy, myofibrillar, desmin-related	DES	AD	1	1	1	1	1	1	0
Smith–Lemli–Opitz syndrome; SLOS	DHCR7	AR	4	6	6	12	3	3	1
Hoyeraal–Hreidarsson syndrome; HHS	DKC1	XL	1	1	1	2	1	1	0
Muscular dystrophy, Duchenne; Becker type; BMD	DMD	XL	33	58	49	96	28	24	4
Dystrophia myotonica 1	DMPK	AD	65	109	91	144	29	24	3
HLA + dystrophia myotonica 1	DMPK	AD	1	2	1	2	1	1	0
Ciliary dyskinesia, primary, 3; CILD3	DNAH5	AR	1	1	1	2	1	1	0
Ectodermal dysplasia, anhidrotic, X-linked	EDA	XL	2	3	3	4	1	1	0
Ectodermal dysplasia, anhidrotic (EDAR)	EDAR	AR	1	1	1	2	1	1	0
Leukoencephalopathy with vanishing white matter; VWM	EIF2B2	AR	1	1	1	2	1	0	0

Emery–Dreifuss muscular dystrophy	EMD	XL	1	2	2	3	1	1	0
Exostoses, multiple, type I	EXT1	AD	8	11	11	21	6	5	0
Hemophilia A;	F8	XL	36	62	51	99	28	26	0
Hemophilia B	F9	XL	3	4	3	3	3	3	0
Tyrosinemia, type I	FAH	AR	1	5	5	9	2	2	0
Fanconi anemia, complementation group A; FANCA	FANCA	AR	1	3	1	2	1	2	0
HLA + FANCA	FANCA	AR	15	45	27	39	8	5	0
Fanconi anemia, complementation group C; FANCC	FANCC	AR	2	5	4	8	1	2	0
HLA + FANCC	FANCC	AR	2	5	5	8	1	1	0
HLA + FANCD2	FANCD2	AR	1	3	2	3	1	1	0
HLA + FANCF	FANCF	AR	1	3	2	3	0	0	0
HLA + FANCI	FANCI	AR	1	2	2	3	0	0	0
HLA + FANCJ	FANCJ	AR	1	3	1	3	0	0	0
Marfan syndrome; MFS	FBN1	AD	15	31	27	56	15	12	2
Kallman syndrome	FGFR1	AD	1	1	1	2	1	1	0
Pfeiffer syndrome	FGFR1	AD	1	1	1	2	1	1	0
Craniofacial dysostosis, type I; (CFD1); (Crouzon)	FGFR2	AD	4	9	8	16	4	3	0
Achondroplasia; ACH	FGFR3	AD	3	4	4	5	3	3	0
Fragile site mental retardation 1	FMR1	XL	151	297	218	370	102	94	7
Blepharophimosis, ptosis, and epicanthus inversus; BPES	FOXL2	AD	2	4	4	4	2	2	0
Immunodysregulation, polyendocrinopathy, and enteropathy, X-linked; IPEX	FOXP3	XL	1	2	2	2	0	0	0
Friedreich ataxia 1; FRDA	FRDA	AR	1	4	4	7	2	2	0
Facioscapulohumeral muscular dystrophy 1A; FSHMD1A	FRG1	AD	12	32	25	48	13	13	0
Glycogen storage disease type II	GAA	AR	4	4	3	4	1	1	0
HLA + Krabbe + aneuploidy	GALC	AR	1	1	1	2	1	2	0
Krabbe	GALC	AR	4	5	5	10	3	3	0

(Continued)

Table 6.1 (Continued) Overall current experience of PGD for single-gene disorders

DISEASE	GENE	Type of Inheritance	No. of Patients	No. of Cycles	No. of ET	No. of Embryos	Pregnancy	Birth	ONGOING
Morquio syndrome, non-keratosulfate-excreting type	GALNS	AR	1	4	4	12	2	2	0
Galactosemia	GALT	AR	1	4	3	4	0	0	0
Gaucher disease, type I	GBA	XL	17	23	21	39	12	10	1
Glutaric acidemia I	GCDH	AR	1	1	1	2	0	0	0
Glutaric aciduria I	GCDH	AR	1	1	1	2	0	0	0
Charcot–Marie–Tooth disease, X-linked, 1; CMTX1	GJB1	XL	4	6	6	12	4	5	0
Deafness, neurosensory, autosomal ecessive 1; DFNB1	GJB2	AR	6	10	9	18	4	4	1
Fabry disease	GLA	XL	5	10	8	13	4	6	0
Gangliosidosis, generalized GM1, type I	GLB1	AR	2	2	2	5	1	1	0
Hyperglycinemia, non-ketotic; NKH	GLDC	AR	3	4	4	7	4	5	1
Non-ketotic hyperglycinemia	GLDC	AR	4	5	5	9	5	8	0
Geroderma osteodysplasticum; GO	GORAB	AR	1	2	2	4	1	3	0
Albinism, ocular, type I; OA1	GPR143	XL	1	12	5	9	4	4	0
Polymicrogyria, bilateral frontoparietal	GPR56	AR	1	1	1	2	0	0	0
Long-chain 3-hydroxyacyl-CoA dehydrogenase deficiency; HADHA	HADHA	AR	2	4	4	13	3	5	0
Hemoglobin-alpha locus 1; HBA1 hemoglobin-beta locus; HBB	HBB	AR	209	329	289	607	112	116	2
HLA + hemoglobin-beta locus; HBB	HBB	AR	61	137	78	121	20	15	1
HLA + sickle cell anemia	HBB	AR	6	9	5	9	1	1	0
Gangliosidosis, GM2 Tay–Sachs disease; TSD	HEXA	AR	12	21	20	41	10	9	0
Sandhoff disease	HEXB	AR	2	4	3	6	2	2	0
Beta-hydroxyisobutyryl CoA deacylase, deficiency	HIBCH	AR	1	1	1	2	0	0	0
Alopecia universalis congenita; ALUNC	HR	AR	1	1	1	2	1	0	0
Huntington's disease; HD	HTT	AD	61	96	74	141	35	35	1
Mucopolysaccharidosis type II (Hunter)	IDS	XL	6	15	11	22	5	5	0

Hurler syndrome	IDUA	AR	3	5	5	10	0	0	0
SMARD1	IGHMBP2	AR	2	3	2	4	1	2	0
Neuropathy, hereditary sensory and autonomic, type III; HSAN3	IKBKAP	AR	5	13	11	21	5	7	0
HLA + ectodermal dysplasia, hypohidrotic, with immune deficiency	IKBKG	XL	2	9	6	8	2	3	0
Incontinentia pigmenti; IP	IKBKG	XL	9	20	13	24	2	3	0
Popliteal pterygium syndrome; PPS	IRF6	AD	1	1	1	2	1	1	0
Van der Woude syndrome; VWS	IRF6	AD	1	1	1	1	1	1	0
HLA + DMD+Glanzmann's thrombastenia	ITGA2B DMD		1	2	2	4	1	0	0
Isovaleric acidemia; IVA	IVD	AR	1	1	1	2	0	0	0
Blood group–Kell–Cellano system	KEL	AR	11	23	16	28	4	5	0
Hydrocephalus, X-linked;	L1CAM	XL	8	12	11	27	4	4	0
Merosin-deficient MD	LAMA2	AR	1	1	1	2	0	0	0
Congenital nephrotic syndrome	LAMB2 NPHS	AR	2	5	5	11	3	1	0
Microcoria–congenital nephrosis syndrome	LAMB2	AR	1	2	2	4	2	1	0
Wolman disease	LIPA	AR	2	2	2	4	2	3	0
Emery–Dreifuss muscular dystrophy, EDMD3	LMNA	AR	4	11	10	19	5	5	0
Nail–patella syndrome; NPS	LMX1B	AD	2	3	2	3	0	0	0
Donnai–Barrow syndrome	LRP2	AR	1	1	0	0	0	0	0
Microtubule-associated protein tau; MAPT	MAPT	AD	1	2	2	4	0	0	0
Ichthyosis follicularis, atrichia, and photophobia syndrome	MBTPS2	XL	2	2	2	5	2	1	0
Rett syndrome; RTT	MECP2	XL	2	1	1	1	0	0	0
Multiple endocrine neoplasia, type I; MEN1	MEN1	AD	4	12	11	18	4	2	0
Charcot–Marie–Tooth disease, axonal, type 2A2; CMT2A2	MFN2	AD	2	6	3	4	1	0	1
Waardenburg syndrome, type 2A; WS2A	MITF	AD	2	3	3	3	1	1	0

(Continued)

Table 6.1 (Continued) Overall current experience of PGD for single-gene disorders

DISEASE	*GENE*	*Type of Inheritance*	*No. of Patients*	*No. of Cycles*	*No. of ET*	*No. of Embryos*	*Pregnancy*	*Birth*	*ONGOING*
Meckel syndrome MKS1; MKS6	MKS1 CC2D2A	AR	3	4	4	8	2	4	0
Currarino syndrome	MNX1	AD	1	1	1	2	1	1	0
Charcot–Marie–Tooth disease, demyelinating, type 1B; CMT1B	MPZ	AD	2	5	2	5	0	0	0
Colon cancer, familial non-polyposis, type 1 & 2	MSH6 MLH1	AD	5	10	9	18	6	7	0
Mthfr deficiency	MTHFR	AR	1	1	1	2	0	0	0
Myotubular myopathy 1; MTM1	MTM1	XL	2	3	1	3	1	2	0
Cardiomyopathy, familial hypertrophic, 4; CMH4	MYBPC3	AD	2	3	2	4	0	0	0
Cardiomyopathy, familial hypertrophic, 4; CMH4 CMH1 CMH7	MYBPC3 MYH7 TNNI3	AD	6	9	8	16	2	1	0
Cardiomyopathy, familial hypertrophic, CMH1	MYH7	AD	1	1	1	1	1	0	0
Norrie disease; NDP	NDP	XL	3	6	4	10	0	0	0
Nemaline myopathy 2; NEM2	NEB	AR	1	1	1	2	1	0	1
Charcot–Marie–Tooth disease, axonal, type 2E	NEFL	AD	1	4	4	7	1	1	1
Neurofibromatosis, type I; NF1	NF1	AD	32	56	52	88	22	22	3
Neurofibromatosis, type II; NF2	NF2	AD	4	7	7	15	5	6	0
Symphalangism, proximal; SYM1	NOG	AD	1	3	3	7	2	2	0
Nephrosis 1, congenital, Finnish type; NPHS1	NPHS1	AR	1	2	2	4	1	0	0
Sotos syndrome	NSD1	AD	1	1	1	1	1	1	0
Optic atrophy 1; OPA1	OPA1	AD	2	4	4	8	0	0	0
Ornithine transcarbamylase deficiency	OTC	XL	8	15	14	26	9	9	0
Phenylketonuria	PAH	AR	1	1	1	4	1	2	0
Propionic acidemia	PCCA, PCCB	AR	2	2	2	3	1	1	0
HLA + PKD1+ aneuploidy	PKD1	AD	1	1	1	2	1	1	0

Polycystic kidney disease 1; PKD1; Polycystic kidney disease 2; PKD2	PKD1 PKD2	AD	16	34	26	49	11	11	1
Polycystic kidney disease, autosomal recessive; ARPKD	PKHD1	AR	8	11	11	20	5	5	0
HLA+ piruvate kinase deficiency	PKLR	AD	1	2	1	1	0	0	0
Pelizaeus–Merzbacher-like disease; PMLD	PLP1	XL	6	10	9	14	6	7	0
Congenital disorder of glycosylation, type IA; CDG1A	PMM2	AR	1	1	1	1	1	1	0
Charcot–Marie–Tooth disease, demyelinating, type 1A; CMT1A	PMP22	AD	16	26	22	30	10	10	0
Alpers' syndrome	POLG	AR	1	1	1	1	1	1	0
Gerstmann–Sträussler disease; GSD	PRNP	AD	1	1	1	2	1	2	0
Pancreatitis, hereditary; PCTT	PRSS1	AD	1	1	1	2	1	2	0
Prosaposin deficiency	PSAP	AR	1	1	0	0	0	0	0
Alzheimer disease 3	PSEN1	AD	2	3	3	6	3	5	0
Early-onset familial Alzheimer disease	PSEN1 PSEN2	AD	2	4	3	6	3	5	0
Basal cell nevus syndrome; BCNS (Gorlin)	PTCH1	AD	4	5	4	7	3	3	0
Retinitis pigmentosa	PTPN11	AD	3	5	1	2	1	2	0
Zellweger syndrome; ZS	PXMP3 PEX1	AR	4	7	6	11	5	7	0
Charcot–Marie–Tooth disease, axonal, type 2B; CMT2B	RAB7A	AD	1	1	1	2	1	2	0
Omenn syndrome	RAG1	AD	2	6	5	12	1	2	0
Retinoblastoma; RB1	RB1	AD	11	19	17	29	8	7	0
Multiple endocrine neoplasia, type IIA; MEN2A	RET	AD	2	3	3	5	2	2	1
Rhesus blood group	RHD	AD	5	6	5	11	3	4	0
Retinitis pigmentosa	RHO	AD	2	3	1	2	1	0	0
Brachydactyly, type B1; BDB1	ROR2	AD	1	3	2	4	2	2	0
DBA	RPS19	AD	1	1	1	2	1	1	0

(Continued)

Table 6.1 (*Continued*) Overall current experience of PGD for single-gene disorders

DISEASE	*GENE*	*Type of Inheritance*	*No. of Patients*	*No. of Cycles*	*No. of ET*	*No. of Embryos*	*Pregnancy*	*Birth*	*ONGOING*
HLA + Diamond–Blackfan anemia; DB	RPS19, RPS24, RPL35A	AD	6	10	7	10	3	3	0
Retinoschisis 1, X-linked, juvenile; RS1	RS1	XL	1	2	1	2	1	1	0
Aicardi–Goutieres syndrome 5; AGS5 + CF	SAMHD1	AR	1	2	2	2	1	1	0
Cardioencephalomyopathy, fatal infantile	SCO2	AR	1	3	3	8	1	1	0
Alpha 1 antitrypsin deficiency	SERPINA1	AR	1	2	2	4	1	0	1
Angioedema, hereditary; HAE	SERPING1	AD	1	2	1	2	0	0	0
Spinocerebellar ataxia, autosomal recessive 1	SETX	AR	1	1	1	1	1	1	0
Sonic hedgehog; SHH	SHH	AD	1	2	2	3	1	1	0
Growth retardation	SHOX	XL	2	2	1	2	1	2	0
Carnitine deficiency, systemic primary; CDSP	SLC22A5	AR	1	2	1	2	1	1	0
Glucose transport defect, blood–brain barrier (Glut1)	SLC2A1	AD	1	2	1	2	0	0	0
Carnitine deficiency, systemic primary; CDSP (tortuosis)	SLC2A10	AR	1	2	2	2	1	1	0
Brain tumor, posterior fossa of infancy, familial	SMARCB1	AD	1	1	1	1	0	0	0
Spinal muscular atrophy, type I	SMN1	AR	47	58	51	91	33	41	1
Niemann–Pick disease, type A	SMPD1	AR	2	4	2	4	2	2	0
Spastic paraplegia 4	SPAST	AD	1	4	2	4	1	2	0
Pseudovaginal perineoscrotal hypospadias	SRD5A2	AR	1	1	0	0	0	0	0
Lipoid congenital adrenal hyperplasia	STAR	AR	1	1	1	2	1	2	0
Peutz–Jeghers syndrome; PJS	STK11	AD	1	3	3	4	2	1	0
Leigh syndrome; LS	SURF1	AR	1	1	1	3	0	0	0
Ulnar–Mammary syndrome; UMS	TBX3	AD	1	3	3	4	1	2	0
Holt–Oram syndrome	TBX5	AD	2	4	4	5	1	2	0

Homocystinuria	TBX5	AD	1	1	1	2	1	0	(2)
Osteopetrosis, autosomal recessive	TCIRG1	AR	5	5	4	9	2	2	0
Treacher Collins–Franceschetti syndrome; TCOF	TCOF1	AD	4	5	5	10	5	6	1
Loeys–Dietz syndrome, type 2B; LDS2B	TGFBR2	AD	2	5	3	4	2	2	0
Ichthyosis, lamellar	TGM1	AD	1	7	3	5	0	0	0
Dyskeratosis congenita, autosomal dominant, 1; DKCA1	TINF2	AD	1	2	2	3	1	1	0
Cardiomyopathy, familial hypertrophic, 7	TNNI3	AD	1	1	1	1	0	0	0
Arthrogryposis, distal, type 2B; DA2B	TNNT3	AD		2	2	3	2	2	0
Torsion dystonia 1, autosomal dominant; DYT1	TOR1A	AD	12	28	26	50	10	8	0
Li–Fraumeni syndrome; LFS	TP53	AD	4	6	5	9	1	1	0
Ceroid lipofuscinosis, neuronal 2, late infantile; CLN2	TPP1	AR	1	2	1	1	0	0	0
Tuberous sclerosis type 1	TSC1	AD	13	19	18	37	11	15	0
Tuberous sclerosis type 2	TSC2	AD	3	5	5	9	0	0	0
Amyloidosis i, hereditary neuropathic	TTR	AD	1	2	1	1	0	0	0
Oculocutaneous albinism, type I; OCA1; type 2; OCA 2	TYR OCA2	AR	4	9	8	17	4	4	0
Familial hemophagocytic lymphohistiocytosis	UNC13D	AR	2	3	3	4	1	1	0
Porphyria, congenital erythropoietic	UROS	AR	1	1	1	1	1	1	0
Von Hippel–Lindau syndrome; VHL	VHL	AD	6	8	7	12	5	6	0
Cohen syndrome; COH1	VPS13B	AR	1	1	1	2	1	2	0
Microphthalmia, isolated 2; MCOP2	VSX2	AR	2	2	1	1	1	1	0
HLA + Wiskott–Aldrich syndrome; WAS	WAS	XL	1	1	0	0	0	0	0
Wiskott–Aldrich syndrome; WAS	WAS	XL	4	7	7	14	5	4	1
Microcephaly 2, primary, autosomal recessive; MCPH2	WDR62	AR	1	1	1	1	0	0	0
Wolfram syndrome	WFS1	AR	1	2	1	1	1	1	0
TOTAL			1685	2982	2396	4419	1095	1118	47

One important factor in avoiding amplification failure in the PCR of single cells is the application of an adequate cell lysis procedure. Several methods, such as the proteinase K treatment, the freeze–thaw technique, and the KOH lysis procedure, have been used to lyse PB1, PB2, blastomeres, and somatic cells.[6] According to our observations, proteinase K treatment is the optimal method of single-cell lysis for PGD. Single cells are placed directly into a lysis solution consisting of 0.5 µl 10 × PCR buffer, 0.5 µl 1% Tween 20, 0.5 µl 1% Triton X-100, 3.5 µl H_2O, and 0.05 µl proteinase K (20 mg/ml in a 0.5-ml PCR tube). After centrifugation at a low speed in a microfuge for a few seconds, the samples are covered with one drop of mineral oil and incubated at 45°C for 15 min in a thermal cycler (a heating block can also be used). Proteinase K is then inactivated at 96°C for 20 min, which is the beginning of the hot-start PCR (see below). In case the samples have to be sent by mail, they are covered with one drop of mineral oil and frozen in vertical position.

The other critical feature of single-cell PCR is preventing DNA contamination. Because standard sterile techniques are not sufficient to avoid DNA contamination, a separate laboratory for preimplantation DNA analysis with its own laminar flow hood, refrigerator, freezer, microcentrifuge, and thermal cyclers is used. To identify possible contamination by extraneous DNA, a multiplex PCR system, involving polymorphic markers, is applied. The following rules are strictly adhered to:

(1) Tubes containing PCR products are never opened in the DNA laboratory.
(2) Gloves are worn at all times.
(3) No traffic is allowed in the DNA laboratory when analysis is being performed.
(4) Positive-displacement pipettes and filter-containing pipette tips are used.
(5) PCR tubes and micromanipulation tools are decontaminated prior to use under ultraviolet light inside a Template Tamer for at least 30 min.
(6) Reagents are stored as small aliquots to minimize the number of times the tubes are opened.
(7) All solutions with the exception of Taq polymerase and dNTPs are millipore filtered.
(8) All reagents, including those used in the embryology laboratory, are tested for DNA contamination prior to every PGD case, as it has been observed that culture media, human serum, and immersion oil can become contaminated with extraneous DNA.

Any PGD assay contains several control assays with no added cells or DNA or false biopsies in fully reconstituted PCR mixtures, in order to ensure that there is no contamination with extraneous DNA sources. Positive controls containing 100 pg of homozygous abnormal, homozygous normal, and heterozygous DNA are also included in each case. Single cells of known origin are used as a positive control, if available.

Pseudo-contamination is eliminated by increasing the stringency of the PCR reaction, lowering concentrations of dNTPs, Mg^{2+}, primers, and Taq polymerase, and increasing annealing temperature. A Template Tamer (ultraviolet decontaminating hood) is used to reduce contamination during the sample preparation for the nested PCR (the list of equipment and reagents used for single-cell DNA analysis is presented in Tables 6.2a and 6.2b).

The sensitivity and specificity of DNA amplification are dramatically improved by using the nested PCR method (Figure 6.2). The larger fragment produced by the first round of PCR is used as a template for the second round of PCR, involving nested PCR primers, i.e., those internal to the first primer pair. This also significantly increases the efficiency of DNA amplification from a single cell. The best results are obtained by using lower stringency, 5% dimethyl sulfoxide (DMSO), and a longer annealing time during the first round of PCR, and higher stringency in the second round. Also, use of a single inside nested primer (hemi-nesting) with the appropriate original outside primer, is as efficient as using two inside primers (full nesting) for the second reaction. In addition, nested PCR allows more reactions to be carried out, especially when multiplex PCR is applied during the first round of amplification (Figure 6.2).

As shown in Figure 6.2, following the first round of PCR containing outside primers for all the genes tested, separate aliquots are amplified using the specific inside primers for each site. Only when both the polymorphic allele and the mutation analysis agree are embryos transferred (Figure 6.3). This dual amplification allows detection of most cases of allele dropout (ADO) and prevents misdiagnosis in PGD (Figures 6.4 and 6.5).

To prevent non-specific annealing of primers and subsequent elongation of spurious DNA fragments, a hot-start PCR is used for the first round of amplification. A hot-start PCR involves withholding one or more of the required reagents of the PCR master mix until the sample has reached a temperature of at least 72°C (Figure 6.2). Lysed samples are placed into a thermal cycler and amplified (first round) at the following thermal cycler program: 45°C for 15 min (1 cycle), 96°C for 15 min (1 cycle); 72°C for 10 min (1 cycle); 94°C for 2 min (1 cycle); 94°C for 30 s, 60°C for 30 s, 55° for 30 s, 50° for 30 s, and 72°C for 30 s (each for 30 cycles); 72°C for 10 min (1 cycle), and 10°C (1 cycle). When the thermal cycler reaches the 72°C step, each sample in a tube is brought up to a final volume of 50 µl, using the first-round PCR master mix, consisting of PCR buffer, dNTPs, $MgCl_2$, DMSO, and the set of outside upstream and downstream primers for the gene tested, under the mineral oil.

After the completion of the first round of amplification the samples are removed from the thermal cycler and spun down in a microcentrifuge to prevent an aerosol splash of PCR product. An aliquot of 1–2 µl of the resulting first-round PCR product is transferred into 0.5-ml tubes with 48 µl of the fresh second-round PCR master mix, containing PCR buffer, dNTPs, $MgCl_2$, Taq polymerase, H_2O, and

Table 6.2a List of equipment for PGD of SGD and 24-chromosome a-CGH testing

Equipment	*Supplier*	*Model*	*Application*
Eppendorf thermal cycler	Eppendorf	Mastercycler Pro	Pre-PCR
Eppendorf thermal cycler	Eppendorf	Mastercycler Nexus eco	Pre-PCR
Thermo electron MBS thermal cycler	Fisher Scientific	HBMBSKIT2, HBMBS02	Pre-PCR
Laminar air flow workstation	Forma Scientific	Model 1849	Pre-PCR
DNA contamination-free workstation	MJR	CleanBox DNA Workstation	Pre-PCR
Microcentrifuge	Thermo Scientific	Legend Micro 17	Pre-PCR
Vortex	LabNet	VX100	Pre-PCR
Capillary DNA sequencer/genotyper	ABI	3130 Genetic Analyzer	Post-PCR
Vertical gel electrophoresis system	Bio Rad	Mini PROTEAN 3 Electrophoresis System	Post-PCR
DC power supply	LabNet	PowerStation 300	Post-PCR
DC power supply	Fisher Brand	FB300-1Q	Post-PCR
Gel documentation system	Fisher Scientific	FD 63020	Post-PCR
Microarray scanner	TECAN	PowerScanner	Microarray
Ozone scrubber	IQAir	GC Series	Microarray
Thermal cycler	Eppendorf	Mastercycler gradient	Microarray
Microarray incubator	SciGene	Hybex Microarray Incubation System	Microarray
SpeedVac centrifuge	ThermoScientific	Savant DNA120 SpeedVac Concentrator	Microarray
Drybath	Baxter	Multi Blok Heater	Microarray

nested upstream and downstream primers for the genes tested. In contrast to the first round, each tube contains singular pairs of specific nested primers. A drop of mineral oil is added in each tube, and the samples are amplified using the thermal cycler program as follows: 94°C for 2 min (1 cycle); then 94°C for 30 s, 55°C for 30 s, and 72°C for 30 s (for 30 cycles); 72°C for 10 min, and 72°C for 1 cycle.

Following nested amplification, PCR products are analyzed either by restriction digestion, real-time PCR, direct fragment size analysis, or minisequencing (Figure 6.2) (see below). Depending on the mutation studied, different primer systems are designed, with special emphasis on the elimination of false priming to possible pseudogenes, such as in PGD for long-chain 3-hydroxyacyl-CoA deficiency (LCHAD) and congenital adrenal hyperplasia, for which purpose the first-round primers are designed to anneal to the regions of non-identity with a pseudogene (Figures 6.6 and 6.7). When breakpoints are known, a similar approach may be used to test for large deletions, such as alpha-thalassemia and large deletion forms of beta-thalassemia (Figure 6.8).

Fluorescence PCR

A direct fragment size analysis of PCR product is performed by fluorescent PCR (F-PCR).[7] Instead of using gel electrophoresis and ethidium bromide staining, F-PCR uses fluorescently labeled primers in the PCR mix, and the sample is analyzed on a fluorescent capillary detector, as shown in Figure 6.9. Because F-PCR is much more sensitive than the standard gel detection, fewer PCR cycles are run, with the multiplex reaction being performed and analyzed in one tube using different color labels on each primer. F-PCR is particularly useful for direct sequencing of the PCR product for detection of point mutations and also for distinguishing preferential amplification from ADO (see below). Examples of the application of F-PCR in parallel with conventional PCR are shown in Figures 6.10 and 6.11.

Because of the possibility of preferential amplification or ADO in single-cell PCR analysis, highly polymorphic linked markers, such as short tandem repeats (STRs), are simultaneously amplified with the gene to which these STRs are strongly linked (Figure 6.12). The conditions of PCR analysis are different for each diagnostic system and require a preliminary work-up.

Real-time PCR

Real-time PCR detects specific nucleic acid amplification products as they accumulate by using a fluorescently labeled oligonucleotide probe, which eliminates the need for post-PCR processing. A reporter fluorescent dye and

Table 6.2b List of reagents for PGD of SGD and aCGH for 24-chromosome testing

Application	*Reagent*	*Vendor*	*Catalog Number*	*Storage*	*Expiration*
Regular PCR	R-Taq DNA polymerase, 5U/μl	Bulls eye	BE200319	–20°C	Manufacturer's
Regular PCR	Standard buffer (Mg free), 10X, 5 ml	Bulls eye	BE200319	–20°C	Manufacturer's
Regular PCR	MgCl2, 50mM, 5ml	Bulls eye	BE200319	–20°C	Manufacturer's
Regular PCR	dNTP Mix, 25mM each, 1ml	Fermentes	R1122	–20°C	Manufacturer's
Regular PCR	dGTP, 100mM	Fermentes	R0162	–20°C	Manufacturer's
Regular PCR	dATP, 100mM	Fermentes	R0142	–20°C	Manufacturer's
Regular PCR	dCTP, 100mM	Fermentes	R0152	–20°C	Manufacturer's
Regular PCR	dTTP, 100mM	Fermentes	R0172	–20°C	Manufacturer's
Regular PCR	DMSO, 250ml	Sigma	D8418-250ml	RT	Manufacturer's
Regular PCR	RapidLoad Buffer, 5X, 5ml	Origene	RL105(5ml)	–20°C	1 year
Regular PCR	1xTE Solution PH 8.0	IDT	11-05-01-10	+4°C	Manufacturer's
Regular PCR	Primers, 25nmole DNA oligo	IDT	NA	–20°C	Manufacturer's
GC-Rich PCR	GC-Melt Reagent	Clontech	639238	–20°C	Manufacturer's
GC-Rich PCR	7-Deaza- dGTP Li-salt	Roche	10-988-537-001	–20°C	Manufacturer's
GC-Rich PCR	ETSSB NE	BioLabs	M2401S	–20°C	Manufacturer's
Lysis Buffer	Tween 20	Amresco	M147-1L	–18°C	Manufacturer's
Lysis Buffer	Triton X 100, 10%	Amresco	M147-1L	–20°C	Manufacturer's
Lysis Buffer	Proteinase K, 20mg/ml	Invitrogen	Proteinase K Solution RNA grade	–20°C	Manufacturer's
Gel Electrophoresis	Acryl/Bis 19:1 Solution 40%	Amresco	0496-500ML	RT	Manufacturer's
Gel Electrophoresis	TBE Buffer 10X Liquid Concentrate	Amresco	0658-4L	RT	Manufacturer's
Gel Electrophoresis	Ammonium Persulfate	Amresco	0486-25G	RT	Manufacturer's
Gel Electrophoresis	TEMED	Amresco	0761-100ML	RT	Manufacturer's
Gel Electrophoresis	DNA Molecular Weight Marker (100–1000bp)	Bioline	HyperLadderIV	–20°C	Manufacturer's
Gel Electrophoresis	Gel Red Nucleic Acid Stain	Phenix	RGB-4103	RT	Manufacturer's
ABI 3130	ROX Size Standard	Applied Biosystem	401735	+4°C	1 year
ABI 3130	Hi-Di Formamide	Applied Biosystem	4311320	–20°C	Manufacturer's
ABI 3130	Polymer 3130 POP-4	Applied Biosystem	4352755	+4°C	Manufacturer's
Other	Water	Irvine Scientific	9307	+4°C	Manufacturer's

a quencher dye are attached to the hybridization probe. In an intact probe, the reporter dye's emission is minimal due to energy transfer to the quencher dye, resulting in negligible fluorescence being observed.

During PCR amplification, the probe anneals to its target sequence on the sample DNA. As the newly synthesized DNA strand reaches the site of probe hybridization, the DNA polymerase cleaves the probe, releasing the reporter dye from the quencher dye. At this point an increase in fluorescence is detected. The replication of the DNA strand continues undisturbed until the amplification cycle is complete. This process is known as TaqMan® chemistry (Figure 6.13). Since the reporter dye molecules are cleaved from the probes during each amplification cycle, the fluorescence intensity of the overall system increases proportionally to the amount of DNA amplified (Figure 6.14). Real-time PCR allows screening for genes with a single base-pair variation between the normal and mutant genotypes, and the detection of sequence changes, deletion, and insertion. Two hybridization TaqMan probes are designed for this purpose: one being a perfect match to the normal sequence and the other containing a mutant sequence. The perfect match probe binds to its target and is cleaved to produce a typical real-time PCR signal. The amplification product from heterozygous cells gives rise to two signals (Figure 6.15).

The fluorescence emission is detected every few seconds, and data are plotted in real time as a function of the cycle number. Rather than monitoring the final amplification product, as is performed in traditional PCR, the real-time PCR reaction is characterized by the point in time when amplification of a PCR product is first detected. This time point is referred to as cycle threshold (Ct). The larger the amount of initial sample, the sooner this threshold value is achieved. Single-cell amplification with TaqMan probes requires at least ten cycles more than extracted genomic DNA amplification (Figures 6.14 and 6.15). The advantage of real-time PCR is that the PCR tubes do not need to be opened after the amplification reaction is complete since all the data have already been collected. This prevents contamination by PCR products and reduces the amount of "false positive" results.

Real-time PCR can also be performed with molecular beacons (MBs). In contrast to the linear probes used in TaqMan systems, MB is a stem-and-loop hairpin structure design with a reporter fluorescent dye on one end and a quencher molecule on the other. The loop portion of the molecule is a probe sequence, which is complementary to a target sequence, and the stem is formed by short complementary sequences located at opposite ends of the molecule (Figure 6.16).

The hairpin structure causes the MB probe to fold when not hybridized. This brings the reporter and quencher molecules into close proximity with little or no fluorescence being emitted. However, when the MB hybridizes to the template, the hairpin structure is broken and the reporter dye is no longer quenched. At this point, the real-time instrument detects fluorescence. The hairpin shape of the probe causes mismatched probe/target hybrids to dissociate easily at a lower temperature than perfectly matched hybrids. The thermal instability of mismatched hybrids increases the specificity of MBs, enabling them to distinguish targets by only a single nucleotide. When conjugated to different fluorophores, two allele-specific MBs can simultaneously discriminate the three possible genotypes (Figure 6.17).

As already mentioned, the PCR product after the second round may also be analyzed by minisequencing (Figure 6.18). As will be described in Chapter 7, the microarray technology at the single-cell level is currently also being applied with the clear prospect of combined PGD for single-gene disorders with simultaneous detection of aneuploidies and surrounding single-nucleotide polymorphisms.

WHOLE GENOME AMPLIFICATION FOR PGD OF SINGLE-GENE DISORDERS TOGETHER WITH 24-CHROMOSOME ANEUPLOIDY TESTING

As whole genome amplification (WGA) is the first key component of the microarray technology recently introduced for PGD of chromosomal disorders, this allows, in addition to a highly improved detection of chromosomally abnormal oocytes and embryos,[8–14] a concomitant testing for single-gene disorders. Of the presently available platforms for 24-chromosome testing, we used the one developed by BlueGnome Ltd, Cambridge, UK, because it can be applied to all biopsy materials, including PB1, PB2, blastomeres, and blastocyst, allows completing the test within 12 h, and provides accurate results in over 90% of samples. The protocol consists of at least five steps, including amplification (2 h), labeling (2.5 h), hybridization (3.5 h), washing (30 min), scanning (30 min), and data analysis (1 h). The technique tests all 24 chromosomes for any gain or loss with the BAC pooling strategy, which coupled with the uniquely designed software enables obtaining straightforward results on aneuploidy in a single cell.

As one of the critical steps of the procedure is whole genome amplification with Super Plex Single Cell Whole Genome Amplification Kit (Rubicon Technologies Inc.), we used the portion of the WGA product for testing single-gene disorders in question, as described above. This approach has opened the possibility of combining aneuploidy testing for 24 chromosomes with PGD for single-gene disorders, which was first performed for GM1 gangliosidosis, an autosomal recessive lysosomal storage disorder.[15] This novel approach was then extended to a variety of genetic conditions, and also applied together with preimplantation HLA typing, to investigate the feasibility of a combined test for 24-chromosome aneuploidy, with PGD for single-gene disorders and preimplantation HLA typing (Table 6.3). The list of 55 conditions for which PGD was performed together with 24-chromosome aneuploidy testing is presented in Table 6.4. The combined test was performed in 138 clinical cycles for 83 couples at risk for producing offspring with any of these 55 genetic disorders. A total of 1054 embryos were tested, including 320 by blastocyst biopsy in 78 cycles, 670 by blastomere biopsy in 53 cycles, and 64 by combined polar body and blastomere biopsy in 4 cycles. Five of these cycles were performed with concomitant HLA typing, including two for chronic granulomatous disease, two for thalassemia, and one for Diamond–Blackfan anemia, by testing for a set of chromosome 6 short tandem repeats throughout the HLA region.

Of these 1054 embryos tested, 434 (41.2%) were predicted to be aneuploidy free and also unaffected. The embryos suitable for transfer were available in all the cycles and were transferred without freezing in 41 of 92 cycles performed by polar body and blastomere biopsy, which resulted in 21 (51.2%) clinical pregnancies and the birth of 24 unaffected children. Embryo freezing was involved in the remaining 51 transfer cycles, performed by blastocyst biopsy, which resulted in 40 (78.4%) clinical pregnancies and 45 unaffected births. In all, concomitant 24-chromosome aneuploidy testing and single gene and HLA analysis resulted in the transfer of 137 embryos in 92 cycles, yielding 61 (66.3%) clinical pregnancies and the birth of 69 unaffected children, suggesting a significant improvement in pregnancy and delivery rates. Thus a combined comprehensive test for 24 chromosomes, single gene disorders, and preimplantation HLA typing is of significant practical value, and may be applied in the framework of ART in efforts to optimize

Table 6.3 Array-CGH 24-chromosome aneuploidy testing combined with PGD for 55 single-gene disorders with or without HLA typing

Cell type	*No. of Patients*	*No. of Cycles*	*No. of Transfers*	*Total no. of Embryos Tested*	*No. of Embryos Suitable for ET*	*No. of Embryos Transferred*	*Frozen Embryos for Future FET*	*Pregnancy*	*Birth*
Trophectoderm	49	78	51	320	134	78 1.5	56	40 78.4%	38 (7)*
Blastomere	31	53	37	670	268	56 1.5	117	20 54%	18 (5)*
Polar body + blastomere	3	7	4	64	32	5 1.25	19	1 25%	1
TOTAL	83	138	92 66.6%	1054	434 41%	139 1.5	192	61 66.3%	57 (12)*

*Ongoing pregnancy with a heartbeat

the pregnancy success of patients of advanced reproductive age who are referred for PGD for Mendelian disorders and preimplantation HLA typing.

DIAGNOSTIC ACCURACY

Because the PGD for single-gene disorders is based on single-cell genetic analysis, its accuracy depends largely on the limitations of single-cell DNA analysis, which may potentially cause misdiagnosis. One of the key contributors to misdiagnosis is the phenomenon of preferential amplification (Figure 6.9), also known as ADO (Figures 6.9 and 6.19), requiring the application of special protocols to ensure the highest ADO detection rate.[16,17] A few previously reported misdiagnoses, involving PGD for beta-thalassemia, myotonic dystrophy (DM), fragile-X syndrome (FMR1) (Figure 6.20), and cystic fibrosis (CF), could have been due to this phenomenon, which initially was not fully recognized.

It has been demonstrated that ADO rates in single cells might be different for different types of heterozygous cells (Figure 6.21).[17] The ADO rate may be as high as between 10% and 20% in blastomeres, compared to the ADO rate in single fibroblasts and PB1, which is under 10%. A high rate of ADO in blastomeres may lead to an obvious misdiagnosis, especially in compound heterozygous embryos. As previously mentioned, most misdiagnoses, especially those at the initial stage of application of PGD for single-gene disorders, have occurred in cases of blastomere biopsy from apparently compound heterozygous embryos. To avoid misdiagnosis due to preferential amplification, a simultaneous detection of the mutant gene together with up to three highly polymorphic markers closely linked to the gene tested was introduced (Figure 6.22).[16] Each additional linked marker may reduce the misdiagnosis rate by approximately half, so that with one linked marker amplified together with mutation a misdiagnosis risk in blastomere

Table 6.4 55 genetic disorders for which PGD was performed combined with 24-chromosome aneuploidy testing by aCGH

Achondroplasia
Aicardi–Goutieres syndrome CFTR
Alpha 1-antitrypsin deficiency
Alzheimer
Arterial tortuosity syndrome
Arthrogryposis
BRCA 1
Cardiomyopathy, familial hypertrophic, 7
Carnitine palmitoyltransferase II deficiency
CFTR
CFTR SMA
CMT 2A
DMD
Ehler–Danlos EDSIV
Emery–Dreifuss
Epidermolysis bullosa
Exostoses, multiple, type I
Exostoses, multiple, type II
Familial hemophagocytic lymphohistiocytosis
Fragile X
G6PD
Gaucher disease
Glycogen storage disease II
Gangliosidosis GM1
Growth retardation
Hemophilia A
HLA
Holt–Oram syndrome
Huntington's disease
Hyperinsulinemic hypoglycemia

Table 6.4 (Continued) 55 genetic disorders for which PGD was performed combined with 24-chromosome aneuploidy testing by aCGH

Marfan syndrome
MEN 2A
MEN I
Mosaic variegated aneuploidy
Myotonic dystrophy
Nail–patella syndrome
Neurofibromatosis type I
Niemann–Pick disease
Noonan syndrome
Norrie disease
OCA 2 & OCA I
Osler–Weber–Rendu syndrome
Osteogenesis imperfecta
PKD AR
PKD I
Retinoblastoma
Retinoschisis
Sandhoff disease
Sickle cell anemia
SMA
THAL B
Torsion dystonia
Tuberous sclerosis 1
Tuberous sclerosis 2
Wiskott–Aldrich syndrome

analysis may be reduced from 20% to 10%, with two from 10% to 5%, and with three from 5% to practically zero. The number of markers required might be reduced with the use of real-time PCR, because of the considerably lower ADO rate observed in real-time PCR (Figure 6.23). Therefore, the most reliable method to date is multiplex nested PCR analysis, with the initial PCR reaction containing all the pairs of outside primers, so that following the first-round PCR, separate aliquots of the resulting PCR product can be amplified using the inside primers specific for each site (Figure 6.24). Only when the polymorphic sites and the mutation agree are embryos transferred. Thus, multiplex amplification allows detection of ADO and prevents the transfer of misdiagnosed affected embryos, as shown in the example of PGD for autosomal dominant early-onset torsion dystonia (DYT) (Figure 6.25).

Another efficient approach to avoid misdiagnosis may be a sequential genetic analysis of the PB1 and PB2 in PGD for maternally derived mutations. Detection of both mutant and normal alleles in the heterozygous PB1, together with the mutant allele in the corresponding PB2, leaves no doubt that the resulting maternal contribution to the embryo is normal, even without testing for the linked markers as a control, as shown in the case of PGD for familial posterior fossa brain tumor (hSNF5) (Figure 6.26). However, as demonstrated in these cases, it is ideal to test simultaneously for at least one linked marker to confirm the diagnosis. Alternatively, mutation-free oocytes can also be predicted when the corresponding PB1 is homozygous mutant, in which scenario the corresponding PB2 should be hemizygous normal, similar to the resulting maternal pronucleus. However, the genotype of the resulting maternal contribution may be quite the reverse, i.e. mutant, if the corresponding PB1 is in fact heterozygous, but erroneously diagnosed as homozygous mutant because of ADO of the normal allele (see Figures 6.3, 6.4 and 6.27). In the above scenario, the extrusion of the normal allele with the PB2 would lead to the mutant allele being left in the resulting oocyte. Therefore, the embryos resulting from the oocytes with homozygous mutant PB1 cannot be acceptable for transfer unless the heterozygous status of the PB1 is excluded by the use of linked markers as described. The example of misdiagnosis due to ADO of the normal allele in PB1 has been described earlier in a PGD cycle performed for FMR1 (Figure 6.20).[18] To avoid misdiagnosis completely, sequential PB1 and PB2 analysis may be required to combine with multiplex PCR to exclude the possibility of an undetected ADO in a heterozygous PB1 (see Figures 6.3, 6.4, and 6.27). The analysis of more than 1000 oocytes tested by sequential PB1 and PB2 analysis showed that more than half of ADOs were detected by sequential analysis of PB1 and PB2, with the remaining cases detected by multiplex PCR.[16] The particular value of linked marker analysis combined with sequential PB1 and PB2 testing is obvious from the presented case of PGD for spinal muscular atrophy (SMA) (Figure 6.28), caused by mutations in survival motor neuron gene (*SMN*), present in two homologous copies (*SMN1* and *SMN2*), the loss of only one of them (*SMN1*) leading to SMA. The accuracy of this approach may also be demonstrated by the reports of PGD for thalassemia and familial dysautonomia (FD), resulting in the transfer of three unaffected embryos in each case, which were confirmed by the birth of the two sets of triplets free from thalassemia and FD (Figures 6.29–6.31).[19]

The other method with the proven potential for the detection and avoidance of misdiagnosis due to preferential amplification is fluorescence PCR (F-PCR), which can allow detection of some of the heterozygous PB1 or blastomeres misdiagnosed as homozygous in conventional PCR, and therefore has the potential to reduce the ADO rates to some extent (Figures 6.9 and 6.23).[16] In addition, the method also allows simultaneous gender determination, DNA fingerprinting, and detection of common aneuploidies (Figures 6.32–6.34). With further improvement and simplification, F-PCR combined with a multiplex system and sequential PB1 and PB2 analysis in cases of maternally derived mutations can almost completely exclude the risk of misdiagnosis due to preferential amplification.

The accuracy of PGD may be further improved with the application of F-PCR with the Expand Long Template (ELT) Kit, which reduces the ADO rate from as high as 30–35% in both conventional and F-PCR to as low as 5% in testing for myotonic dystrophy (DM).[20] Another development to improve the accuracy of single-cell PCR analysis involves the application of real-time PCR, which reduces the ADO rate almost by half, as shown in Figure 6.23, compared to conventional or F-PCR. The application of these approaches, together with simultaneous testing for the causative mutation along with at least one or two linked markers, can reliably eliminate the risk of misdiagnosis.

Finally, because of the high rate of aneuploidies in oocytes and embryos, including mosaicism at the cleavage stage, testing for the chromosome in which the gene in question is mapped is of obvious value in ruling out a missing or extra mutant allele caused by monosomy or trisomy of this chromosome in the biopsied blastomere (Figures 6.35–6.38). As shown in Figures 6.32, 6.34, and 6.39, aneuploidy testing is technically feasible and can be performed by adding primers for chromosome-specific microsatellite markers (Figure 6.40) to the multiplex PCR protocols worked out for specific genetic disorders, although this is currently performed by microarray-based analysis, as described above (Tables 6.3 and 6.4). The development of multiplex nested PCR systems will also allow PGD to be performed simultaneously for different conditions, as attempted for CFTR or SMN mutations, together with aneuploidy testing and gender determination (Figures 6.32, 6.34, 6.36, 6.41), as well as for mutation testing together with HLA typing (see below), for which purpose different strategies may be chosen (Figure 6.42). For example, HLA typing demonstrated an approximately 6% aneuploidy rate for chromosome 6, which has a clear impact on correct HLA typing, as shown in Figure 6.43. There is a strong indication for aneuploidy testing in PGD for patients of advanced reproductive age, such as in many cases of preimplantation HLA typing. The relevance of aneuploidy testing in HLA typing for patients of advanced reproductive age is demonstrated in Figure 6.33. Experience shows that the average maternal age of couples requesting PGD with HLA typing is significantly higher than of PGD couples overall, so a concomitant testing for aneuploidy may appear useful. According to our observation of PGD for HLA typing, the pregnancy rate in 151 couples without aneuploidy testing was 23%, in contrast to over 40% in 91 couples for whom a concomitant aneuploidy testing was applied.[21]

Owing to the requirement to develop a custom-made PGD design for each mutation and each couple, preparatory work has become an integral part of PGD for single-gene disorders to ensure that potential misdiagnoses are avoided. For example, in some cases a particular set of outside primers has to be designed to eliminate false priming to a pseudogene, as described in PGD for long-chain 3-hydroxyacyl-CoA dehydrogenase deficiency and also (as presented above) for congenital adrenal hyperplasia (Figures 6.6 and 6.7).[22] Furthermore, the preparatory work can frequently involve single-sperm typing, which is required for establishing paternal haplotypes, so that linked marker analysis can be performed in addition to mutation analysis, especially in cases of paternally derived dominant conditions. The availability of the parental haplotypes allows not only the absence of the mutant gene to be confirmed, but also the presence of both maternal and paternal wild alleles in PGD by blastomere analysis (Figure 6.44), especially when only one informative marker is available (Figure 6.45).[23] Finally, haplotype analysis allows PGD for those conditions for which no exact causative gene status is available, such as autosomal dominant polycystic kidney disease type 1 and 2 (PKD1 and PKD2), the first experience of which is presented in Figures 6.46 and 6.47.[24] This may have implications for PGD of other, similar conditions that, to date, cannot be performed by traditional approaches.

In fact, we have now an experience of a total of 28 PGD cycles for two or more genetic disorders at the same cycle (Table 6.5). Eleven of these PGD cycles were performed for CF in six couples at risk for producing offspring with other genetic conditions, including facioscapulohumeral muscular dystrophy (FSHD) (Figure 6.48), Darrier disease (Figure 6.49), SMA (Figure 6.50), Aicardi–Goutieres syndrome, hereditary hemochromatosis, and Robertsonian translocations. Unaffected embryos were available for transfer in all the cycles, and the transfer of a total of 14 embryos resulted in 7 pregnancies and birth of 6 children free of both CF and all of the above conditions. The other concomitant PGD has been performed for Charcot–Marie–Tooth (CMT) and Fabry diseases in a couple with both partners carrying Fabry mutation and the male partner with CMT disease. The testing was performed by a sequential PB1 and PB2 analysis of Fabry disease, followed by embryo biopsy and testing for CMT, which allowed the identification and transfer of an unaffected embryo, resulting in a triplet pregnancy and birth of three healthy children, which appear to be monozygotic triplets (see below).

A similar approach was used for other concomitant PGD cycles for BRCA1 and SMA, BRCA1 and BRCA2, BRCA2 and PSEN (see below), and BRCA2 and MEN12. Testing for both mutations in these cycles allowed identification of unaffected embryos for transfer in each of the cases. Three cycles were performed for the patient at risk for alpha 1-antitrypsin deficiency and translocation, one for CMT 1A combined with brain tumor, two for Glanzmann's thrombastenia and DMD, one for Kell and RHD, one for SMA and Hurler syndrome, two for hemophilia and Huntington's disease, one for CMT2A and Dejerine–Sottas syndrome, and one for NF1 and CMT1A. Overall, of 28 PGD cycles performed for 18 at-risk patients, 32 unaffected embryos were transferred

Table 6.5 Combined PGD for two and more genetic disorders

Disease	*Number of Patients*	*Number of Cycles*	*Number of Transfers*	*Number of Embryos Transferred*	*Pregnancy*	*Birth*
Aicardi–Goutières syndrome CFTR	1	2	1	1	1	1
Alpha 1-antitrypsin deficiency +translocation	1	3	2	4	1	0
BRCA 1 SMA	1	1	1	2	1	2
BRCA 2 MEN 1	1	4	2	3	0	0
CFTR Robertsonian translocation	1	1	1	3	1	2
CFTR SMA	1	3	2	3	1	2
CMT 1A, brain tumor	1	1	1	1	0	0
FSHD CFTR	1	1	1	2	1	1
HLA Glanzmann's thrombasthenia DMD	1	2	2	3	1	0
PKD 1 PKD2	1	1	1	2	1	1
PSEN BRCA2	1	1	1	2	0	0
Hereditary hemochromatosis CFTR	1	1	1	1	0	0
Fabry disease CMT1A	1	1	1	2	1	3
BRCA1 BRCA2	1	1	1	1	1	1
NF1 CMT1A	1	1	0	0	0	0
CMT2A (MFN2) Dejerine–Sottas syndrome	1	1	0	0	0	0
CFTR Darier disease	1	1	1	1	1	1
Hemophilia A+ Huntington	1	2	1	1	1	1
	18	28	20	32	12	15

in 20 cycles, resulting in 12 pregnancies and birth of 15 healthy children, with no misdiagnosis (Table 6.5).

As mentioned, the experience presented below is the result of the world's largest series of PGD for Mendelian disorders, comprising 2982 PGD cycles, which clearly shows an extremely high accuracy and reliability (Table 6.1). Only three misdiagnoses (0.27%) occurred during this time, while 1095 clinical pregnancies and the birth of 1118 healthy children occurred during the period of over 20 years (with 47 pregnancies still ongoing at the time of the review). All three misdiagnoses were due to ADO: one in PGD for CFTR involving a misdiagnosis of compound heterozygote embryos as heterozygous at the beginning of the introduction of PGD, when the phenomenon of ADO was not yet appreciated, and the other two in PGD for FRM1 and myotonic dystrophy, involving the transfer of the embryos with the predicted 5% risk of misdiagnosis, which the couple decided to transfer in addition to others with 100% accuracy to improve their chances of becoming pregnant. Assuming that the overall experience has involved the genetic testing of tens of thousands of oocytes and embryos, which resulted in preselection and transfer of 4419 unaffected embryos in 2396 cycles in all, the technique may be applied in clinical practice with a high accuracy.[25]

It is of note that at least one-third of these cycles were performed by PB analysis only, which was sufficient for high accuracy. This included a PB-based PGD series of 938 PGD cycles, which included PB testing in over 9000 oocytes, resulting in preselection and transfer of 1578 unaffected embryos originating from mutation-free oocytes in 790 of 938 cycles (84%), demonstrating the safety, reliability, and extremely high accuracy of the procedure (99.7%).[25] PB analysis is obviously the method of choice in PGD for X-linked disorders, as well as for maternally derived autosomal recessive disorders, because preselection of oocytes free of X-linked disorders allows avoiding any micromanipulation of the embryo. The PB-based approach is an integral part of PGD, which makes it possible to perform preselection of mutation-free oocytes and complete PGD prior to fertilization. This provides the possibility for pre-embryonic diagnosis for couples who object to embryo biopsy because of their social or religious attitudes. Although the approach is currently limited to PGD for autosomal recessive conditions, X-linked disorders, and dominant mutations of maternal origin, the future progress in the testing of paternal mutations prior to fertilization may allow performing pre-embryonic diagnosis for any disease. The presented results demonstrate that the PB approach is highly efficient and reliable, providing an extremely high accuracy of PGD for Mendelian disorders. Along with the application of embryo biopsy, this technique provides a comprehensive diagnostic package for an efficient and reliable, and extremely accurate PGD.

PB sampling was sufficient for making decisions about embryo transfer in one-quarter of the cycles, while additional blastomere and/or blastocyst biopsy was required in the remaining cases involved. A total of 9036 oocytes were tested, of which 7841 (86.8%) were with both PB1 and PB2, with the results of sequential PB1 and PB2 testing obtained in 97.6% of these oocytes. This made it possible to preselect for transfer as many as 1578 embryos originating from these oocytes (1.99 on the average) in 790 (84.2%) cycles, resulting in 329 pregnancies (41.6%) and the birth of 353 healthy children.

So, clearly, the other alternative approaches, such as single blastomere removal at the cleavage stage and blastocyst biopsy, should be available to ensure PGD application in complex cases, and to avoid the transfer of affected embryos with paternally derived mutations. In addition, these methods also provide a confirmatory diagnosis following the PB testing. The choice of additional methods will differ depending on circumstances, and a reliable diagnosis may require using two or even three different methods, especially when there is more than one indication for PGD, such as PGD for single-gene disorders together with HLA typing, or PGD for one or two conditions together with aneuploidy testing (see Figures 6.48–6.50). Additional embryo biopsy was applied in 701 of these cases, to confirm the diagnosis when necessary, or identify unaffected embryos for transfer in the absence of embryos originating from mutation-free oocytes, such as heterozygous carrier embryos originating from mutant oocytes. As demonstrated above, the combined PGD is also required to include 24-chromsome aneuploidy testing in couples of advanced reproductive age who are referred for HLA typing and testing for single-gene disorders. As seen from Tables 6.3 and 6.4, these cases can presently be done by microarray technology, because 24-chromosome testing requires WGA anyway, so providing WGA product in this first step, applicable for testing for any number of alleles in question (see Figure 6.50).

Similar high accuracy was reported as well from the center with the world's second most-extensive PGD experience for monogenic disorders, which documented only a 0.6% misdiagnosis rate in PGD of 1443 PGD cycles: one misdiagnosis in PGD for muscular dystrophy and three in PGD for Charcot–Marie–Tooth disease (CMT1A), due to errors in linkage analysis in preparation for PGD.[26]

PGD FOR SPECIFIC GENETIC DISORDERS

The list of disorders for which PGD has been applied currently comprises over 300 different conditions and is being extended beyond the traditional indications of prenatal diagnosis, although the most frequent ones are still CF and hemoglobin disorders, the conditions for which PGD was applied from the very beginning.[27–31] As seen from Table 6.1, the most frequent indications for PGD were CF and hemoglobin disorders, followed by DM and FMR1, similar to the experiences in other active centers.[1–3] Our experience of 2982 PGD cycles has currently resulted in the transfer of 4419 unaffected embryos in 2396 (80%) cycles (1.84 embryos per transfer on the average), yielding 1095 (45.7%) unaffected pregnancies and the birth of 1118 apparently healthy children, with 47 pregnancies still ongoing.

Specific diagnosis for X-linked diseases

More than half of PGD cases for single-gene disorders have been performed by gender determination for X-linked conditions, which has been the most straightforward application from the very beginning, using either PCR or FISH techniques.[1–3] This was not only because the sequence information was not always available, but also because it was technically easier to identify female embryos by DNA analysis or FISH, despite the obvious cost of discarding 50% of the healthy embryos because they were male. On the other hand, testing for X-linked genetic disorders may be limited entirely to oocytes, because the mutations involved are fully maternally derived. Therefore, testing of oocytes for maternally derived specific mutations makes it possible to avoid further testing of the resulting embryos, which may be transferred irrespective of gender or any contribution from the father. Initially this approach was applied for ornithine transcarbamylase deficiency (OTC)[32]; it was then extended to specific diagnoses of other X-linked disorders[18] and presently comprises the experience of specific diagnoses in dozens of cycles performed for OTC (Figure 6.51), FMR1 (Figure 6.20), myotubular myotonic dystrophy, Alport syndrome, Charcot–Marie–Tooth disease X-linked type, hemophilia A, hemophilia B, Hunter syndrome, incontinentia pigmenti, Duchenne muscular dystrophy (DMD), Becker-type muscular dystrophy (BMD), Norrie disease, Pelizaeus–Merzbacher disease, retinitis pigmentosa, Wiskott–Aldrich syndrome, X-linked adrenoleukodystrophy, X-linked hyper-IgM syndrome, X-linked incontinentia pigmenti, and X-linked hydrocephalus, to mention only a few of the most important examples. This resulted in the transfer of mutation-free embryos in most of the cycles and births of unaffected children, demonstrating an extremely high accuracy and the clinical usefulness of the specific polar body testing for X-linked disorders to replace PGD by gender determination, which is no longer acceptable in many centers.

Couples with a homozygous affected partner

PGD has also been provided for couples with one homozygous or double-heterozygous partner affected with thalassemia, cystic fibrosis, or phenylketonuria (PKU), resulting in an unaffected pregnancy and the birth of healthy children (Figures 6.34, 6.52–6.54).[33,34]

Although the risk of producing an affected child in such couples is as high as 50%, irrespective of the maternal or paternal affected status, the strategy of PGD in such cases will depend on whether the father or mother is affected. In couples with affected fathers, PGD may concentrate on the preselection of mutation-free oocytes, while with affected mothers, cleavage-stage PGD is required to identify those few embryos containing the normal gene. The testing is particularly complicated if the parents carry different mutations.

In our experience, the largest group for which PGD was provided for couples with one affected partner was the group of homozygous or double heterozygous CF patients (Table 6.6). A total of 44 PGD cycles were performed, which were based on the testing for two or even three mutations simultaneously, as demonstrated in Figures 6.34 and 6.53. PGD for these cases seems to be the only choice, as the male or female partners are double heterozygous for two different mutations, while the healthy partners are carriers of the Delta F508 or other mutation in the CFTR gene. To avoid testing for two different mutations simultaneously in the same blastomere—taking into consideration up to 20% risk of ADO for each of the alleles tested,[17] potentially leading to a misdiagnosis—a sequential PB1 and PB2 analysis was performed in those cases when the healthy heterozygous partner was the mother, thus to identify the mutation-free oocytes as the first step (Figure 6.53). As a result, mutation-free oocytes were detected in both of these cycles, with PGD resulting in the birth of healthy children confirmed to be unaffected carriers of the parental mutation.[34]

So PGD is of special value for couples with homozygous and double heterozygous affected partners, with only a 50% chance of having an unaffected child, which is also the case with PGD for the thalassemia patient presented in Figure 6.54, in which the female partner was affected double heterozygous (IVSI-110; IVSI-1-6), and the male partner a heterozygous carrier of the third mutation (IVSII-745).

With progress in the treatment of some genetic disorders, PGD will have an increasing impact on the decision of the affected and well-treated patients to reproduce. For example, life expectancy has been significantly improved for such common conditions as CF and thalassemia, both representing the most frequent indications in the PGD practice. In each of such cases the strategy depends on whether the affected partner is male or female, because testing may be entirely limited to the oocyte if a male partner is affected, in contrast to embryo testing, which will be required if the female partner is affected.

In couples where one of the partners is homozygous affected, PGD is actually the only hope to reproduce with the real chance of having unaffected children of their own.

PGD for conditions determined by *de novo* mutations

PGD has recently become applicable to couples who may themselves be non-carriers of the mutation, with no family history of the genetic disease, but *de novo* mutation (DNM) may be found in their gonads, with the disease first diagnosed in one of the parents or their affected children. (Our current experience on PGD for *de novo* mutations is summarized in Table 6.7.) As neither origin nor relevant haplotypes are available for tracing the inheritance of such mutations in single cells biopsied from embryos or in oocytes, the main emphasis is on the identification of mutation and/or relevant haplotypes to be able to trace the mutation.[35]

The PGD strategy was developed for a total of 152 families with various genetic disorders, determined by 134 dominant, 6 recessive, and 12 X-linked DNM (the list of DNM for which this PGD strategy was performed is presented in Table 6.8). The majority of these families (134 of 152) were with dominant mutations, of which 69 were of paternal origin, 57 of maternal origin, and

Table 6.6 PGD for affected cystic fibrosis patients

Number of Mutations Between Partners	*Number of Patients*	*Number of Cycles*	*Number of Transfers**	*Number of Embryos Transferred*	*Pregnancy*	*Birth*
1	122 (119 – delta 508; 2 – W1282X; 1 – 3120G-A)	180	159	317	81 (4) 50.9%	84
2	131	199	164	314	84 51.2 %	95
3	25 (18P + 7M)	44	36	72	17 (2) 47.2%	13 (3 affected mothers; 10 affected fathers)
Total	278	423	359	703	182 (6) 50.7%	192

*FET pending for trophectoderm samples

Table 6.7 PGD for *de novo* mutations

Type of Inheritance	*Mutation Origin*			*Number of Patients*	*% Cycle*	*ET*	*Number of Embryos Transferred*	*Pregnancy*	*Birth*
	PATERNAL	MATERNAL	DETECTED IN CHILD						
Dominant	69	57	8	134	251	214	363	106	112
Recessive	3	1	2	6	11	11	16	6	5
X-linked	0	7	5	12	17	14	24	7	7
TOTAL	72	65	15	152	279	239 (86%)	403 (1.7)	119 (50%)	124 (52%)

Table 6.8 Outcome of PGD for *de novo* mutation causing different genetic disorders with different origin

Disease	*Inheritance*	*Gene*	*De novo Mutations Origin*			*Number of Patients had PGD*	*Cycle*	*ET*	*Number of Embryos*	*Pregnant*	*Birth*
			PAT	MAT	CHILD						
Achondroplasia	AD	FGFR3	1	0	0	1	3	1	3	2	1
Blepharophimosis	AD	FOXL2	1	0	0	1	1	1	1	0	0
Brachydactyly	AD	ROR2	1	0	0	1	3	3	4	2	2
BRCA1	AD	BRCA1	0	1	0	1	1	1	1	0	0
Brain tumor	AD	SMARC B1	0	0	1	1	1	1	0	0	0
Cardiomyopathy 7	AD	TNNI3	1	0	0	1	1	1	0	0	0
Cmt1a	AD	PMP22	3	0	0	3	5	5	8	4	5
Cmt2a	AD	MFN2	2	0	0	2	4	4	4	1	1
Crouzon syndrome	AD	FGFR2	1	3	0	4	5	5	10	3	2
Darier disease	AD	ATP2A2	0	1	0	1	1	1	2	1	1
DBA	AD	RPS19 RPL35A RPS10	0	2	5	7	11	8	12	4	4
Dystrophia myotonica 1	AD	DMPK	1	0	0	1	2	2	3	1	1
Ehlers–Danlos syndrome	AD	COL5A1	0	1	0	1	2	2	3	2	2
Emery–Dreifuss	AD	LMNA	2	0	0	2	5	4	9	2	3
Exostoses, multiple	AD	EXT1	3	0	0	3	6	6	12	3	3
FAP	AD	APC	0	4	0	4	9	8	17	2	2
FSHD	AD	FRG1	4	0	0	4	13	8	16	4	6
Glanzmann's thrombasthenia	AR		0	1	0	1	2	2	2	1	0
Gorlin syndrome	AD	FGFR2	4	1	0	5	6	5	9	3	3
HNPCC2	AD	MLH1	1	0	0	1	1	1	2	1	1
Holt–Oram syndrome	AD	TBX5	0	1	0	1	3	3	3	1	2

Table 6.8 (*Continued*) Outcome of PGD for *de novo* mutation causing different genetic disorders with different origin

Disease	*Inheritance*	*Gene*	*De novo Mutations Origin*			*Number of Patients had PGD*	*Cycle*	*ET*	*Number of Embryos*	*Pregnant*	*Birth*
Hypertrophic cardiomyopathy	AD	TNNI3	1	0	0	1	2	1	2	0	0
Kallmann syndrome	AD	FGFR1	0	1	0	1	1	1	2	1	1
Li–Fraumeni syndrome	AD	TP53	1	0	0	1	1	0	0	0	0
Loyes–Dietz syndrome	AD	TGFBR2	0	1	0	1	2	2	4	2	1
Marfan	AD	FBN1	4	5	0	9	20	17	31	9	6
MEN 1	AD	MEN1	1	0	0	1	2	2	4	1	1
MEN2b	AD	RET	1	0	0	1	2	2	4	1	2
Metaphyseal dysplasia	AD	COL10A1	1	0	0	1	1	1	2	1	1
Myotonia congenita	AD	CLCN1	1	0	0	1	1	2	4	1	1
NF1	AD	NF1	8	12	1	21	37	33	57	14	17
NF2 (mosaic)	AD	NF2	1	1	0	2	3	3	5	3	5
Noonan's syndrome	AD	PTPN	2	0	0	2	4	2	3	2	2
OPA1	AD	OPA1	1	0	0	1	1	2	0	0	0
Osteogenesis imperfecta I	AD	COL1A1 COL1A2	6	5	0	11	26	17	30	7	8
Peutz–Jeghers syndrome	AD	STK11	0	1	0	1	2	2	3	2	1
Pfeiffer syndrome	AD	FGFR1	0	1	0	1	1	1	2	1	1
PKD1	AD	PKD1	3	3	0	6	14	12	19	5	5
Retinoblastoma	AD	RB1	4	2	1	7	12	11	16	2	2
SCA6	AD	CACNA1A	0	1	0	1	2	1	2	0	0
Sotos syndrome	AD	NSD1	0	1	0	1	1	1	1	1	1
Stickler syndrome	AD	COL2A1	0	1	0	1	1	1	3	0	0
Treacher–Collins	AD	TCOF1	1	1	0	2	2	2	4	2	2
Torsion dystonia 1 (DYT1)	AD	TOR1A	4	1	0	5	9	8	14	6	6
TSC1	AD	TSC1	2	3	0	5	10	9	17	4	5
TSC2	AD	TSC2	0	1	0	1	2	2	4	0	0
Ulnar–mammary syndrome	AD	TBX3	0	1	0	1	3	3	4	1	2
VHl	AD	VHL	2	0	0	2	4	4	5	3	3
Subtotal (AD-48)			69	57	8	134	251	214	363	106	112
Fanconi anemia A	AR	FANCA	1	0	0	1	2	2	2	1	1
Fanconi anemia I	AR	FANCI	0	0	1	1	2	2	3	0	0
Cystic fibrosis	AR	CFTR	0	0	1	1	1	1	2	1	2
SMA	AR	SMN1	1	0	0	1	1	1	2	1	1

(Continued)

Table 6.8 *(Continued)* Outcome of PGD for *de novo* mutation causing different genetic disorders with different origin

Disease	*Inheritance*	*Gene*	*De novo Mutations Origin*			*Number of Patients had PGD*	*Cycle*	*ET*	*Number of Embryos*	*Pregnant*	*Birth*
Ataxia–telangiectasia	AR	ATM	1	0	0	1	3	3	3	2	1
Thrombasthenia of Glanzmann and Naegeli	AR	ITGA2B	0	1	0	1	2	2	4	1	0
Subtotal (6-AR)			3	1	2	6	11	11	16	6	5
Atypical Rett syndrome (epileptic encephalopathy)	XL	CDKL5	0	0	1	1	1	1	2	1	1
Chronic granulomatosis	XL	CYBB	0	1	0	1	4	4	6	1	0
DMD	XL	DMD	0	0	1	1	1	1	2	1	1
Incontinentia pigmenti	XL	IKBKG	0	5	0	5	8	5	9	3	4
Pelizeaus–Merzbacher	XL	PLP1	0	1	0	1	1	1	1	1	1
Wiskott–Aldrich syndrome	XL	WAS	0	0	1	1	2	2	4	0	0
Rett syndrome	XL	MECP2	0	0	2	2	2	1	1	0	0
Subtotal (7-XL)			0	7	5	12	17	14	24	7	7
			PAT	MAT	CHILD						
Subtotal (AD-48)			69	57	8	134	251	214	363	106	112
Subtotal (6-AR)			3	1	2	6	11	11	16	6	5
Subtotal (7-XL)			0	7	5	12	17	14	24	7	7
TOTAL			72	65	15	152	279	239	403	119	124

8 detected for the first time only in the affected children. Three DNM of autosomal recessive inheritance were of paternal origin, including cystic fibrosis (CFTR), spinal muscular atrophy (SMA), and Fanconi anemia (FA), one of maternal (thrombasthenia of Glansmann and Naegeli), and two detected in the affected child (FA and CFTR). Of 12 PGD for X-linked DNM, seven were of maternal origin (including PGD for chronic granulomatosis, Pelizeaus–Menzbacher, and five cases of incontinentia pigmenti), and five were detected in the affected children (Wiskott–Aldrich syndrome, chronic granulomatosis, atypical Rett syndrome, and two cases of Rett syndrome).

Accordingly, PGD strategies for *de novo* mutations depend on their origin, and thus the DNA analysis of the parents and affected children prior to PGD is required for verification of the mutation and polymorphic markers through single sperm testing and PB analysis, providing the normal and mutant haplotypes to trace the mutation. In case of the paternal origin of the mutation, it is first confirmed on the paternal DNA from blood and total sperm, and then by single sperm typing to determine the proportion of sperm with DNM and relevant normal and mutant haplotypes. It is also useful to test the relevant linked markers for the partner to exclude misdiagnosis caused by possible shared maternal and paternal markers. In cases of the maternal origin of the mutation, PB testing is the method of choice to provide the normal and mutant maternal haplotypes. Again to exclude misdiagnosis caused by possible shared paternal and maternal markers, the relevant paternal haplotypes are established through a single sperm typing. Accordingly, if the mutation was first detected in children, both the maternal and paternal haplotypes are established as above. The examples of PGD for *de novo* mutations are presented in Figures 6.55–6.57.

It is of interest that some of the embryos may appear unaffected, despite determining the mutant haplotype, which, however, misses the mutant gene. This phenomenon was not known previously, and the decision on the transfer of such embryos is controversial. According to our preliminary experience, these embryos may be considered for transfer with the parents' consent if no other unaffected embryos are available. With the accumulation of data on the outcome of such embryo transfers, parents may be provided information on the percentages of risk.

The other important phenomenon detected in PGD for *de novo* mutation is gonadal mosaicism, which has been detected as being of both maternal and paternal origin. Although the strategies may differ depending on the type of DNM inheritance, the general approach involves the identification of DNM origin and the search for a possible gonadal mosaicism and relevant parental haplotypes. Despite the complexity, the overall clinical outcome of PGD for DNM showed as high as 86% success rate for identifying unaffected embryos for transfer (239 of 279 initiated cycles), with the average 1.7 embryos per transfer (403 embryos transferred in 239 cycles) resulting in 50% pregnancy rate (119 clinical pregnancies) and the birth of 124 unaffected children.

The world's most extensive PGD experience with this group of conditions shows that despite the complexity of PGD for *de novo* mutations, no misdiagnoses were observed, suggesting that the above strategies may be applied in the clinical practice of PGD with extremely high accuracy, without the traditional requirement of family data, which are not always available.

PGD for common disorders with genetic predisposition

Cancer predisposition

Traditionally, cancer predisposition has not been considered an indication for prenatal diagnosis, as this might lead to a pregnancy termination, something that can hardly be justified on the basis of genetic predisposition alone. However, the possibility of choosing embryos for transfer free from the genetic predisposition would obviate the need to consider pregnancy termination, as only potentially normal pregnancies would be established. PGD for such conditions appears to be acceptable on ethical grounds because only a limited number of the embryos available from hyperstimulation are selected for transfer.

The first PGD for inherited cancer predisposition was performed in a couple carrying p53 tumor-suppressor gene mutations, which are known to determine a strong predisposition for the majority of cancers.[36] The couple had the paternally derived missense mutation due to a transversion of a G to an A in exon 5 of the p53 tumor-suppressor gene (Figure 6.58). The carrier was a 38-year-old proband with Li–Fraumeni syndrome (LFS), diagnosed with rhabdomyosarcoma of the right shoulder at the age of 2 years followed by right upper extremity amputation. At the age of 31, he was also diagnosed with a high-grade leiomyosarcoma of the bladder and underwent a radical cystoprostatectomy. His mother was diagnosed with leiomyosarcoma at the age of 37.

PGD was performed by blastomere biopsy and multiplex nested PCR analysis with simultaneous testing for the p53 tumor-suppressor gene mutation and linked polymorphic markers, allowing the preselection and transfer back to the patient of only mutation-free embryos. This resulted in a singleton pregnancy and the birth of a mutation-free child with no risk of developing the disease.

PGD has also been applied for other cancers, including familial adenomatous polyposis coli (FAP) (Figure 6.59), von Hippel–Lindau syndrome (Figure 6.60), retinoblastoma, breast cancer (Figure 6.61), neurofibromatosis type I and II (Figures 6.62 and 6.63), and hSNF5 (Figure 6.26).[37] Overall, 315 PGD cycles have been performed for 159 couples, resulting in the preselection and transfer of 448 mutation-free embryos, which to date have yielded 112 unaffected clinical pregnancies and 120 births of healthy children (Table 6.9). Despite the controversy of PGD use for late-onset disorders, the data demonstrate the usefulness of this approach as the only acceptable option for at-risk couples to avoid the birth of children with an inherited predisposition to cancer and instead have a healthy child.

Predisposition to inherited cardiac disorders

Inherited cardiac diseases may be included with those conditions that have no current prospect of effective treatment, and that may manifest despite pre-symptomatic diagnosis and follow-up. For these PGD may provide the only possibility for at-risk couples to reproduce.

The first case of PGD for inherited cardiac disease was described for a couple at risk for producing offspring with Holt–Oram syndrome (HOS), which is an autosomal dominant condition determined by mutation in the TBX5 gene.[38] HOS is characterized by atrial septal defect and cardiac conduction disease, together with upper extremity malformations, although these clinical manifestations may be extremely variable, not usually being presented at birth, or presented with a sinus bradycardia as the only clinical sign, which also might go unnoticed. The PGD case for HOS is presented in Figure 6.64, which was performed together with 24-chromosome aneuploidy testing because of the advanced reproductive age of the maternal partner.

As in PGD for other common disorders, the fact that inherited cardiac disorders may not be realized even during a lifetime makes the application of PGD controversial, perhaps explaining the limited application of PGD for inherited cardiac diseases at the present time. The majority of inherited cardiac disorders are dominant, for which no cure may be administered because their first

Table 6.9 PGD for cancer predisposition

Disease	*Number of Patients*	*Number of Cycles*	*Number of Transfers*	*Number of Embryos Transferred*	*Pregnancy*	*Birth*
AT	1	3	2	3	1	1
BCNS (GORLIN)	5	6	5	9	3	3
Brain tumor	1	1	1	1	0	0
BRCA 1	25	40	31	54	18	27
BRCA 2	14	36	23	39	10	13
FANC	20	62	37	60	11	9(2)*
FAP	10	23	21	38	5	3
HNPCC 1	1	2	2	4	2	2
HNPCC 2	3	7	7	14	3	4
LFS	4	6	5	9	2	2
MEN1	4	12	11	18	4	2(2)*
MEN2	2	3	3	5	2	2(1)*
NF1	32	56	52	88	22	21(3)*
NF2	4	7	7	15	5	7
RB1	11	19	17	32	8	7
TSC1	13	19	18	37	11	15
TSC2	3	5	5	9	0	0
VHL	6	8	7	13	5	6
TOTAL	159	315 (1.98)	254	448 (1.76)	112 (44%)	120(8)* (50%)

*Ongoing pregnancy with a heartbeat

and only clinical occurrence may be premature or sudden death. One of such conditions is familial hypertrophic cardiomyopathy (HCM), which clinically manifests at various ages, with no symptoms observed for years until provoked by one or more of a number of factors, such as excessive exercise. Various conditions leading to HCM have been reported, two of which are HCM4 and HCM7. HCM4 is caused by mutation in the gene *MYBPC3* located on chromosome 11 (11p11.2), which encodes the cardiac isoform of myosin-binding protein C, exclusively in heart muscle. HCM7 is caused by a mutation in the *TNNI3* gene located on chromosome 19 (19q13.4), leading to an asymmetric ventricular hypertrophy and defect in the interventricular septum, with high risk of cardiac failure and sudden death.

The other condition, for which PGD is strongly indicated, is dilated cardiomyopathy (CMD), which is an autosomal dominant disease caused by different mutations in the *LMNA* gene located on chromosome 1 (1q21.2). This cardiac disease is characterized by ventricular dilation and impaired systolic function, resulting in heart failure and arrhythmia, which causes premature or sudden death. While the large phenotypic variability of patients may be determined by different mutations in the *LMNA* gene, differences from one family to another may be observed within the same mutation, with possible involvement of skeletal muscles that leads to muscle weakening similar to that in Emery–Dreifuss muscular dystrophy (EMD), an X-linked disease also characterized by cardiomyopathy, although presenting within the first year after birth.

Table 6.10 presents our cumulative experience of PGD for 19 cycles of inherited cardiac disorders that resulted in the birth of 7 healthy children free of the above predisposing gene mutations.[39] These PGD cycles were performed for couples at risk for producing an affected progeny with inherited cardiac disease, including 9 cycles for CMD, 1 for CMH1 (Figure 6.65), 3 for CMH4, 1 for CMH7, 3 for cardioencephalomyopathy, and 2 for EDMD. The couples at risk for producing a progeny with CMD requested PGD prospectively, with no previous pregnancies attempted because of one of the partners being a carrier of the mutation predisposing to CMD.

Our results show that PGD is a realistic option for couples at risk for producing offspring with an inherited predisposition for cardiac disease. Inheritance of such susceptibility factors places the individual at risk of developing serious cardiac disease, clinically manifested from as early as the first year of life, such as in cardioencephalopathy, to late in life, with the only clinical realization being premature or sudden death, as in CMD and CMH.

Table 6.10 PGD for inherited cardiac diseases

Disease	*Gene (Mutation)*	*Patient/ Cycle*	*Embryos*				*Number of Transfers*	*Number of Embryos Transferred*	*Pregnancy*	*Birth*
			Total Received/ Amplified	Normal/ Carrier	Abnormal*	Inconclusive				
Cardioencephalomyopathy (AR)	SCO2 *(R262delCA; E140K)*	1 / 3	33 / 32	16	13	3	3	7	2	1
Cardiomyopathy dilated; CMD1 (AD)	LMNA *(K270K)*	1 / 4	51 / 47	20	26	1	4	9	2	3
	LMNA *(R335T)*	1 / 1	11 / 11	7	2	2	1	2	1	1
	LMNA *(R189P)*	1 / 1	2 / 2	1	1	0	1	1	0	0
	LMNA *(T528K)*	1 / 3	44 / 34	9	19	6	2	3	1	0
Cardiomyopathy familial, hypertrophic 4; CMH4 (AD)	MYBPC3 *(D1076fs)*	1 / 1	7 / 6	3	3	0	1	2	0	0
	MYBPC3 *(IVS11-10 C-A)*	1 / 2	10 / 8	1	6	1	0	0	0	0
Cardiomyopathy, familial, hypertrophic, 1; CMH1 (AD)	MYH7 *(E1142K/N)*	1 / 1	3 / 3	1	2	0	1	1	1	0
Cardiomyopathy familial,hypertrophic, 7; CMH7 (AD)	TNNI3 *(A157V)*	1 / 1	11 / 11	3	8	0	1	2	0	0
Emery–Dreifuss muscular dystrophy 1, X-linked	EMD	1 / 2	31 / 31	17	14	0	2	5	3	2
TOTAL		10 / 19	193 / 185 (96%)	78	94	13	16 (84%)	32 (1.68)	10 (52.6%)	7 (37%)

*Including aneuploidies

Among the conditions in the family history of the couples at risk that may indicate a possible need for PGD are heart attack and sudden death at a young age and family members with pacemakers or internal cardiac defibrillators, and who have arrhythmia or have undergone heart surgery. The chances that the offspring of these parents will develop the same heart disease will differ depending on the mode of inheritance, but penetrance is difficult to predict because many inherited cardiac conditions are difficult to diagnose, as they develop with age and may be induced by certain medications or activities, such as excessive exercise, which may lead to cardiac arrest or sudden death. Such possibilities justify parents requesting PGD. In fact, in some cases a common, apparently "milder" disease-susceptibility gene may contribute to premature death, major disability, or hardship in a family. However, only the personal experience may alter a family's perception of severity of the condition as the basis for their decision to undertake PGD. Many couples already going through IVF for fertility treatment may have questions about the implications of genetic susceptibility factors for offspring, the option to test embryos, and the appropriateness of using PGD in testing for susceptibility to inherited cardiac disease.

Because the symptoms of inherited cardiac disease may be easily overlooked, as in the cases above, family history may be the only reason to test for the presence of predisposing gene mutations and to consider the need for PGD, which may come to be a life-saving procedure for individuals at risk. With the future identification of the genes predisposing to inherited cardiac disease, PGD might appear as a useful tool for couples at risk for producing offspring with inherited cardiac diseases with high probability of premature or sudden death.

Alzheimer disease and dimentia

One of the first experiences of PGD for late-onset disorders was PGD for genetic predisposition to one form of Alzheimer disease (AD)[40] caused by an autosomal dominant familial predisposition to the presenile form of dementia and determined by a nearly completely penetrant autosomal dominant mutation in the amyloid precursor protein gene (*APP*), for which no treatment is available despite a possible predictive diagnosis. A 30-year-old woman had no signs of AD, but was a carrier of V717L mutation, resulting from G to C substitution in exon 17 of the *APP* gene (Figure 6.66). Predictive testing in the patient was performed because of the early onset of AD in her sister, who also carried this mutation and developed symptoms of AD at the age of 38. At the time of publication, this sister was still alive, but her cognitive problems had progressed to the point that she was placed in an assisted living facility (Figure 6.67). Her father had died at the age of 42 and also had a history of psychological difficulties and marked memory problems. The V717L mutation was also detected in one of her brothers, who had experienced mild short-term memory problems as early as age 35, with a moderate decline in memory, new learning, and sequential tracking over the next 2–3 years. The other family members, including one brother and two sisters, were asymptomatic, although predictive testing was performed only in the sisters, who appeared to be free from the *APP* gene mutation.

PGD was performed by DNA analysis of the PB1 and PB2 (Figure 6.66). Based on both mutation and the linked marker analysis, unaffected embryos resulting from mutation-free oocytes were preselected for transfer back to the patient, resulting in a singleton clinical pregnancy and the birth of an unaffected mutation-free child in the first PGD cycle and healthy twins in the second PGD cycle (Figure 6.67). Our present experience of PGD for AD and other dementias is presented in Table 6.11. The other example of PGD for AD is presented in Figure 6.68.

Therefore, PGD provides a non-traditional option for patients who may wish to avoid the transmission of the mutant gene predisposing to late-onset disorders in their potential children. Because such diseases that present beyond early childhood and even later may not be expressed in 100% of the cases, the application of PGD for this group of disorders is still controversial. However, for diseases with no current prospect for treatment, manifesting despite presymptomatic diagnosis and follow-up, PGD may be offered as the only relief for at-risk couples.

Inherited neurological diseases

The other large group of mental illness included 312 PGD cycles for mental retardation, with over 90% represented by fragile-X syndrome (Table 6.12), mentioned above in the section on X-linked disorders and presented in Figure 6.20. The remaining 15 cycles were 7 for Alport syndrome, 6 for Smith–Lemi–Opitz syndrome, and 2 for Rett and Sotos syndromes. PGD resulted in birth of unaffected children in all but one couple.

As seen from Table 6.13, the neuromuscular disorders were one of the major PGD indications, with a total of 376 PGD cycles performed, including 240 cycles for myopathies (muscular dystrophies, metabolic myopathies, and muscle channelopathy), 73 cycles for motor neuron diseases, and 63 cycles for hereditary neuropathies, including Charcot–Marie–Tooth disease (CMT) axonal type 2A2 (CMT2A2), CMT2B, CMT2E, CMT1A, CMT1, and CMTX1, hereditary sensory and autonomic neuropathy Type III (HSAN3), hereditary neuropathic amyloidosis I, and prion diseases, such as Gerstmann–Sträussler–Scheinker syndrome (Figure 6.69).

As a special group, muscular dystrophies are the third most frequent indications for PGD. As summarized in Table 6.13, over 200 PGD cycles were performed for this indication, including Duchenne and Becker type (58 cycles), Emery–Dreifuss (15 cycles), myotonic dystrophy types 1 and 2 (110 cycles), facioscapulohumeral (32 cycles),

Table 6.11 PGD for Alzheimer disease and dementia

Disease	*Gene*	*Number of Patients*	*Number of Cycles*	*Number of Transfers*	*Number of Embryos Transferred*	*Pregnancy*	*Birth*
Microtubule-associated protein TAU; MAPT	MAPT	1	2	2	4	0	0
Early-onset familial Alzheimer disease	PSEN1 PSEN2	2	4	3	6	3	5
Gerstmann–Sträussler disease; GSD	PRNP	1	1	1	2	1	2
TOTAL		4	7	6	12	4	7

*Ongoing pregnancy with a heartbeat

Table 6.12 PGD for mental retardation

Disease	*Gene*	*Number of Patients*	*Number of Cycles*	*Number of Transfers*	*Number of Embryos Transferred*	*Pregnancy*	*Birth*
Alport syndrome, X-linked; ATS	AMMECR1	3	7	7	11	3	3
Smith–Lemli–Opitz syndrome; SLOS	DHCR7	4	6	6	12	3	3 (1)*
Fragile X site mental retardation 1	FMR1	151	297	218	370	102	94 (7)*
Rett syndrome; RTT	MECP2	1	1	1	1	0	0
Sotos syndrome	NSD1	1	1	1	1	1	1
TOTAL		160	312	233 (74.6%)	395 (1.7)	109 (46.7%)	101 (43.3%)

*Ongoing pregnancy with a heartbeat

Table 6.13 PGD for neuromuscular diseases

	Disease	*Gene*	*Number of Patients*	*Number of Cycles*	*Number of Transfers*	*Number of Embryos Transferred*	*Pregnancy*	*Birth*
MYOPATHIES	***Muscular dystrophies***							
	Muscular dystrophy, Duchenne type; BMD & Becker type; BMD	DMD	33	58	49	96	28(4)*	24
	Emery–Dreifuss muscular dystrophy, autosomal recessive; EDMD3	LNMA	5	13	11	20	6	6
	Emery–Dreifuss muscular dystrophy, X-linked; EDMD	EMD	1	2	2	3	1	1
	Myotonic dystrophy 1; DM1	DMPK	65	109	91	144	29(3)*	24
	Myotonic dystrophy 2; DM2	CNBP	1	1	1	2	1	1
	Facioscapulohumeral muscular dystrophy 1a; FSHMD1a	FRG1	12	32	25	48	13	13
	Muscular dystrophy–dystroglycanopathy	FKTN	1	1	1	2	1	1
	Muscular dystrophy, congenital merosin-deficient, 1a; MDC1a	LAMA2	1	1	1	2	0	0

(Continued)

Table 6.13 (*Continued*) PGD for neuromuscular diseases

	Disease	*Gene*	*Number of Patients*	*Number of Cycles*	*Number of Transfers*	*Number of Embryos Transferred*	*Pregnancy*	*Birth*
	Nemaline myopathy 2; NEM2	NEB	1	1	1	2	(1)*	0
	Myopathy, myofibrillar, 1; MFM1	DES	1	1	1	1	1	1
	Metabolic myopathies							
	Glycogen storage disease II	GAA	4	4	3	7	1	1
	Carnitine palmitoyltransferase II deficiency, lethal neonatal	CPT2	1	1	1	1	1	1
	Acyl-CoA dehydrogenase, very long-chain	ACADVL	5	5	5	10	1	1
	Long-chain 3-hydroxyacyl-CoA dehydrogenase deficiency	HADHA	2	4	3	5	3	5
	Acyl-CoA dehydrogenase, medium-chain, deficiency	ACADM	1	5	5	12	1	1
	Leigh syndrome; LS	SURF1	1	1	1	2	0	0
	Muscle channelopathy							
	Myotonia congenita, autosomal dominant	CLCN1	1	1	1	2	1	1
SUBTOTAL		*17*	*136*	*240*	*202*	*359*	*89 (8)**	*80*
MOTOR NEURON DISEASES	Kennedy spinal and bulbar muscular atrophy	AR	1	2	2	2	1	0
	Spinal muscular atrophy, type I; SMA1	SMN1	47	62	52	91	34(2)*	43
	Spinal muscular atrophy, distal, autosomal recessive	IGHMBP2	2	3	2	4	1	2
	Spastic paraplegia 4, autosomal dominant; SPG4	SPAST	1	4	2	4	1	2
	Amyotrophic lateral sclerosis 4; ALS4	SETX	1	1	1	2	1	1
	Amyotrophic lateral sclerosis 1; ALS1	SOD1	1	1	1	1	1	0
SUBTOTAL		*6*	*53*	*73*	*60*	*104*	*39*	*48*
HEREDITARY NEUROPATHY	Charcot–Marie–Tooth disease, axonal, type 2A2; CMT2A2	MFN2	2	6	3	4	1(1)*	0
	Charcot–Marie–Tooth disease, axonal, type 2B; CMT2B	RAB7A	1	1	1	2	1	2
	Charcot–Marie–Tooth disease, axonal, type 2E	NEFL	1	4	4	7	1	1
	Charcot–Marie–Tooth disease, demyelinating, type 1A; CMT1A	PMP22	16	26	22	30	10	10

Table 6.13 (*Continued*) PGD for neuromuscular diseases

Disease	Gene	Number of Patients	Number of Cycles	Number of Transfers	Number of Embryos Transferred	Pregnancy	Birth
Charcot–Marie–Tooth disease, demyelinating, type 1B; CMT1B	MPZ	2	5	2	5	0	0
Charcot–Marie–Tooth disease, X-linked, 1; CMTX1	GJB1	4	6	6	12	4	5
Neuropathy, hereditary sensory and autonomic, type III; HSAN3	IKBKAP	5	13	11	21	5	7
Amyloidosis I, hereditary neuropathic	TTR	1	2	1	1	0	0
SUBTOTAL	*8*	*32*	*63*	*50*	*82*	*22(1)**	*25*
TOTAL	31	221	376	312 (83%)	545 (1.74)	150(10)* (48.1%)	153 (48.8%)

*Ongoing pregnancy with a heartbeat

Table 6.14 PGD for hereditary ataxias

Disease	*Gene*	*Number of Patients*	*Number of Cycles*	*Number of Transfers*	*Number of Embryos Transferred*	*Pregnancy*	*Birth*
Spinocerebellar ataxia 1; SCA1	ATXN1	1	2	2	4	1	1
Spinocerebellar ataxia 2; SCA2	ATXN2	6	13	13	26	5	7
Machado–Joseph disease; MJD	ATXN3	1	3	2	3	2	3
Spinocerebellar ataxia 6; SCA6	CACNA1A	1	2	1	1	0	0
Spinocerebellar ataxia 7; SCA7	ATXN7	2	3	3	7	2	1
Spinocerebellar ataxia, autosomal recessive 1	SETX	1	1	1	1	1	1
Joubert syndrome 3; JBTS3 Joubert syndrome 6; JBTS6	AHI1 TMEM67	2	2	1	2	0	0
TOTAL		14	26	23	44	11	13

*Ongoing pregnancy with a heartbeat

and muscular dystrophy dystroglycanopathy and congenital merosin deficient (2 cycles). One of the most frequent PGD indications was myotonic dystrophy type 1, for which a total of 109 cycles were performed from 65 couples at risk, with embryos transferred in 91 cycles, resulting in 29 unaffected pregnancies and the birth of 24 healthy children, with 3 pregnancies still ongoing. Overall, approximately 2 cycles for each couple at risk for producing offspring with muscular dystrophies were performed (219 cycles for 121 couples), with unaffected embryos available for transfer in 183 (83.6%) cycles. Despite transferring 1.75 embryos per transfer on average (320 unaffected embryos in 183 cycles), 44% pregnancy rate was observed (81 pregnancies), with 70 unaffected children born as a result of the procedure, with 8 pregnancies still ongoing. As shown in Figure 6.48, in some cases muscular dystrophy was an additional indication to other genetic disorders, and 24-chromosome aneuploidy testing and HLA typing were also performed.

Finally, Table 6.14 presents our experience of PGD for hereditary ataxias, which was highly efficient, resulting in healthy unaffected children born to 11 of 14 patients. A total of 44 unaffected embryos were detected for transfer in 23 of 26 PGD cycles performed for these patients, resulting in 11 clinical pregnancies and 13 children born.

Congenital malformations

Congenital malformations are highly prevalent (29.3/1000 live births) and are usually sporadic. However, with the progress of the human genome project, an increasing number of inherited forms are being described, which, therefore, may be avoided through PGD. For example, sonic hedgehog (*SHH*) gene mutation, for which the first PGD was performed,[41] causes failure of the cerebral hemispheres to separate into distinct left and right halves and leads to holoprosencephaly (HPE), which is one of the most common developmental anomalies of forebrain and midface. Although the majority of HPE are sporadic, familial cases are not rare, with clear autosomal dominant inheritance.

Wide intrafamilial clinical variability of HPE, from alobar HPE and cyclopia to cleft lip and palate, microcephaly, ocular hypertelorism, and even normal phenotype, suggests the interaction of the *SHH* gene with other genes expressed during craniofacial development and the possible involvement of environmental factors. This may explain the fact that almost one-third of carriers of *SHH* mutations may be clinically unaffected. Therefore, even in familial cases, the detection of *SHH* mutations in prenatal diagnosis might not justify pregnancy termination, making PGD a more attractive option for couples at risk for producing progeny with HPE, as demonstrated by the first PGD for this mutation mentioned.[23]

A couple presented for PGD because of their previous two children, who had the clinical signs of HPE (Figure 6.45). One of them, a female, with severe HPE and cleft lip and palate, died shortly after birth. Both the child and the parents were chromosomally normal, but DNA analysis of the child's autopsy material demonstrated the presence of *SHH* nonsense mutation due to GAG>TAG sequence change leading to premature termination of the protein at position 256 (Glu256stop). The same mutation was found in their 5-year-old son, who was born after a full-term normal pregnancy. This child had less severe facial dysmorphisms, which included microcephaly, Rathke's pouch cyst, single central incisor and choanal stenosis. There was also clinodactyly of the fifth fingers and incurved fourth toes bilaterally. The child's growth was slow during the first 2 years, but after that time he maintained reasonably good growth.

PGD was performed by blastomere biopsy and multiplex nested PCR analysis, involving specific mutation testing simultaneously with linked marker analysis (Figure 6.70). Of nine tested embryos four embryos were free of the mutant gene, two of which were transferred back to the patient, resulting in a singleton pregnancy and the birth of a healthy child following confirmation of the mutation-free status by amniocentesis. A similar approach was used for PGD of Crouzon syndrome (9 cycles) (Figure 6.27) and Currarino triad, representing inherited congenital malformations for which PGD may be an attractive approach to ensure that at-risk couples can have an unaffected offspring (Table 6.15). Nine PGD cycles were performed for four couples with Crouzon syndrome, resulting in transfer of 16 embryos in 8 cycles, yielding four unaffected pregnancies and birth of three healthy children. Only one cycle was performed for Currarino syndrome, which resulted in the birth of an unaffected child.[41] The data suggest that PGD for familial cases of congenital malformations is clinically useful. Because of the high prevalence of congenital anomalies, the approach may have practical implications for at-risk couples as a preventive measure to be employed in genetic practice.

In addition to the above congenital disorders PGD was performed for a large group of heterogeneous bone disorders (109 clinical cycles) (Table 6.16); ectodermal disorders 75 cycles (Table 6.17); hereditary nephrotic syndromes, 53 cycles (Table 6.18); inherited ophthalmic disorders, 57 cycles (Table 6.19); and hereditary hearing loss, 15 cycles (Table 6.20).

Table 6.15 PGD for congenital malformations

Disease	*Number of Patients*	*Number of Cycles*	*Number of Transfers*	*Number of Embryos Transferred*	*Pregnancy*	*Birth*
Currarino syndrome	1	1	1	2	1	1
Sonic hedgehog; SHH	1	2	2	3	1	1
Craniofacial dysostosis, type I; (CFD1); (Crouzon)	4	9	8	16	4	3
Treacher Collins–Franceschetti syndrome	4	5	5	10	5	6(1)*
Noonan syndrome	3	5	1	2	1	2
Van der Woude syndrome; VWS	1	1	1	1	1	1
Blepharophimosis, ptosis, and epicanthus inversus; BPES	2	4	4	4	2	2
Cohen syndrome; COH1	1	1	1	2	1	2
Donnai–Barrow syndrome	1	1	0	0	0	0
Hydrocephalus, X-linked; L1CAM	7	11	10	25	3	4
TOTAL	25	40	33	65	19	22(1)*

*Ongoing pregnancy with a heartbeat

Table 6.16 PGD for congenital bone disorders

Disease	*Gene*	*Number of Patients*	*Number of Cycles*	*Number of Transfers*	*Number of Embryos Transferred*	*Pregnancy*	*Birth*
Hypophosphatasia, infantile	ALPL	5	5	4	7	3	4
Hyalinosis, infantile systemic	ANTXR2	1	1	1	2	1	1
Chondrodysplasia punctata 1, X-linked recessive; CDPX1	ARSE	1	2	2	3	0	0
Metaphyseal chondrodysplasia, schmid type; MCDS	COL10A1	1	1	1	2	1	1
Stickler syndrome, type I; STL1	Col11A1 Col2A1	3	8	6	17	0	0
Osteogenesis imperfecta congenita; OIC	COL1A1 PPIB	17	44	35	59	12	13(2)*
Ehlers–Danlos syndrome, type IV, autosomal dominant	COL3A1 COL5A1 PLOD1	4	5	4	6	4	5
Epiphyseal dysplasia, multiple, 1; EDM1	COMP	1	2	1	3	0	0
Exostoses, multiple, type I	EXT1	8	11	11	21	6	5
Pfeiffer syndrome	FGFR1	1	1	1	2	1	1
Kallman syndrome	FGFR1	1	1	1	2	1	1
Achondroplasia; ACH	FGFR3	3	4	4	5	3	3
Geroderma osteodysplasticum; GO	GORAB	1	2	2	4	1	3
Nail–patella syndrome; NPS	LMX1B	2	3	2	3	0	0
Symphalangism, proximal; SYM1	NOG	1	3	3	7	2	2
Brachydactyly, type B1; BDB1	ROR2	1	3	2	4	2	2
Growth retardation	SHOX	2	2	1	2	1	2
Holt–Oram syndrome	TBX5	2	4	4	5	1	2
Osteopetrosis, autosomal recessive	TCIRG1	5	5	4	9	2	2
Arthrogryposis, distal, type 2B; DA2B	TNNT3	1	2	2	3	2	2
TOTAL		61	109	91 (83.4%)	166 (1.82)	43 (47.2%)	49 (2)* (53.8%)

*Ongoing pregnancy with a heartbeat

Of special interest is PGD for severe metabolic disorders, including mucopolysaccaridoses and lysosomal storage diseases, some of which are endemic in certain ethnic groups. As seen from Table 6.21, 94 such PGD cycles were performed, the majority being Gaucher (23 cycles), Tay–Sachs (21 cycles), Hunter (15 cycles), and Fabry (10 cycles) diseases, which resulted in the birth of 41 unaffected children. Overall, our experience shows that, with few exceptions, the majority of PGD cycles resulted in the transfer of unaffected embryos and birth of healthy children with no misdiagnosis in any of these cases.

Hematologic diseases

This is the largest group of conditions for which PGD was performed, including 663 cycles for 371 couples at risk, with the most widespread being thalassemias and sickle cell disease, followed by coagulopathies, such as hemophilia, and aplastic anemias (Table 6.22).

Hemoglobinopathies

Hemoglobinopathies are a major indication for PGD. Available experience includes PGD for sickle-cell disease and alpha- and beta-thalassemias, highly prevalent in the Eastern Mediterranean and Southeast Asia. Initially, PGD was offered to those at-risk couples who had undergone prenatal diagnosis but had to terminate the pregnancy with the affected fetus in repeated attempts.[30] PGD then became a primary option for patients with infertility problems, and for those who could not accept the risk for a negative prenatal diagnosis and termination of pregnancy. PGD is presently available as well for

Table 6.17 PGD for ectodermal disorders

Disease	*Gene*	*Number of Patients*	*Number of Cycles*	*Number of Transfers*	*Number of Embryos Transferred*	*Pregnancy*	*Birth*
Darier–white disease; DAR	ATP2A2	1	1	1	1	1	1
Hoyeraal–Hreidarsson syndrome; HHS	DKC1	1	1	1	2	1	1
Ectodermal dysplasia, anhidrotic, X-linked	EDA	2	3	3	4	1	1
Ectodermal dysplasia, anhidrotic (EDAR)	EDAR	1	1	1	2	1	1
Ectodermal dysplasia, hypohidrotic, with immune deficiency	IKBKG	2	9	6	8	2	3
Incontinentia pigmenti; IP	IKBKG	9	20	13	24	2	3
Ichthyosis follicularis, atrichia, and photophobia syndrome	MBTPS2	2	2	2	5	2	1
Basal cell nevus syndrome; BCNS (Gorlin)	PTCH1	4	5	4	7	3	3
Ichthyosis, lamellar	TGM1	1	7	3	5	0	0
Dyskeratosis congenita, autosomal dominant, 1; DKCA1	TINF2	1	2	2	3	1	1
Oculocutaneous albinism, type I; OCA1; type 2; OCA 2	TYR	4	9	8	17	4	4
Epidermolysis bullosa dystrophica	COL7A1 LAMB3 PLEC1 LAMA3	11	15	11	19	5	6
TOTAL		39	75	55 (73.3%)	97 (1.37)	23 (41.8%)	25 (45.4%)

Table 6.18 PGD for hereditary nephrotic syndromes

Disease	*Gene*	*Number of Patients*	*Number of Cycles*	*Number of Transfers*	*Number of Embryos Transferred*	*Pregnancy*	*Birth*
Congenital nephrotic syndrome	LAMB2 NPHS	2	5	5	11	3	1
Polycystic kidney disease 1; PKD1; Polycystic kidney disease 2; PKD2	PKD1 PKD2	16	34	26	49	11	11(1)*
PKD1 + HLA	PKD1	1	1	1	2	1	1
Polycystic kidney disease, autosomal recessive; ARPKD	PKHD1	8	11	11	20	5	5
Nephrosis 1, congenital, Finnish type; NPHS1	NPHS1	1	2	2	4	1	0
TOTAL		28	53	45 (85%)	86 (1.9)	21 (46.4%)	18 (40%)

*Ongoing pregnancy with a heartbeat

couples objecting to any embryo biopsy procedures, and for whom preselection of unaffected embryos is done through identification of mutation-free oocytes prior to embryo formation. PGD is also presently used for affected patients and for couples with existing children with hemoglobinopathies who require HLA-compatible bone marrow transplantation.[42]

The results of PGD for hemoglobinopathies are presented in Table 6.22, representing the most extensive experience available in one center. At the present time,

Table 6.19 PGD for inherited ophthalmic disorders

Disease	*Gene*	*Number of Patients*	*Number of Cycles*	*Number of Transfers*	*Number of Embryos Transferred*	*Pregnancy*	*Birth*
Choroideremia; CHM	CHM	2	4	2	7	3	4
Stickler syndrome, type I; STL1	Col11A1 Col2A1	3	8	6	17	0	0
Norrie disease; NDP	NDP	3	6	4	10	0	0
Optic atrophy 1; OPA1	OPA1	2	4	4	8	0	0
Retinitis pigmentosa	RHO	2	3	1	2	1	0
Retinoschisis 1, X-linked, juvenile; RS1	RS1	1	2	1	2	1	1
Retinoblastoma; RB1	RB1	11	19	17	29	8	7
Microphthalmia, isolated 2; MCOP2	VSX2	2	2	1	1	1	1
Oculocutaneous albinism, type I; OCA1; type 2; OCA 2	TYR OCA2	4	9	8	17	4	4
TOTAL		30	57	46 (80.7%)	93 (2.0)	18 (39%)	17 (36.9%)

Table 6.20 PGD for hereditary hearing loss

Disease	*Gene*	*Number of Patients*	*Number of Cycles*	*Number of Transfers*	*Number of Embryos Transferred*	*Pregnancy*	*Birth*
Deafness, neurosensory, autosomal recessive 1; DFNB1	GJB2	6	10	9	18	4	4(1)*
Wolfram syndrome	WFS1	1	2	1	1	1	1
Waardenburg syndrome, type 2A; WS2A	MITF	2	3	3	3	1	1
TOTAL		9	15	13	22	6	6(1)*

*Ongoing pregnancy with a heartbeat

PGD for hemoglobinopathies is more than 15% of our overall experience of 2982 PGD cycles performed for single-gene disorders, and involves testing of over two dozen different HBB gene mutations. Of 475 clinical cycles performed, unaffected embryos for transfer were detected in 372 (78.3%) of them, resulting in 133 (30.8%) clinical pregnancies and the birth of 132 hemoglobinopathy-free children. As many as one-quarter of the PGD cycles were performed for IVS I-110 mutation, which is the most common thalassemia mutation in the Eastern Mediterranean region, and approximately one-fifth for sickle cell disease, prevalent in African Americans in the USA.

Of 146 PGD cycles performed together with HLA typing, 83 (57%) resulted in transfer of 130 unaffected HLA matched embryos, with the average number of transferred embryos being 1.57.[42] Over 90% of tested embryos were with conclusive results, of which one-quarter, as expected, were predicted to be abnormal. Approximately 15% of the embryos were HLA identical to the affected siblings and were transferred, resulting in unaffected HLA-compatible pregnancies and birth of healthy children as potential donors for their affected siblings.

With the current progress in treatment of hemoglobinopathies, PGD may have an increasing impact on the decision of well-treated patients to reproduce. In fact, the life expectancy of patients with hemoglobin disorders has been dramatically improved over the last 10 years through the success of radical treatment by stem cell transplantation, so PGD for hemoglobinopathies is already a practical option and available for a wider application in those communities where these genetic diseases are prevalent. It may be expected that a combined PGD and preimplantation HLA testing will in the future be more widely used for further improvements in radical therapy of hemoglobinopathies by stem cell transplantation.

Other hematologic conditions

Among other hematological disorders for which PGD was applied, hemophilia A is the most frequent. Overall, 62 PGD cycles were performed, resulting in the transfer of 99 unaffected embryos in 51 cycles, with over 50% pregnancy rate and the birth of 26 healthy children. The other coagulopathies were much rarer, including hemophilia B (4 cycles), thrombasthenia (2 cycles), and congenital thrombotic thrombocytopenic purpura and Wiskott–Aldrich syndrome (8 cycles). PGD for some with the latter two

Table 6.21 PGD for mucopolysaccharidoses and other lysosomal storage disorders

Disease	*Gene*	*Number of Patients*	*Number of Cycles*	*Number of Transfers*	*Number of Embryos Transferred*	*Pregnancy*	*Birth*
Cystinosis, nephropathic; CTNS	CTNS	1	1	1	1	0	0
Morquio syndrome, non-keratosulfate-excreting type	GALNS	1	4	4	12	2	2
Fabry disease	GLA	5	10	8	13	4	6
Gangliosidosis, generalized GM1, type I	GLB1	2	2	2	5	1	1
Gaucher disease, type I	GBA	17	23	21	39	12	10 (1)*
Gangliosidosis, GM2 Tay–Sachs disease; TSD	HEXA	12	21	20	41	10	9
Sandhoff disease	HEXB	2	4	3	6	2	2
Mucopolysaccharidosis type II (Hunter)	IDS	6	15	11	22	5	5
Hurler syndrome	IDUA	3	5	5	10	0	0
Wolman disease	LIPA	2	2	2	4	2	3
Congenital disorder of glycosylation, type Ia; CDG1A	PMM2	1	1	1	1	1	1
Ceroid lipofuscinosis, neuronal 2, late infantile; CLN2	TPP1	1	2	1	1	0	0
Niemann–Pick disease, type A	SMPD1	2	4	2	4	2	2
TOTAL		55	94	81 (86.1%)	159 (1.96)	41 (50.6%)	41 (50.6%) (1)*

*Ongoing pregnancy with a heartbeat

conditions was performed together with preimplantation HLA typing (Table 6.22).

Concomitant HLA typing was also performed for some of the hemolytic anemias (2 of 32 cycles), most of aplastic anemias, such as Fanconi anemias (61 of 64 PGD cycles), and Diamond–Blackfan anemia (10 of 11 PGD cycles). The majority of PGD for hemolytic anemias were represented by maternal fetal incompatibility, as determined by Rhesus and Kell blood groups.

The first PGD for maternofetal incompatibility resulting in a healthy pregnancy outcome was performed for the Kell (K1) genotype, which is one of the major antigenic systems in human red blood cells, comparable in importance to RhD, causing maternofetal incompatibility and leading to severe hemolytic disease of the newborn (HDN) in sensitized mothers.[43,44] The K1 allele is present in 9% of the population, in contrast to its highly prevalent allelic variant K2. The gene is located on chromosome 7 (7q33), consisting of 19 exons, with only C to T base substitution in exon 6 in K1, compared to the K2 antigen.

In the case of a pregnancy with a K1 fetus in a K2 mother, antibodies to K1 can develop leading to maternofetal incompatibility that causes severe HDN. Although prenatal diagnosis is available for identification of pregnancies at risk for HDN, this cannot always prevent potential complications for the fetus, including stillbirth and neonatal death, making PGD a possible option for preventing both Kell and Rhesus hemolytic diseases.

PGD for Kell disease was first performed for two at-risk couples with a history of neonatal death in previous pregnancies due to HDN. The preselection and transfer of the embryos free from the K1 allele of the KEL gene was possible in each case, yielding a clinical pregnancy and the birth of healthy twins confirmed to be free of the K1 allele (Figures 6.71 and 6.72).

In all, 23 PGD cycles for the Kell blood group were performed, resulting in the transfer of 28 compatible embryos in 16 cycles and the birth of 5 healthy children. Much smaller numbers of cycles were undertaken for the Rhesus blood group, with PGD for 5 couples resulting in the birth of compatible healthy children in 3 of them. Both of these conditions are quite prevalent, taking into consideration the approximately 15% frequency for the RhD and 9% for the KEL antigen, presenting a risk for alloimmunization that may lead to HDN in some of the at-risk couples. Therefore, PGD may be a useful option for these couples to avoid the establishment of an RhD or K1 pregnancy in sensitized mothers.

Although the at-risk pregnancies detected by prenatal diagnosis may be treated by intrauterine transfusion, potential complications for the fetus cannot be completely ruled out even after this procedure. Pregnancy termination in such cases is unacceptable, as the antibodies to K1, for example, are developed in 5% of those obtaining incompatible blood. On the other hand, some of the at-risk couples have had the unfortunate experience of HDN resulting in neonatal death, as had both of our couples, so that they

Table 6.22 PGD for congenital hematologic diseases

Disease	*Gene*	*Number of Patients*	*Number of Cycles*	*Number of Transfers*	*Number of Embryos Transferred*	*Pregnancy*	*Birth*
Hemoglobinopathies (congenital abnormality of the hemoglobin molecule or of the rate of hemoglobin synthesis)							
Hemoglobin-alpha locus 1; HBA1 Hemoglobin-beta locus; HBB	HBA1 HBB	148	237	206	437	78	86
HLA + hemoglobin-beta locus; HBB	HBB	61	137	78	121	20	15
Sickle cell anemia	HBB	61	92	83	170	34	30
Sickle cell anemia + HLA	HBB	6	9	5	9	1	1
SUBTOTAL		276	475	372	737	133	132
Anemias (lack of red blood cells or hemoglobin)							
Hemolytic anemias (destruction of red blood cells)							
Pyruvate kinase deficiency of red cells + HLA	PKLR	1	2	1	1	0	0
Rhesus blood group	RHD	5	6	5	11	3	4
Blood group–Kell–Cellano system	KEL	11	23	16	28	4	5
Porphyria, congenital erythropoietic	UROS	1	1	1	1	1	1
SUBTOTAL		18	32	23	41	8	9
Aplastic anemia							
Diamond–Blackfan anemia; DBA	RPS19	1	1	1	2	1	1
HLA + Diamond–Blackfan anemia; DBA	RPS19, RPS24, RPL35A	6	10	7	10	3	3
Fanconi anemia, complementation group A; FANCA	FANCA	1	3	1	2	1	2
FANCA + HLA	FANCA	15	45	27	39	8	5
FANCC + HLA	FANCC	2	5	5	8	1	1
FANCD2 + HLA	FANCD2	1	3	2	3	1	1
FANCF + HLA	FANCF	1	3	2	3	0	0
FANCI + HLA	FANCI	1	2	2	3	0	0
FANCJ + HLA	FANCJ	1	3	1	3	0	0
SUBTOTAL		29	75	48	73	15	13
Coagulopathies (disorders of bleeding and coagulation)							
Hemophilia A	F8	36	62	51	99	28	26
Hemophilia B	F9	3	4	3	3	3	3
Thrombasthenia of glanzmann + HLA + DMD	ITGA2B DMD	1	2	2	4	1	0
Thrombotic thrombocytopenic purpura, congenital; TTP + HLA	ADAMTS13	1	2	2	4	1	1
Wiskott–Aldrich syndrome; WAS	WAS	4	7	7	14	5	4
Wiskott–Aldrich syndrome; WAS + HLA	WAS	1	1	0	0	0	0
SUBTOTAL		46	78	65	124	38	34

(Continued)

Table 6.22 (*Continued*) PGD for congenital hematologic diseases

Disease	*Gene*	*Number of Patients*	*Number of Cycles*	*Number of Transfers*	*Number of Embryos Transferred*	*Pregnancy*	*Birth*
Miscellaneous							
Hemophagocytic lymphohistiocytosis, familial, 3; FHL3	UNC13D	2	3	3	4	1	1
TOTAL		371	663	511 (77%)	979 (1.91)	195 (38.1%)	189 (37%)

*Ongoing pregnancy with a heartbeat

regard PGD as their only option in planning another pregnancy. This makes PGD attractive for patients at risk for alloimmunization, although such conditions have rarely been an indication for prenatal diagnosis.

PREIMPLANTATION HLA TYPING

Preimplantation HLA matching was first introduced in combination with mutation analysis for Fanconi anemia, with the objective of establishing an unaffected pregnancy yielding potential donor progeny for transplantation into an affected sibling.[45] This resulted in a clinical pregnancy and the birth of an unaffected child, whose cord blood was transplanted into the affected sibling, which saved her life.

This strategy would probably not be clinically acceptable using traditional prenatal genetic diagnosis because of a possible clinical pregnancy termination after HLA typing. However, PGD for such a purpose should be acceptable as usually only a limited number of the embryos are preselected for transfer, which in this case will be unaffected embryos with a perfect match for affected siblings in need of a transplant. Since the multiplex single-cell PCR used in PGD presents the opportunity for combined PGD and HLA testing, it has become a useful way to preselect an embryo that may be an HLA match to the affected sibling requiring stem cell transplantation.[46–49] HLA genes were tested simultaneously using the short tandem repeats in the HLA region by applying a multiplex hemi-nested PCR system involving only closely linked polymorphic short tandem repeat (STR) markers located throughout the HLA region, including D6S426, D6S291, Ring 3 CA, TAP1, G51152, D6S2447, LH1, DN, D6S273, 9N-2, TNF a,b,c,d; 62, MIC A, MIB, D6S276, D6S439, D6S1624, D6S265, D6S510; D6S248, RF, MOG a,b,c,d, D6S 258, D6S306, D6S464, D6S299, and D6S461 (Figure 6.73). The choice of alleles and markers was based on the information they provide about the presence of maternal and paternal matching or non-matching chromosomes. For each family, heterozygous alleles and markers not shared by the parents were selected. Such markers provided information about the origin of chromosome 6.

As can be seen from Figure 6.74, recombination within the HLA region was detected in 4.3% of cases and can lead to misdiagnosis in the preselection of HLA-matched embryos. To avoid this, a haplotype analysis for father, mother, and the affected child was performed for each family prior to preimplantation HLA typing. This allowed detecting and avoiding misdiagnosis due to preferential amplification and ADO (exceeding 10% in PCR of single blastomeres), potential recombination within the HLA region (see below), and a possible aneuploidy or uniparental disomy of chromosome 6, which may also affect the diagnostic accuracy of HLA typing of the embryo. The applied strategy provided a 100% HLA match, because the embryos with the same paternal and maternal chromosome 6 as in the affected siblings were preselected.

We applied this method for the HLA genotyping in 374 cycles, including 265 in combination with PGD for 23 different conditions, and 109 without PGD (Table 6.23). Overall, 351 HLA-matched unaffected embryos were detected and transferred in 230 cycles, resulting in 72 clinical pregnancies and the birth of 59 HLA-matched children as potential donors for their siblings (three pregnancies still ongoing). The largest group was PGD with HLA typing for thalassemia (Figures 6.75–6.77) and sickle cell disease (Figure 6.78), including 146 cycles that resulted in the transfer of 130 unaffected HLA-matched embryos in 83 cycles, yielding 21 clinical pregnancies and the birth of 16 unaffected HLA-matched children.

Severe congenital immunodeficiencies (SCID) are the other important group of conditions requiring PGD for HLA typing, as without compatible bone marrow transplantation these patients cannot survive. HLA-matched stem cell transplantation improves or completely replenishes the immune system, so PGD is an obvious alternative for inherited forms of SCID to ensure the birth of unaffected children who may then also serve as potential stem cell donor progeny for affected siblings.

Our experience with PGD for SCID is presented below, including PGD for ataxia–telangiectasia (AT), Omenn syndrome (OMS), FANCA, hyperimmunoglobulin M syndrome (HIGM), X-linked agammaglobulinemia type 1, X-linked chronic granulomatous disease (CGD), X-linked immunodysregulation, polyendocrinopathy, and enteropathy (IPEX), Wiskott–Aldrich syndrome (WAS), and X-linked hypohidrotic ectodermal displasia with immune

Table 6.23 PGD for HLA and combined testing

Disease	*Gene*	*Number of Patients*	*Number of Cycles*	*Number of Transfers*	*Number of Embryos Transferred*	*Pregnancy*	*Birth*
HLA + adrenoleukodystrophy	ABCD1	2	5	1	1	0	0
HLA + Diamond–Blackfan anemia; DBA	RPS19, RPS24, RPL35A	6	10	7	10	3	3
HLA + DMD + Glanzmann's thrombasthenia	ITGA2B, DMD	1	2	2	4	1	0
HLA + dystrophia myotonica 1	DMPK	1	2	1	2	1	1
HLA + ectodermal dysplasia, hypohidrotic, with immune deficiency	IKBKG	2	9	6	8	2	3
HLA + FANCA	FANCA	16	46	28	40	9	6
HLA + FANCC	FANCC	3	6	6	9	2	2
HLA + FANCD2	FANCD2	1	3	2	3	1	1
HLA + FANCF	FANCF	1	3	2	3	0	0
HLA + FANCI	FANCI	1	2	2	3	0	0
HLA + FANCJ	FANCJ	1	3	1	3	0	0
HLA + granulomatous disease, chronic, X-linked; CGD	CYBB	4	10	7	10	3	2
HLA + hemoglobin-beta locus; HBB	HBB	61	137	78	121	20	15
HLA + immunodeficiency with hyper-IgM, type 1; HIGM1	CD40LG	6	11	7	11	4	3
HLA + Krabbe + aneuploidy	GALC	1	1	1	2	1	2
HLA + sickle cell anemia	HBB	6	9	5	9	1	1
HLA + thrombotic thrombocytopenic purpura, congenital; TTP	ADAMTS13	1	2	2	4	1	1
HLA + Wiskott–Aldrich syndrome; WAS	WAS	1	1	0	0	0	0
HLA + PKD1 + aneuploidy	PKD1	1	1	1	2	1	1
HLA genotyping		46	109	70	105	22	18
HLA + pyruvate kinase deficiency	PKLR	1	2	1	1	0	0
TOTAL	23	163	374	230 (61.5%)	351 (1.52%)	72 (31.3%)	59 (3)* (25.6%)

*Ongoing pregnancy with a heartbeat

deficiency (HED-ID) (Table 6.24).[50] Because finding the HLA-identical stem cell donor is the key for achieving the success in stem cell transplantation, a complete cure was observed in the cases of stem cell transplantation in siblings with Fanconi anemia, hyper IgM (Figure 6.79), and HEDIP (Figure 6.80).

Finally, 58 PGD cycles were performed for leukodystrophies, listed in Table 6.25, resulting in the birth of 26 unaffected children. The majority of these children born as a result of PGD were also an HLA match to their affected siblings requiring stem cell transplantation treatment.

The presented data show the usefulness of PGD for SCID, as there are no effective treatments for these conditions other than stem cell transplantation. PGD provides the couples at risk with the option of avoiding an affected pregnancy and of having progeny free of SCID, and this also makes HLA identical stem cell transplantation possible through selection and transfer of those unaffected embryos that have been HLA matched to the sibling. Preimplantation HLA matching is useful as part of PGD for immunodeficiencies to facilitate stem cell transplantation treatment of inherited conditions requiring an HLA-compatible donor for bone marrow transplantation.

Table 6.24 PGD for immunodeficiencies

Disease	*Gene*	*Number of Patients*	*Number of Cycles*	*Number of Transfers*	*Number of Embryos Transferred*	*Pregnancy*	*Birth*
Ataxia–telangiectasia; AT	ATM	1	3	2	3	1	1
Agammaglobulinemia, X-linked, type 1	BTK	3	5	5	11	2	3
HLA + immunodeficiency with hyper-IgM, type 1; HIGM1	CD40LG	6	11	7	11	4	3
Immunodeficiency with hyper-IgM, type 1; HIGM1	CD40LG	4	9	9	13	3	3
HLA + granulomatous disease, chronic, X-linked; CGD	CYBB	4	10	7	10	3	2
Immunodysregulation, polyendocrinopathy, and enteropathy, X-linked; IPEX	FOXP3	1	2	2	2	0	0
HLA + ectodermal dysplasia, hypohidrotic, with immune deficiency	IKBKG	2	9	6	8	2	3
Incontinentia pigmenti; IP	IKBKG	9	20	13	24	2	3
Omenn syndrome	RAG1	2	6	5	12	1	2
Wiskott–Aldrich syndrome; WAS	WAS	4	7	7	14	5	4(1)*
TOTAL		36	82	63 (71.4%)	108 (1.71)	23 (36.5%)	24 (38.0%) (1)*

*Ongoing pregnancy with a heartbeat

Table 6.25 PGD for leukodystrophies

Disease	*Gene*	*Number of Patients*	*Number of Cycles*	*Number of Transfers*	*Number of Embryos Transferred*	*Pregnancy*	*Birth*
Metachromatic leukodystropy	ARSA	1	2	2	2	0	0
Canavan disease	ASPA	1	2	2	4	2	2
Adrenoleukodystrophy; ALD	ABCD1	10	22	14	23	5	4
HLA + adrenoleukodystrophy	ABCD1	2	5	1	1	0	0
Leukoencephalopathy with vanishing white matter; VWM	EIF2B2	1	1	1	2	1	0
HLA + Krabbe + aneuploidy	GALC	1	1	1	2	1	2
Krabbe	GALC	4	5	5	10	3	3
Pelizaeus–Merzbacher-like disease; PMLD	PLP1	6	10	9	14	6	7
Prosaposin deficiency	PSAP	1	1	0	0	0	0
Zellweger syndrome; ZS	PXMP3 PEX1	4	7	6	11	5	7
Aicardi-Goutieres syndrome 5; AGS5 + CF	SAMHD1	1	2	2	2	2	1
TOTAL		32	58	43 (74.1%)	71 (1.65)	25 (58.1%)	26 (60.4%)

Initially, preimplantation HLA typing was done only in combination with PGD; however, it has become extremely useful for the sole purpose of identifying HLA-matched embryos for acquired bone marrow disorders in order to have a potential donor for stem cell transplantation for siblings with these disorders.[51] Although this is still a controversial issue, it appears to be very attractive for the couples who need an HLA-matched bone marrow transplantation for siblings with such disorders.

A total of 109 clinical cycles were performed for preimplantation HLA typing only, in which 105 HLA matched embryos were preselected for transfer in 70 cycles, resulting in 22 singleton clinical pregnancies and 18 HLA-matched children born (Table 6.23). These results suggest that testing of an available number of embryos per cycle allows preselecting a sufficient number of the HLA-matched embryos for transfer to achieve clinical pregnancies and birth of HLA-matched progeny. Thus couples with affected children requiring HLA-compatible stem cell transplantation have a realistic option of undergoing IVF and PGD for HLA typing in order to have an HLA-matched child as potential donor of compatible stem cells for a sibling.

Despite ethical issues involved in preimplantation HLA typing, there is an increase of the attractiveness of this option for the couples with affected children requiring HLA-compatible stem cell transplantation, providing a practical option for those couples who would like to have another child anyway. This and other new indications above make preimplantation testing a genuine alternative to conventional prenatal diagnosis, providing patients with an important prospect not only of avoiding an inherited risk and the possibility of termination of pregnancy, but also of establishing a pregnancy with particular genetic parameters that may also benefit the affected member of the family.

CONCLUSIONS

PGD has become an established procedure for avoiding the birth of affected children with single-gene disorders and having healthy unaffected offspring. PGD is performed through PB or embryo biopsy, which has no deleterious effects on pre- and post-implantation development. At present, PGD experience includes approximately 10,000 clinical cycles performed for single-gene defects, with the majority of these cycles resulting in embryo transfer, and more than one-quarter resulting in clinical pregnancy and the birth of unaffected and apparently healthy children. Therefore, PGD for single-gene disorders may be considered to be a safe, accurate, and reliable technique, with growing value for the prevention of genetic disorders.

Available experience provides the basis for the wider application of PGD for any genetic disease currently diagnosed by prenatal diagnosis, and also for indications for which prenatal diagnosis thus far has not been used, such as late-onset and complex disorders, congenital malformations, and blood group incompatibility. With its utility being no longer limited to the prevention of single-gene disorders, this extends the practical value of PGD to the treatment of siblings requiring stem cell transplantation.

REFERENCES

1. Preimplantation Genetic Diagnosis International Society (PGDIS). Guidelines for good practice in PGD: program requirements and laboratory quality assurance. *Reprod Biomed Online* 2008; 16:134–47.
2. Kuliev A. *Practical Preimplantation Genetic Diagnosis*. New York, London, Heidelberg: Springer, 2012.
3. ESHRE Preimplantation Genetic Diagnosis (PGD) Consortium. Best practice guidelines for preimplantation genetic diagnosis/screening (PGD/PGS). *Hum Reprod* 2011; 26:14–46.
4. Verlinsky Y, Rechitsky S, Cieslak J, et al. Preimplantation diagnosis of single gene disorders by two-step oocyte genetic analysis using first and second polar body. *Biochem Molec Med* 1997; 62:182–87.
5. Saiki R, Scharf S, Faloona F, et al. Enzymatic amplification of beta-globin genomic sequences and restriction site analysis for diagnosis of sickle cell anemia. *Science* 1985; 230:1350–54.
6. Li H, Cui X, Arnheim N. Analysis of DNA sequence variation in single cells. *Meth Enzymol* 1991; 2:49–59.
7. Findlay I, Quirke P. Fluorescent polymerase chain reaction: Part I. A new method allowing genetic diagnosis and DNA fingerprinting of single cells. *Hum Reprod Update* 1996; 2:137–52.
8. Schoolcraft WB, Fragouli E, Stevens J, Munné S, Katz-Jaffe MG, Wells D. Clinical application of comprehensive chromosomal screening in the blastocyst stage. *Fertil Steril* 2010; 94:1700–1706.
9. Geraedts J, Montag M, Magli C, et al. Polar body array CGH for prediction of the status of the corresponding oocyte. Part I: clinical results. *Hum Reprod* 2011; 26:3172–80.
10. Treff NR, Northrop LE, Kasabwala K, Su J, Levy B, Scott RT. Single nucleotide polymorphism microarray-based concurrent screening of 24-chromosome aneuploidy and unbalanced translocations in preimplantation human embryos. *Fertil Steril* 2011; 95:1606–1612.
11. Fragouli E, Alfarawati S, Daphnis DD, et al. Cytogenetic analysis of human blastocyst with the use of FISH, CGH, and aCGH: scientific data and technical evaluation. *Hum Reprod* 2011; 26:480–90.
12. Scott RT Jr., Ferry K, Su J, Tao X, Scott K, Treff NRT. Comprehensive chromosome screening is highly predictive of the reproductive potential of human embryos: a prospective, blinded, nonselection study. *Fertil Steril* 2012; 97:870–75.
13. Colls P, Escudero T, Fischer J, et al. Validation of array comparative genome hybridization for diagnosis of translocations in preimplantation human embryos. *Reprod Biomed Online* 2012; 24:621–29.
14. Yang Z, Liu J, Collins GS, Salem SA, Liu X, Lyle SS, Peck AC, Sills ES, Salem RD. Selection of single blastocysts for fresh transfer via standard morphology assessment alone and with array CGH for good prognosis IVF patients: results from a randomized pilot study. *Mol Cytogenet* 2012; 5:24–29.

15. Brezina PR, Benner A, Rechitsky S, Kuliev A, Pomerantseva E, Pauling D, Kearns WG. Single-gene testing combined with single nucleotide polymorphism microarray preimplantation genetic diagnosis for aneuploidy: a novel approach in optimizing pregnancy outcome. *Fertil Steril* 2011; 95:1786.
16. Rechitsky S, Verlinsky O, Amet T, et al. Reliability of preimplantation diagnosis for single gene disorders. *Mol Cell Endocrinol* 2001; 183:S65–68.
17. Rechitsky S, Strom C, Verlinsky O, et al. Allele drop out in polar bodies and blastomeres. *J Assist Reprod Genet* 1998; 15:253–57.
18. Verlinsky Y, Rechitsky S, Verlinsky O, et al. Polar body based preimplantation diagnosis for X-linked genetic disorders. *Reprod Biomed Online* 2002; 4:38–42.
19. Rechitsky S, Verlinsky O, Kuliev A, et al. Preimplantation genetic diagnosis for familial dysautonomia. *Reprod Biomed Online* 2003; 6:488–93.
20. Sermon K, Seneca S, De Rycke M, et al. PGD in the lab for triplet diseases – myotonic dystrophy, Huntington's disease and fragile-X syndrome. *Mol Cell Endocrinol* 2001; 183:S77–85.
21. Rechitsky S, Kuliev A, Sharapova T, et al. Preimplantation HLA typing with aneuploidy testing. *Reprod Biomed Online* 2006; 12:81–92.
22. Verlinsky Y, Rechitsky S, Verlinsky O, et al. Preimplantation diagnosis for long-chain 3-hydroxyacyl-CoA dehydrogenase deficiency. *Reprod Biomed Online* 2001; 2:17–19.
23. Verlinsky Y, Rechitsky S, Verlinsky O, et al. Preimplantation diagnosis for sonic hedgehog mutation causing familial holoprosencephaly. *N Engl J Med* 2003; 348:1449–54.
24. Verlinsky Y, Rechitsky S, Verlinsky O, Ozen S, Beck R, Kuliev A. Preimplantation diagnosis for polycystic kidney disease. *Fertil Steril* 2004; 82:926–29.
25. Kuliev A, Rechitsky S. Polar body-based preimplantation genetic diagnosis for Mendelian disorders. *Molec Hum Reprod* 2011; 17(No.5): 275–85.
26. Liebaers I, Desmyttere S, Verpoest W, De Rycke M, Staessen C, Sermon K, Devroey P, Haentjens P, Bonduelle M. Report on a consecutive series of 581 children born after blastomere biopsy for preimplantation genetic diagnosis. *Hum Reprod* 2010; 25:275–82.
27. Handyside AH, Lesko JG, Tarin JJ, et al. Birth of a normal girl after in vitro fertilization and preimplantation diagnosis testing for cystic fibrosis. *N Engl J Med* 1992; 327:905–09.
28. Verlinsky Y, Kuliev AM, eds. *Preimplantation Diagnosis of Genetic Diseases: A New Technique in Assisted Reproduction.* New York: Wiley-Liss, 1993.
29. Xu K, Shi ZM, Veeck LL, et al. First unaffected pregnancy using preimplantation genetic diagnosis for sickle cell disease. *J Am Med Assoc* 1999; 281:1701–06.
30. Kuliev A, Rechitsky S, Verlinsky O, et al. Birth of healthy children after preimplantation diagnosis of thalassemias. *J Assist Reprod Genet* 1999; 16:207–11.
31. Goossens V, Sermon K, Lissens W, et al. Clinical application of preimplantation genetic diagnosis for cystic fibrosis. *Prenat Diagn* 2000; 20:571–81.
32. Verlinsky Y, Rechitsky S, Verlinsky O, et al. Preimplantation diagnosis for ornithine transcarbamylase deficiency. *Reprod Biomed Online* 2000; 1:45–47.
33. Verlinsky Y, Rechitsky S, Verlinsky O, et al. Preimplantation diagnosis for PKU. *Fertil Steril* 2001; 76:346–49.
34. Rechitsky S, Verlinsky O, Kuliev A. PGD for cystic fibrosis patients and couples at risk of an additional genetic disorder combined with 24-chromsome aneuploidy testing. *Reprod Biomed Online* 2013; 26:420–30.
35. Rechitsky S, Pamerantseva K, Pakhalchuk T, Pauling D, Verlinsky O, Kuliev A. First systematic experience of preimplantation genetic diagnosis (PGD) for de-novo mutations. *Reprod Biomed Online* 2011; 22:350–361.
36. Verlinsky Y, Rechitsky S, Verlinsky O, et al. Preimplantation diagnosis for p53 tumor suppressor gene mutations. *Reprod Biomed Online* 2001; 2:102–55.
37. Rechitsky S, Verlinsky O, Chistokina A, et al. Preimplantation genetic diagnosis for cancer predisposition. *Reprod Biomed Online* 2002; 5:148–55.
38. He J, McDermont DA, Song Y, Gilbert F, Kligman I, Basson C. Preimplantation genetic diagnosis of human congenital heart disease and Holt-Oram syndrome. *Amer J Med Genet* 2004; 126A:93–98.
39. Kuliev A, Pomerantseva E, Polling D, Verlinsky O, Rechitsky S. PGD for inherited cardiac diseases. *Reprod Biomed Online* 2001; 24(4):443–53.
40. Verlinsky Y, Rechitsky S, Verlinsky O, Masciangelo C, Lederer K, Kuliev A. Preimplantation diagnosis for early onset Alzheimer disease caused by V717L mutation. *J Am Med Assoc* 2002; 287:1018–21.
41. Verlinsky Y, Rechitsky S, Schoolcraft W, Kuliev A. Preimplantation diagnosis for homeobox gene HLXB9 mutation causing Currarino syndrome. *Am J Med Genet* 2005; 134A:103–04.
42. Kuliev A, Pakhalchuk T, Verlinsky O, Rechitsky S. Preimplantation genetic diagnosis for hemoglobinopathies. *Hemoglobin* 2011; 35:547–55.
43. Verlinsky Y, Rechitsky S, Verlinsky O, et al. Preimplantation diagnosis for Kell genotype. *Fertil Steril* 2003; 80:1047–51.
44. Van Den Veyver IB. Prenatal and preimplantation genetic diagnosis for RhD alloimmunization. 10th International Conference on Prenatal Diagnosis and Therapy, Barcelona (Spain), June 19–21, 2000; Barcelona: University of Barcelona, 2000; 181–85.
45. Verlinsky Y, Rechitsky S, Verlinsky O, et al. Preimplantation diagnosis for Fanconi anemia combined with HLA matching. *J Am Med Assoc* 2001; 285:3130–33.
46. Rechitsky S, Kuliev A, Tur-Kaspa I, Morris R, Verlinsky Y. Preimplantation HLA typing with preimplantation genetic diagnosis. *Reprod Biomed Online* 2004; 6: 488–493.
47. Kuliev A, Rechitsky S, Verlinsky O, Kalakoutis G, Angastiniotis M, Verlinsky Y. Preimplantation diagnosis and HLA typing for haemoglobin disorders. *Reprod Biomed Online* 2005; 11:362–70.
48. Rechitsky S, Kuliev A, Sharapova T, et al. Preimplantation HLA typing with aneuploidy testing. *Reprod Biomed Online* 2006; 12:81–92.
49. Kuliev A, Packalchuk T, Verlinsky O, Rechitsky S. Preimplantation diagnosis: efficient tool for human leukocyte antigen matched bone marrow transplantation for thalassemia. *Thalassemia Rep* 2011; 1:1–3.
50. Verlinsky Y, Rechitsky S, Sharapova T, Laziuk K, Barsky I, Verlinsky O, Tur-Kaspa I, Kuliev A. Preimplantation diagnosis for immunodeficiencies. *Reprod Biomed Online* 2007; 14:214–223.
51. Verlinsky Y, Rechitsky S, Sharapova T, et al. Preimplantation HLA typing. *J Am Med Assoc* 2004; 291:2079–85.

7 Future perspectives for preimplantation diagnosis

With the expanding indications for preimplantation genetic diagnosis (PGD) and its wider application to assisted reproduction practices, the annual number of PGD cycles performed in the past few years has almost equaled all previous experience. To date, thousands of unaffected children have been born following PGD, indicating a further improvement in the accuracy and reliability of this relatively novel procedure.[1]

Introduced initially as an alternative to prenatal diagnosis, PGD has now become an important complement to the currently available approaches for the prevention of genetic disorders, which can allow some couples at risk to attempt pregnancy only because an unaffected pregnancy can be established. As previously described, PGD has also stimulated improvements in the accuracy of single cell genetic analysis. A major breakthrough been achieved in PGD for aneuploidies and translocations through the introduction of novel and improved techniques of microarray technology, and next generation sequencing (NGS).

IMPROVING ACCURACY OF PGD FOR SINGLE-GENE DISORDERS

More than 12,000 PGD cycles have been performed for single-gene disorders, including 2982 resulting in the birth of 1118 unaffected children[1–3] in our center. Among the new groups of disorders for which PGD has been performed since the Second Edition of the Atlas are the conditions determined by *de novo* mutations, some important late-onset disorders with a genetic predisposition, such as inherited cardiac diseases and breast cancer, and wider application of PGD for HLA (human leukocyte antigen) typing.[4–13] The accumulated experience shows that some of the problems previously known to lead to misdiagnosis of single-cell genetic analysis, such as contamination by extraneous DNA, failed amplification, and ADO, can now be well controlled by reliable methods currently available.[1,3] Moreover, some centers are presently concentrating on the development of completely novel PGD protocols, including microarray technology and next generation sequencing.[14–21] Array CGH is already used practically for PGD of aneuploidies and translocations.[14–18] Despite these new developments, the available experience still suggests that PGD protocols for single-gene disorders may not be appropriate for clinical practice without the use of a set of closely linked polymorphic markers being tested simultaneously with the causative gene, even with the current prospect of the use of next generation sequencing.[22]

Because the availability of a sufficient number of closely linked informative markers cannot be predicted, especially in certain populations or ethnic groups, the introduction of single nucleotide polymorphisms (SNPs) as linked markers has considerably improved the chances of finding such markers, including the use of SNP arrays. Because of the observed high rate of a crossover within the HLA area, the sufficient number of markers is being used to identify a possible crossover in the proband, as there is little probability of finding the appropriate HLA match in such cases.[6,8] It is also of clinical importance to detect any possible crossover in the process of the actual procedure of preimplantation HLA, because the outcome of transplantation is very poor in cases of undetected crossover in some key areas of HLA cluster, which has not previously been fully appreciated.[8,9]

There is also no doubt that the accuracy of PGD may be compromised by the copy number of the chromosome(s) in which the causative gene tested is localized, which is particularly important in PGD for single-gene disorders offered to patients of advanced reproductive age, when the same biopsied single cell has to be simultaneously tested for the causative gene and specific chromosome number. In our data on the preimplantation HLA typing of 371 embryos, as many as 6.4% of tested cells were aneuploid for chromosome 6, with 2.2% trisomic and 4.2% monosomic embryos, which without evaluating the copy number of chromosome 6 may have led to the misdiagnosis of HLA alleles.[8] The data suggest that reliable HLA typing, as well as PGD for single-gene disorders, should involve testing for the copy number and the origin of the missing or extra chromosomes in which the genes tested are localized. The introduction of microarray technology for aneuploidy testing, which uses whole genome amplification as the first step of the technique, made it possible to perform PGD for single-gene disorders in the same biopsy material, which has become increasingly applied in PGD for single-gene disorders and HLA typing in patients of advanced reproductive age (see Chapter 6).

PRECONCEPTION DIAGNOSIS FOR GENETIC DISORDERS AND PRODUCTION OF MALE AND FEMALE GAMETES FROM HUMAN SOMATIC CELLS

As previously described in the Second Edition, the genetic composition of the oocyte can be reliably tested before conception through removal and testing of the first and second polar bodies. However, no method is yet available for testing the outcome of male meiosis, as genetic analysis destroys the sperm, making it useless for fertilization. As described in Chapter 3, a new technique has been introduced that allows the duplication of a sperm before genetic analysis, so that one of the duplicated sperm can be used for testing and the other for fertilization with the consequent transfer of the resulting embryos.[23,24] The technique was tested using mouse recipient oocytes, and appeared to produce identical haploid pairs in 97% of cases. Preliminary data on using human oocytes as recipient cells for duplication revealed higher aneuploidy rates, so more research is needed to explore whether human oocytes are able to duplicate sperm as faithfully as murine oocytes before the technique can be implemented in the practice of PGD for paternally derived conditions.

This may soon be facilitated by the developments in stem cell technology, as the individually specific stem cells may now be derived from adult somatic cells, such as skin fibroblasts, through the induced pluripotent stem cell (iPSC) technique, which then may be differentiated into sperm, as described in animal models.[25] Primordial germ cells have been differentiated from fetal and adult-derived human iPSCs,[26,27] and haploid cells resulting from meiosis are consistently obtained from iPSC lines generated from different tissues.[28] However, the use of such cells in clinical practice is still controversial, so the other approach is to use the oogonial stem cells that have been identified in human ovarian cortical biopsies.[29]

DEVELOPMENTS IN SAMPLING PROCEDURES

There have also been developments in the biopsy procedures applied for removing samples from oocytes and embryos, which may be required to improve the accuracy of PGD. For example, current PGD practice frequently requires the removal of a sample from both the oocyte and the resulting embryo, such as in PGD combined with preimplantation HLA typing, and in a combined PGD for single-gene and chromosomal disorders. It is of interest that the evaluation of the outcome of such a double biopsy appeared to have no effect on the viability of the embryos.[30,31] The approach has been applied on a regular basis as a tool for avoiding misdiagnosis due to mosaicism.

With the current progress in vitrification procedures and increasing use of blastocyst transfer, blastocyst biopsy is becoming one of the major approaches for PGD. As described in Chapter 3, blastocyst biopsy improves PGD accuracy, as instead of a single cell, a number of cells are used for analysis, lowering the ADO rates in PGD for single-gene disorders and overcoming to some extent the problem of mosaicism in PGD for aneuploidy. Blastocyst biopsy and vitrification, coupled with microarray-based testing, have also simplified the organization of PGD, as the samples may be processed without a time limitation for genetic analysis, and may be shipped to specialized centers for more sophisticated testing. Blastocyst biopsy may also be required for additional testing to confirm the polar body or blastomere diagnosis.

DEVELOPMENT OF A COMPREHENSIVE APPROACH FOR CONCOMITANT PGD OF SINGLE-GENE AND CHROMOSOMAL DISORDERS

As described in Chapter 6, it is currently possible to perform PGD for single-gene disorders with preimplantation HLA typing and aneuploidy testing in the same biopsy material, as the first step of array CGH or SNP array involves whole genome amplification. However, this still requires the development of PGD designed for a particular family, because the DNA of WGA product for single-gene disorders is analyzed according to the traditional approach described in Chapter 6. There have been attempts to detect multiple conditions in the same reaction, using "next generation sequencing" (NGS), which, however, is highly dependent on equipment-assisted technology and is extremely expensive at the present time. NGS provides base pair resolution data with the unique opportunity to evaluate multiple customized genomic loci and multiple samples on the same run and one chip,[19] so DNA from PB and blastomeres from different couples may be analyzed simultaneously, which will decrease the cost.

Although the technique has not been validated for PGD, the principle of the use of NGS for testing single cells has been demonstrated.[32,33] Also there was a recent attempt to evaluate the applicability of NGS for PGD and develop a specific protocol that could evaluate DNA from trophectoderm biopsy with the use of semiconductor-based NGS[19] with direct comparison with the results of the same embryos obtained by conventional standard PGD methods. Although this study demonstrated perfect consistency of NGS results with two independent conventional PGD methodologies, the major concern with NGS is that it is also prone to ADO, because WGA must be first performed to generate an adequate amount of DNA for analysis, which is still extremely inefficient for recovering all genomic sequences. So without simultaneous testing of the sufficient number of linked markers, false negative results cannot be excluded, which may lead to misdiagnosis, especially in PGD for dominant diseases. It can therefore be predicted that the technique may be upgraded to perform NGS with the use of SNP analysis for this purpose, or to work out the level of deep sequencing that can overcome the problem of ADO or develop more efficient WGA.[22]

There has been also progress in the development of the techniques for examining the gene-expression profiles of individual human oocytes and embryos, although, to date, no reliable correlation has been identified between molecular markers and the developmental competence of oocytes and preimplantation embryos. By testing the expression profile of over 8000 genes examined in single oocytes and embryos, using Affymetrix GeneChip Microarrays, differences in expression were evident even between oocytes of the same developmental stage, which could be due to underlying genetic differences that contribute to the patient's phenotype.[34,35] Comparison of embryos at different stages of development revealed large divergences in gene expression, so microarray technology may help to reveal genes that play a critical role in specific infertile conditions and normal preimplantation development, thus providing potential targets for diagnosis.

It may also be expected that the invasive approaches to PGD based on biopsy of oocytes and embryos may in future be replaced by non-invasive methods that determine the genetic status of oocytes and embryos by testing the products of their metabolism obtained from spent culture media, or by testing cumulus cells. By comparing the gene expression patterns of cumulus cells removed from normal and aneuploid oocytes, it was shown that cumulus cells of abnormal oocytes are less proliferative and transcriptionally quiescent, with certain genes exhibiting highly significant differences in their expression.[36,37] Analyzing the relationship between human preimplantation embryo metabolism and aneuploidy rates during development *in vitro* by testing 18 amino acid turnovers in spent media using high-performance chromatography also demonstrated that some of the amino acids were significantly different in aneuploid embryos.[38] Mitochondrial activity was also correlated with the turnover of these particular amino acids. The fact that amino acid profiling can distinguish oocytes with different competence in maturing to metaphase II *in vitro* was also demonstrated.[39] The possibility of selecting healthy oocytes was also tested in preliminary studies of mitochondrial metabolic efficiency and chromosomal analysis in oocytes and their corresponding polar bodies from couples with advanced reproductive age.[40] Research is underway on morphokinetic analysis of early human embryos, as a possibility for non-invasive detection of aneuploid embryos, but prognostic value of a time-lapse imaging is still questionable.[41]

STEM CELL TRANSPLANTATION AND AVAILABILITY OF HUMAN EMBRYONIC STEM CELLS

Preimplantation HLA matching has been used during the past 13 years for the preselection of mutation-free embryos that may also be potential donor progeny for bone marrow transplantation.[6–9] Preimplantation HLA genotyping in combination with PGD was applied in more than 1000 cycles, resulting in the preselection and transfer of the HLA-matched unaffected embryos in 17.5% of the embryos tested, as expected. Overall, the number of requests to perform PGD in combination with HLA typing has been increasing, with the recent emergence of a considerable proportion of cases involving preimplantation HLA typing without PGD. The currently available experience in our center includes more than 3000 PGD cycles performed for more than 300 different conditions, including single-gene defects, dynamic mutations, and some medically relevant genetic variations, of which over 12% of cycles have been performed for HLA typing. While the majority of these cases were undertaken for preimplantation HLA genotyping in combination with PGD for causative genes, including thalassemia, Fanconi anemia, hyperimmunoglobulin M syndrome, X-linked adrenoleukodystrophy, and Wiskott–Aldrich syndrome, to mention only a few, an increasing number of clinical cycles are being performed for HLA typing without PGD, i.e., with the only objective of preselecting HLA-matched progeny for transplantation treatment of siblings with bone marrow disorders.[42] As described in Chapter 6, the present experience of preimplantation HLA typing as the sole indication has already resulted in the birth of dozens of HLA-matched healthy children who are potential HLA-compatible donors for siblings requiring bone marrow transplantation. The data provide a realistic option for couples desiring to establish a pregnancy with the potential to provide an HLA-matched progeny for the treatment of an affected family member, and there is the prospect of applying the approach to other inherited or acquired conditions that also require HLA-compatible donors for bone marrow transplantation.

Although preimplantation HLA typing is still controversial in some social settings and is not allowed in certain countries, it appears to be so attractive for couples in need that they are prepared to achieve their goal to provide the affected sibling with HLA-matched donor progeny even by traveling out of the country. For example, PGD for genetic disease combined with HLA typing has generally been allowed, while HLA typing in the absence of high-risk genetic transmissible disease is still not allowed in some social settings. The couples from such communities usually request preimplantation HLA typing outside their countries, with examples already available in achieving the goal of producing the birth of HLA-matched progeny for siblings with a number of diseases. Similarly, the law in some countries condones the use of embryos for stem cell research and therapeutic cloning, though this is still the subject of intense discussion.

In addition to the provision of HLA-matched stem cells for bone marrow disorders, PGD provides a novel source for the establishment of embryonic stem cell (ESC) lines,[41,42] (see Chapter 1). These ESC lines, as well as numerous other ESC lines established from spare human blastocysts obtained after PGD for chromosomal disorders, were characterized as typical pluripotent ESCs and were shown to spontaneously differentiate *in vitro* into a variety of cell types, including neurons and contracted cardiocytes. The established repository of ESC lines is currently used for research purposes.

The prospect of obtaining individually specific ESC lines has been overcome by the discovery of the induced pluripotent stem cells (iPSC), which makes it possible to develop a custom-made hESC for future cell therapy.[43,44] This involves the induction of overexpression of four main genes responsible for stemness, *Oct-3/4*, *Sox2*, *Klf4*, and *c-Myc*, which result in pluripotency and differentiation characteristics similar to hESCs. However, it is still not clear whether these iPSCs may provide an alternative to hESC, as they are not identical in DNA microarray analysis, and it is not known whether they are safe, because of significant gene modification and possible tumorigenic potential. The prospect of clinical therapies derived from hESC lines will likely hold true for many congenital and acquired diseases. Our repository, with its large collection of hESC lines, provides a unique opportunity to screen available hESC lines for polymorphisms associated with susceptibility and/or resistance to diseases in humans, which may prove invaluable to the future stem cell therapy of severe disorders for which there is no available treatment.

INTRODUCTION OF PGD AS THE FUTURE IVF STANDARD

An increasing number of centers have been involved in PGD for chromosomal disorders, including translocations and aneuploidies. As previously mentioned, significant reproductive improvements have been demonstrated following the use of PGD for chromosomal translocations. The experience accumulated to date further confirms the previous observations of more than a five-fold reduction in the spontaneous abortion rate in translocation carriers, making PGD a preferred option for chromosomal translocations over traditional prenatal diagnosis (see Chapter 5).

Despite present controversy, further evidence amounting to the dozens of thousands of cycles has been accumulated on the positive clinical impact of PGD for aneuploidy, which is currently performed for advanced reproductive age, repeated IVF failures, and repeated spontaneous abortions. The improvement in reproductive outcome was particularly obvious from the analysis of the reproductive history of PGD patients.[45,46] From the outcomes of the transfer of 318 FISH-normal embryos, an implantation rate of 65.1% was observed, with a total of 161 clinical pregnancies generated, which resulted in the birth of 153 children from 125 couples, and 26 spontaneous abortions, giving a take-home baby rate of 82.3%. Of the 161 couples involved in the study, 41 were in their first cycle, and 14 had experienced 31 spontaneous pregnancies with 29 abortions and two deliveries, with only one birth occurring in the remaining 27 couples. A total of 367 cycles were performed in 120 of these couples before undertaking PGD, with 30 pregnancies, five term and 25 aborted. These couples had also experienced 50 spontaneous pregnancies, three term and 47 aborted. The overall implantation rate derived from their reproductive experience was 13.0% and the take-home baby rate was 6.8%. This makes obvious the clinical usefulness of PGD for aneuploidy for IVF patients with poor reproductive performance.

The potential of preselecting euploid embryos for transfer is supported by the fact that more than half of the oocytes and embryos tested by PGD for poor-prognosis IVF patients were shown to have chromosomal abnormalities.[47–51] At least half of chromosomally abnormal embryos have mosaicism, which is the major challenge in improving the accuracy of PGD for aneuploidies. As the overall prevalence of chromosomal abnormalities in oocytes and embryos seems to be comparable, suggesting that mosaic embryos may originate from the aneuploid oocytes through the process known as "trisomy rescue," the further improvement of PGD accuracy may, in the future, require testing of both the oocyte and the resulting embryo. As previously mentioned, this can be achieved by a sequential biopsy of both the polar bodies and the embryo (blastocyst) from the resulting embryo, so that both meiotic and mitotic errors can be excluded. In addition, the information from both the oocyte and the embryo chromosome sets will make it possible to detect potential uniparental disomy cases, which may be expected from the detection of normal disomic embryos originating from trisomic oocytes. Because more than half of IVF patients are 35 years or older, and more than half of their oocytes have aneuploidies, avoiding the transfer of the embryos resulting from these oocytes through PGD for aneuploidies should also be useful—in addition to potentially improving implantation and pregnancy rates—in avoiding the transfer of embryos with potential uniparental disomies as possible contributors to imprinting disorders.

Although randomized controlled studies may, of course, still be useful in quantifying the clinical impact of preselection of aneuploidy-free zygotes for genetic counseling purposes, it is also obvious that in order to achieve the expected benefit, the testing should first of all not damage embryo viability and be performed accurately according to the available standards. In other words, despite the present controversy about the uselessness of aneuploid embryo transfer, the major issue is the safety and reliability of aneuploidy testing, which will no doubt be further improved in the near future.

In light of these data, the current IVF practice of selection of embryos for transfer based on morphologic criteria may hardly be an acceptable procedure for poor-prognosis IVF patients. In addition to an extremely high risk of establishing an affected pregnancy from the onset, this will significantly compromise the very poor chances of these patients to become pregnant, especially with the current tendency of limiting the number of transferred embryos to only two, leaving only a single embryo on the average with a potential chance of reaching term.

The current switch of aneuploidy testing from FISH to microarray technology and possibly to NGS (the first baby has already been born following NGS-based aneuploidy testing[52]) coupled with blastocyst biopsy, further confirmed the positive impact of excluding aneuploid embryos from transfer.[14,16,18,53–63] In addition to testing all 24 chromosomes at the blastocyst stage, when only established anomalies are tested, the embryos are transferred after freezing in a subsequent cycle, when uterine receptivity is much higher than in stimulated cycles.

It may, therefore, be predicted that, with the future improvement of the safety and accuracy, PGD should definitely contribute to improving the overall standards of the assisted reproduction practices by replacing the presently practiced selection of embryos for transfer using morphologic parameters with the preselection of chromosomally normal embryos with the higher potential to result in pregnancy.

The presented data provide strong evidence that PGD is currently an important alternative to prenatal diagnosis, as it widens the options available for couples wishing to avoid the birth of an affected child, while providing the possibility of having children for those who would otherwise remain childless because of their objection to termination of pregnancy following prenatal diagnosis. At the same time, PGD is also becoming an integral part of assisted reproduction, allowing avoidance of the transfer of chromosomally abnormal and potentially non-viable embryos, which will clearly contribute to a significant increase in the implantation and pregnancy rates in IVF and to a general improvement in the standards of assisted reproduction practices.

REFERENCES

1. Preimplantation Genetic Diagnosis International Society (PGDIS). Guidelines for good practice in PGD: program requirements and laboratory quality assurance. *Reprod Biomed Online* 2008; 16:134–47.
2. Kuliev A. *Practical Preimplantation Genetic Diagnosis*. New York, London, Heidelberg: Springer, 2012.
3. ESHRE Preimplantation Genetic Diagnosis (PGD) Consortium. Best practice guidelines for preimplantation genetic diagnosis/screening (PGD/PGS). *Hum Reprod* 2011; 26:14–46.
4. Rechitsky S, Verlinsky O, Chistokina A, et al. Preimplantation genetic diagnosis for cancer predisposition. *Reprod Biomed Online* 2002; 5:148–55.
5. Verlinsky Y, Rechitsky S, Verlinsky O, et al. Preimplantation diagnosis for early onset Alzheimer disease caused by V717L mutation. *J Am Med Assoc* 2002; 287:1018–21.
6. Rechitsky S, Kuliev A, Tur-Kaspa I, Morris R, Verlinsky Y. Preimplantation HLA typing with preimplantation genetic diagnosis. *Reprod Biomed Online* 2004; 6: 488–93.
7. Kuliev A, Rechitsky S, Verlinsky O, Kalakoutis G, Angastiniotis M, Verlinsky Y. Preimplantation diagnosis and HLA typing for haemoglobin disorders. *Reprod Biomed Online* 2005; 11:362–70.
8. Rechitsky S, Kuliev A, Sharapova T, et al. Preimplantation HLA typing with aneuploidy testing. *Reprod Biomed Online* 2006; 12:81–92.
9. Kuliev A, Packalchuk T, Verlinsky O, Rechitsky S. Preimplantation diagnosis: efficient tool for human leukocyte antigen matched bone marrow transplantation for thalassemia. *Thalassemia Rep* 2011; 1:1–3.
10. Rechitsky S, Pamerantseva K, Pakhalchuk T, Pauling D, Verlinsky O, Kuliev A. First systematic experience of preimplantation genetic diagnosis (PGD) for de-novo mutations. *Reprod Biomed Online* 2011; 22:350–61.
11. Kuliev A, Rechitsky S. Polar body-based preimplantation genetic diagnosis for Mendelian disorders. *Molec Hum Reprod* 2011; 17:275–85.
12. Kuliev A, Pomerantseva E, Polling D, Verlinsky O, Rechitsky S. PGD for inherited cardiac diseases. *Reprod Biomed Online* 20012; 24:443–53.
13. Rechitsky S, Verlinsky O, Kuliev A. PGD for cystic fibrosis patients and couples at risk of an additional genetic disorder combined with 24-chromsome aneuploidy testing. *Reprod Biomed Online* 2013; 26:420–30.
14. Treff NR, Northrop LE, Kasabwala K, Su J, Levy B, Scott RT. Single nucleotide polymorphism microarray-based concurrent screening of 24-chromosome aneuploidy and unbalanced translocations in pre-implantation human embryos. *Fertil Steril* 2011; 95:1606–12.
15. Fragouli E, Alfarawati S, Daphnis DD, et al. Cytogenetic analysis of human blastocyst with the use of FISH, CGH, and aCGH: scientific data and technical evaluation. *Hum Reprod* 2011; 26:480–90.
16. Scott RT Jr., Ferry K, Su J, Tao X, Scott K, Treff NRT. Comprehensive chromosome screening is highly predictive of the reproductive potential of human embryos: a prospective, blinded, nonselection study. *Fertil Steril* 2012; 97:870–75.
17. Colls P, Escudero T, Fischer J, et al. Validation of array comparative genome hybridization for diagnosis of translocations in preimplantation human embryos. *Reprod Biomed Online* 2012; 24:621–29.
18. Yang Z, Liu J, Collins GS, Salem SA, Liu X, Lyle SS, Peck AC, Sills ES, Salem RD. Selection of single blastocysts for fresh transfer via standard morphology assessment alone and with array CGH for good prognosis IVF patients: results from a randomized pilot study. *Mol Cytogenet* 2012; 5:24–29.
19. Treff N, Fedic A, Xin T, et al. Evaluation of targeted next-generation sequencing-based preimplantation genetic diagnosis of monogenic disorders. *Fertil Steril* 2013; 99:1377–84.
20. Treff N, Scott RT. Four-hour quantitative real-time polymerase chain reaction-based comprehensive chromosome screening and accumulating evidence of accuracy, safety, predictive value, and clinical efficiency. *Fertil Steril* 2013; 99:1049–53.
21. Martin J, Cervero A, Mir P, Martinez JAC, Pollicer A, Simon C. The impact of next-generation sequencing technology on preimplantation genetic diagnosis and screening. *Fertil Steril* 2013; 99:1054–61.
22. Simpson JL, Rechitsky S, Kuliev A. Next generation sequencing for preimplantation genetic diagnosis. *Fertil Steril* 2013; 99:1203–04.
23. Willadsen S, Munné S, Schmmel T, Cohen J. Applications of nuclear sperm duplication. Fifth International Symposium on Preimplantation Genetics, 5–7 June, Antalya, Turkey, 2003:35.

24. Munné S, Willadsen S, Schmmel T, Cohen J. Nuclear sperm duplication as a tool to study mosaicism. Fifth International Symposium on Preimplantation Genetics, 5–7 June, Antalya, Turkey, 2003:55–56.
25. Nayernia K, Nolte J, Michelmann HW, et al. In vitro-differentiated embryonic stem cells give rise to male gametes that can generate offspring mice. *Develop Cell* 2006; 11:1–8.
26. Park TS, Galic Z, Conway AE, et al. Derivation of primordial germ cells from human embryonic and induced pluripotent stem cells is significantly improved by coculture with human fetal gonadal cells. *Stem Cells* 2009; 27:783–95.
27. Panula S, Medrano JV, Kee1 K, et al. Human germ cell differentiation from fetal- and adult-derived induced pluripotent stem cells. *Hum Mol Genet* 2011; 20(4):752–62.
28. Eguizabal C, Montserrat N, Vassena R, et al. Complete meiosis from human induced pluripotent stem cells. *Stem Cells* 2011; 29:1186–95.
29. Woods DC, Tilly JL. The next (re)generation of ovarial biology and fertility in women: is current science tomorrow's practice? *Fertil Steril* 2012; 98:3–10.
30. Magli MC, Ferraretti A, Gianaroli L, et al. The combination of polar body and embryos biopsy does not affect embryo viability. Fifth International Symposium on Preimplantation Genetics, 5–7 June, Antalya, Turkey, 2003:24.
31. Cieslak J, Tur-Kaspa I, Ilkevitch Y, Bernal A, Morris R, Verlinsky Y. Multiple micromanipulations for preimplantation genetic diagnosis do not affect embryo development to the blastocyst stage. *Fertil Steril* 2006; 85:1826–29.
32. Navin N, Kendall J, Troge J, et al. Tumour evolution inferred by single-cell sequencing. *Nature* 2011; 472:90–94.
33. Wang J, Fan HC, Behr B, Quake SR. Genome-wide single-cell analysis of recombination activity and de novo mutation rates in human sperm. *Cell* 2012; 150:402–12.
34. Steuerwald N, Bermudes MG, Wells D, et al. The use of microarray technology to examine the gene expression profiles of individual human oocytes and embryos. Fifth International Symposium on Preimplantation Genetics, 5–7 June, Antalya, Turkey, 2003:14.
35. Bermudes MG, Wells D, Malter H, et al. Expression profiles of individual human oocytes using microarray technology. *Reprod Biomed Online* 2004; 8:325–37.
36. Gasca S, Pellestor F, Assou S, et al. Identifying new human oocyte marker genes: a microarray approach. *Reprod Biomed Online* 2007; 14:175–83.
37. Fragouli E, Bianchi V, Obradors A, et al. Transcriptional profiling of human oocytes: association of meiotic aneuploidy and altered oocyte gene expression. *Mol Hum Reprod* 2010; 16:570–82.
38. Picton HM, Elder K, Houghton FD, et al. Association between amino acid turnover and chromosome aneuploidy during human preimplantation embryo development in vitro. *Mol Hum Reprod* 2010; 16:557–69.
39. Hemmings KE, Maruthini D, Vyjayanthi S, et al. Amino acid turnover by human oocytes is influenced by gamete developmental competence, patient characteristics and gonadotrophin treatment. *Hum Reprod* 2013; 28:1031–44.
40. Gardner DK, Phil D, Wales PL. Analysis of metabolism to select viable human embryos for transfer. *Fertil Steril* 2013; 99:1062–72.
41. Montag M. Morphokinecs and embryo aneuploidy: has time come or not yet? *Reprod Biomed Online* 2013; 23:528–35.
42. Verlinsky Y, Strelchenko N, Kukharenko V, Shkumatov A, Rechitsky S, Verlinsky O, Kuliev A. Repository of human embryonic stem cell lines and development of individual specific lines using stembrid technology. *Reprod Biomed Online* 2006; 13:547–50.
43. Takahashi KK, Tanabe K, Ohnuki M, Narita M, Ishisaka T, Tomoda K, Jamanaka S. Induction of pluriopotent stem cells from adult human fibroblasts by defined factors. *Cell* 2007; 131:861–72.
44. Park IH, Zhao R, West JA, Jabuuchi A, Huo H, Ince TA, Lerou PH, Lensch MW, Daley GQ. Reprogramming of human somatic cells to pluripotency with defined factors. *Nature* 2008; 451:141–45.
45. Gianaroli L, Magli MC, Tabanelli C, Trengia V, Farfalli V, Cavallini G. The beneficial effects of preimplantation genetic diagnosis for aneuploidy support extensive clinical application. *Reprod Biomed Online* 2005; 10:633–40.
46. Verlinsky Y, Tur-Kaspa I, Cieslak J, Bernal A, Morris R, Taranissi M, Kaplan B, Kuliev A. Preimplantation diagnosis for chromosomal disorders improves reproductive outcome of poor-prognosis patients. *Reprod Biomed Online* 2005; 11: 219–25.
47. Munné S. Preimplantation genetic diagnosis of numerical and structural chromosome abnormalities. *Reprod Biomed Online* 2000; 4:183–96.
48. Gianaroli L, Magli MC, Ferraretti AP. The in vivo and in vitro efficiency and efficacy of PGD for aneuploidy. *Mol Cell Endocrinol* 2001; 183:S13–18.
49. Munné S, Sandalinas M, Escudero T, et al. Improved implantation after preimplantation genetic diagnosis of aneuploidy. *Reprod Biomed Online* 2003; 7:91–97.
50. Kuliev A, Cieslak J, Ilkevitch Y, Verlinsky Y. Nuclear abnormalities in series of 6733 human oocytes. *Reprod Biomed Online* 2003; 6:54–59.
51. Kuliev A, Zlatopolski Z, Kirillova I, Spivakova J, Cieslak-Jansen J. Meiosis errors in over 20,000 oocytes studied in the practice of preimplantation aneuploidy testing. *Reprod Biomed Online* 2011; 22:2–8.
52. Wells D, Kaur K, Grifo J, et al. A novel embryo screening provides new insights into embryo biology and yields the first pregnancies following genome sequencing. *Hum Reprod.* 2013; 28 (suppl 1):i25-i27. doi: 10.1093/humrep/det143
53. Munné S, Wells D, Cohen J. Technology requirements for preimplantation genetic diagnosis to improve ART outcome. *Fertil Steril* 2010; 94:408–30.
54. Scott RT, Tao X, Taylor D, Ferry KM, Treff NR. A prospective randomized controlled trial demonstrating significantly increased clinical pregnancy rates following 24 chromosome aneuploidy screening: biopsy and analysis on day 5 with fresh transfer. *Fertil Steril* 2010; 94:S2(0–05).
55. Schoolcraft WB, Fragouli E, Stevens J, Munné S, Katz-Jaffe MG, Wells D. Clinical application of comprehensive chromosomal screening at the blastocyst stage. *Fertil Steril* 2010; 94:1700–06.
56. Harton G, Surrey M, Grifo J, Kaplan B, Munné S. Implantation and miscarriage rates following array CGH analysis at the cleavage and blastocyst stages. *Fertil Steril* 2011: 95(Suppl 1):0–6.
57. Schoolcraft WB, Treff NR, Stevens JM, Ferry K, Katz-Jaffe M, Scott RT. Live birth outcome with trophectoderm biopsy, blastocyst vitrification, and single-nucleotide polymorphism microarray–based comprehensive chromosome screening in infertile patients. *Fertil Steril* 2011; 96:638–40.
58. Forman EJ, Tao X, Ferry KM, Taylor D, Treff NR, Scott RT Jr. Single embryo transfer with comprehensive chromosome

screening results in improved ongoing pregnancy rates and decreased miscarriage rates. *Hum Reprod* 2012; 27:1217–22.
59. Treff NR, Ferry KM, Zhao T, Su S, Forman EJ, Scott RT. Cleavage stage embryo biopsy significantly impairs embryonic reproductive potential while blastocyst biopsy does not: a novel paired analysis of cotransferred biopsied and non-biopsied sibling embryos. *Fertil Steril* 2011; 95 (suppl 1);0–4.
60. Scott RT Jr., Ferry K, Su J, Tao X, Scott K, Treff NRT. Comprehensive chromosome screening is highly predictive of the reproductive potential of human embryos: a prospective, blinded, nonselection study. *Fertil Steril* 2012; 97:870–5.
61. Yang Z, Liu J, Collins GS, Salem SA, Liu X, Lyle SS, Peck AC, Sills ES, Salem RD. Selection of single blastocysts for fresh transfer via standard morphology assessment alone and with array CGH for good prognosis IVF patients: results from a randomized pilot study. *Mol Cytogenet* 2012; 5:24.
62. Ata B, Kaplan B, Danzer H, Glassner M, Opsahl M, Tan SL, Munné S. Array CGH analysis shows that aneuploidy is not related to the number of embryos generated. *Reprod Biomed Online* 2012; 24:614–20.

SECTION II PREIMPLANTATION GENETIC DIAGNOSIS ILLUSTRATED

1 Normal and abnormal human preimplantation development in relation to preimplantation genetic diagnosis and establishment of embryonic stem cell lines

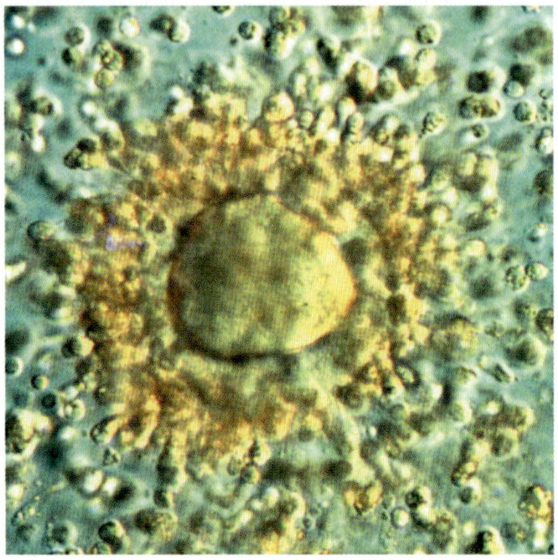

Figure 1.1 Oocyte–corona–cumulus complex 1 h after retrieval with an apparently immature oocyte. Surrounding corona cells are compact around the oocyte, which is irregular in shape. Maturation *in vitro* can be achieved for a proportion of immature oocytes in culture, although the fertilization rate and viability of embryos resulting from these oocytes are reduced (x200).

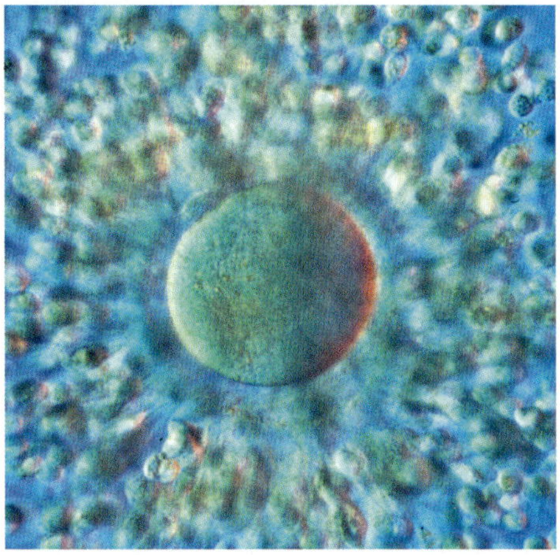

Figure 1.2 Oocyte–corona–cumulus complex 1 h after retrieval with a mature oocyte. Corona and cumulus cells are well dispersed, allowing easy visualization of this round oocyte that has completed the first meiotic division, which is evident by the presence of the first polar body at the 11 o'clock position.

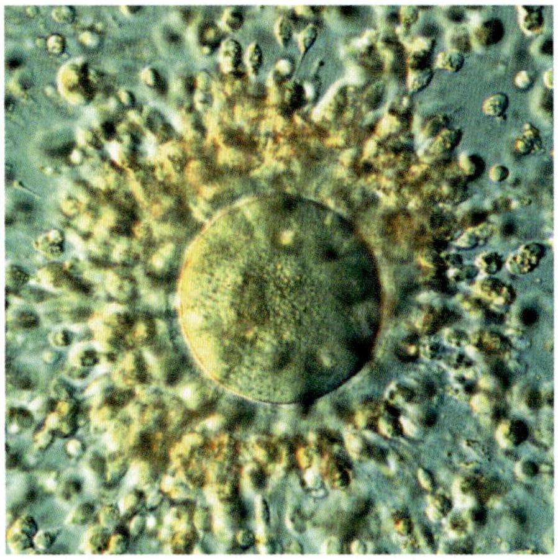

Figure 1.3 Oocyte–corona–cumulus complex 1 h after retrieval with an apparently normal oocyte. Cumulus cells are well dispersed. However, corona cells remain compact in some areas around the oocyte. The oocyte is round in shape, but the first polar body is not visible. Removal of corona cells is required to verify the exact stage of maturation (x200).

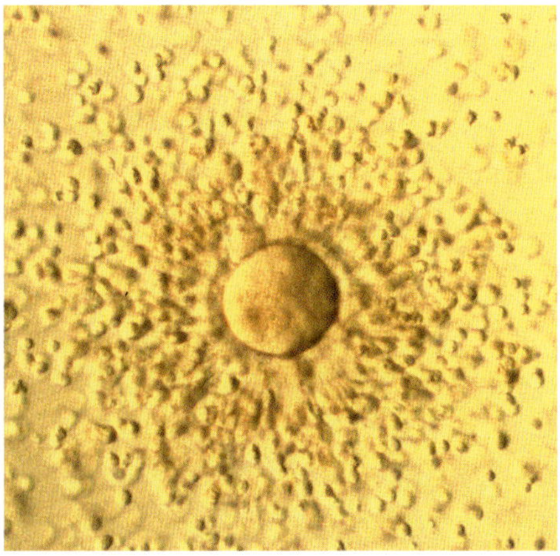

Figure 1.4 Oocyte–corona–cumulus complex 1 h after retrieval with an apparently normal oocyte. Cumulus cells are well dispersed. Corona cells form a "sun-ray" appearance around the oocyte, which is round in shape (x100).

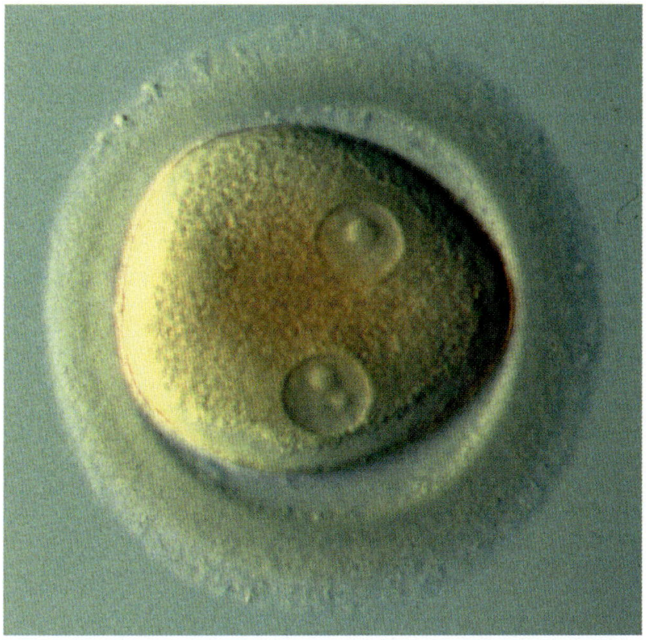

Figure 1.5 Binuclear prophase I oocyte, an extremely rare abnormality observed in human oocytes. The oocyte, 40 h after injection of human chorionic gonadotropin, is slightly irregular in shape and significantly larger than the rest of the oocytes from the same cohort. The cytoplasm is coarse, with a dark area in the center often seen in prophase I oocytes. Two germinal vesicles are located on opposite sides at the periphery of the cytoplasm containing one and two nuclear organizers. The perivitelline space is clear and the zona pellucida is intact and evenly thick along the circumference (x200).

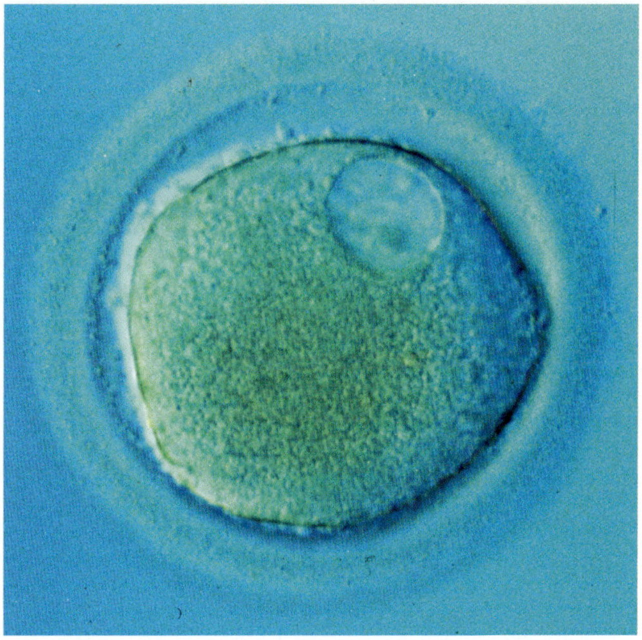

Figure 1.6 Early prophase I oocyte, 40 h after injection of human chorionic gonadotropin, is slightly irregular in shape and regular in size. The cytoplasm is coarse. A germinal vesicle is located at the periphery of the cytoplasm and contains one nuclear organizer. The perivitelline space is without debris, and the zona pellucida is intact and evenly thick along the circumference (x400).

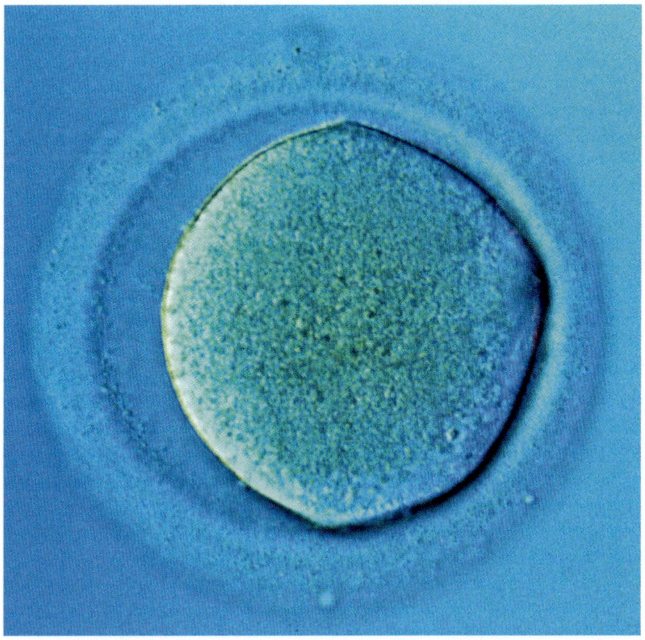

Figure 1.7 Early metaphase I oocyte, 40 h after injection of human chorionic gonadotropin, is slightly irregular in shape and regular in size. The cytoplasm is less coarse than is usually observed at the germinal vesicle stage. The perivitelline space is clear. Neither a first polar body nor a germinal vesicle is present (x400).

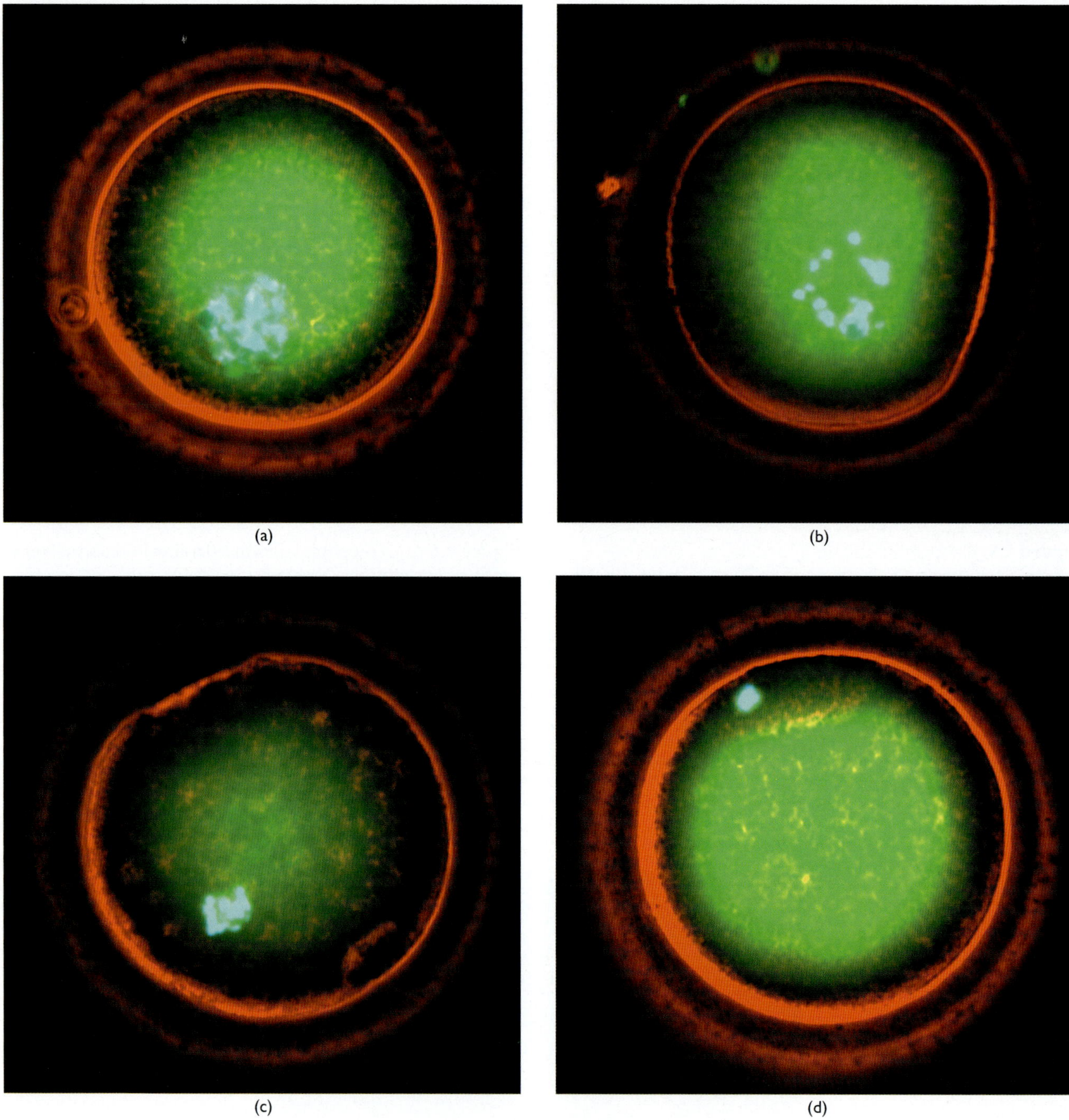

Figure 1.8 Germinal vesicle breakdown (GVBD): immunocytochemical staining (bright-field view of the oocyte is shown in red, tubulin in green, chromatin in blue). (a) Germinal vesicle. (b) GVBD: disappearance of nucleoli. (c) GVBD: chromatin compaction. (d) GVBD: early metaphase I stage: chromatin is compacted but no spindle is formed.

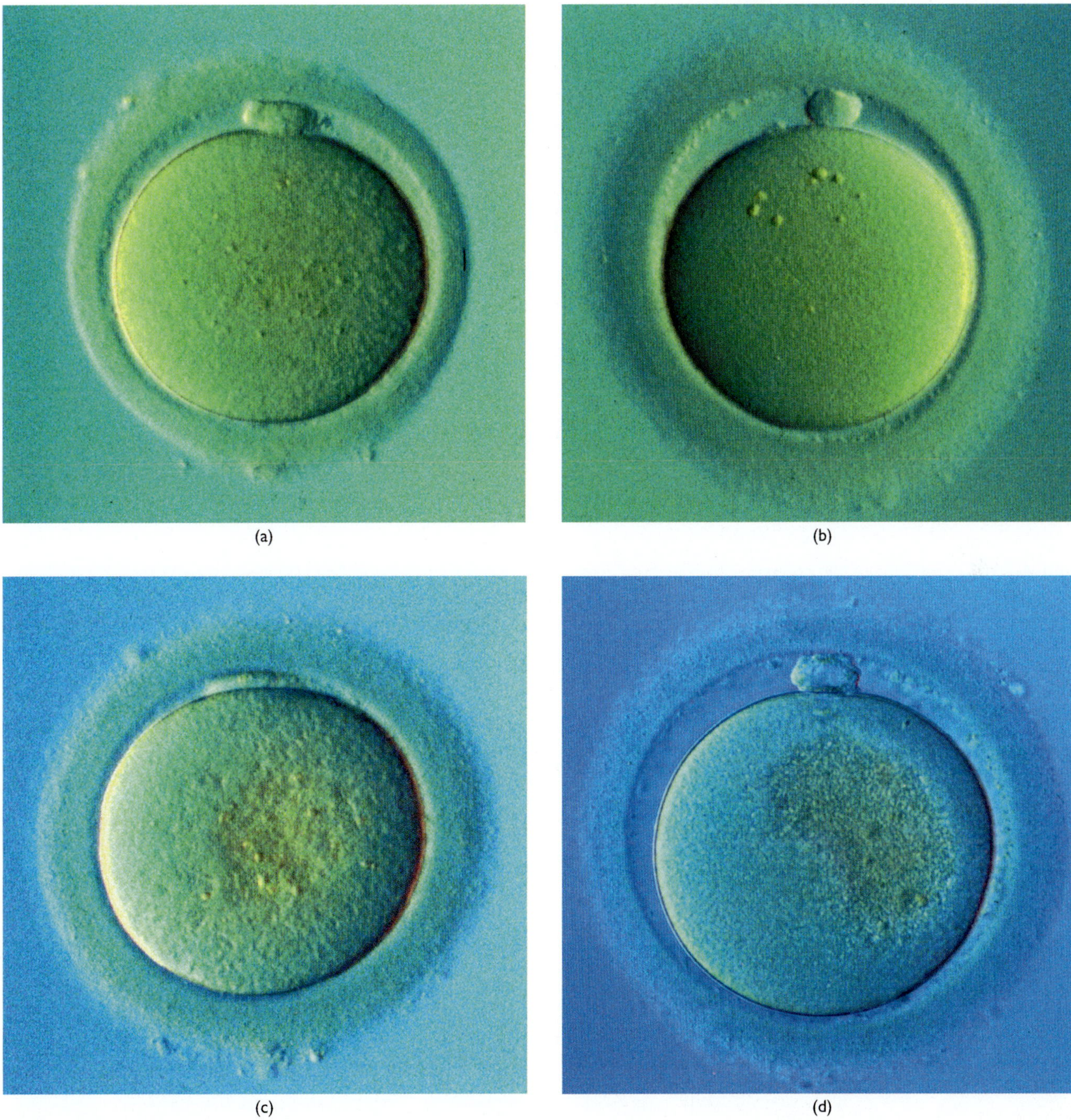

Figure I.9 Metaphase II oocytes with an apparently normal first polar body. Oocytes are round in shape and regular in size. The cytoplasm is homogeneous (a) or contains a few cytoplasmic inclusions (b) and (c) or a coarse-appearing region (d). The perivitelline space is even, except in the area where the first polar body is located. One oval, round or flattened, non-fragmented polar body is visible at the 12 o'clock position in each. For preconception genetic diagnosis, the flattened polar body (c) is removed in culture medium containing 0.1 mol/l sucrose solution in order to increase the perivitelline space by slight shrinkage of the ooplasm (×200).

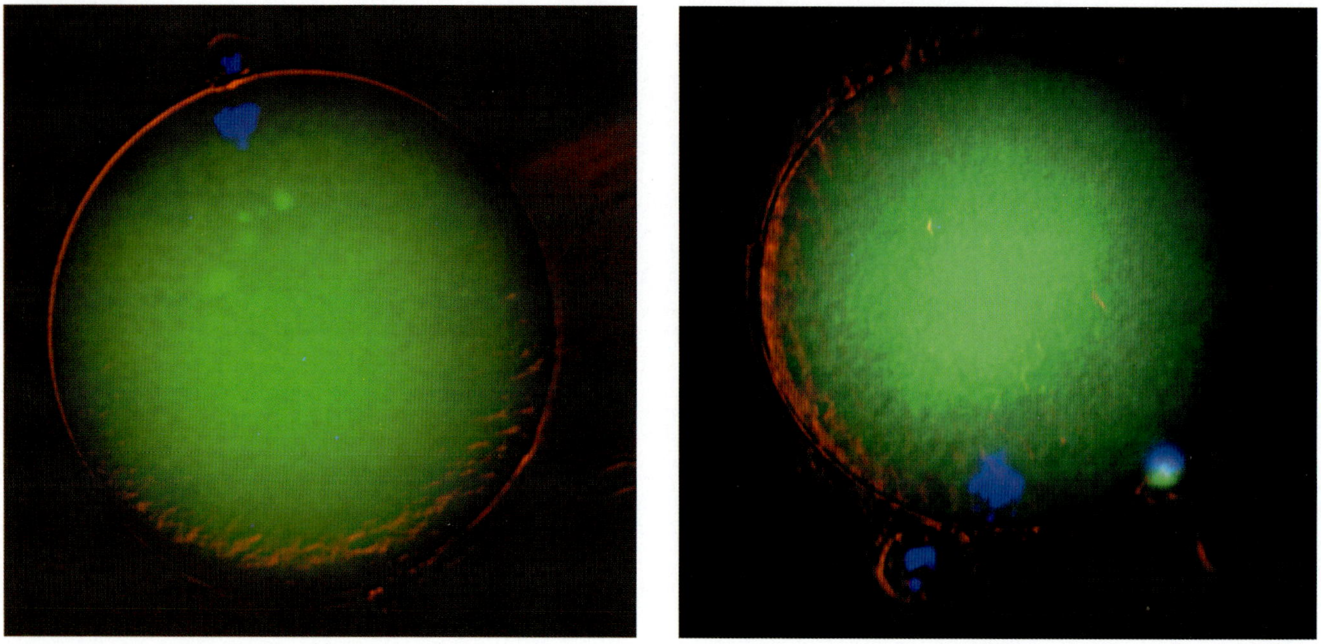

(a) (b)

Figure 1.10 Distribution of mitochondria in metaphase II oocytes: rhodamine staining (bright-field view of the oocyte is shown in red, mitochondria in green, chromatin in blue). (a) The first polar body does not have a significant number of mitochondria detectable at the light microscopy level. (b) A cumulus cell attached to the oocyte serves as a control that the observed phenomenon is not due to an artifact of the staining procedure or due to the polar body size.

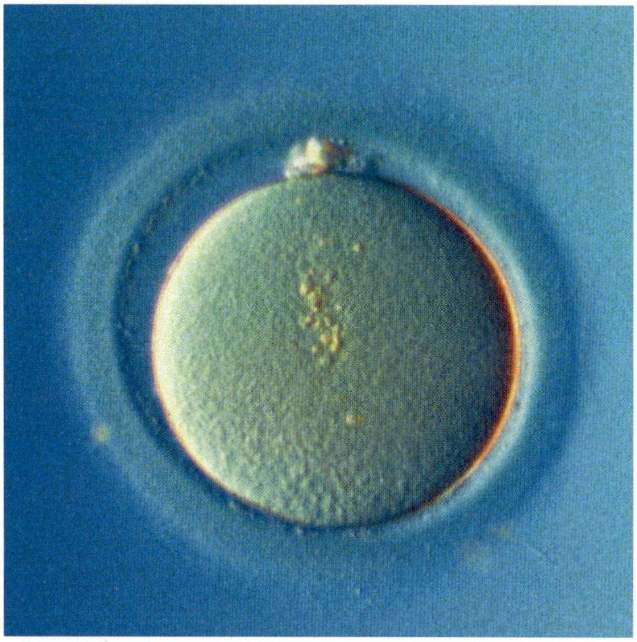

Figure 1.11 Metaphase II oocyte with a fragmented first polar body. The oocyte is round in shape and regular in size. The cytoplasm is granular and contains multiple inclusions tightly positioned in the center of the ooplasm. The perivitelline space is clear. The first polar body, consisting of a cluster of fragments, is visible at the 12 o'clock position (×200).

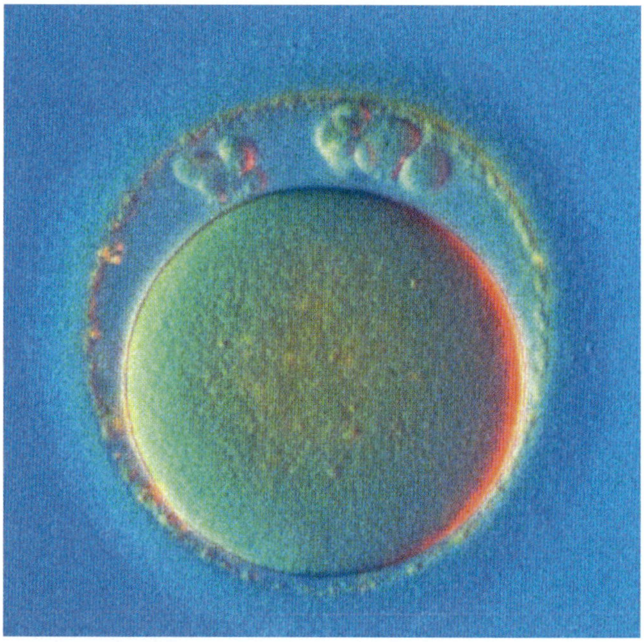

Figure 1.12 Metaphase II oocyte with a fragmented first polar body and additional cytoplasmic fragments. The oocyte is round in shape and regular in size. The cytoplasm has a slightly coarse area in the center of the oocyte. The perivitelline space has a grainy appearance and is enlarged in the area of the fragmented first polar body and the additional cytoplasmic fragments. The zona pellucida is intact and evenly thick along the circumference (×200).

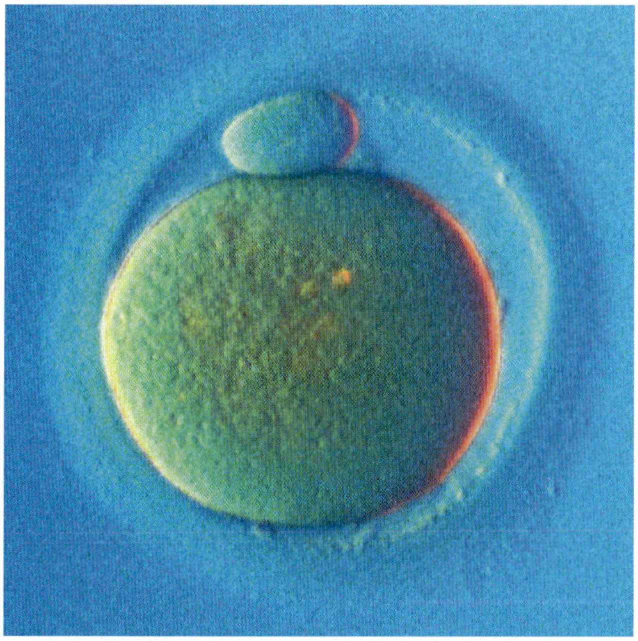

Figure 1.13 Metaphase II oocyte with an enlarged first polar body. The oocyte is round in shape and slightly smaller in size. The cytoplasm is coarse and the perivitelline space is enlarged. One large non-fragmented polar body is visible at the 12 o'clock position (×200).

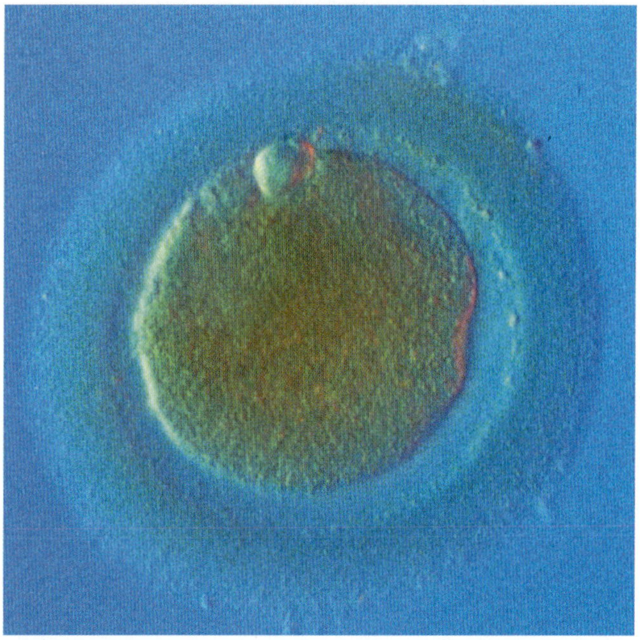

Figure 1.15 Atretic metaphase II oocyte, 40 h after injection of human chorionic gonadotropin, is irregular in shape and reduced in size. The plasma membrane is rough; the cytoplasm is grainy and dark brown in color. The perivitelline space is without debris, and an intact first polar body is visible at the 11 o'clock position. The zona pellucida is intact (×200).

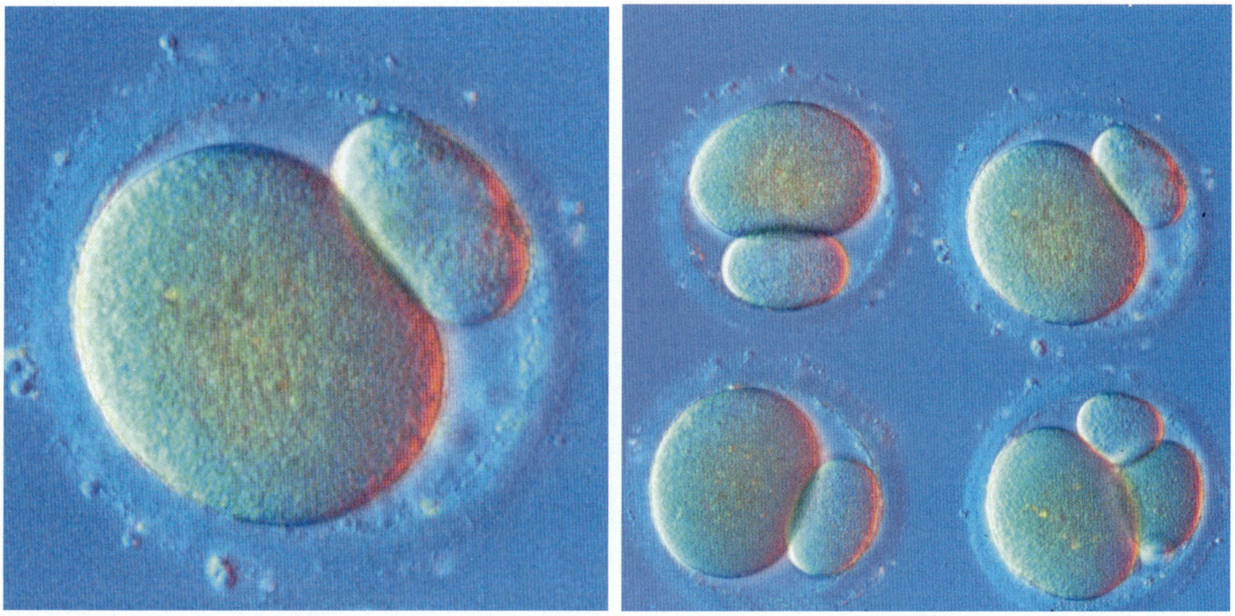

(a) (b)

Figure 1.14 Metaphase II oocytes with abnormal first polar bodies (a) and (b). Oocytes from a harvest of 11, retrieved 36 h after injection of human chorionic gonadotropin. Three of the 11 oocytes were at prophase I, while the remaining eight were with large cytoplasmic structures almost four times the size of a normal first polar body. In two oocytes these structures were divided into two parts. The structures were removed from all oocytes with the aid of a large pipette and analyzed by FISH, revealing chromatin contents similar to those of the first polar body. Sixteen hours after ICSI the oocytes were unevenly divided into two, three, or four fragments with varying numbers of nuclei, suggesting abnormalities in cytokinesis ((a) ×200; (b) ×100).

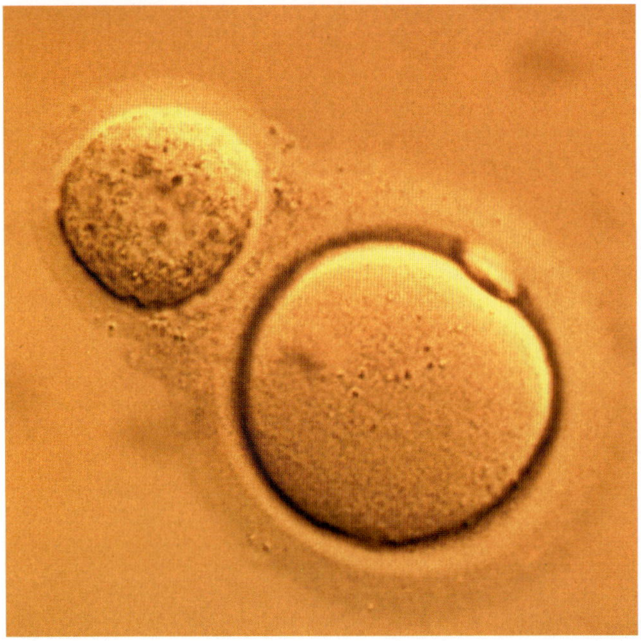

Figure 1.16 Binovular complex with one mature metaphase II and one immature oocyte. The smaller oocyte is at the germinal vesicle stage, and has coarse cytoplasm. The other oocyte is of normal size, with homogeneous cytoplasm with a few inclusions and the first polar body at the 1 o'clock position. Both oocytes are surrounded by a conjoined zona pellucida of an '8-shape' appearance and do not share the same perivitelline space (×200).

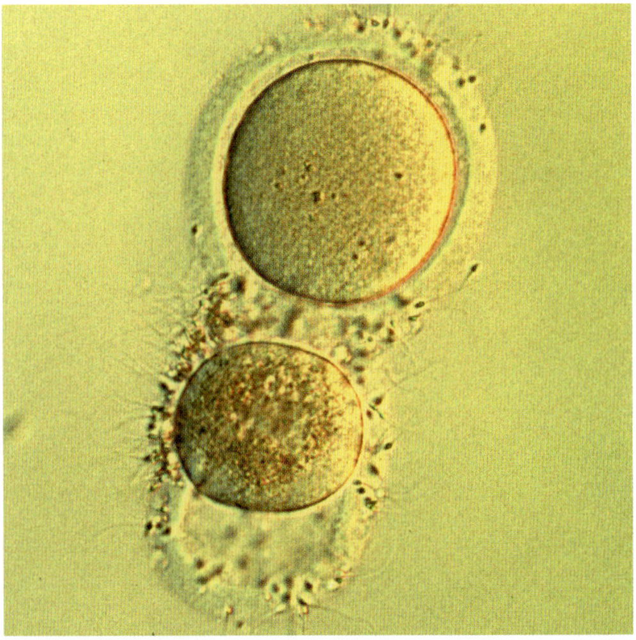

Figure 1.17 Binovular complex following insemination. The smaller oocyte is at the germinal vesicle stage and has coarse, dark cytoplasm. The second, metaphase I, oocyte has a normal size and homogeneous cytoplasm with a few inclusions. No polar body is visible in the perivitelline space. Both oocytes are surrounded by a conjoined zona pellucida, each with a separate perivitelline space. Multiple spermatozoa are seen attached to the zona pellucida (×200).

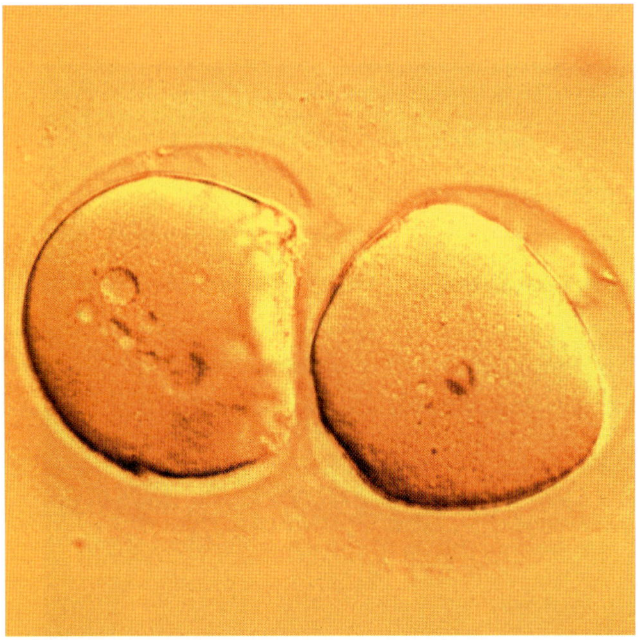

Figure 1.18 Binovular complex consisting of an immature metaphase I and a mature metaphase II oocyte. Both oocytes are irregular in shape, but have a normal size. The oocyte on the left contains several vacuoles and appears to be at metaphase I, since no polar body can be seen. The oocyte on the right has a few inclusions and has completed the first meiotic division, evident by the presence of a polar body at the 1 o'clock position. Both oocytes are surrounded by a conjoined zona pellucida (×200).

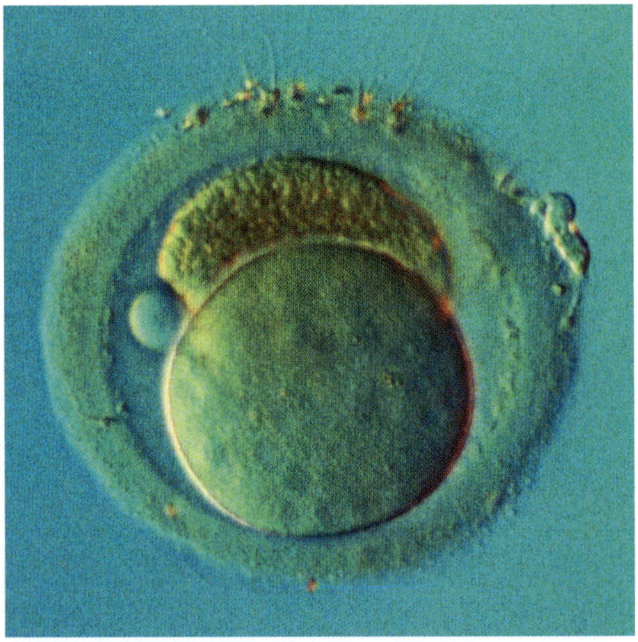

Figure 1.19 Apparently mature oocyte following insemination. The metaphase II oocyte is small and round, containing vacuole-like structures. A round first polar body (PB1) is visible at the 10 o'clock position. There is a dark cytoplasmic structure occupying one-quarter of the subzonal space next to the PB1 and is intimately attached to the plasma membrane of the oocyte. The zona pellucida is intact, unevenly thick along the circumference with multiple spermatozoa attached (×200).

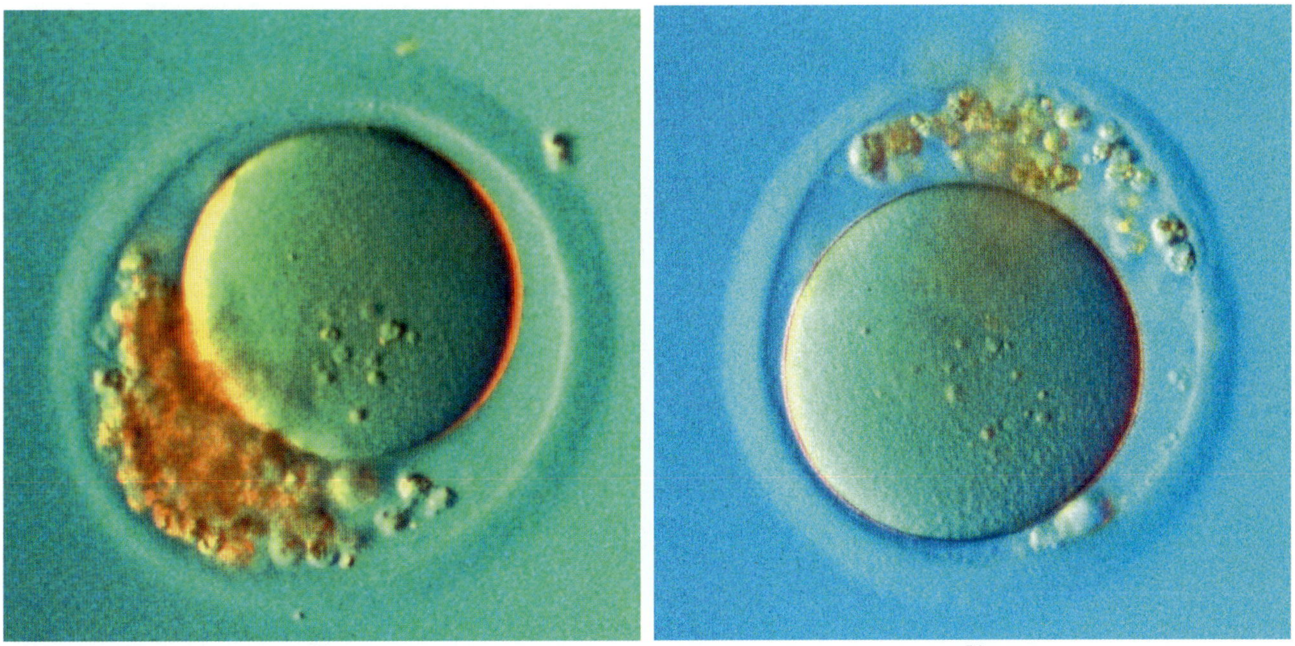

(a) (b)

Figure 1.20 Metaphase II oocytes (a) and (b) with multiple cumulus cells within the perivitelline space. The oocytes are round in shape and small in size. The cytoplasm is homogeneous with several inclusions. The perivitelline space is significantly enlarged, containing multiple cumulus cells. The presence of the first polar body cannot be determined, making the oocytes useless for preconception genetic testing. The zona pellucida is intact, slightly irregular in shape and unevenly thick along the circumference (×200).

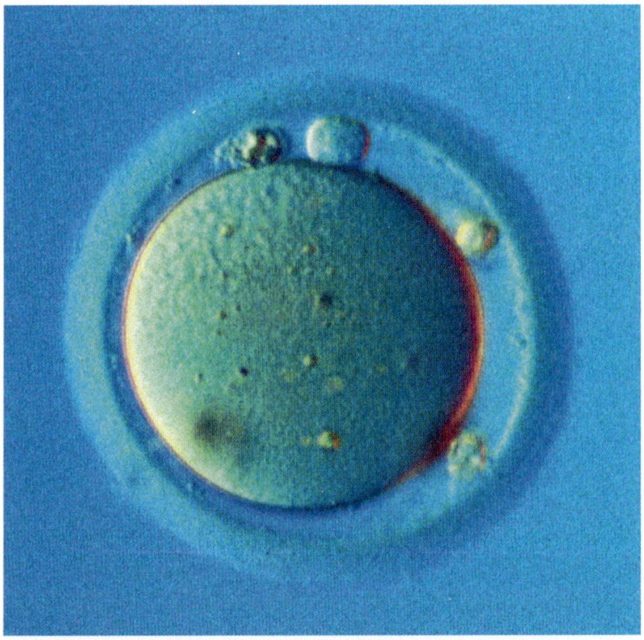

Figure 1.21 Metaphase II oocyte with a few cumulus cell inclusions in the perivitelline space (PVS). The oocyte is round in shape and regular in size. The cytoplasm appears coarse, with several cytoplasmic inclusions. The PVS is slightly enlarged, containing at least four cumulus cells attached to the internal surface of the zona pellucida. The first polar body can be identified at the 12 o'clock position (×200).

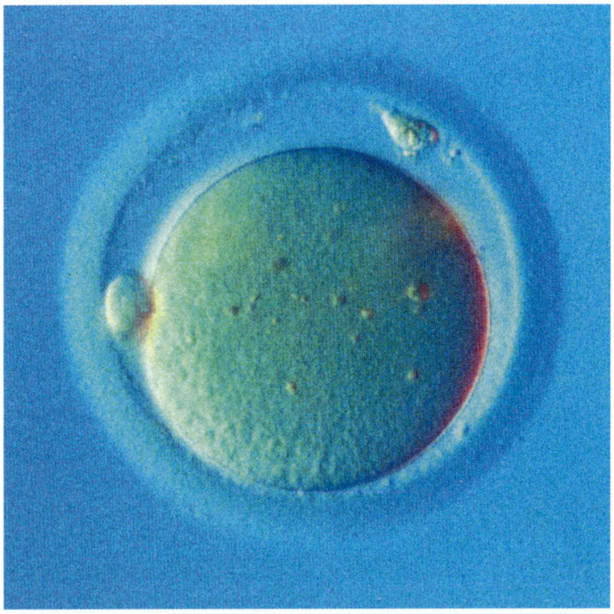

Figure 1.22 Metaphase II oocyte with single cumulus cell inclusion in the perivitelline space (PVS). The oocyte is round in shape and regular in size. The cytoplasm appears coarse and granular along the periphery, with several cytoplasmic inclusions. The first polar body can be identified at the 9 o'clock position. The PVS is slightly enlarged containing one cumulus cell attached to the internal surface of the zona pellucida (×200).

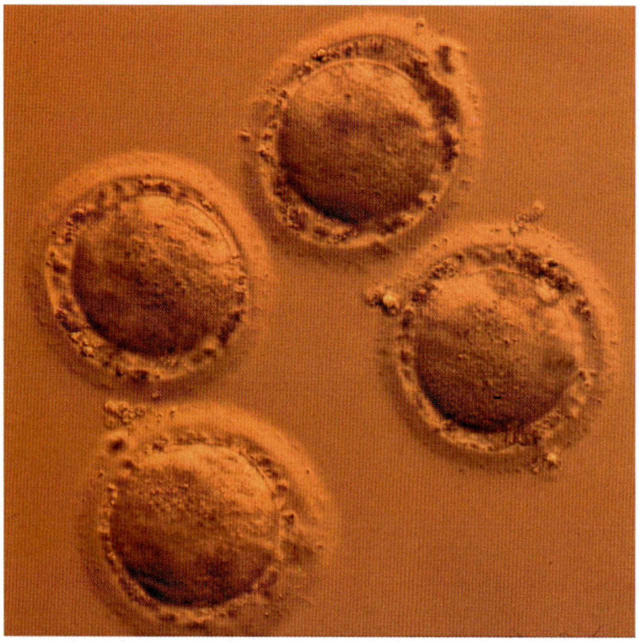

Figure 1.23 Apparently mature metaphase II oocytes with granularity of the perivitelline space (PVS). The oocytes are round in shape. The cytoplasm appears coarse, with many inclusions. One polar body can be identified with difficulty. The PVS is slightly enlarged, containing multiple dark granules and debris, possibly the remnants of corona cells or an extracellular matrix comprising granules and filaments. Although this has no effect on fertilization, cleavage rate and embryo quality, the first polar body removal is complicated in such oocytes, making them of little value for genetic testing (x100).

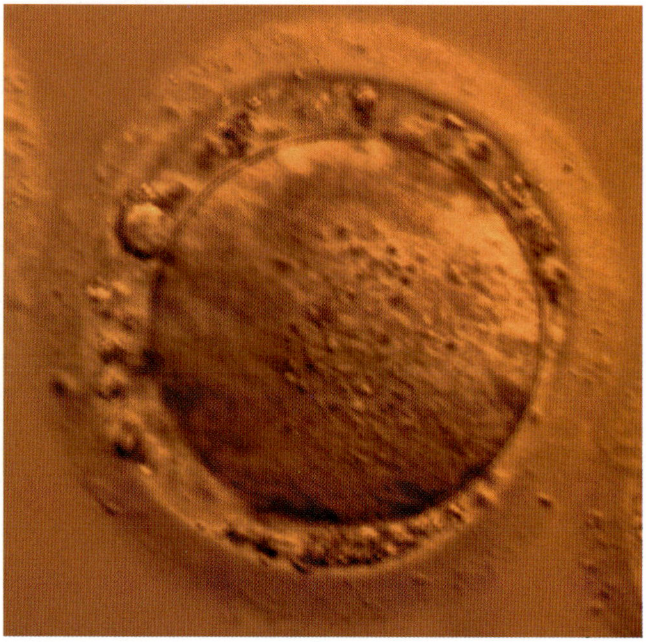

Figure 1.24 Enlarged view of one of the metaphase II oocytes from Figure 1.23.

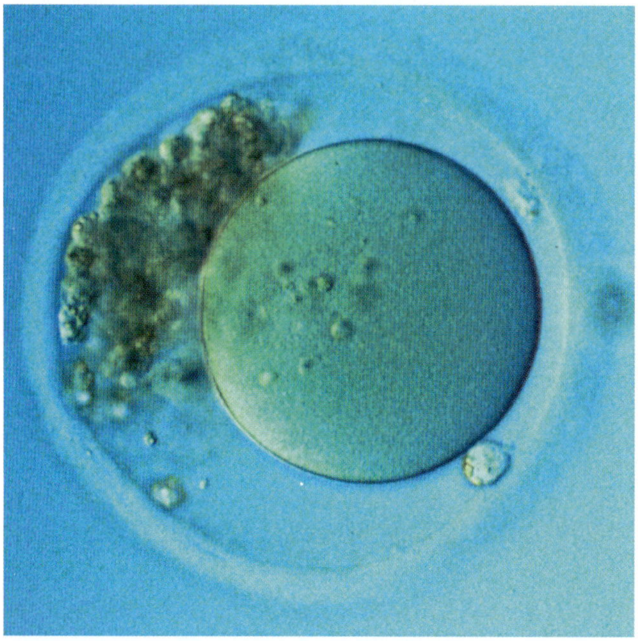

Figure 1.25 Apparently mature metaphase II oocyte with multiple cumulus cells in the perivitelline space (PVS). The oocyte is round in shape and small in size. The cytoplasm is homogeneous with a few inclusions. A questionable first polar body can be seen at the 4–5 o'clock position. The PVS is significantly enlarged, containing multiple cumulus cells, which can be a source of DNA contamination in genetic testing. The zona pellucida is intact and slightly irregular in shape (x400).

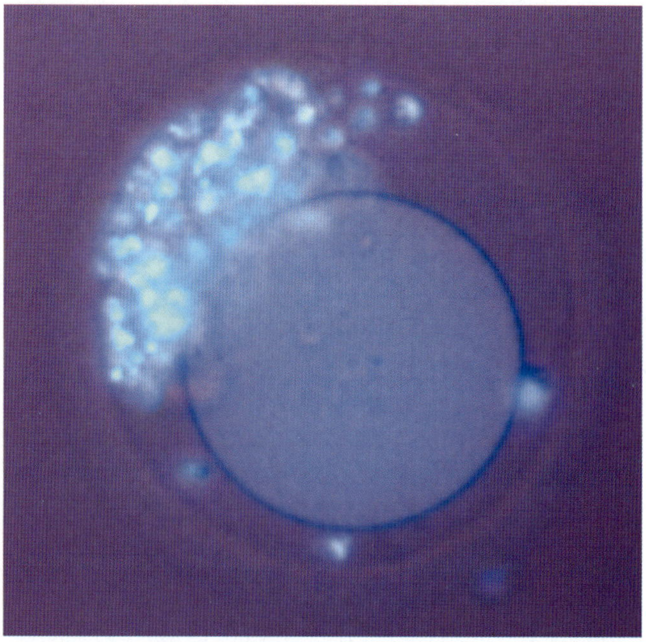

Figure 1.26 Apparently mature metaphase II oocyte with multiple cumulus cells (fluorescent DNA staining). The fluorescence analysis confirms the presence of DNA in multiple cell inclusions localized in the perivitelline space, which can lead to misdiagnosis in genetic testing (x400).

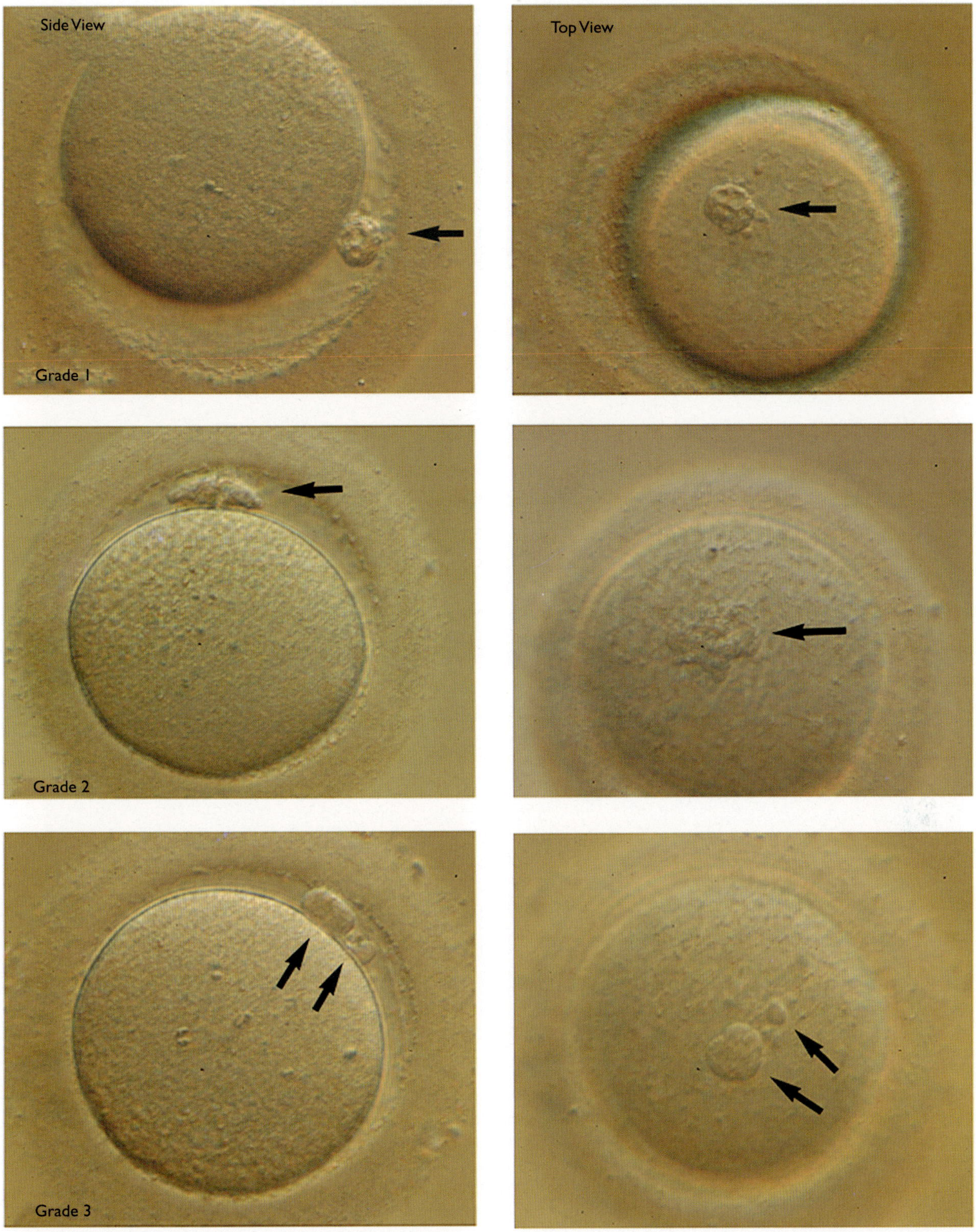

Figure 1.27 Three categories of first polar body (PB1) morphology at day 0 oocyte recovery. Grade 1, an intact, round or oval-shaped PB1; grade 2, an intact (non-fragmented) irregularly shaped PB1; grade 3, a partially or totally fragmented PB1. Observations were made using Hoffman phase-contrast optics at a magnification of ×200. Images of both the side and top view positions were captured.

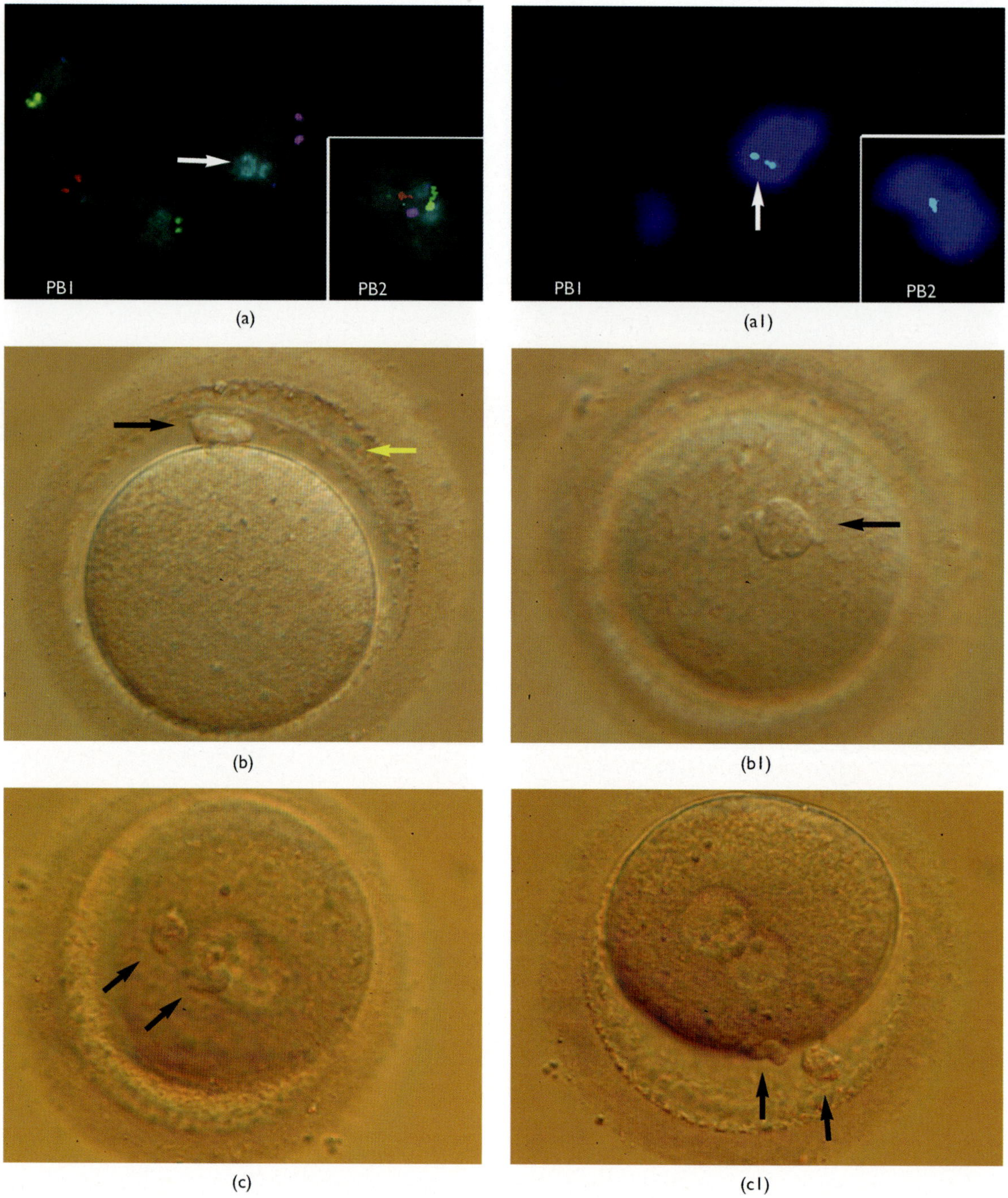

Figure 1.28 Fluorescence *in situ* hybridization (FISH) images of grade 2, slightly irregularly shaped first polar body (PB1). (a) FISH images of PB1 and second polar body (PB2) after a 3-h hybridization with MultiVysion PB panel probe for autosomes 13 (red), 16 (aqua), 18 (violet blue), 21 (green), and 22 (gold), removed simultaneously on day 1 at the pronuclear stage of development (c) following fertilization assessment of an oocyte retrieved from a 40-year-old woman. A normal number of signals are present for four of the five autosomes tested in PB1 with the exception of chromosome 16, in which one of two signals in close proximity is split (white arrow). PB2 contains a normal number of signals with the exception of chromosome 16, about which no conclusion can be made owing to two areas of diffuse aqua background, necessitating a second round of testing. (a1) Rehybridization of PB1 and PB2 for chromosome 16 targeting a different locus using sub-telomeric 16p (green) in which two signals are present in PB1 (white arrow) and one signal in PB2 indicating a normal chromosome complement in the oocyte. (b) Mature metaphase II oocyte with a grade 2 PB1 (black arrow) corresponding to the FISH images in (a) and (a1). A bilayer defect in the zona pellucida can be seen at the top right (yellow arrow). The oocyte is round with a homogeneous cytoplasm. (b1) Top view of the slightly irregular-shaped PB1 (black arrow). (c) The same oocyte as shown in (b), 18 h post-intracytoplasmic sperm injection (ICSI). Top view of PB1 and PB2 (black arrows) located in close proximity to one another and both of which are irregular in shape. (c1) Two pronuclei, both of which consist of partially aligned nucleoli of differing sizes, are visible along with two polar bodies (black arrows).

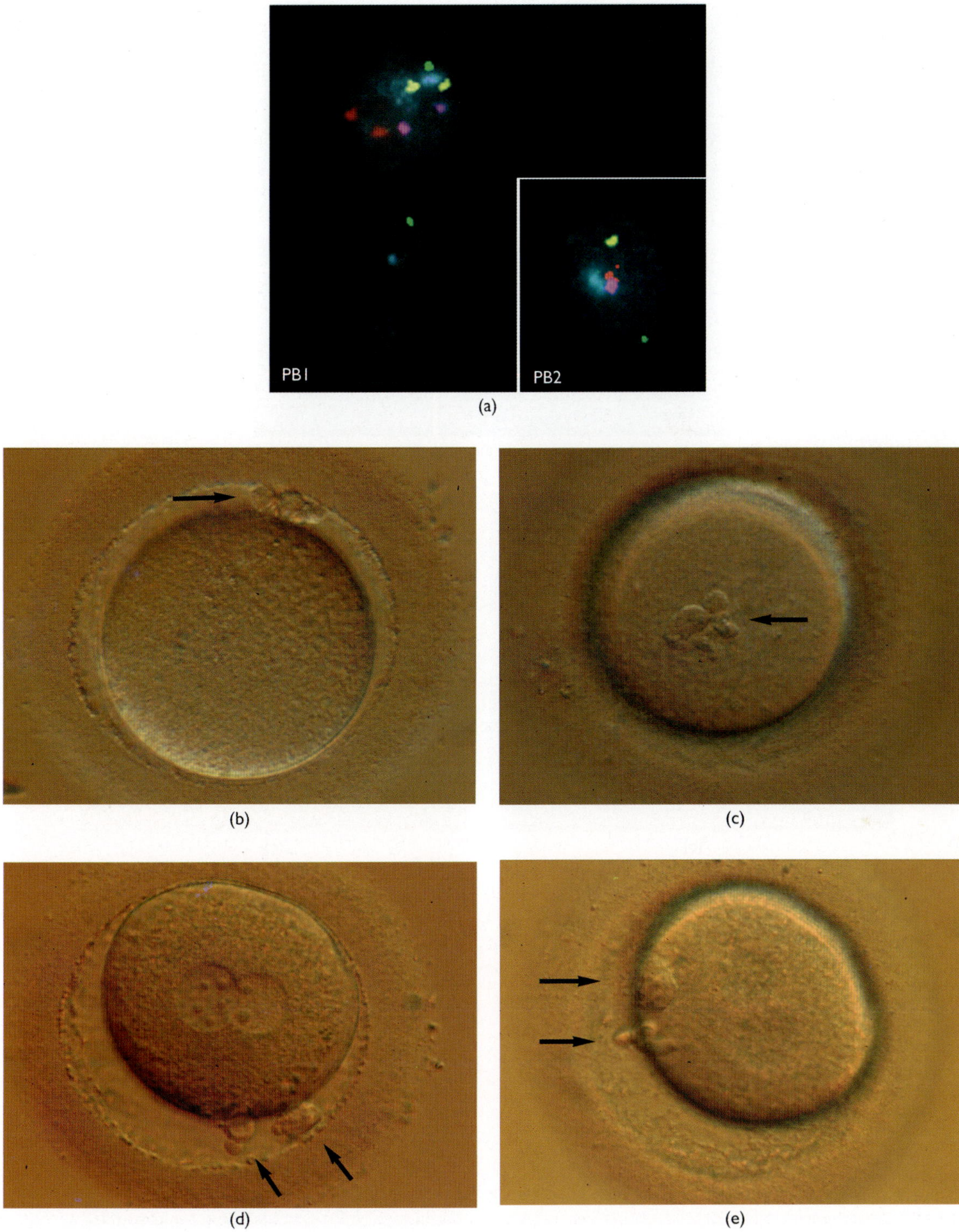

Figure 1.29 Fluorescence *in situ* hybridization (FISH) images of a grade 3 (fragmented) first polar body (PB1). (a) FISH images of PB1 and second polar body (PB2) after a 3-h hybridization with MultiVysion PB panel probe for autosomes 13 (red), 16 (aqua), 18 (violet blue), 21 (green), and 22 (gold), removed simultaneously on day 1 at the pronuclear stage of development (d) and (e) following fertilization assessment of an oocyte retrieved from the same 40-year-old woman as in Figure 1.28, showing a normal number of signals in both PB1 and PB2. (b) Mature metaphase II oocyte with a grade 3 PB1 (black arrow) corresponding to the FISH image in (a). The oocyte is round with a homogeneous cytoplasm surrounded by a thick zona pellucida. (c) Top view of the fragmented PB1 appearing as a grape-like cluster (black arrow). (d) The same oocyte shown in (b), 18 h post-intracytoplasmic sperm injection (ICSI). Two pronuclei with non-aligned nucleoli are visible along with PB1 and PB2 at 5 o'clock (black arrows). (e) Top view of PB1 and PB2. PB2 has an irregular 'S' type shape; a faint outline of the pronuclei can be seen in the center.

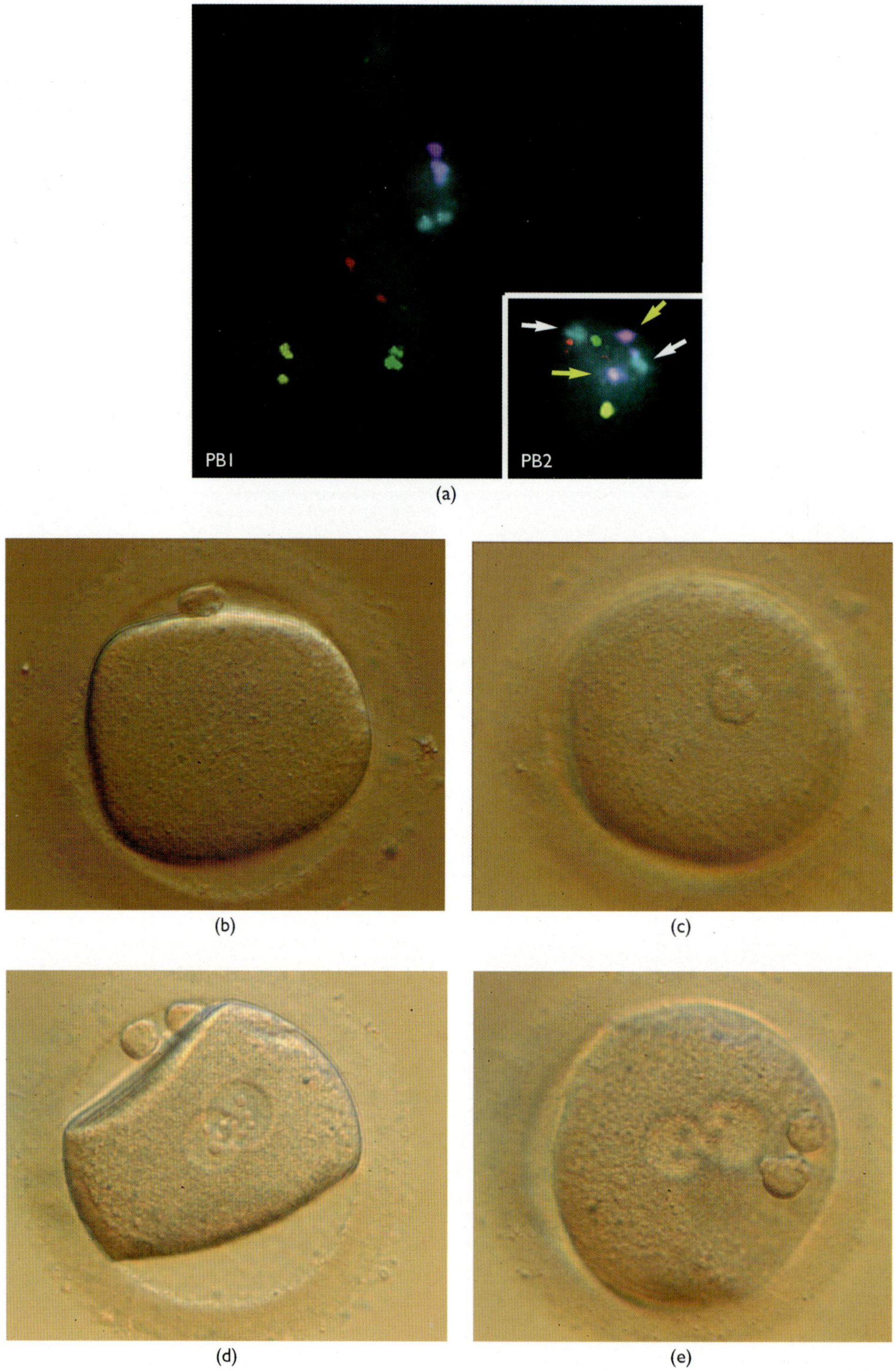

Figure 1.30 Fluorescence *in situ* hybridization (FISH) images of a grade 1 (round) first polar body (PB1). (a) FISH images of PB1 and second polar body (PB2) after a 3-h hybridization with MultiVysion PB panel probe for autosomes 13 (red), 16 (aqua), 18 (violet blue), 21 (green), and 22 (gold), removed simultaneously on day 1 at the pronuclear stage of development (d) and (e) following fertilization assessment of an oocyte retrieved from the same 40-year-old woman as in Figure 1.28, showing a normal number of signals in PB1, but additional signals for chromosomes 16 (white arrows) and 18 (yellow arrows) in PB2 indicating a nullisomic oocyte for chromosomes 16 and 18, which will result in a double monosomic embryo. (b) Mature metaphase II oocyte with a grade 1 PB1 corresponding to the FISH image in (a). The oocyte is irregular in shape with a homogeneous cytoplasm surrounded by a thick zona pellucida. (c) Top view of the grade 1 PB1. (d) Side view of PB1 and PB2, both appearing to be round, while the fertilized oocyte containing two pronuclei with scattered nucleoli is grossly irregular in shape. (e) Top view of both polar bodies in close proximity to one another.

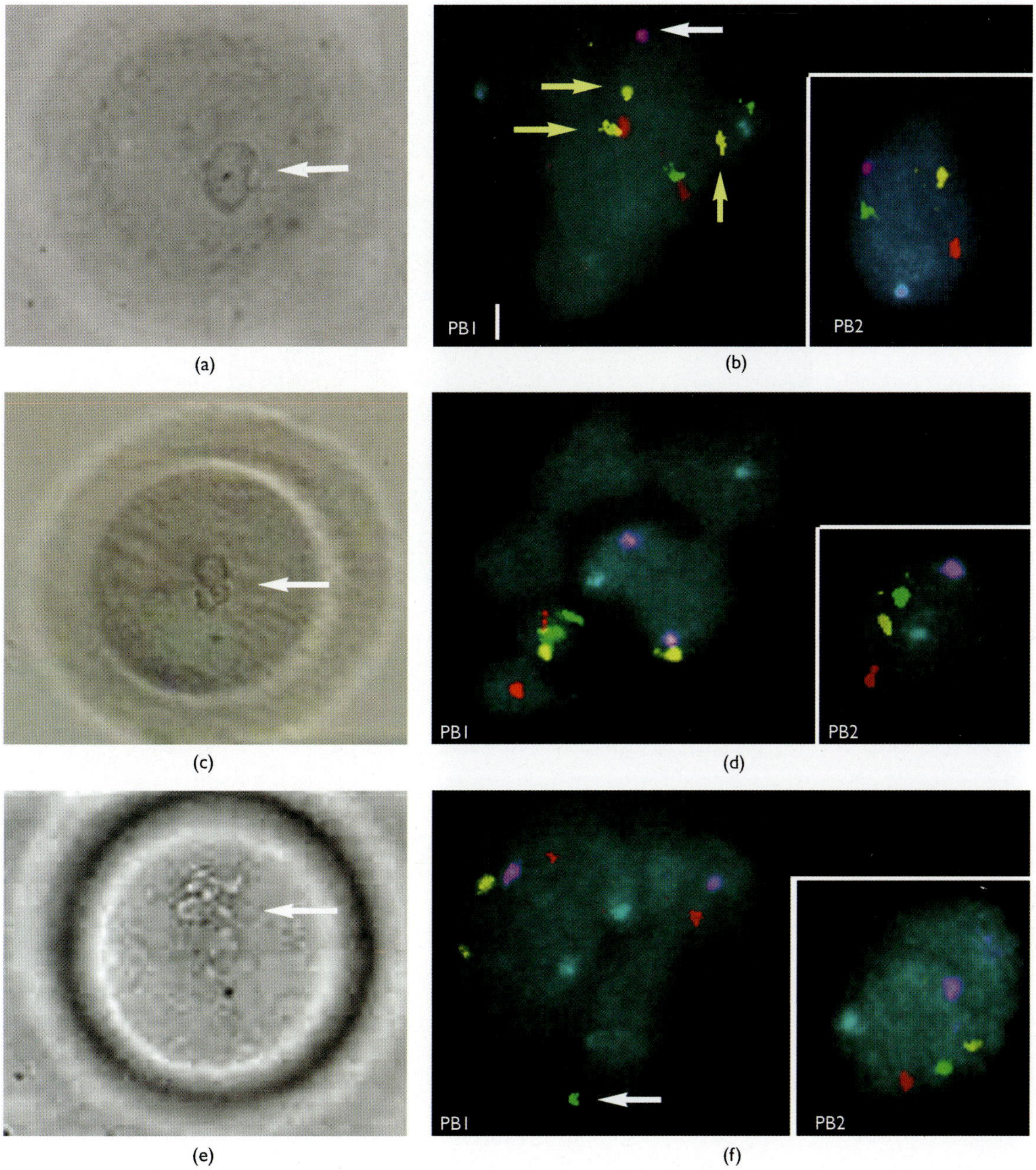

Figure 1.31 First polar body (PB1) morphology with corresponding fluorescence *in situ* hybridization (FISH) results. (a) Phase-contrast image of a mature metaphase II oocyte with a grade 2 PB1 (slightly irregular in shape) (white arrow) retrieved from a 42-year-old patient. (b) FISH image of the same PB1 chromatin and corresponding PB2 nucleus obtained on day 1, following fertilization. Hybridization was performed using MultiVysion PB panel probe for chromosomes 13, 16, 18, 21, and 22, showing complex errors evident from an additional signal for chromosome 22 (yellow arrows) and only one signal for chromosome 18 (white arrow) in PB1. A normal number of signals (one for each chromosome) is present in PB2. Based on the PB findings the resulting oocyte is expected to be nullisomic for chromosome 22 and disomic for chromosome 18, which will result in an embryo with a trisomy 18 and monosomy 22. (c) Phase-contrast image of a mature metaphase II oocyte with a grade 3 PB1 (fragmented) (white arrow) obtained from a 37-year-old woman. (d) FISH image of this PB1 chromatin and the corresponding PB2 nucleus obtained on day 1, following fertilization. Hybridization was performed using MultiVysion PB panel probe for chromosomes 13, 16, 18, 21, and 22, showing a normal number of signals for each of the autosomes tested in both PB1 and PB2. (e) Phase-contrast image of a mature metaphase II oocyte with a grade 3 PB1 (fragmented) (white arrow) retrieved from a 38-year-old woman. (f) FISH image of this PB1 chromatin and corresponding PB2 nucleus obtained on day 1 following fertilization. Hybridization was performed using MultiVysion PB panel probe for chromosomes 13, 16, 18, 21, and 22, showing a normal number of signals for four of the five chromosomes tested with the exception of chromosome 21, in which only one signal is seen (white arrow). Based on this and also a normal number of signals present in the PB2 nucleus, this oocyte is predicted to contain an extra chromatid 21 leading to trisomy 21 in the embryo.

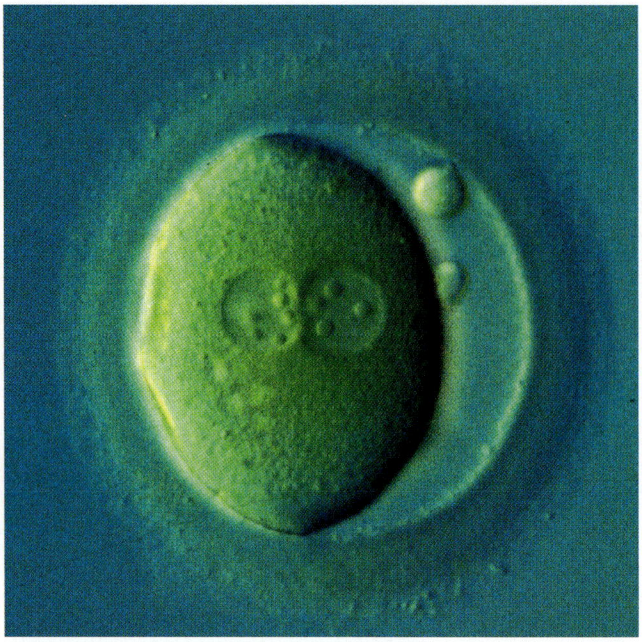

Figure 1.32 Normal fertilization after ICSI. A prezygote of smaller size and irregular shape 18h after ICSI. The cytoplasm contains a few inclusions. Two equal-sized pronuclei are visible in the cytoplasm. Six nucleoli can be counted inside the left pronucleus and approximately four in the right pronucleus. The perivitelline space (PVS) is slightly enlarged, containing two polar bodies at the 1–2 o'clock position. The first polar body is larger and round, and lies freely in the PVS, completely separated from the plasma membrane. The second polar body is almost half as small, round in shape, and attached to the plasma membrane (x200).

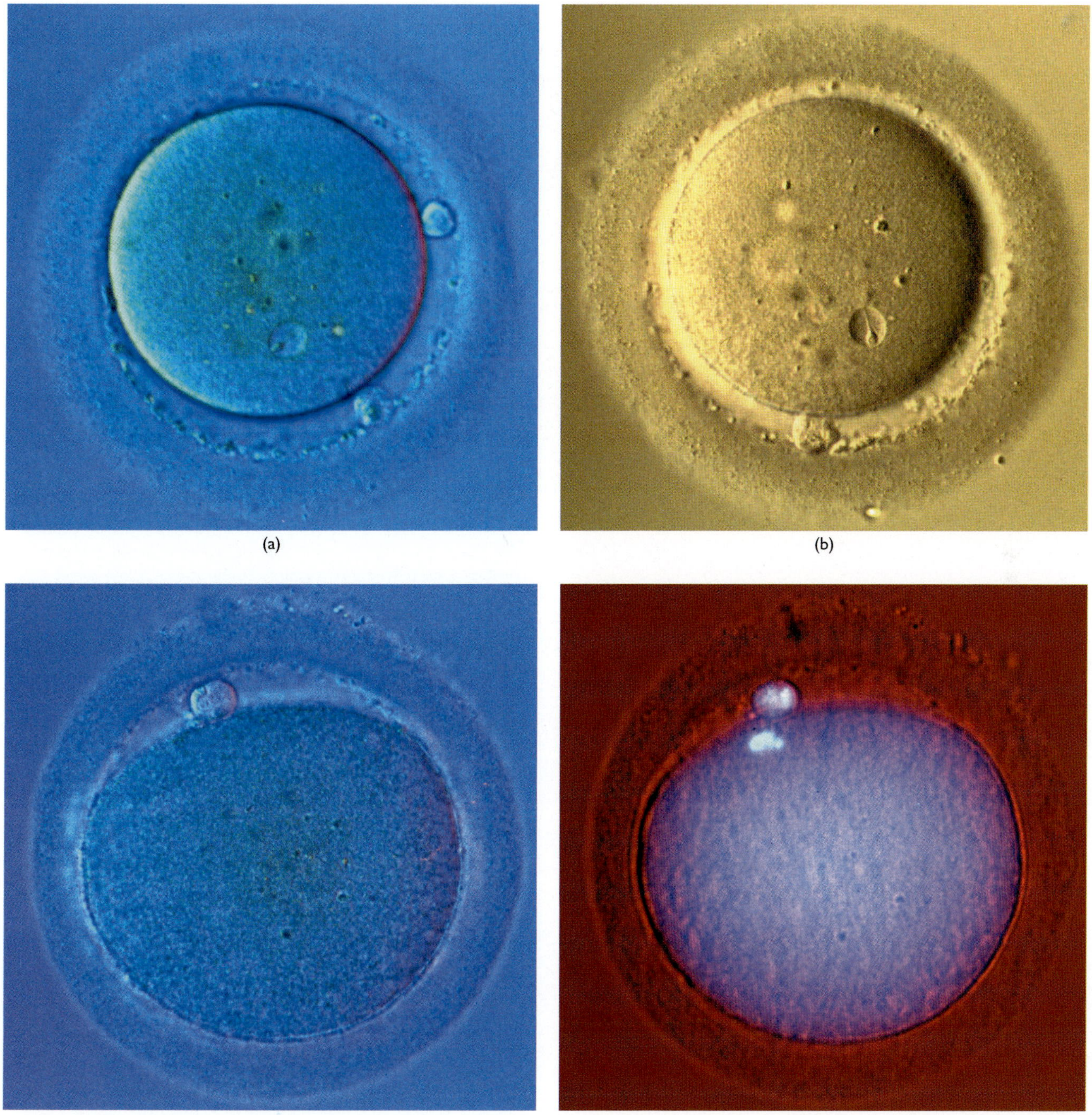

(a) (b) (c) (d)

Figure 1.33 Fertilization failure after insemination or ICSI. Metaphase II oocytes 18 h after ICSI or insemination; no pronuclei are visible. A round vacuole containing an intact spermatozoon can be seen just inside the periphery (a) and (b), which suggests that the plasma membrane of these oocytes was not broken during ICSI. Only one polar body is visible in each oocyte, corresponding to inactivation of the oocyte. A cumulus cell inclusion is visible at the 5 o'clock position (a) in the perivitelline space. Fluorescence DNA analysis (Hoechst staining) (d) of the same oocyte shown in (c) confirms the presence of the first polar body chromatin juxtaposed to the chromosomes of the oocyte. There is no additional fluorescence corresponding to the presence of spermatozoa (×400).

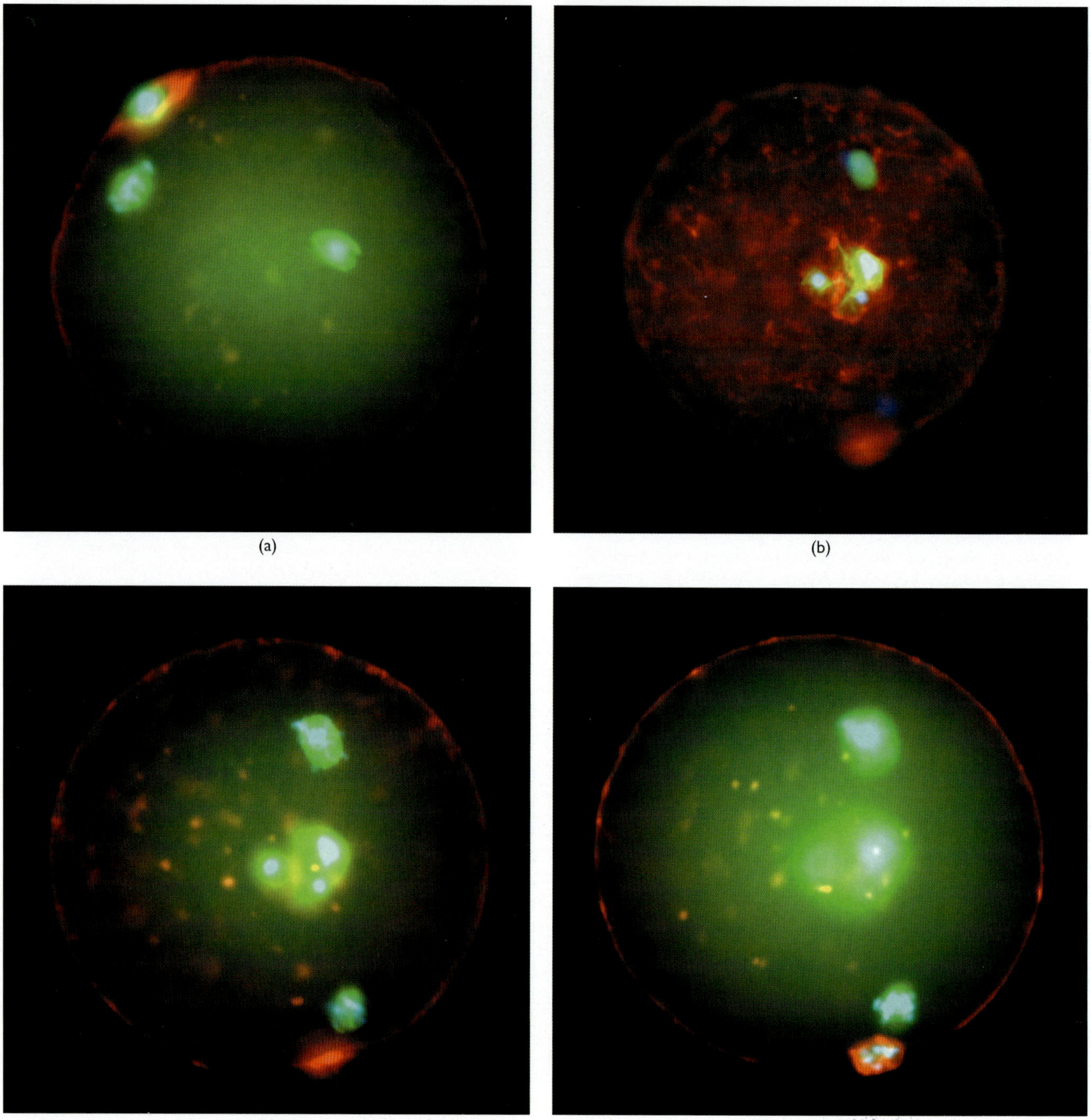

(a) (b) (c) (d)

Figure 1.34 Fertilization failure following initial activation and extrusion of the second polar body (PB2) (actin is seen as red, tubulin as green, and chromatin as blue). (a) First polar body (PB1), oocyte metaphase, and spindle around prematurely condensed sperm chromatin (PCC) can be seen. After activation and decondensation of the sperm head, the oocyte returns to its initial metaphase II-like state (metaphase III phase) without extruding the PB2. (b–d) Three focal planes of an oocyte, which extruded the PB2 body after activation, before entering the metaphase III state. (b) Focal plane at the PB1. (c) Focal plane at the metaphase III spindle and sperm PCC spindle. (d) Focal plane at the PB2.

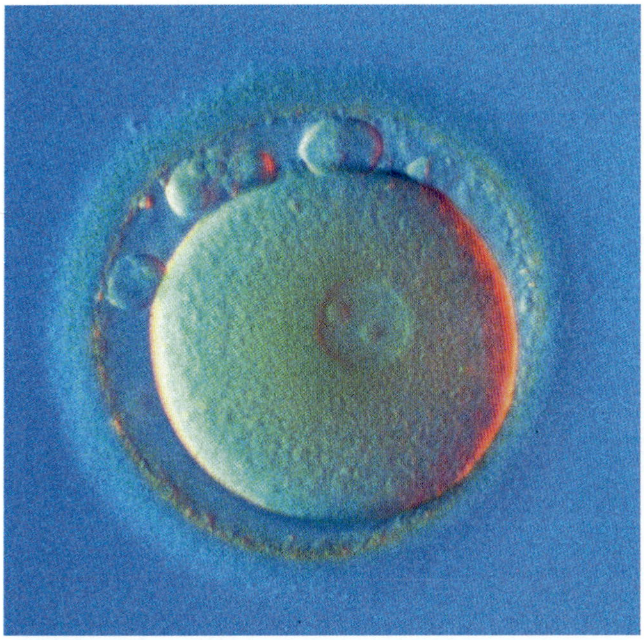

Figure 1.35 Abnormal fertilization after ICSI. An oocyte 18 h after ICSI is of regular size and shape. A single, large pronucleus is present with three visible nucleoli. The cytoplasm appears grainy around the pronucleus and in the center of this abnormal zygote. The perivitelline space is slightly enlarged, containing multiple small granules. Five or six different-sized cytoplasmic extrusions including polar bodies are visible at the 11–12 o'clock position. Prior to ICSI, an intact first polar body was seen (x200).

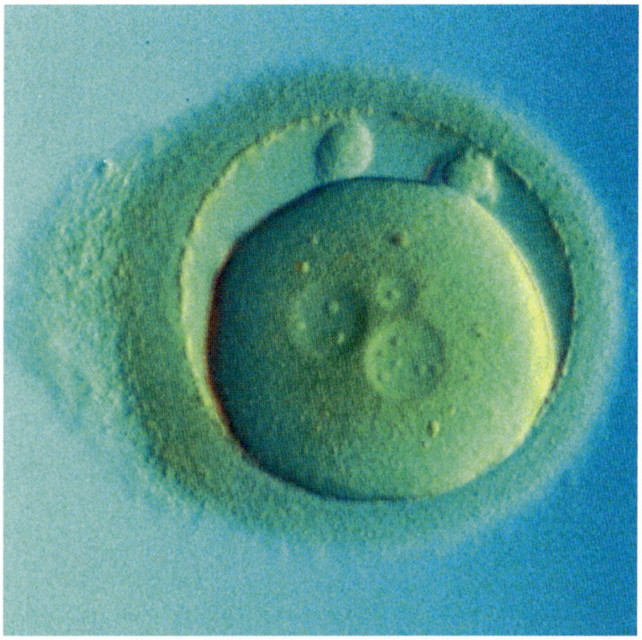

Figure 1.36 Abnormal fertilization after ICSI. An abnormal prezygote of smaller size 18 h after ICSI. The cytoplasm is homogeneous, containing a few inclusions. Three pronuclei are present: two pronuclei of regular and equal size and one small pronucleus. Different numbers of nucleoli are visible in each pronucleus. The perivitelline space is slightly enlarged, with two polar bodies visible at the 12–1 o'clock position. Both intact polar bodies are of equal size and round, and seem attached to the plasma membrane. The zona pellucida is intact, unevenly thick along the circumference with significant deformation on the left side (x200).

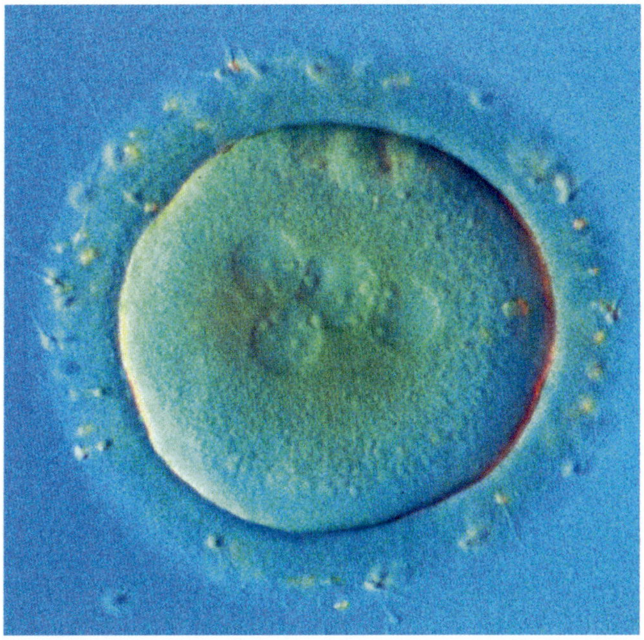

Figure 1.37 Abnormal fertilization after insemination. An abnormal prezygote, 18 h after insemination, has four regular pronuclei of equal size. Different numbers of nucleoli are visible within each pronucleus. The perivitelline space is almost absent. One fragmented polar body is present at the 12 o'clock position (out of focus). The zona pellucida is intact and evenly thick along the circumference, with multiple spermatozoa attached (x400).

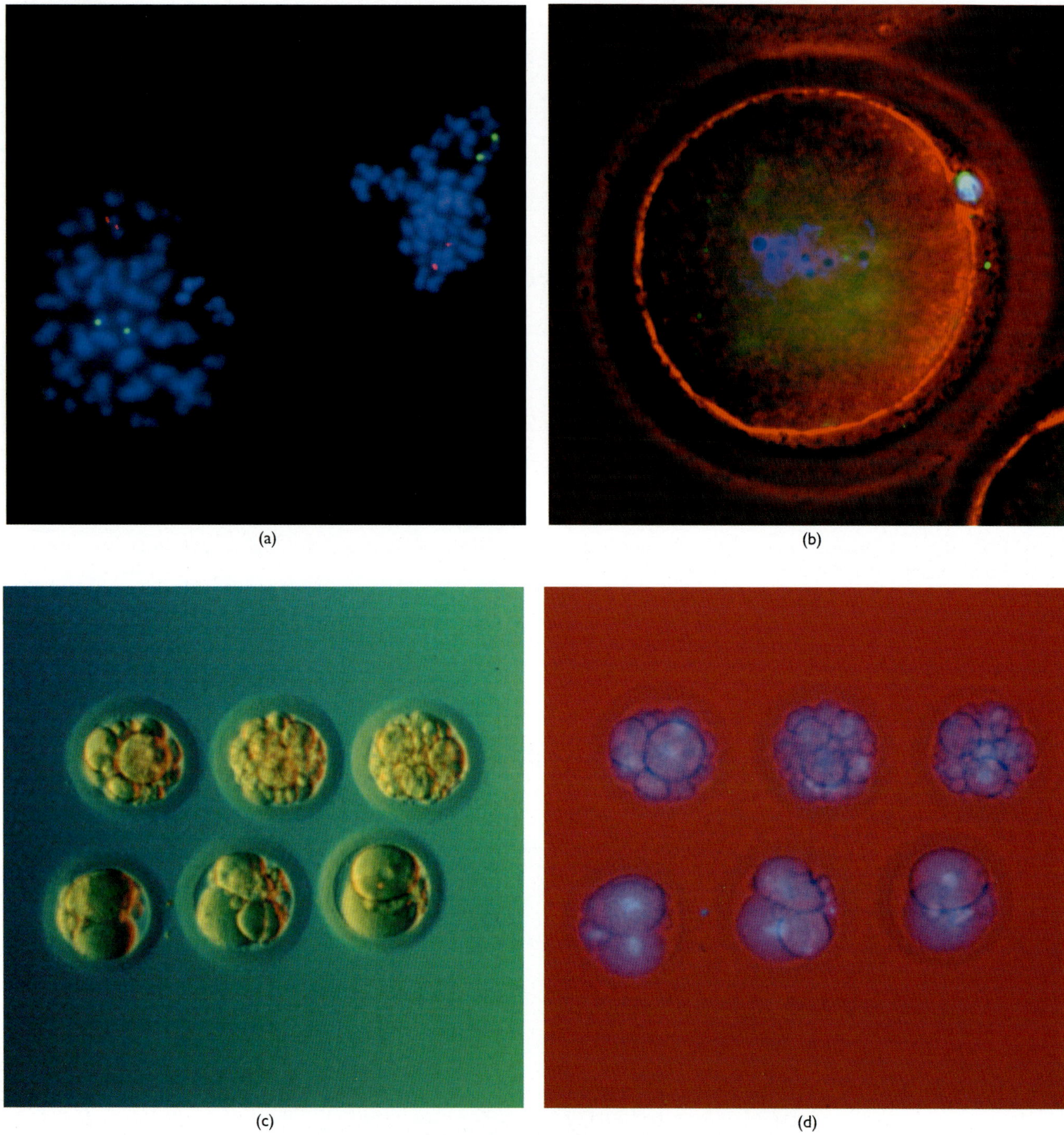

Figure 1.38 Fertilization and development of oocytes matured *in vitro* for 24–48 h from the germinal vesicle or metaphase I stages. (a) Fluorescence *in situ* hybridization of *in vitro*-matured metaphase II oocyte (chromosome 18, CEP aqua; chromosome 21, LSI red). Euploid metaphase II oocyte with paired red and aqua signals is seen on the left, and the corresponding euploid first polar body chromosomes with an identical number of signals are seen on the right. (b) Normal fertilization of *in vitro*-matured metaphase II oocytes after ICSI, resulting in a perfectly normal diploid zygote (tubulin is immunostained in green, and chromatin DAPI in blue). (c) Poor *in vitro* development of zygotes resulting from *in vitro*-matured metaphase II oocytes. These embryos are extremely sensitive to suboptimal *in vitro* conditions. (d) The same embryos after chromatin visualization with Hoechst stain. Anucleate fragments are seen.

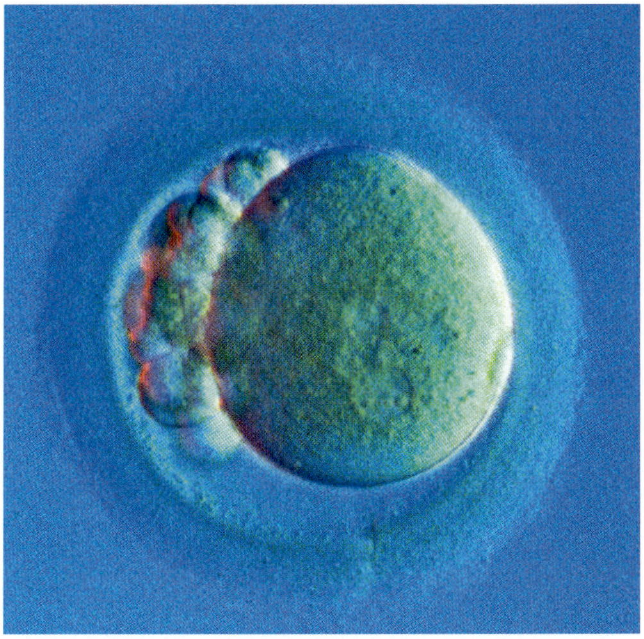

Figure 1.39 Day-2 embryo with failed first cleavage. Uneven distribution of zygote cytoplasm is seen in this embryo originating from a two-pronucleate zygote. A single, larger multinucleated blastomere, containing five small nuclei, is present along with multiple cytoplasmic fragments. Further development of such an embryo is unlikely (×200).

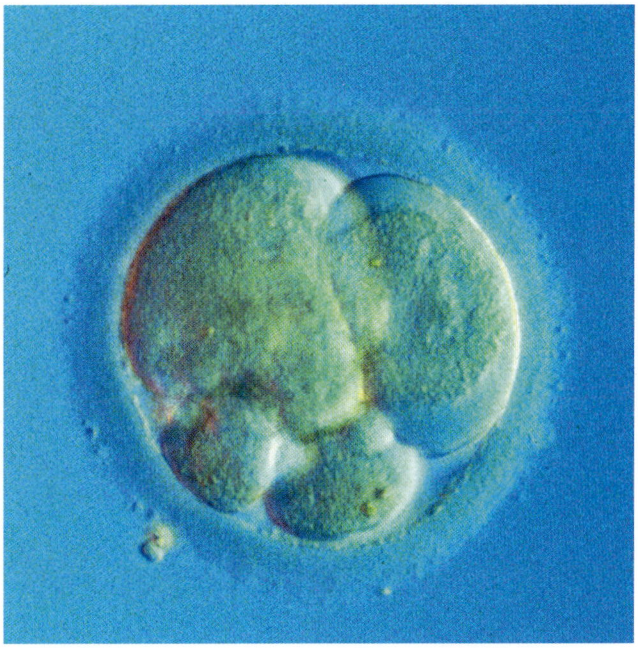

Figure 1.40 Day-2 embryo with asymmetric first cleavage. The day-2 embryo is still in process of the first cleavage, with uneven distribution of zygote cytoplasm. Further development of this embryo is unlikely (×200).

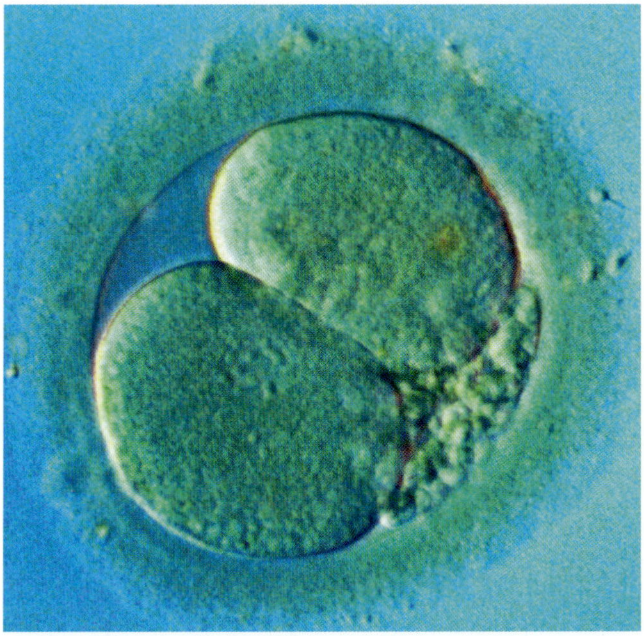

Figure 1.41 Two-cell embryo with slightly asymmetric division and fragmentation. Slightly uneven distribution of zygote cytoplasm is seen in this day-2 embryo, consisting of two blastomeres, one slightly larger than the other, with an additional fragmented portion. No nuclei are visible in the blastomeres (×200).

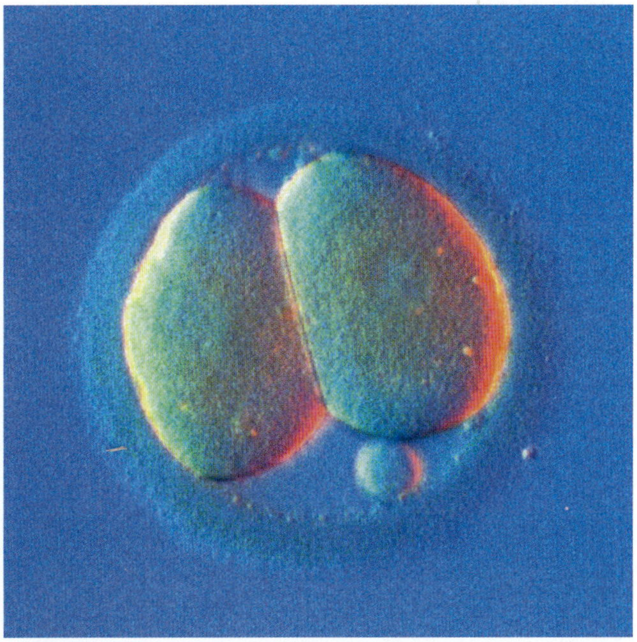

Figure 1.42 Typical two-cell embryo. Two equal-sized blastomeres are present in this day-2 embryo resulting from an even distribution of zygote cytoplasm. A first polar body is visible at the 5 o'clock position. The other polar body is obscured by the blastomere. Each of the blastomeres contains one nucleus (×200).

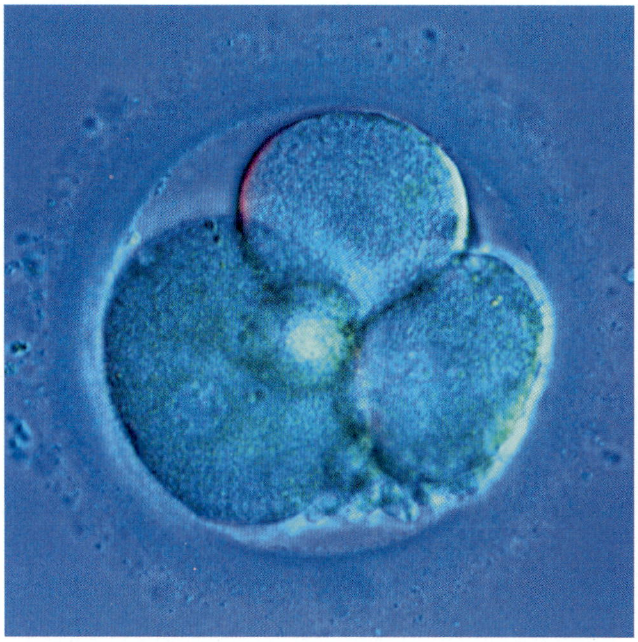

Figure 1.43 Three-cell embryo exhibiting asynchronous division and multinucleation. Three blastomeres, one large and two of equal size, are seen in this day-2 embryo with slight fragmentation at the 5 o'clock position. Three nuclei are visible in the larger blastomere, while no visible nuclei are present in the others. This may be the result of asynchrony in the cell cycle between two original blastomeres in which the second division was completed by only one (×200).

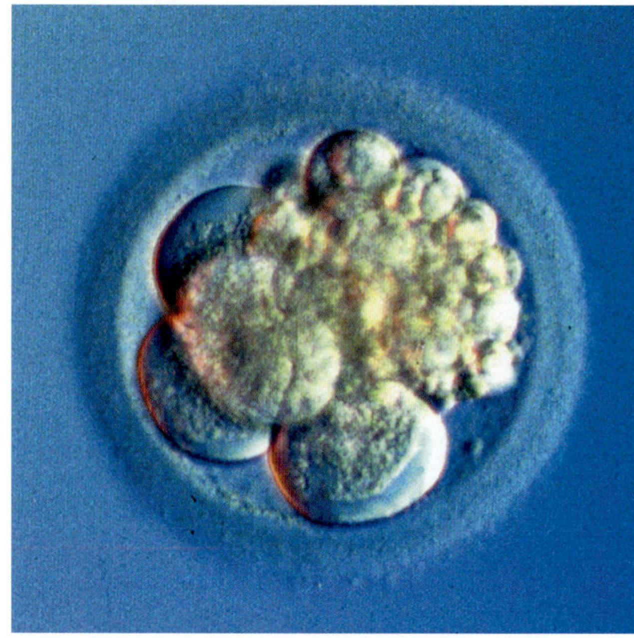

Figure 1.44 Morphologically abnormal four-cell embryo with fragmentation. Four round blastomeres, slightly different in size, are observed in this day-2 embryo with an extensive cytoplasmic fragmentation occupying nearly half of the subzonal space. The viability of such embryos is extremely poor; they usually undergo developmental arrest (×200).

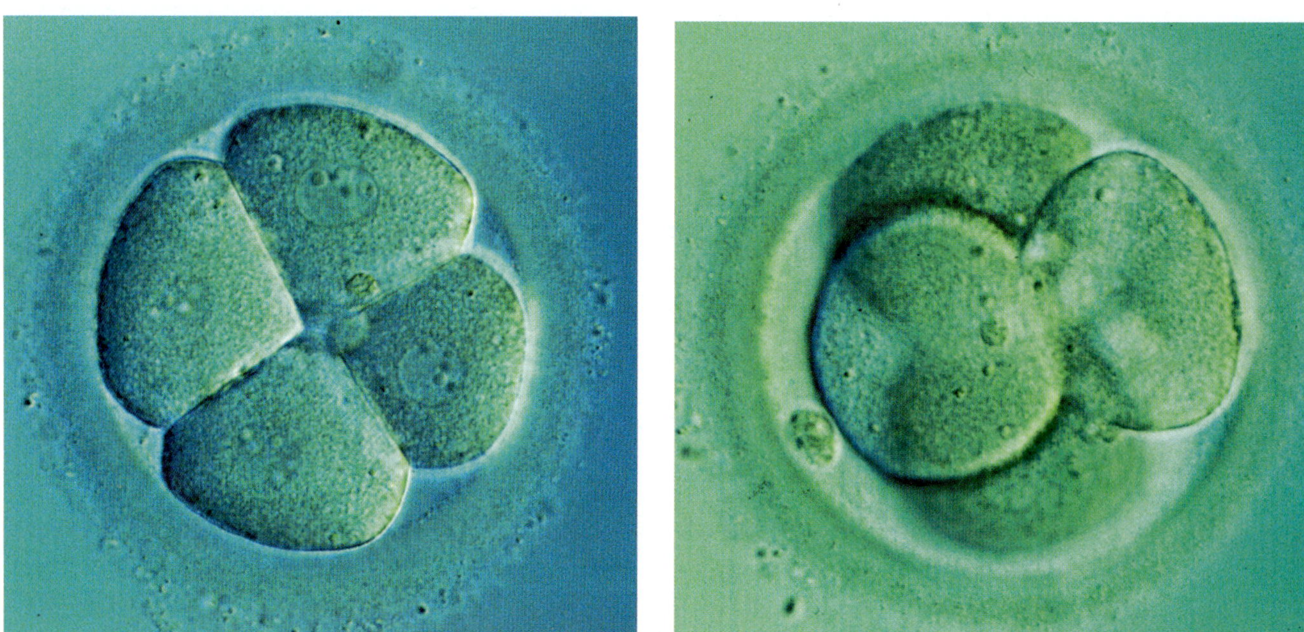

(a) (b)

Figure 1.45 Morphologically normal four-cell embryos (a) and (b). Four equal-sized blastomeres are seen in these day-2 embryos. All blastomeres have nuclei, with a polar body visible at the 8 o'clock position (b). Although both embryos seem to be normal, they differ considerably in cleavage symmetry (×400).

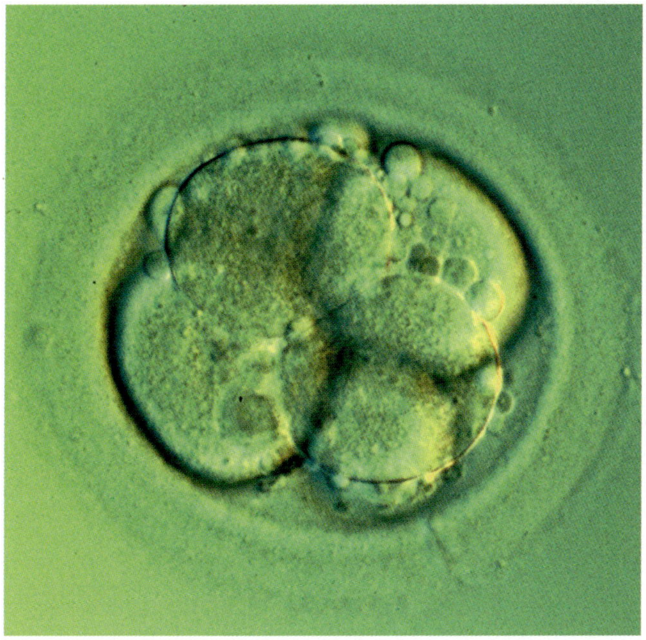

Figure 1.46 Slow five-cell embryo with cytoplasmic blebs. Four round equal-sized blastomeres and one smaller blastomere are visible in this day-3 embryo. A few small, round cytoplasmic blebs are also present. The odd number of blastomeres present suggests asynchronous cleavage and/or cytoplasmic fragmentation. In many instances such slow embryos undergo developmental arrest (×400).

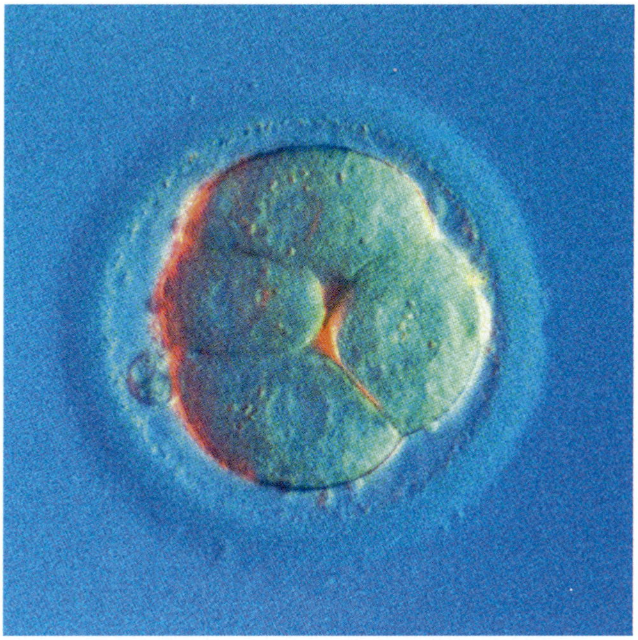

Figure 1.47 Compacting of a four-cell embryo. Four stretched blastomeres, each with a visible nucleus, are seen in this day-3 embryo. Tight contacts between blastomeres indicate the beginning of compaction. Compaction on day 3 of embryo development is not uncommon, particularly in the commercially available G1.1 medium. Compacting embryos pose a problem when performing blastomere biopsy, because of tight gap junctions. An attempt at removal of one blastomere may result in loss of the whole embryo; therefore decompaction is necessary and performed by exposure of the embryo to medium devoid of calcium and magnesium prior to biopsy (×400).

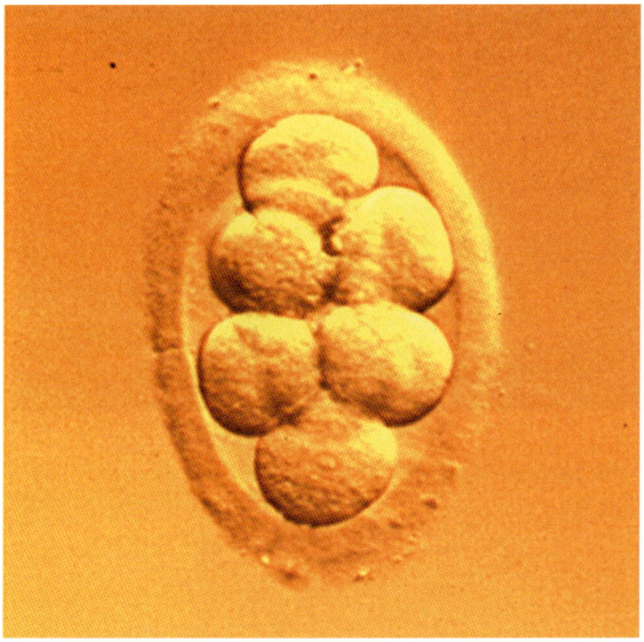

Figure 1.48 Irregular-shaped eight-cell embryo. Eight round, equal-sized blastomeres are seen in this day-3 embryo. The embryo and zona pellucida are oblong. Development of embryos with this abnormal morphology is compromised and such embryos usually undergo developmental arrest. Blastomere biopsy is also complicated by the irregular shape (×200).

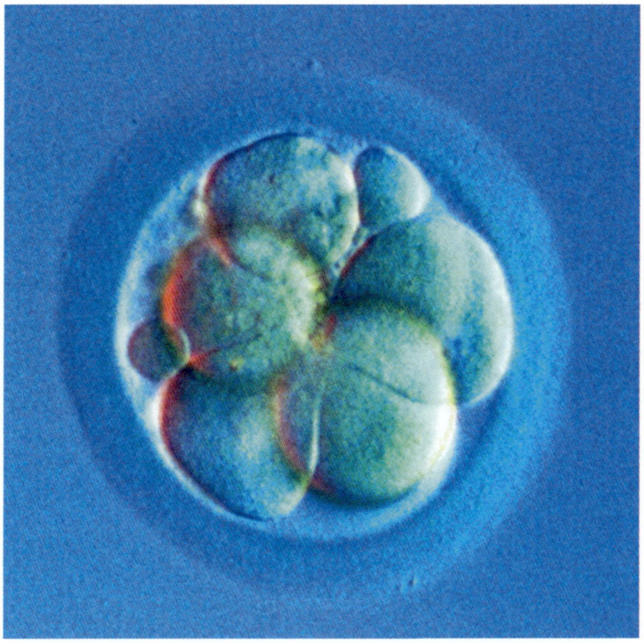

Figure 1.49 Six-cell embryo with cytoplasmic fragments. Six round, slightly unequal-sized blastomeres are seen in this day-3 embryo. At least two large cytoplasmic fragments are visible at the 1 and 9 o'clock positions, which usually have no chromatin and may not interfere with further development of the embryo (×200).

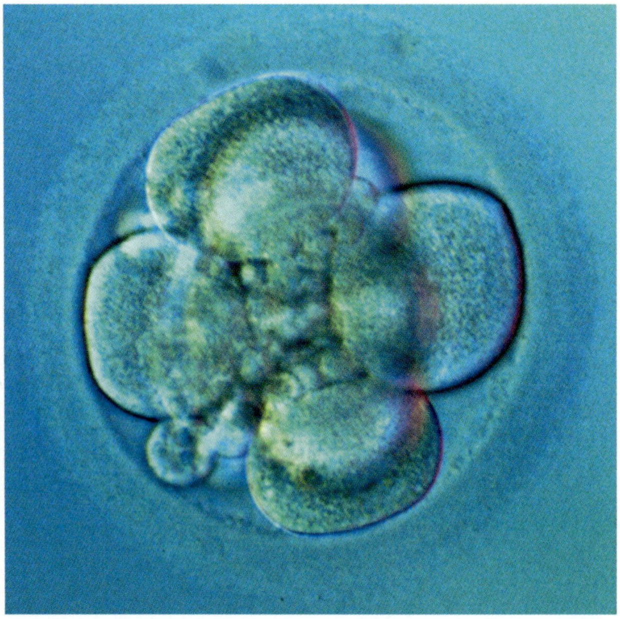

Figure 1.50 Six-cell embryo with cytoplasmic blebs. Six round, equal-sized blastomeres are present in this day-3 embryo with cytoplasmic blebs between blastomeres located in the center of the embryo. Cytoplasmic blebs can distort contacts among blastomeres and mechanically prevent compaction of the embryo (×400).

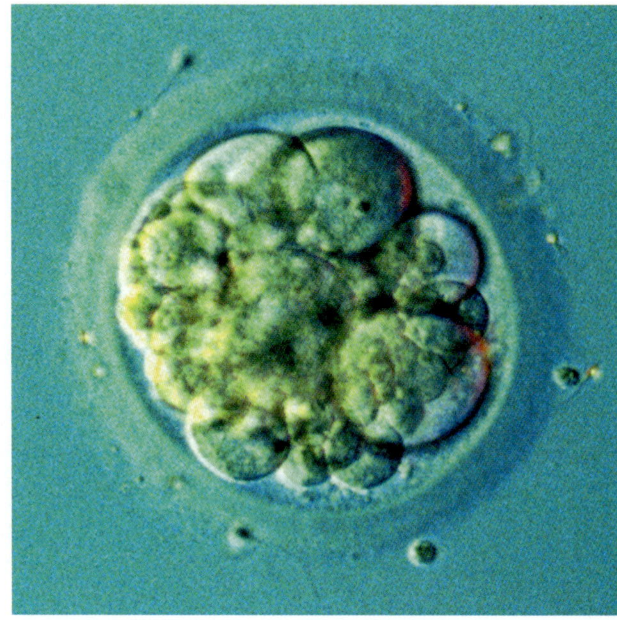

Figure 1.51 Extensive cytoplasmic fragmentation comprising 50% of the subzonal space is seen in this day-3 embryo. Five to six round blastomeres, which vary in size, are present. Embryos with a similar abnormality usually undergo developmental arrest (×200).

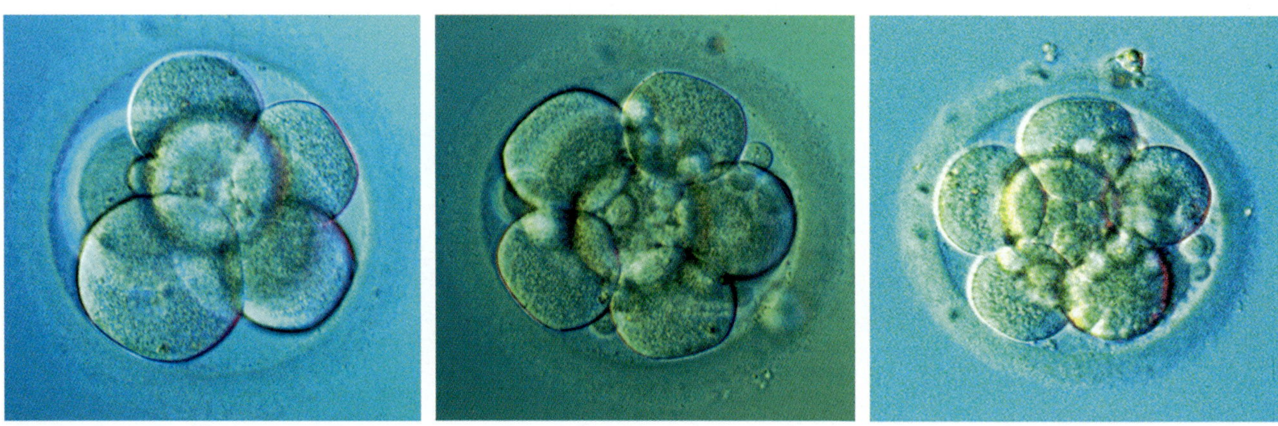

(a) (b) (c)

Figure 1.52 Eight-cell embryos (a), (b), and (c) with a few cytoplasmic blebs. Eight round, equal-sized blastomeres are seen in each of these day-3 embryos. A few small cytoplasmic blebs present do not affect development and compaction of the embryo ((a) and (b) ×400; (c) ×200).

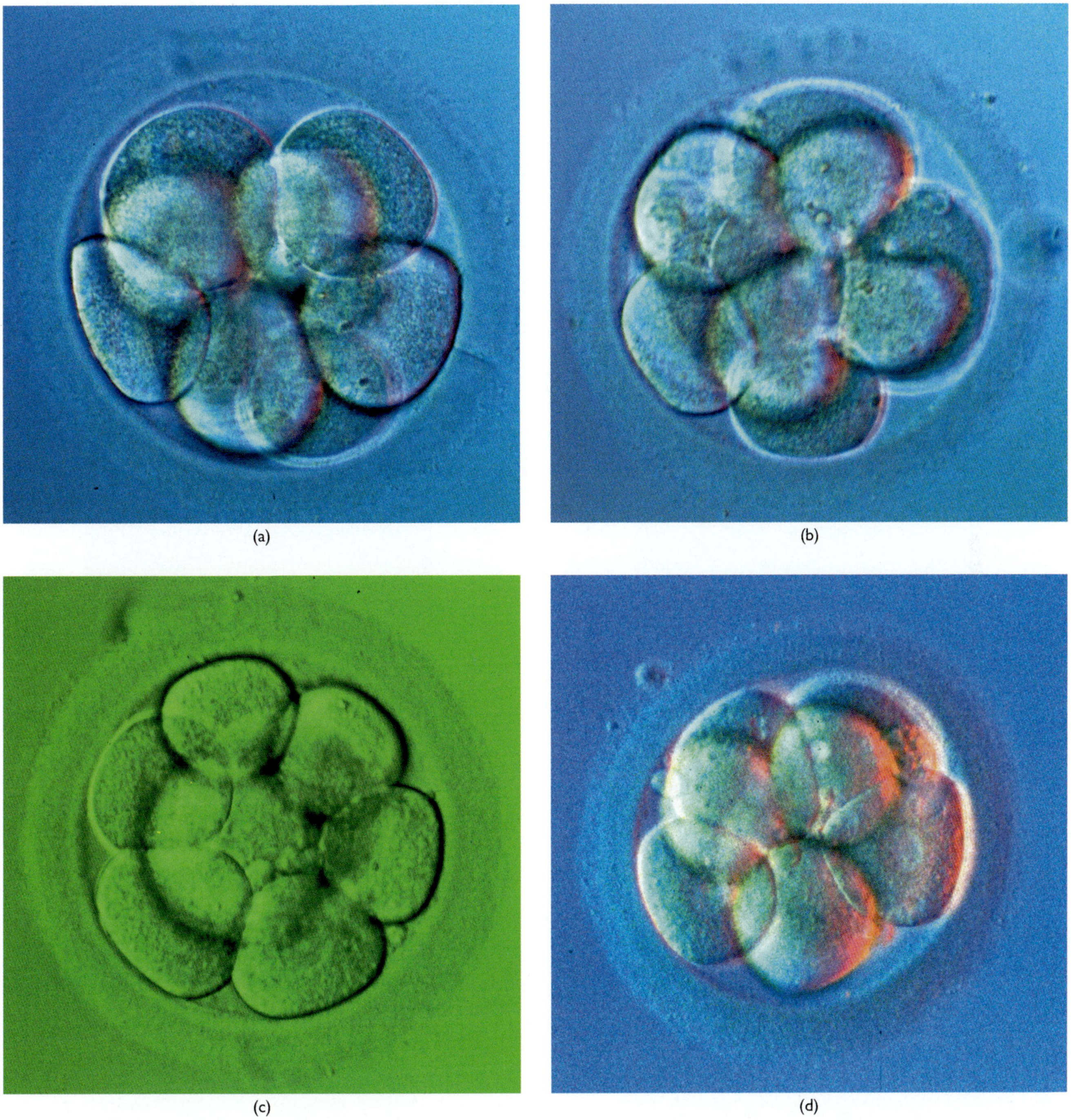

Figure 1.53 Morphologically normal day-3 embryos. Eight round, equal-sized blastomeres are seen in the embryos. Cytoplasm is homogeneous. Their morphology is considered of grade 1 quality, since no fragmentation or cytoplasmic blebs are present in any of these embryos. Loose contacts between the blastomeres and their symmetrical positioning provide acceptable material for performing blastomere biopsy. One of two slit openings after removal of first and second polar bodies can be seen at the 4 o'clock position in (a) (×400).

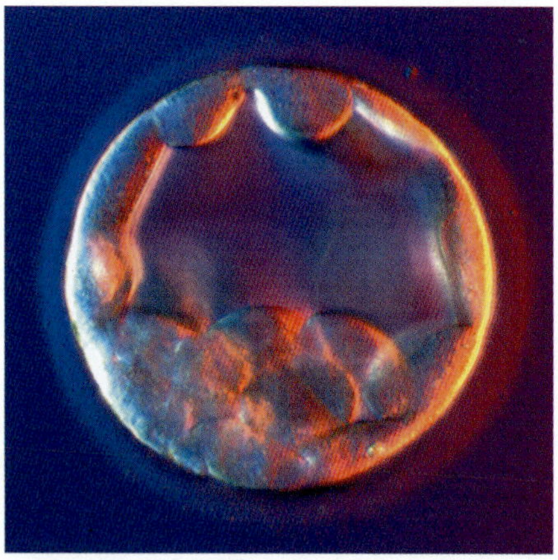

Figure 1.54 Day-5 early blastocyst, 120 h after insemination, with a well-defined blastocele formed by the large oval cells of the developing trophoblast. Round cells accumulating in the lower pole are involved in the formation of the inner cell mass. There is no perivitelline space present. The zona pellucida is thinning (x400).

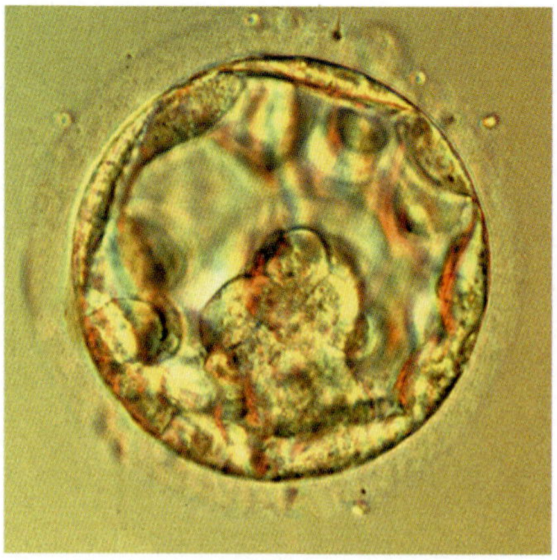

Figure 1.55 Day-5 early blastocyst, 120 h after insemination, in which the blastocele comprises one-half of the conceptus. Trophectoderm cells are flattened and stretched to accommodate the expansion. The inner cell mass is distinguishable inside the blastocele cavity (x400).

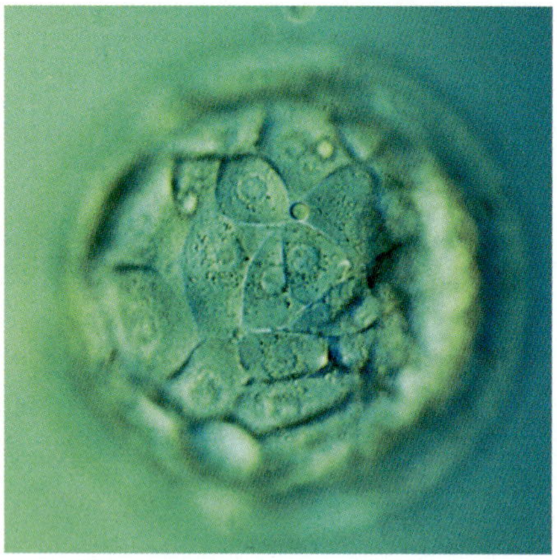

Figure 1.56 Day-5 early blastocyst. Cells are polygonal and tightly connected to the neighboring cells in this conceptus, 120 h after insemination. Nuclei are visible in the majority of cells (x400).

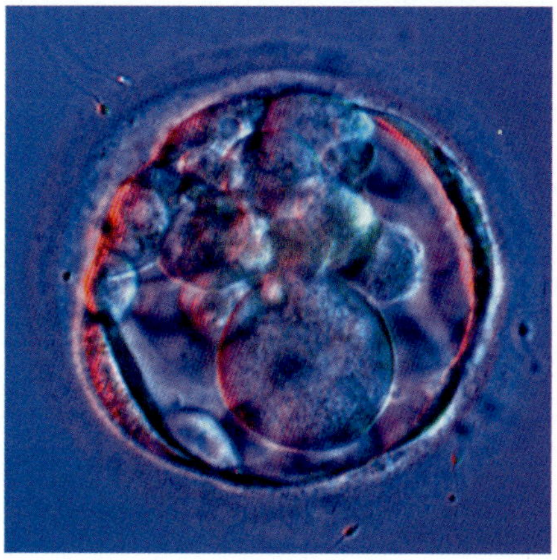

Figure 1.57 Apparently abnormal day-5 early blastocyst, 120 h after insemination, consists of a small blastocele formed by a reduced number of large, flattened cells. Round cells, different in size, are scattered inside the blastocele and are not participating in formation of the blastocyst. A perivitelline space is still visible. Normal development of this blastocyst is unlikely (x400).

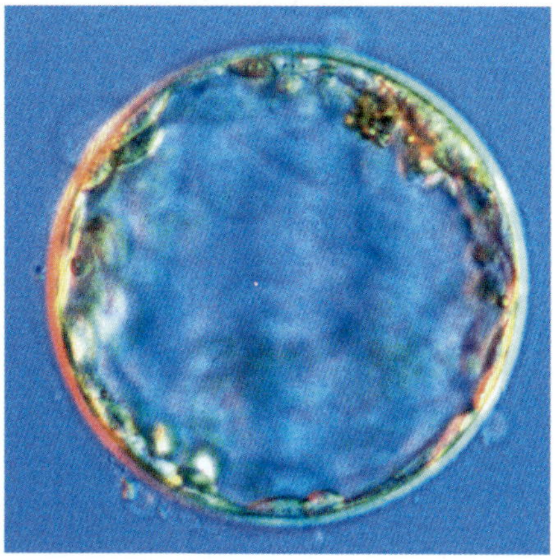

Figure 1.58 Abnormal embryo development, day 6. The trophoblastic vesicle, 144 h after insemination, consists of a large blastocelic cavity formed by a single layer of trophectoderm cells. There is no identifiable inner cell mass. The zona pellucida is very thin (x400).

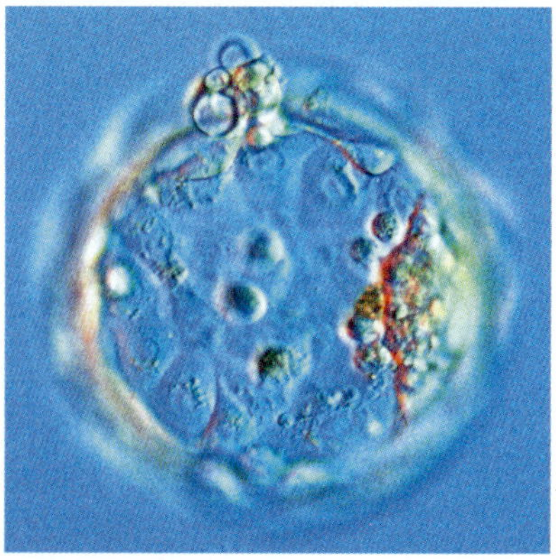

Figure 1.59 Day-6 blastocyst. The very beginning of the hatching process is seen in this fully expanded blastocyst. A few trophectoderm cells are present outside the zona pellucida at the 12 o'clock position. The inner cell mass is also visible on the left (x400).

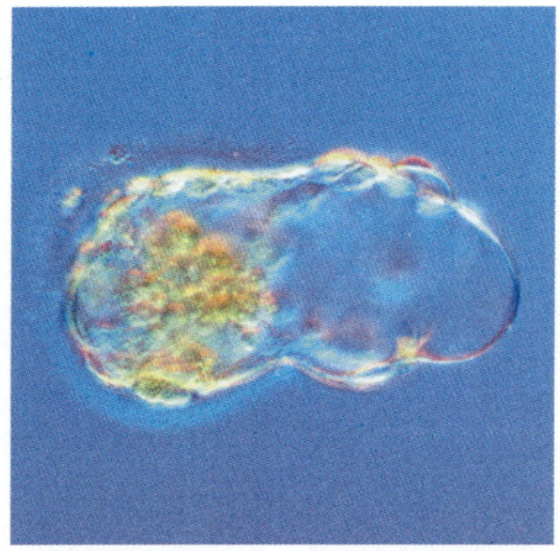

Figure 1.60 Hatching of an expanded blastocyst 130 h after insemination through the V-shaped opening created in the zona pellucida prior to blastomere biopsy. Hatching of embryos with the opening in the zona pellucida occurs earlier than in embryos with intact zonae pellucidae (×200).

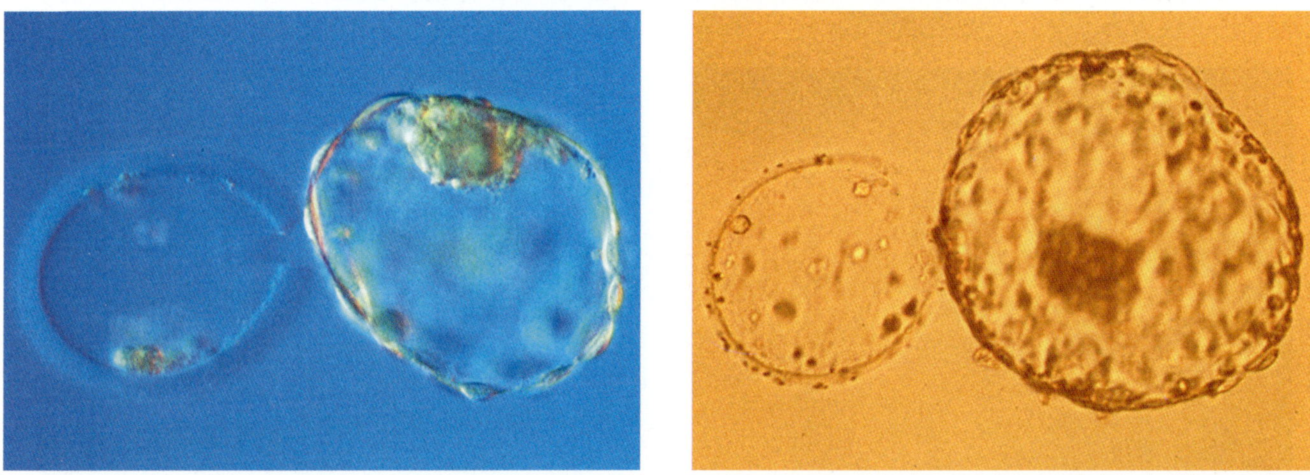

(a) (b)

Figure 1.61 Completely hatched, morphologically normal blastocysts, 130–140 h after insemination (a) and (b). The V-shaped opening was created in the zonae pellucidae prior to blastomere biopsy. An inner cell mass is clearly seen in each blastocyst (×200).

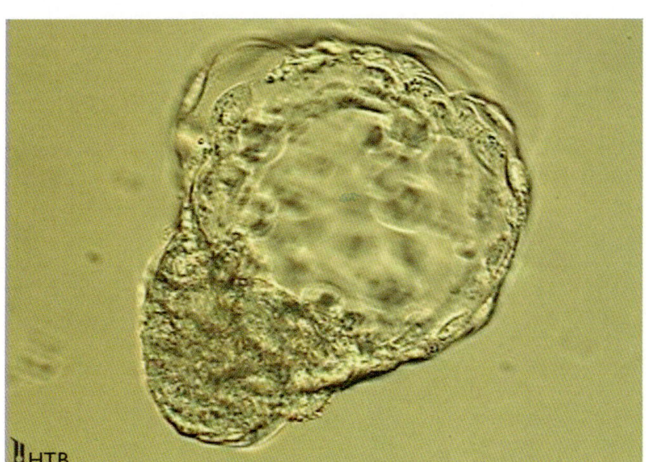

Figure 1.62 Contracted normal blastocyst mimicking an abnormal inner cell mass position.

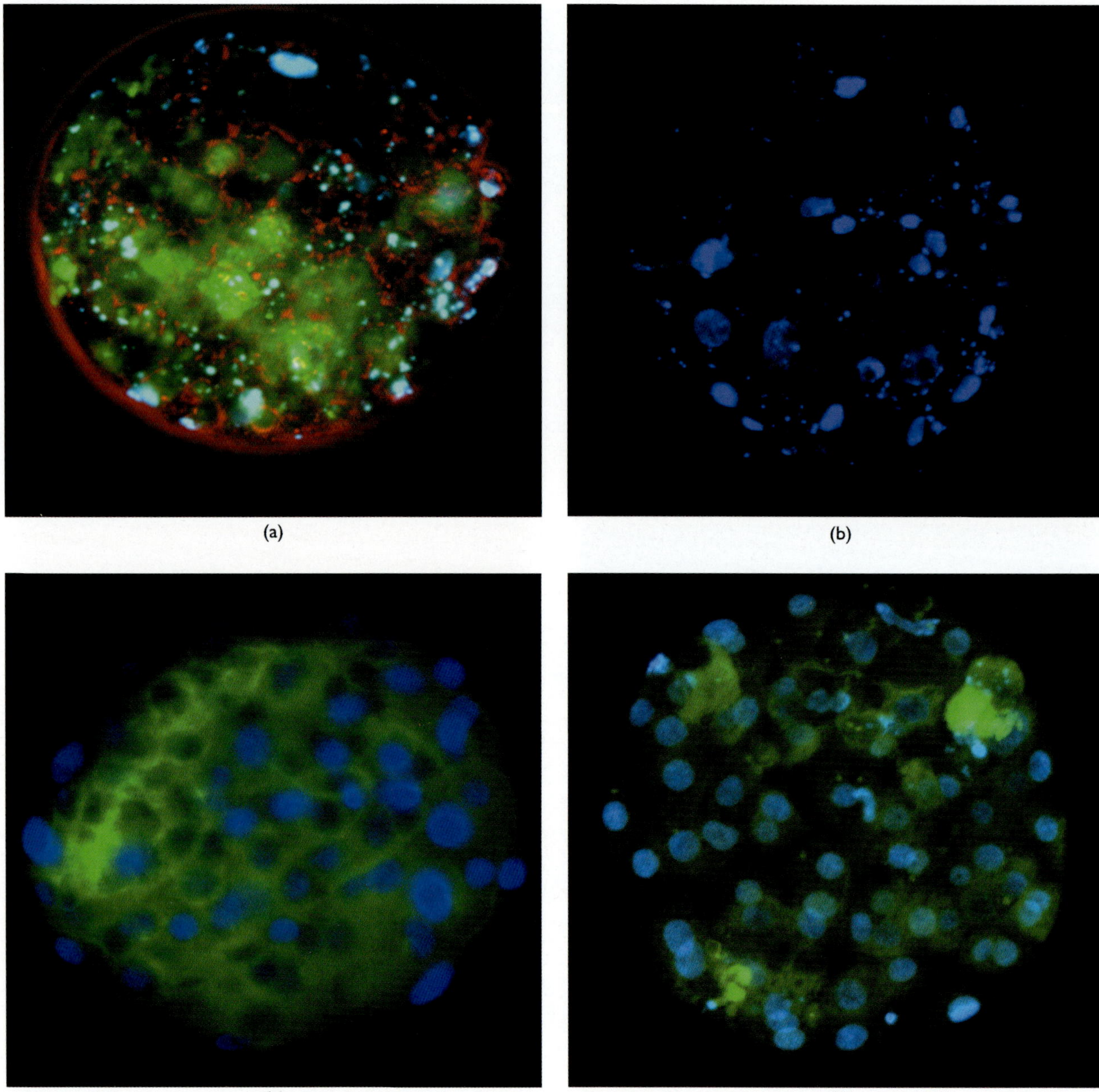

(a) (b) (c) (d)

Figure I.63 Human blastocysts stained for tubulin and chromatin. (a) Human blastocyst with abnormal nuclei and cytoskeleton initially graded as normal on the basis of morphological appearance under the bright-field optics. Tubulin stained green, nuclei blue, bright-field view of the blastocyst red. (b) Analysis of the same blastocyst after fixation and nucleus staining (blue) demonstrates the abnormal development of the embryos resulting from 'chaotic cleavage.' (c) and (d) Normal human blastocysts. Nuclei are blue, tubulin microfilaments green.

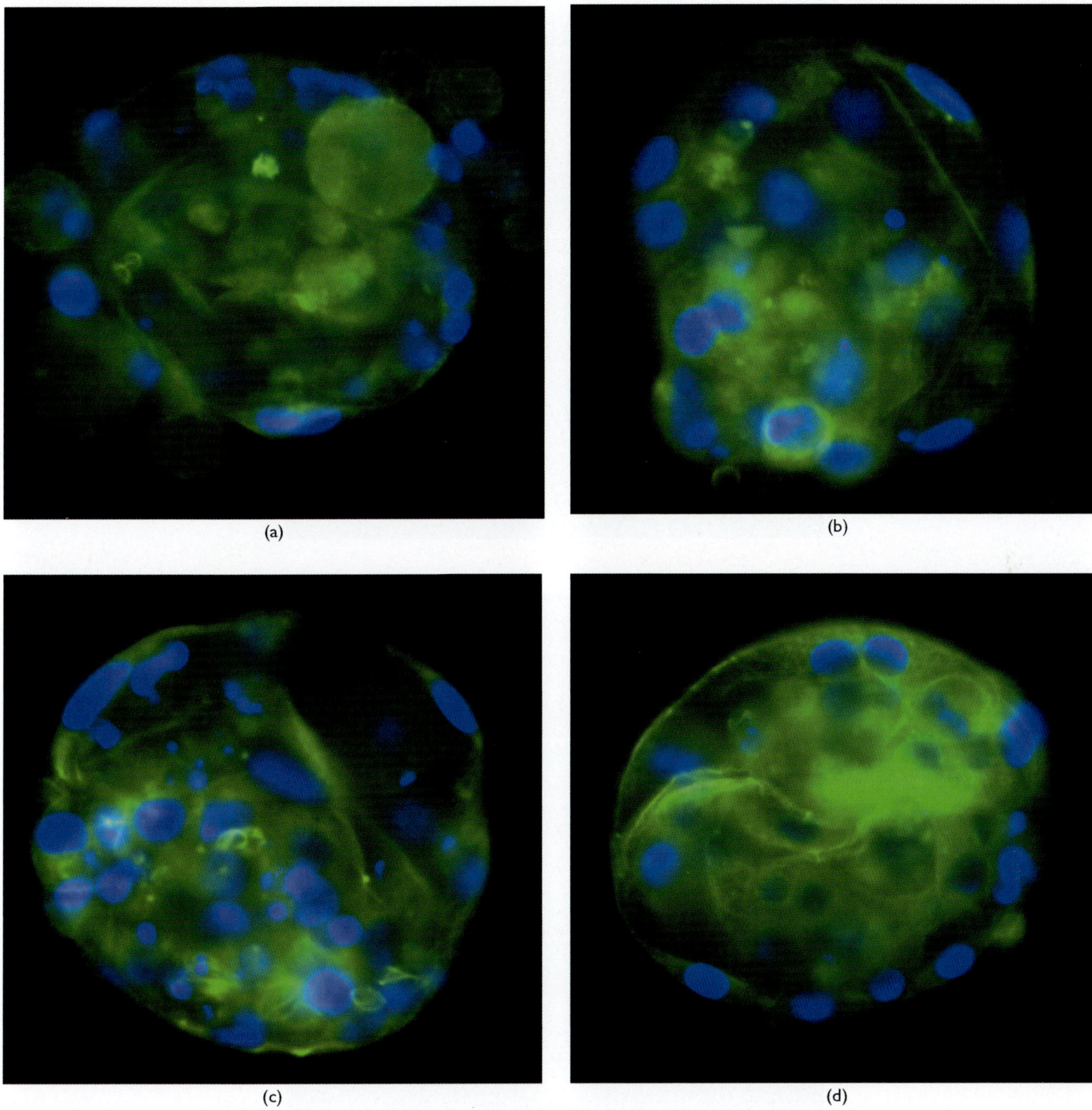

Figure 1.64 Human blastocysts stained for tubulin and chromatin. (a) Apparently abnormal blastocyst with a few cells extruded into the perivitelline space and not included in the process of blastocyst formation (nuclei are stained blue, tubulin microfilaments green). (b–d) Morphologically normal blastocysts.

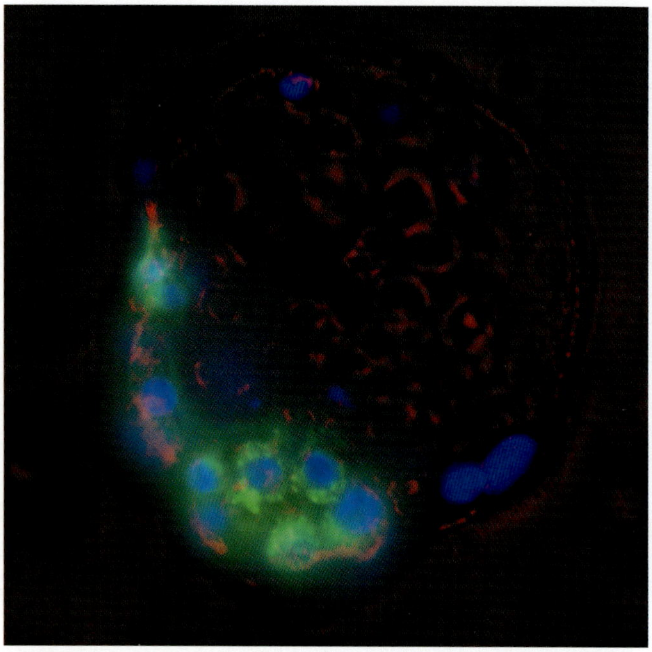

(a)

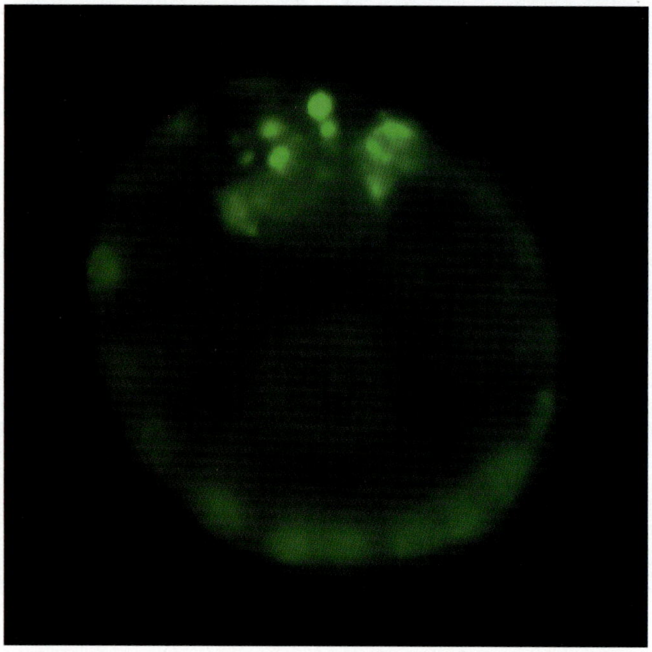

(b)

Figure 1.65 Distribution of mitochondria in the human blastocyst (rhodamine stain in green). (a) Inner cell mass in focus. Mitochondria are stained green, chromatin stained with DAPI in blue. (b) Trophectoderm in focus. Trophectoderm cells have a similar number of mitochondria to the inner cell mass cells.

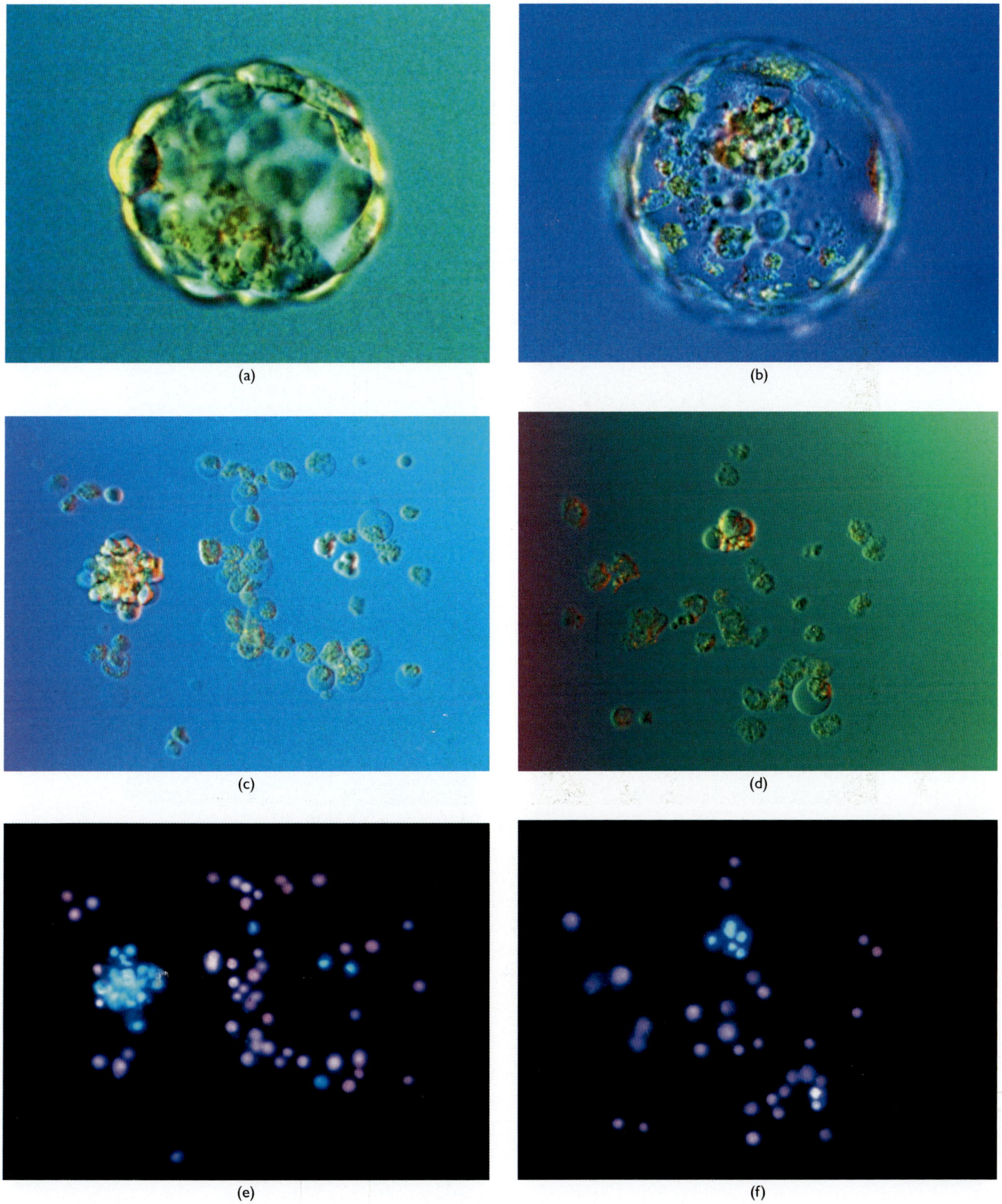

Figure 1.66 Separation of the inner cell mass and trophectoderm by blastocyst immunosurgery. (a) and (b) Blastocysts before immunosurgery, after zona pellucida removal. (c) and (d) Bright-field view of the dissociated blastocyst cells after immunosurgery. (e) and (f) The same embryos, under epifluorescence. The inner cell mass cell nuclei are stained blue compared to lysed trophectoderm cell nuclei stained pink.

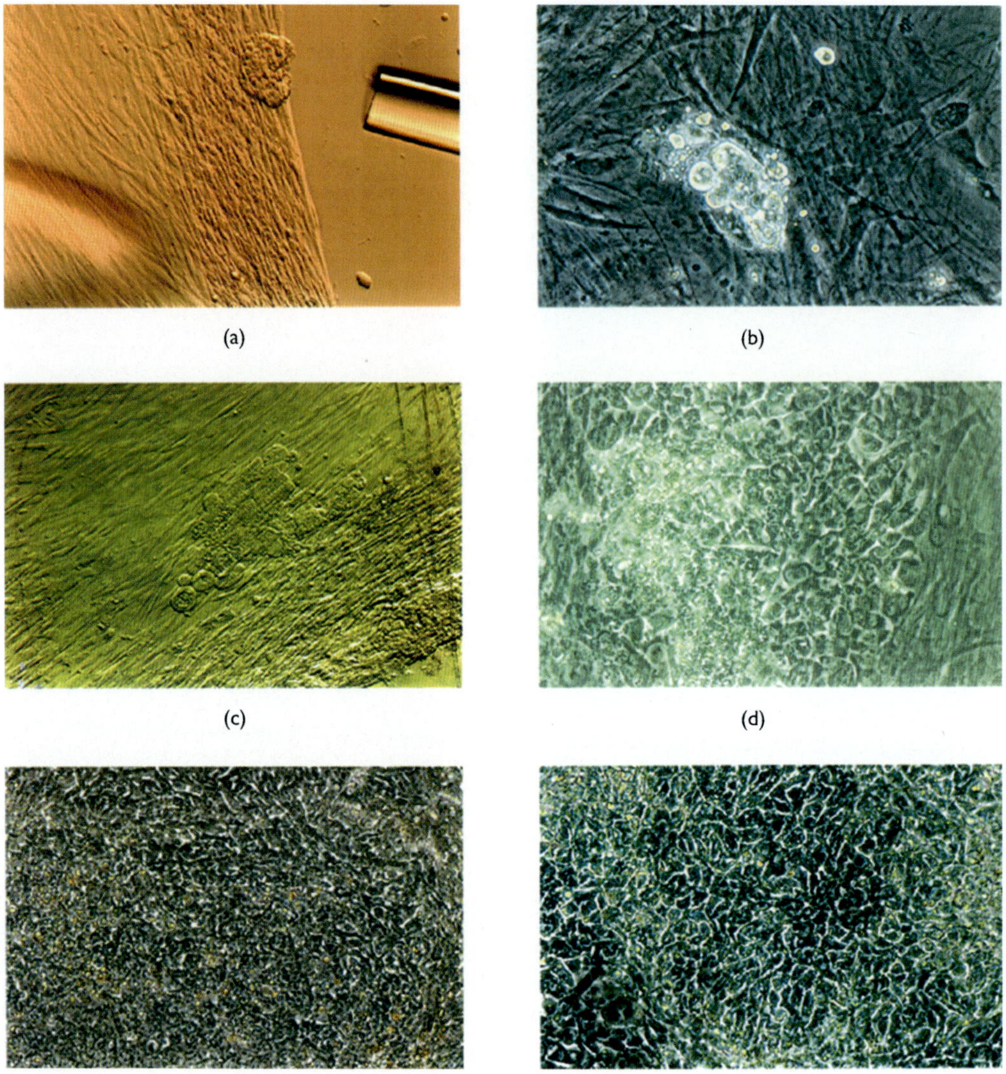

(a) (b) (c) (d) (e) (f)

Figure 1.67 Establishment of embryonic stem (ES) cells from morula and blastocyst. (a) Human embryo at morula stage is placed under mouse embryonic fibroblasts to establish ES cells (x10). (b) Initial growth of morula cells under feeder layer (x10). (c) Morphology of human morula-derived ES cells (x10). (d) Initial outgrowth of ES cells from isolated inner cell mass (ICM) (x20). (e) Primary colony of ES cells derived from ICM (x20). (f) Morphology of human ICM-derived ES cells (x10).

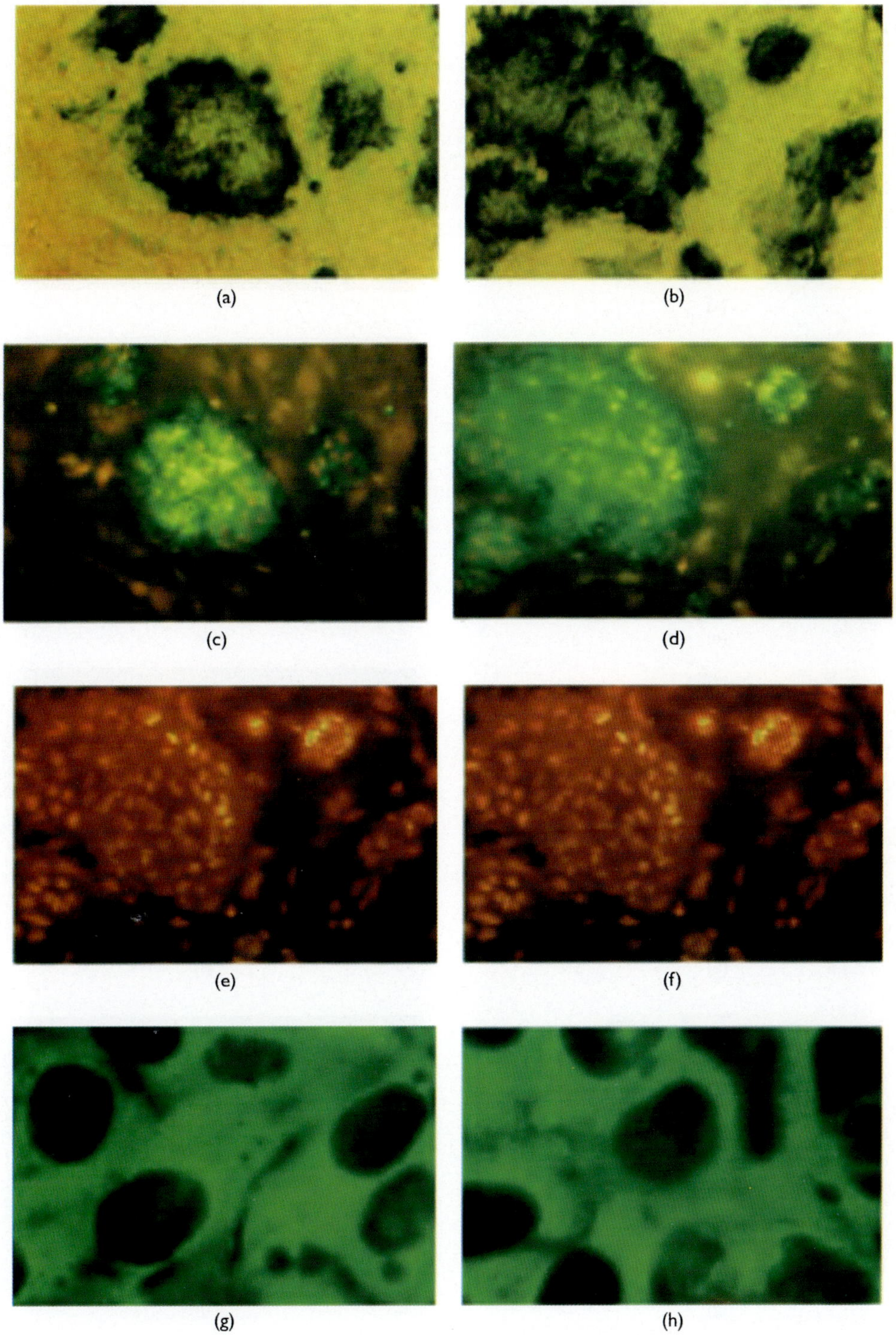

Figure 1.68 Expression of markers in embryonic stem cell lines derived from morula (left column) and inner cell mass (ICM) (right column): generic enzymatic activity of alkaline phosphatase (a) and (b); human embryonic carcinoma L-alkaline phosphatase, primary antibodies TRA-2-39 against epitope 2102 (b) and (e); Oct-4 (e) and (f); and beta-tubulin (g) and (h). (a) Enzymatic activity of alkaline phosphatase in morula-derived ES cells growing on the murine feeder layer (x20). (b) Matched fluorescein isothiocyanate (FITC): immunofluorescence cell surface staining of TRA-2-39 detected by monoclonal antibodies in the same colonies of morula-derived ES cells growing on the murine feeder layer (x20). (c) Tetramethyl rhodamine isothiocyanate (TRITC): immunofluorescence cell-surface staining of Oct-4 expression in the same colonies of morula-derived ES cells growing on the murine feeder layer (x20). (d) Enzymatic activity of alkaline phosphatase in ICM-derived ES cells growing on the murine feeder layer (x20). (e) Matched FITC: immunofluorescence cell-surface staining of TRA-2-39 detected by monoclonal antibodies labeled with FITC in the same colonies of ICM-derived ES cells growing on the murine feeder layer (x20). (f) TRITC: immunofluorescence cell surface staining of Oct-4 expression in the same colonies of ICM-derived ES cells growing on the murine feeder layer (x20). (g) Expression of beta-tubulin in morula-derived ES cell line (x40). (h) Expression of beta-tubulin in ICM-derived ES cell line (x40).

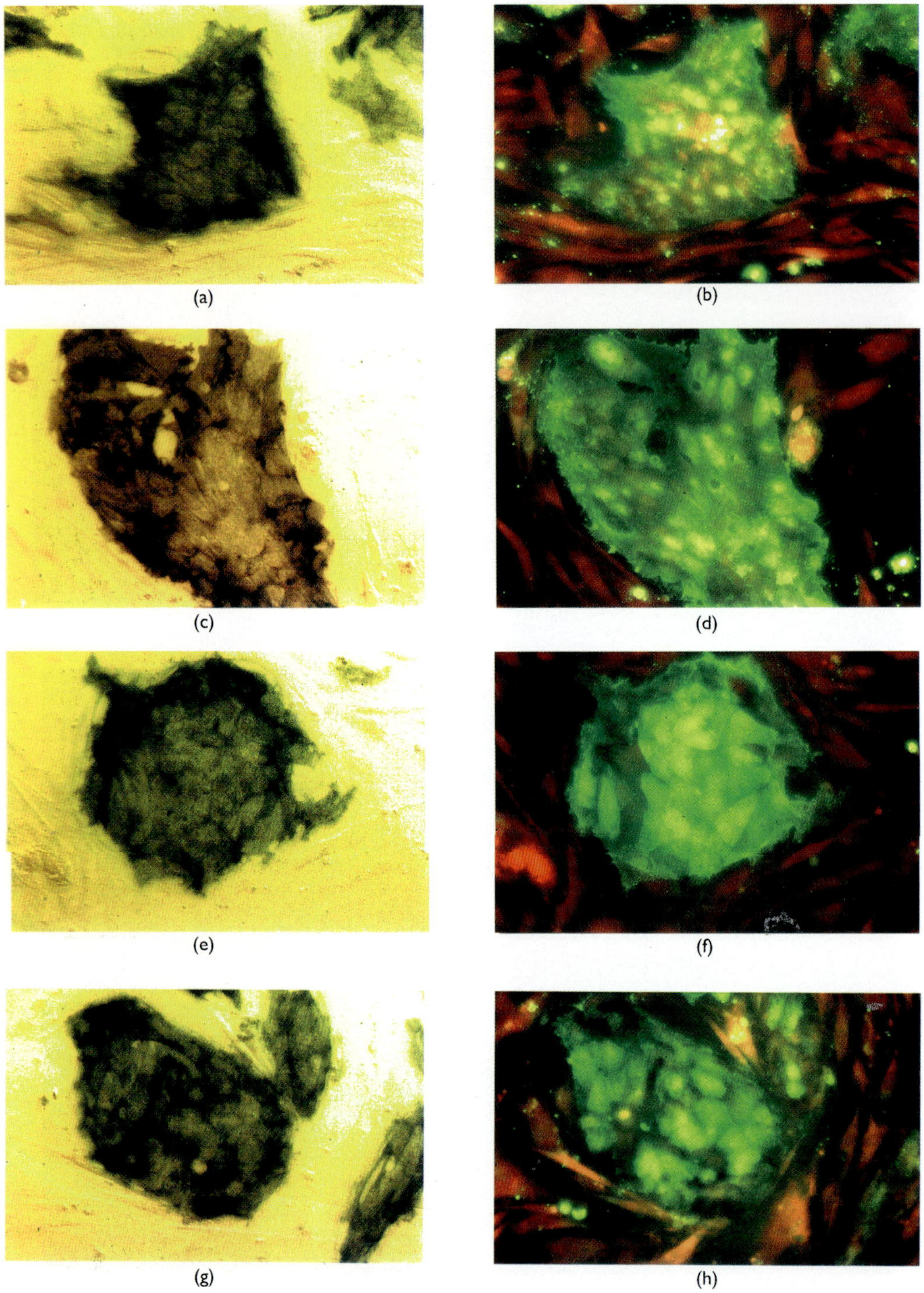

Figure 1.69 Expression of markers SSEA-3, SSEA-4, TRA-1-60, TRA-1-81, and corresponding enzymatic activity of alkaline phosphatase (AP) in a morula-derived embryonic stem (ES) cell line. (a) Expression of enzymatic activity of alkaline phosphatase in colony of ES cells growing on the murine feeder layer (×20). (b) Corresponding immunofluorescence cell-surface staining of SSEA-3 detected by monoclonal antibodies labeled with fluorescein isothiocyanate (FITC) in the same colony of ES cells as (a) growing on the murine feeder layer. (c) Expression of enzymatic activity of alkaline phosphatase in colony of ES cells growing on the murine feeder layer. (d) Corresponding immunofluorescence cell-surface staining of SSEA-4 detected by monoclonal antibodies labeled with FITC in the same colony of ES cells as (c) growing on the murine feeder layer. (e) Expression of enzymatic activity of alkaline phosphatase in colony of ES cells growing on the murine feeder layer. (f) Corresponding immunofluorescence cell-surface staining of TRA-1-60 detected by monoclonal antibodies labeled with FITC in the same colony of ES cells as (e) growing on the murine feeder layer. (g) Expression of enzymatic activity of alkaline phosphatase in colony of ES cells growing on the murine feeder layer. (h) Corresponding immunofluorescence cell-surface staining of TRA-1-80 detected by monoclonal antibodies labeled with FITC in the same colony of ES cells as (g) growing on the murine feeder layer (×20).

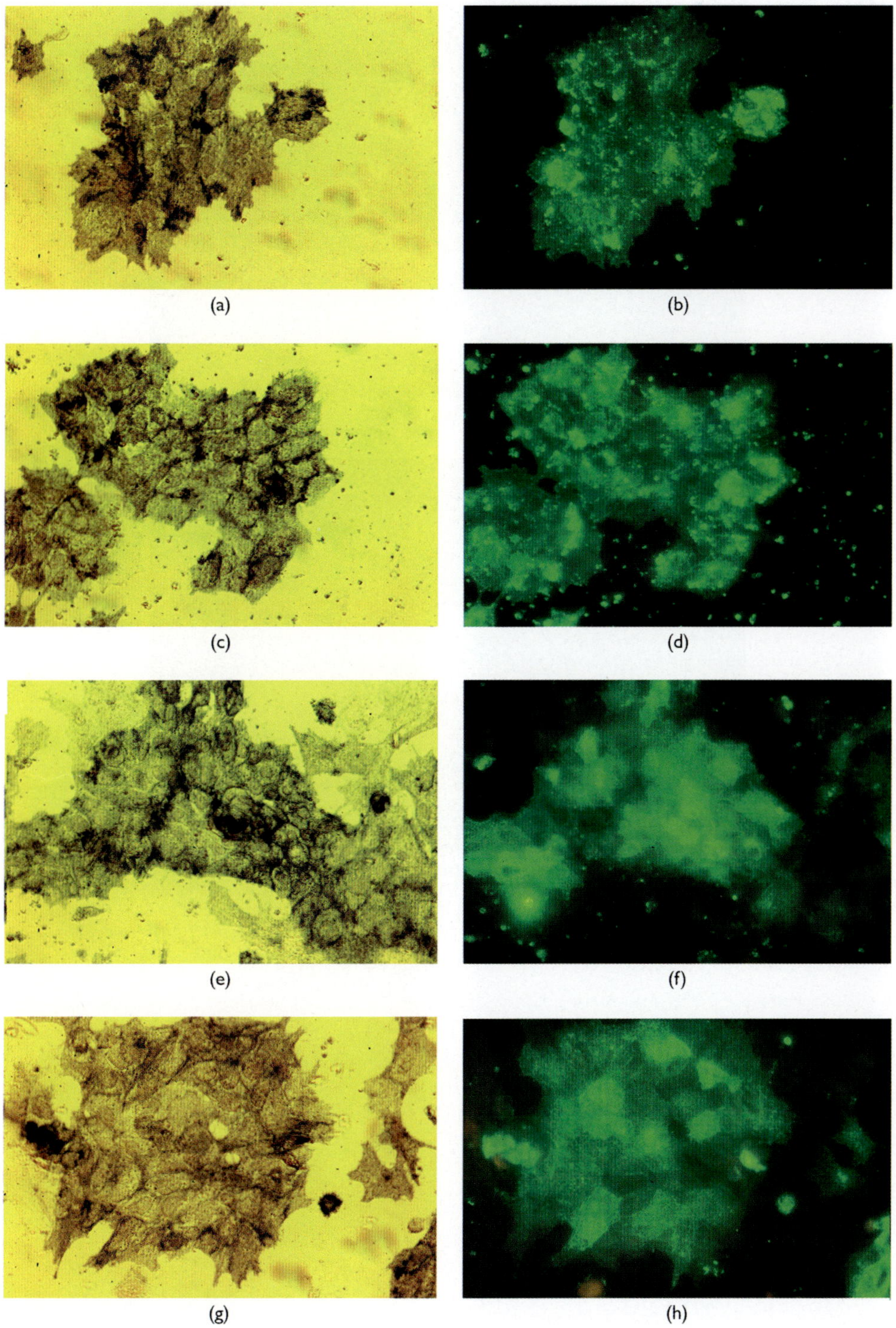

Figure 1.70 Expression of markers SSEA-3, SSEA-4, TRA-1-60, TRA-1-80, and corresponding enzymatic activity of alkaline phosphatase (AP) in morula-derived embryonic stem (ES) cell line growing on feeder-free system. (a) Expression of enzymatic activity of alkaline phosphatase in the colony of ES cells growing on the feeder-free system (Matrigel) (×20). (b) Corresponding immunofluorescence cell-surface staining of SSEA-3 detected by monoclonal antibodies labeled with FITC in the same colony of ES cells as (a) growing on the feeder-free system (Matrigel). (c) Expression of enzymatic activity of alkaline phosphatase in the colony of ES cells growing on the feeder-free system (Matrigel). (d) Corresponding immunofluorescence cell-surface staining of SSEA-4 detected by monoclonal antibodies labeled with FITC in the same colony of ES cells as (c) growing on the feeder-free system (Matrigel). (e) Expression of enzymatic activity of alkaline phosphatase in the colony of ES cells growing on the feeder-free system (Matrigel). (f) Corresponding immunofluorescence cell-surface staining of TRA-1-60 detected by monoclonal antibodies labeled with FITC in the same colony of ES cells as (e) growing on the feeder-free system (Matrigel). (g) Expression of enzymatic activity of alkaline phosphatase in the colony of ES cells growing on the feeder-free system (Matrigel). (h) Corresponding immunofluorescence cell-surface staining of TRA-1-80 detected by monoclonal antibodies labeled with FITC in the same colony of ES cells as (g) growing on the feeder-free system (Matrigel) (×20).

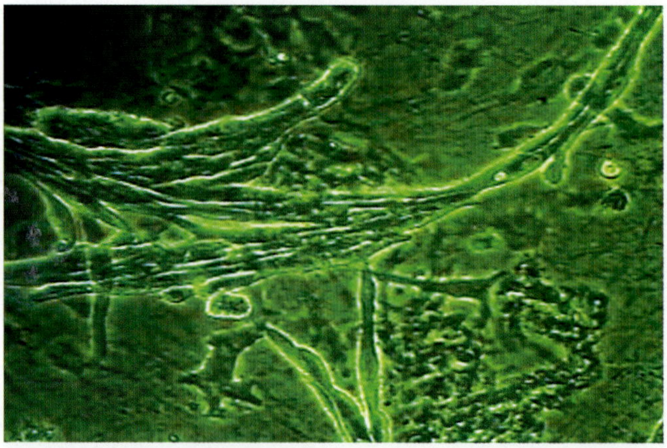

(a)

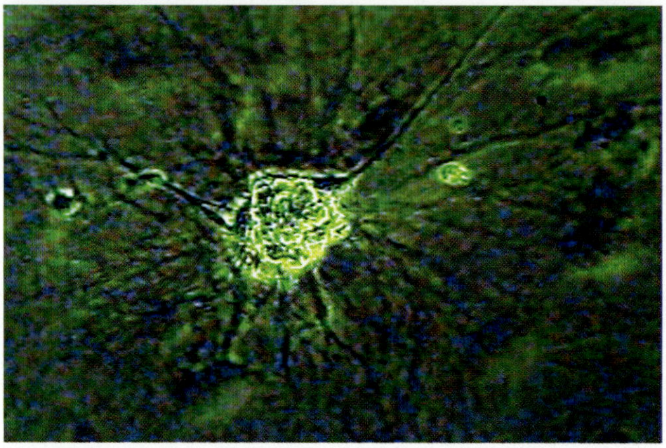

(b)

Figure 1.71 Differentiation of morula-derived embryonic stem (ES) cells into cardiocyte-like cells (a) and neuron-like cells (b). (a) Differentiation *in vitro* of human ES cells into contracting primitive cardiocyte-like cells (×20; captured frame from video file). (b) Differentiation *in vitro* of human ES cells into neuron-like cells (×20; captured frame from video file).

2 Micromanipulation and biopsy of polar bodies, blastomeres, and blastocysts

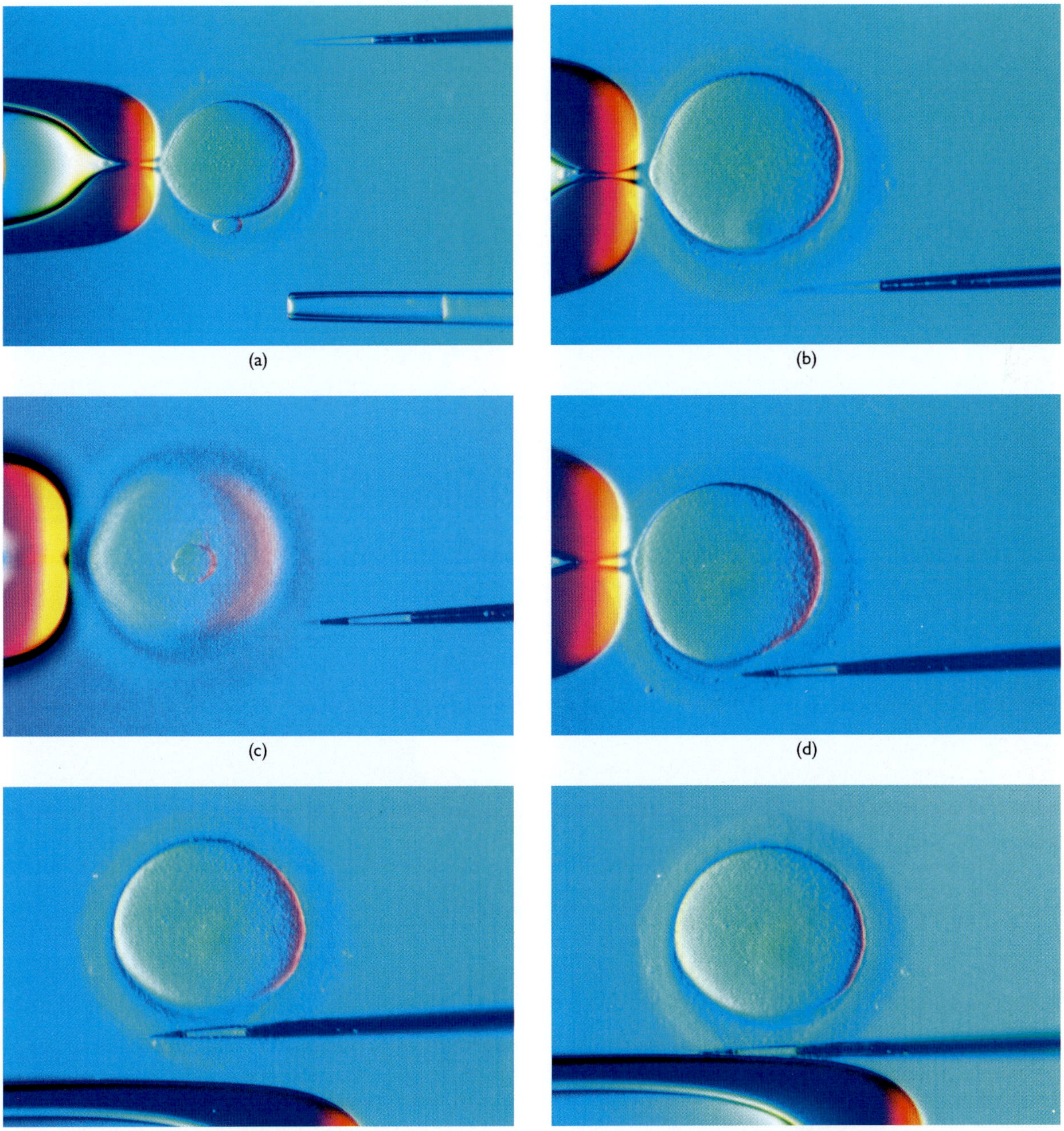

(a) (b) (c) (d) (e) (f)

Figure 2.1 First polar body (PB1) removal. (a) Once the oocyte has been secured by the holding pipette by gentle suction, the oocyte is oriented using the microneedle so that the PB1 is visualized at the 6 o'clock position. (b) and (c) Using the microneedle, the oocyte is rotated horizontally until the polar body is visualized directly in the center of the oocyte, facing the operator. This orientation of the oocyte, prior to creating the opening, is important when performing ICSI afterwards. (d) A slit is made in the zona pellucida at the 4–5 o'clock position, passing tangentially through the perivitelline space and out at the 7–8 o'clock position. (e) The oocyte is released from the holding pipette and held by the microneedle. (f) The partial zona dissection microneedle with the oocyte is brought to the top of the holding pipette and pressed to it, pinching a portion of the zona pellucida. By gently rubbing the microneedle against the holding pipette, with a sawing motion, partial zona dissection is accomplished.

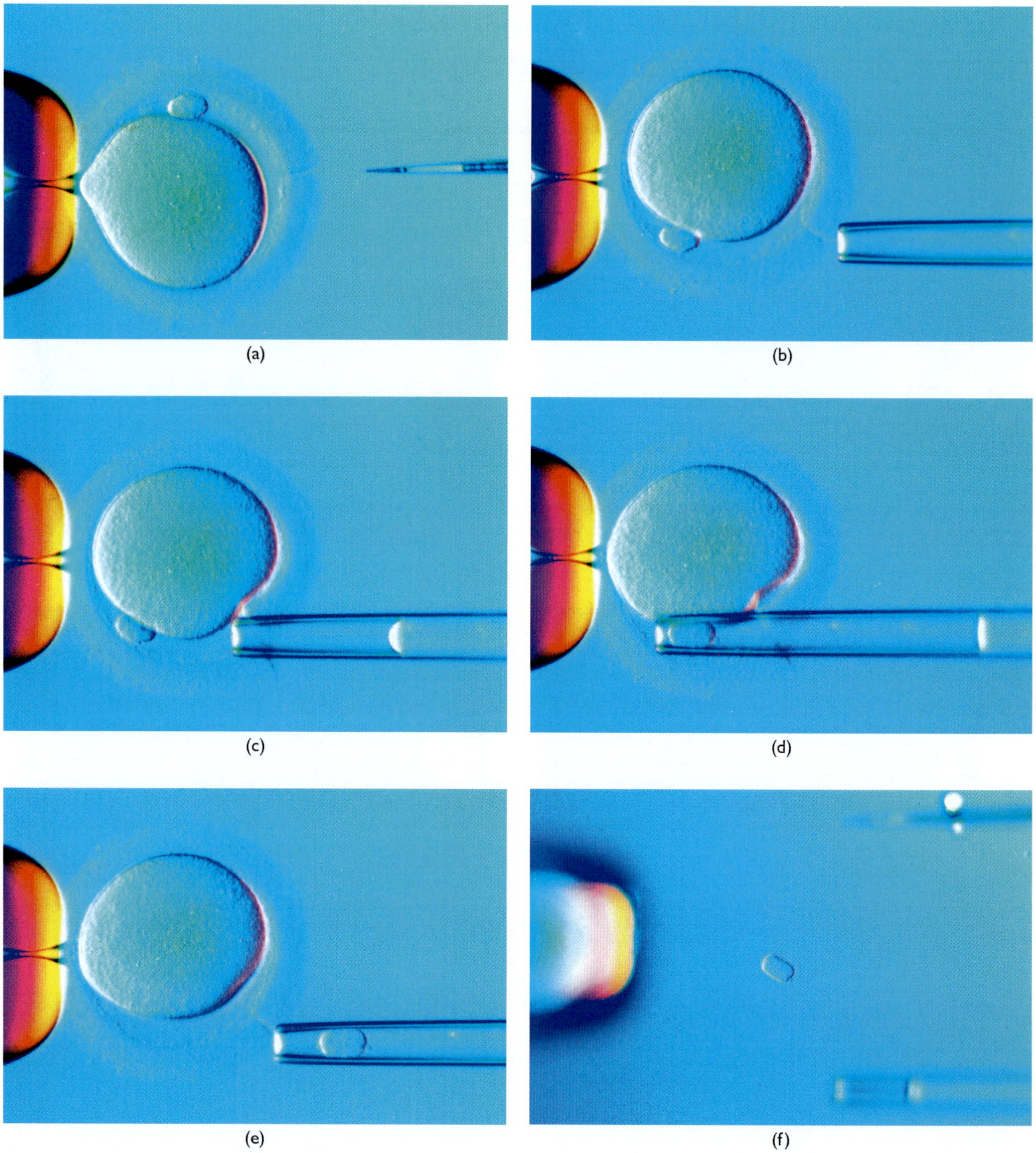

Figure 2.2 First polar body (PBI) removal (continued). (a) The oocyte is positioned so that the slit opening in the zona pellucida (3 o'clock) and the PBI (6 or 12 o'clock) are clearly seen. (b) The oocyte is rotated so that the opening in the zona pellucida is at the 5 o'clock position and the polar body is in focus. In some cases, sucrose (0.05 mol/l) is added to the medium to increase the size of the perivitelline space by shrinkage of the ooplasm. (c) The aspirating micropipette is passed through the opening to the polar body. (d) and (e) Gentle suction is applied to aspirate the polar body into the micropipette. Pressure from the hydraulic system is equilibrated prior to the withdrawal of the aspirating micropipette to avoid oocyte damage. Removal of the PBI is postponed when it is still attached to the oocyte in order to prevent possible enucleation of the oocyte. (f) The oocyte is released from the holding pipette, and all the microtools are raised slightly from the bottom of the dish. The microscope stage is moved so that another drop of medium at the 6 o'clock position is visualized. The micropipette containing the polar body is lowered to the bottom of the dish, and the PBI is expelled into the drop of medium.

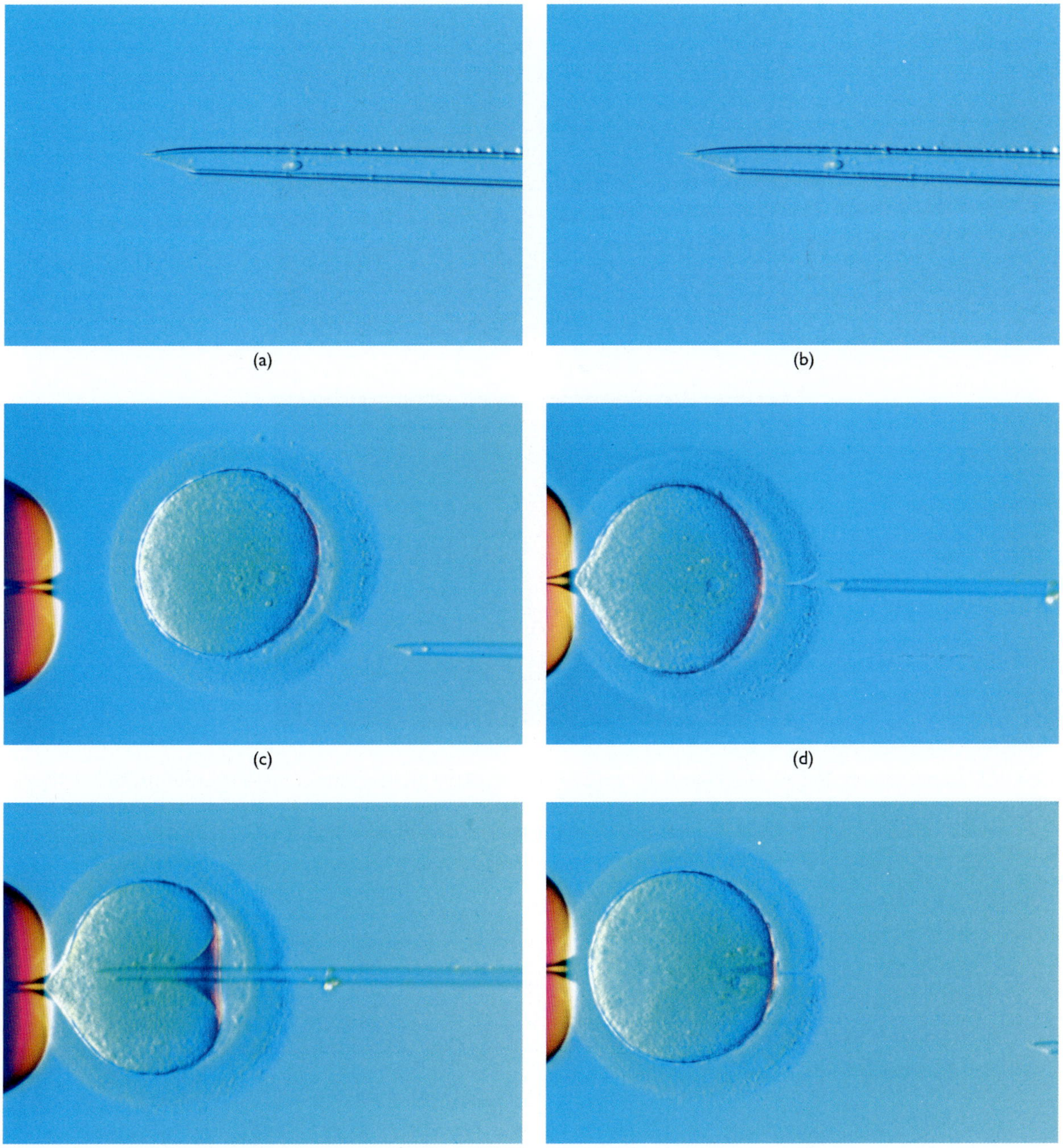

(a) (b) (c) (d) (e) (f)

Figure 2.3 ICSI after polar body removal. (a) A morphologically normal spermatozoon is chosen and immobilized by being pressed against the bottom of the dish with the injection needle, and the membrane of the tail is broken after a few sawing movements with the needle. (b) The spermatozoon is aspirated into the injection needle and then raised above the bottom of the dish. (c) The microscope stage is moved so that one of the drops of medium containing an oocyte appears in view. The holding pipette is lowered to the bottom, next to the oocyte. Using the injection needle, the oocyte is rotated until the slit opening in the zona pellucida is visible. (d) The oocyte is positioned and held by the holding pipette with the slit opening at the 3 o'clock position. In this position, the first polar body, prior to its removal, would have been located at the 6 or 12 o'clock position. (e) The injection needle is passed through the opening in the zona pellucida and slowly continued to almost three-quarters of the oocyte's diameter deep into the ooplasm. At this point, movement has stopped, and a small amount of the ooplasm is aspirated until a sign is visible of plasma membrane breakage. Contents of the injection needle with the spermatozoon are gently expelled into the ooplasm. (f) After the spermatozoon has been deposited into the ooplasm, the injection needle is slowly withdrawn.

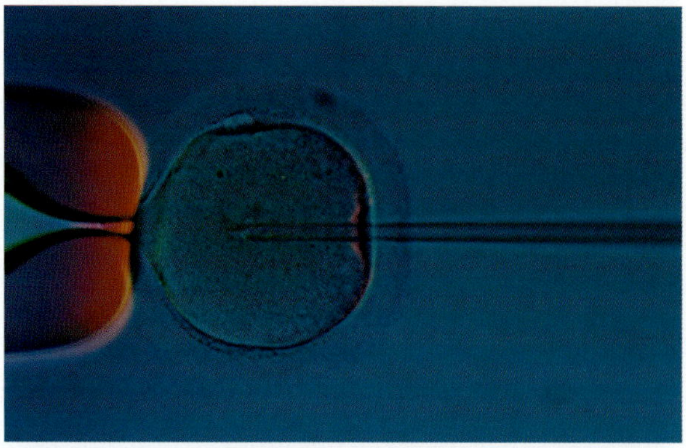

(a)

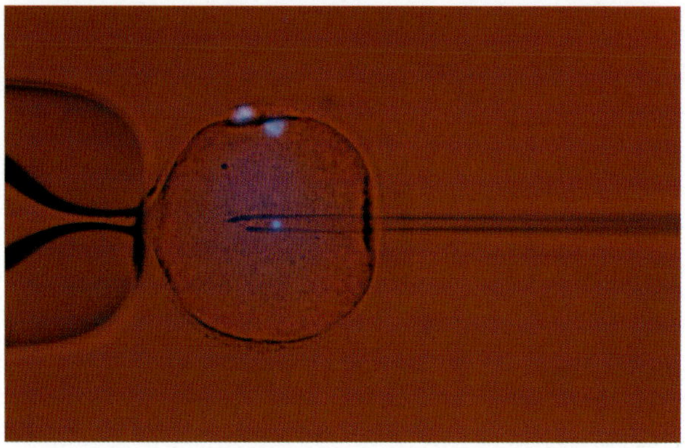

(b)

Figure 2.4 ICSI (continued). (a) Bright-field (Nomarski) optics. Entrance of the micropipette containing a spermatozoon. The first polar body (PB1) is located at the 11 o'clock position. (b) Epifluorescence after chromatin staining with Hoechst. Three areas of fluorescence can be seen: the PB1 chromatin; the oocyte chromosomes near the area of the PB1; and the sperm chromatin.

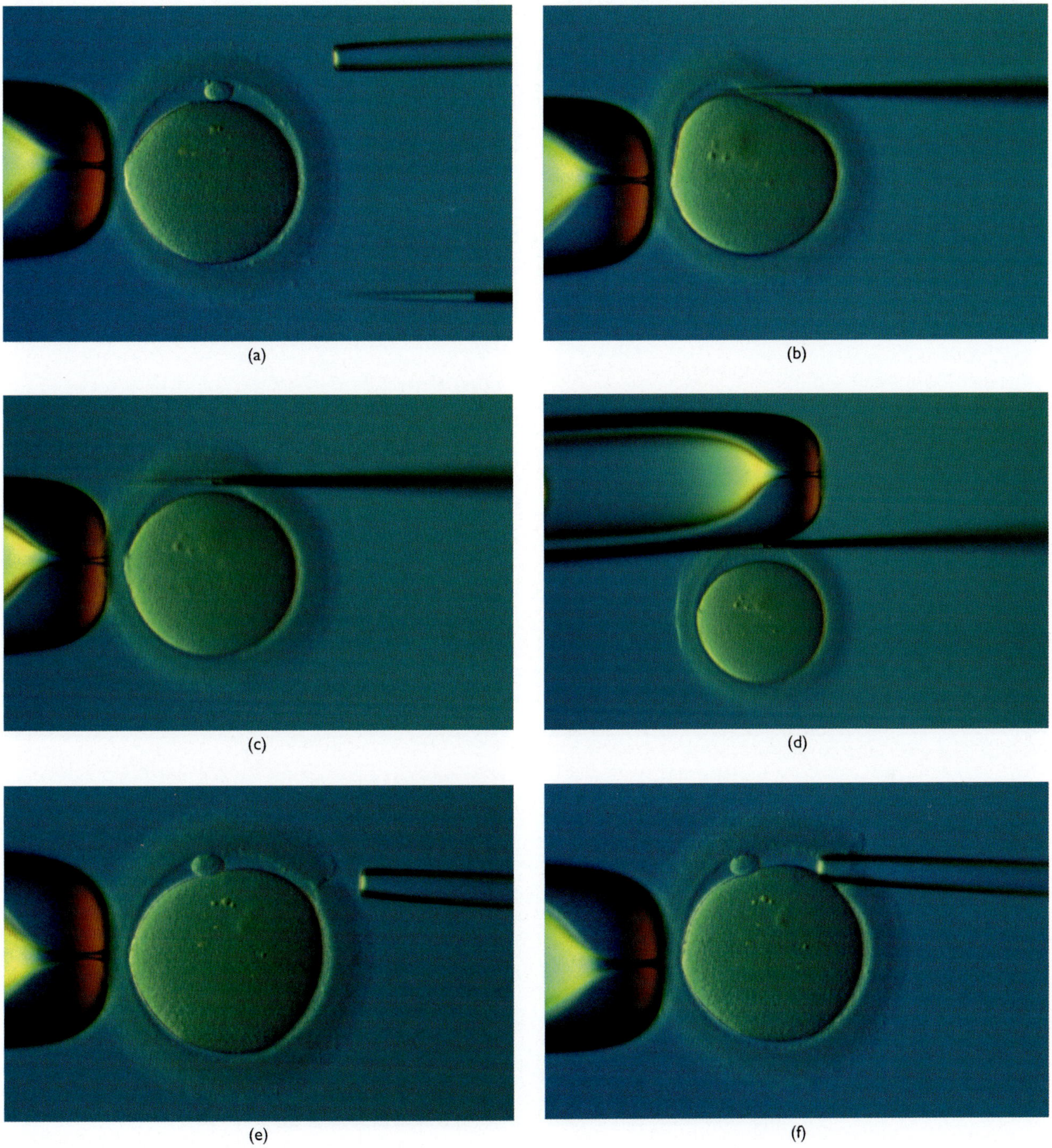

Figure 2.5 First polar body (PBI) removal after ICSI. (a) Once secured by the holding pipette, the oocyte is oriented by means of the microneedle so that the PBI is visualized at the 12 o'clock position. (b) and (c) By means of the microneedle, the oocyte is rotated horizontally until the PBI is slightly out of focus. In this case, the slit in the zona pellucida is located closer to the PBI, providing easier access to it. If the zona pellucida is cut right above the PBI, it will lead to deformation or damage of the polar body by the biopsy pipette when it passes through the opening. The microneedle is passed through the zona pellucida at the 1–2 o'clock position, tangentially through the perivitelline space and out at the 10–11 o'clock position. (d) The oocyte is released from the holding pipette and held by the microneedle. The microneedle with the oocyte is brought to the bottom of the holding pipette and pressed to it, pinching a portion of the zona pellucida. By gently rubbing the microneedle against the holding pipette with a sawing motion, partial zona dissection is performed and the oocyte is released. (e) The oocyte is rotated so that the opening in the zona pellucida is at the 2 o'clock position and the polar body is in focus. (f) The aspirating micropipette is passed through the opening to the PBI.

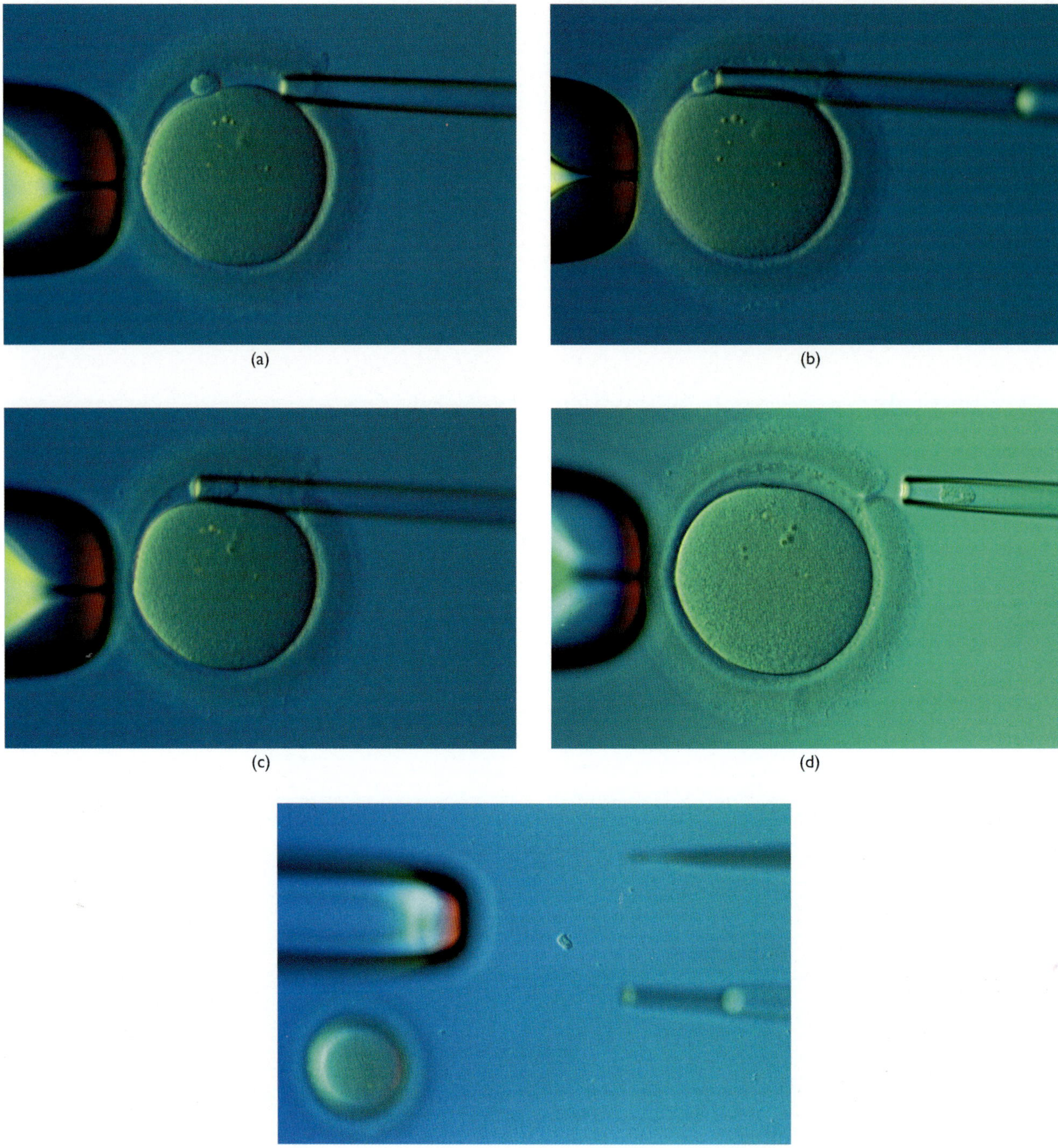

(a) (b) (c) (d) (e)

Figure 2.6 First polar body (PB1) removal after ICSI (continued). (a) The aspirating micropipette is further passed through the opening to the PB1. (b), (c), and (d) Gentle suction is applied to aspirate the polar body into the micropipette. Pressure from the hydraulic system is equilibrated prior to withdrawal of the aspirating micropipette to avoid damage to the oocyte. (e) The oocyte is released from the holding pipette, and all the microtools are raised slightly from the bottom of the dish. The microscope stage is moved so that another drop of medium at the 6 o'clock position is visualized. The micropipette containing the polar body is lowered to the bottom of the dish, and the PB1 is expelled to the middle of the drop of medium. In this picture, however, the polar body was expelled immediately for demonstration and can be seen in the center.

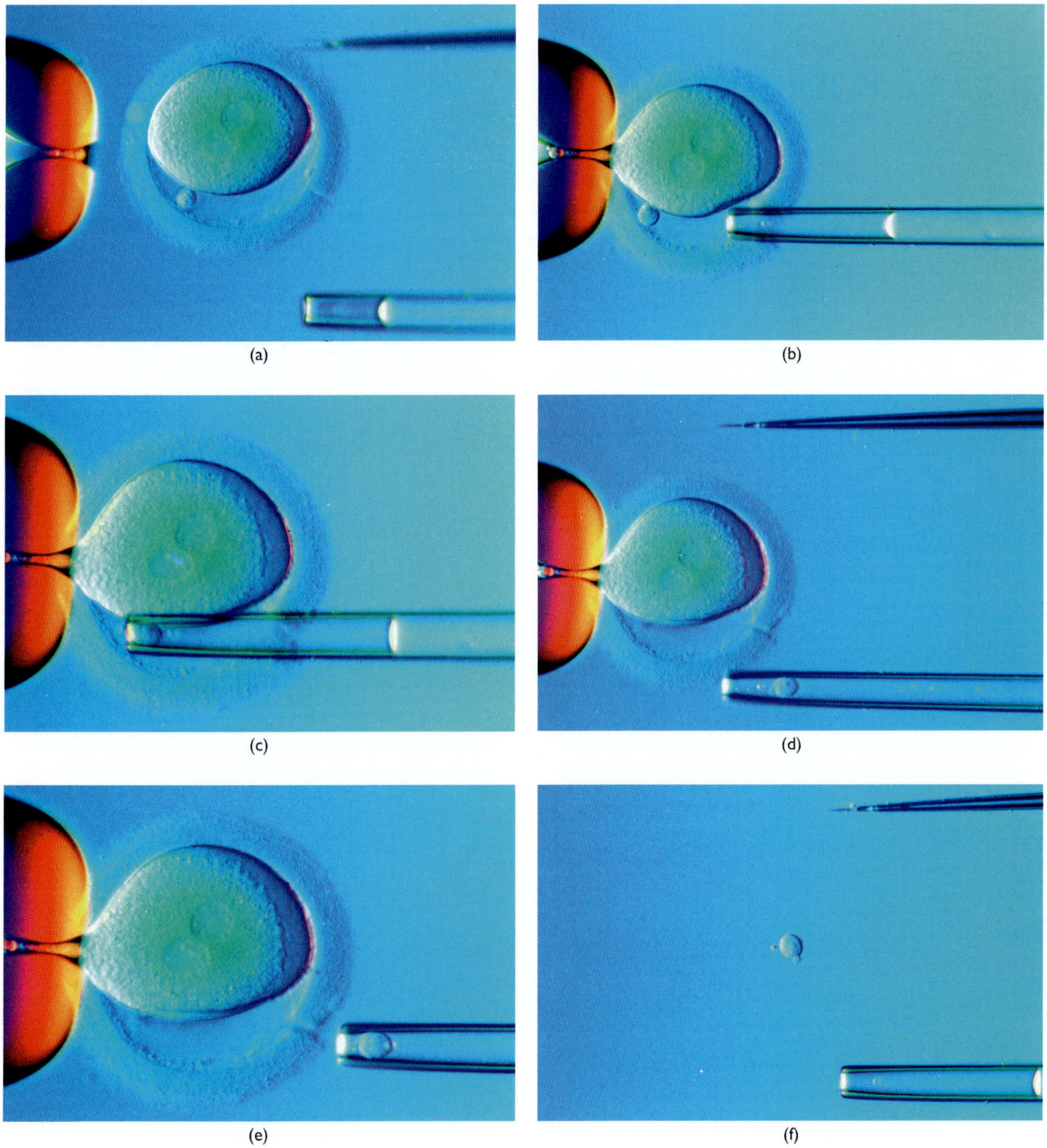

Figure 2.7 Second polar body (PB2) removal. (a) Since an opening has already been created in the zona pellucida prior to the first polar body removal, the prezygote is rotated so that the opening in the zona pellucida is positioned conveniently enough to access the PB2. (b) The opening should be in focus when passing the micropipette into the perivitelline space (PVS). (c) Once in the PVS the PB2 is brought into focus and the micropipette is advanced to the polar body. With gentle suction the polar body is aspirated into the micropipette. (d) and (e) At this point, the micropipette with the PB2 is withdrawn from the PVS. Because the PB2 is almost always attached by a cytoplasmic bridge to the prezygote, positive pressure in the micropipette is maintained during withdrawal until the cytoplasmic bridge is pinched off. (f) The prezygote is released from the holding pipette, and all the microtools are raised slightly from the bottom of the dish. The microscope stage is moved so that another drop of medium at the 6 o'clock position is visualized. The micropipette containing the second polar body is lowered to the bottom of the dish, and the PB2 is expelled to the middle of the drop of medium. For demonstration, the PB2 can be seen in the center; the prezygote is out of focus.

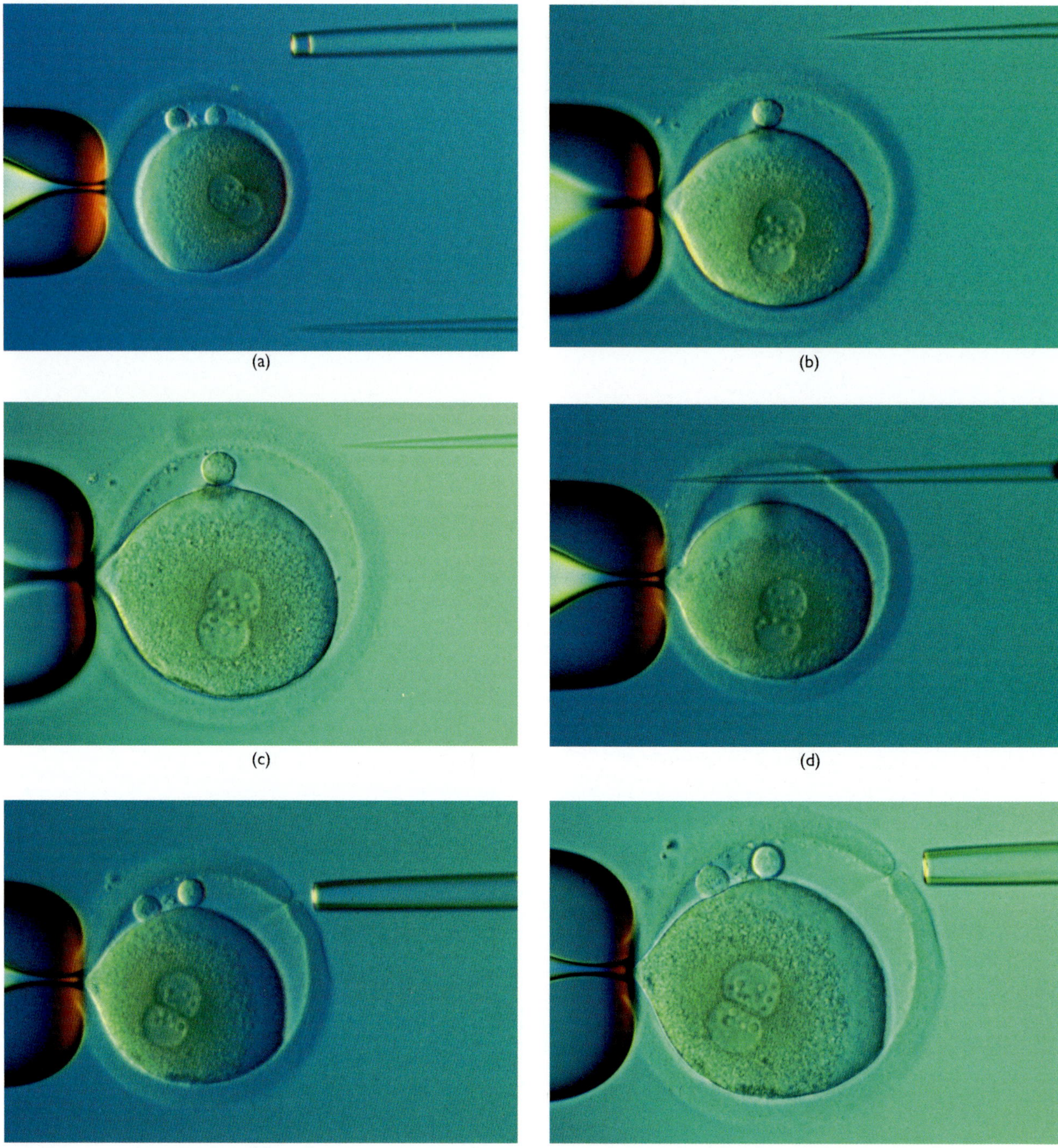

Figure 2.8 Simultaneous first (PB1) and second (PB2) polar body removal. (a) Once secured by the holding pipette, the prezygote is oriented by the microneedle to visualize the PB1 and PB2 side by side at the 12 o'clock position. At this position, the morphology and number of polar bodies are evaluated. (b) and (c) The prezygote is released and gently rotated so that both polar bodies are still at the 12 o'clock position, one behind the other. (d) The prezygote is rotated until the polar bodies are slightly out of focus. A slit is made by entering the zona pellucida with the partial zona dissection needle at the 1–2 o'clock position, passing tangentially through the perivitelline space and out at the 10–11 o'clock position. The opening in the zona pellucida is made similarly to the PB1 removal procedure. The prezygote is released from the holding pipette and held by the microneedle. The microneedle with the prezygote is brought to the bottom of the holding pipette and pressed to it, pinching a portion of the zona pellucida. By gently rubbing the microneedle against the holding pipette with a sawing motion, a partial zona dissection is performed and the prezygote is released. (e) and (f) The prezygote is oriented by the microneedle to visualize both polar bodies at the 12 o'clock position, side by side, and the opening in the zona pellucida. In this position, both polar bodies and slit opening in the zona pellucida are positioned on the same straight line so that the polar bodies are easily accessed by the aspirating pipette.

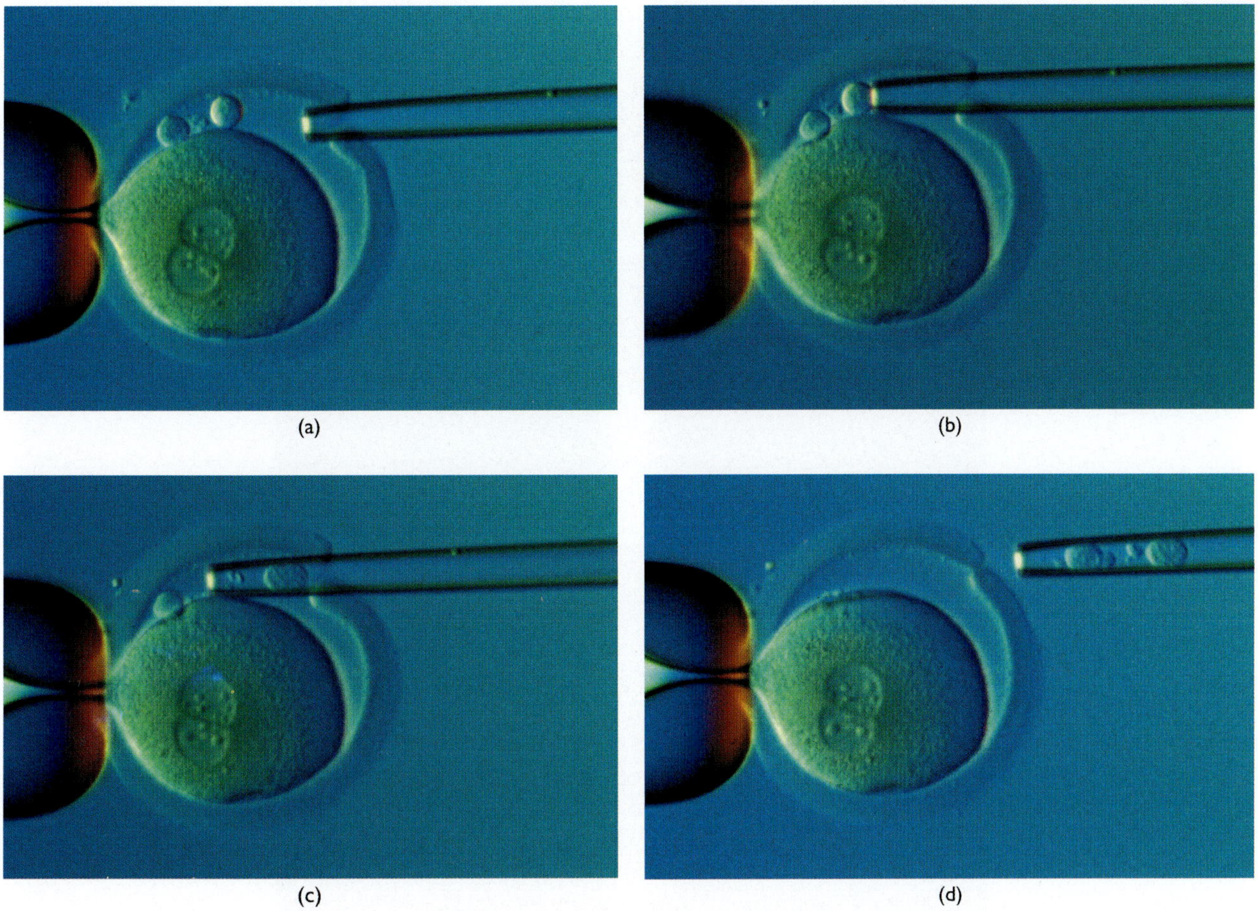

Figure 2.9 Simultaneous first and second polar body removal (continued). (a) and (b) The aspirating micropipette is passed through the opening to one of the polar bodies. (c) and (d) Gentle suction is applied to aspirate the first available polar body into the micropipette. Once pressure from the hydraulic system has been equilibrated, the micropipette is moved forward to the remaining polar body, gentle suction is applied, and the second polar body is aspirated. If one or both polar bodies are fragmented, all of the fragments are removed in similar fashion, focusing on the target object and redirecting the position of the micropipette towards it. Pressure from the hydraulic system is equilibrated prior to the withdrawal of the aspirating micropipette to avoid damage to the prezygote. The prezygote is released from the holding pipette, and all the microtools are raised slightly from the bottom of the dish. The microscope stage is moved so that another drop of medium at the 6 o'clock position is visualized. The micropipette containing all the polar bodies is lowered to the bottom of the dish, and the polar bodies are expelled in the middle of the drop of medium.

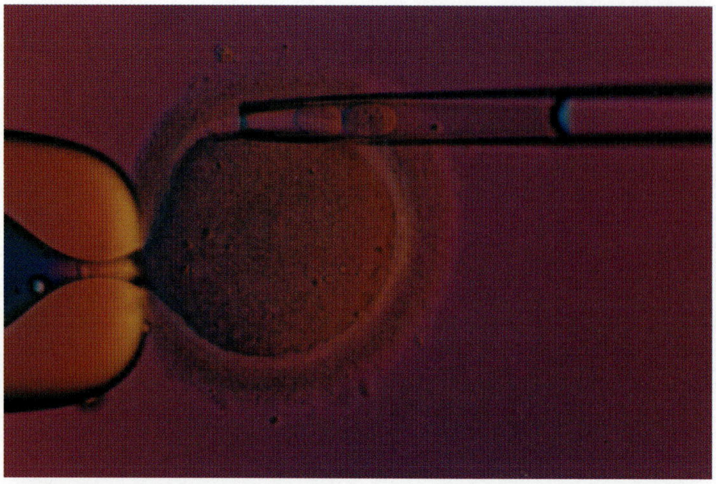

(a)

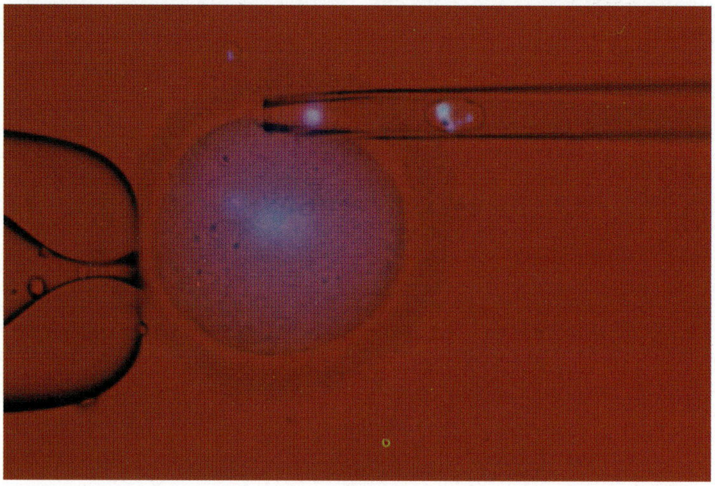

(b)

Figure 2.10 Simultaneous first (PB1) and second (PB2) polar body removal (continued). (a) Bright-field (Nomarski) optics. Simultaneous PB1 and PB2 removal from an abnormally fertilized prezygote. (b) Epifluorescence after chromatin staining with Hoechst DNA stain.

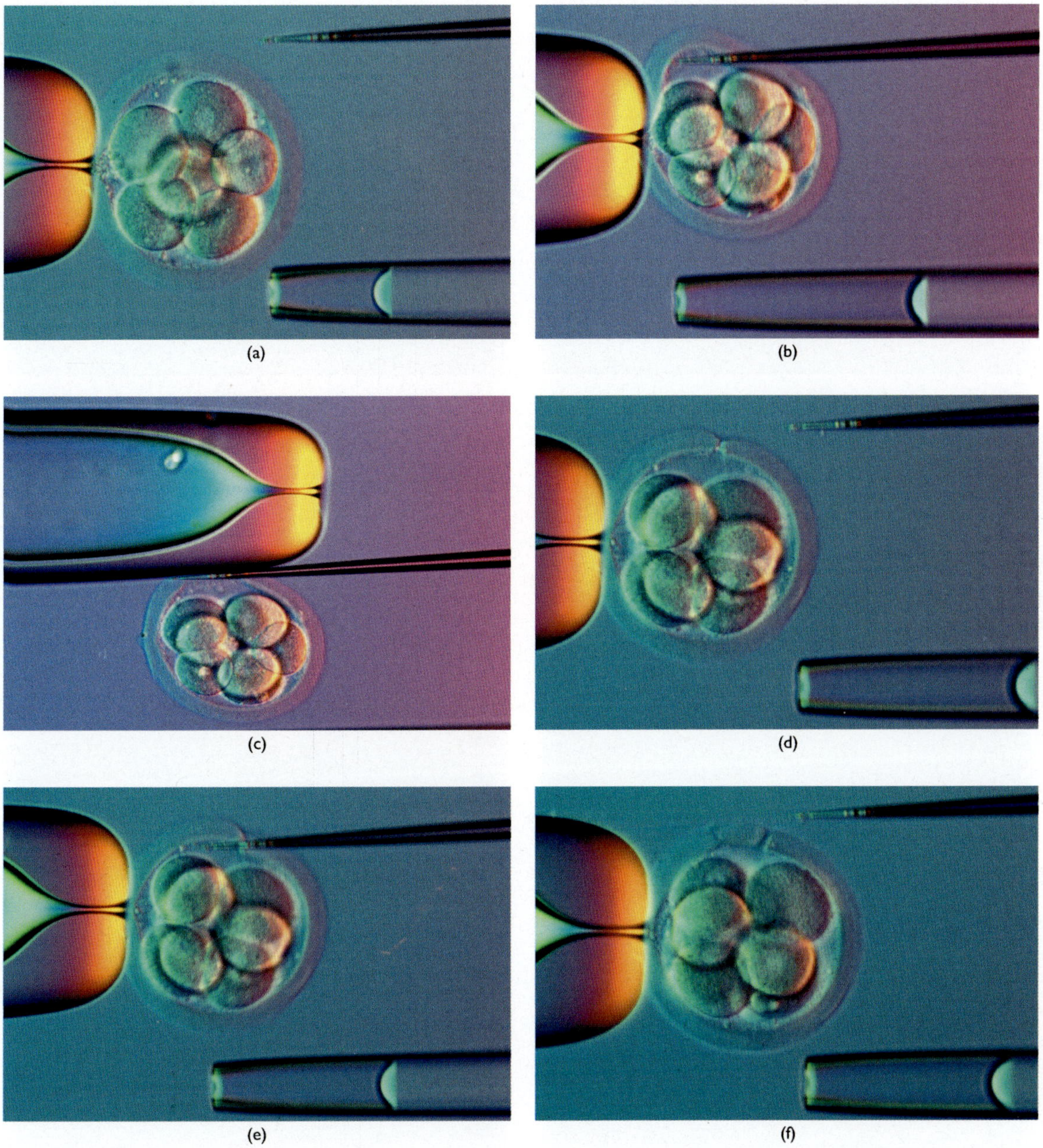

Figure 2.11 Embryo biopsy following the making of a square opening in the zona pellucida. (a) The embryo is held loosely by gentle suction from the holding pipette and rotated using the microneedle until the area with the largest perivitelline space (PVS) is visible at the 12 o'clock position. (b) Additional suction is applied to hold the embryo firmly in this position. The microneedle is passed through the zona pellucida starting at the 1–2 o'clock position and advanced tangentially through the PVS and out the other side at the 10–11 o'clock position. (c) The embryo is released from the holding pipette and held by the microneedle. The microneedle is brought to the bottom of the holding pipette and pressed to it, pinching a portion of the zona pellucida. By gently rubbing the microneedle against the holding pipette with a sawing motion, the cut is accomplished and the embryo is released. (d) and (e) To perform the second cut, the embryo is rotated vertically until the slit is clearly visible at the 12 o'clock position and then rotated horizontally backwards until the slit is slightly out of focus, reaching the end of the slit, which is now at the 12 o'clock position. The second intersecting cut is positioned at the end of the first cut to create the V-shaped opening. This cut is completed by entry into the first slit, advancing tangentially through the PVS and ending at the 10–11 o'clock position. The embryo is released from the holding pipette and held by the microneedle. After the second cut is accomplished, the embryo is again rotated vertically until the new slit is visible at the 12 o'clock position and then rotated horizontally backwards until the slit is slightly out of focus, reaching the end of the slit. The microneedle is passed through the slit opening, through the PVS, and out at the 10–11 o'clock position. The third intersecting cut makes up the third side of the square. (f) To complete the square and create a hole in the zona pellucida, the fourth intersecting cut is made by rotating the embryo vertically until two slits are visible at the 12 o'clock position. The embryo is rotated horizontally backwards until both slits are slightly out of focus, and the final cut is made by entering the first slit, passing through the PVS and out at the 11 o'clock position. The embryo is released from the holding pipette and is held by the microneedle. The microneedle is brought to the bottom of the holding pipette, pressed slightly and, with a sawing motion, the final cut is accomplished.

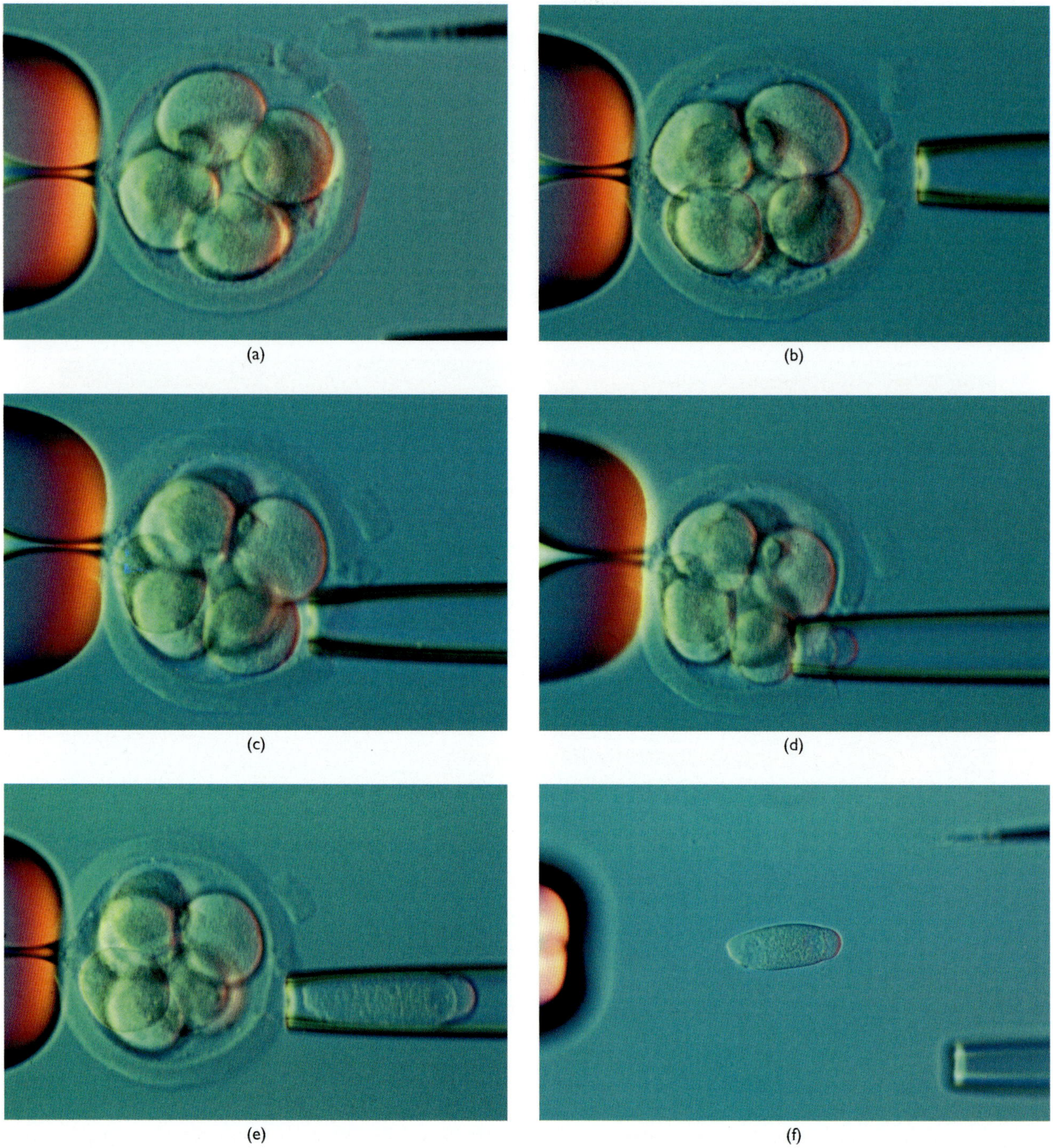

Figure 2.12 Embryo biopsy following the making of a square opening in the zona pellucida (continued). (a) An opening in the shape of a square can be seen after removal of the cut-out portion using the microneedle. The size of the hole created is dependent on the length of the first two cuts. (b) The embryo is positioned and held by the holding pipette with the opening in the zona pellucida at the 3 o'clock position. A square piece can be seen adhering to the zona pellucida above the opening. (c) The blastomere biopsy needle is freely passed through the opening towards the nearest blastomere. (d) The blastomere is slowly aspirated into the pipette. (e) Aspiration is continued slowly until the whole blastomere is inside the aspiration needle. The micropipette containing the blastomere is withdrawn from the perivitelline space. (f) The embryo is released from the holding pipette, and all the microtools are raised slightly from the bottom of the dish. The microscope stage is moved so that the drop of medium at the 6 o'clock position is visualized. The micropipette containing the blastomere is lowered to the bottom of the dish, and the blastomere is expelled to the middle of the drop of medium.

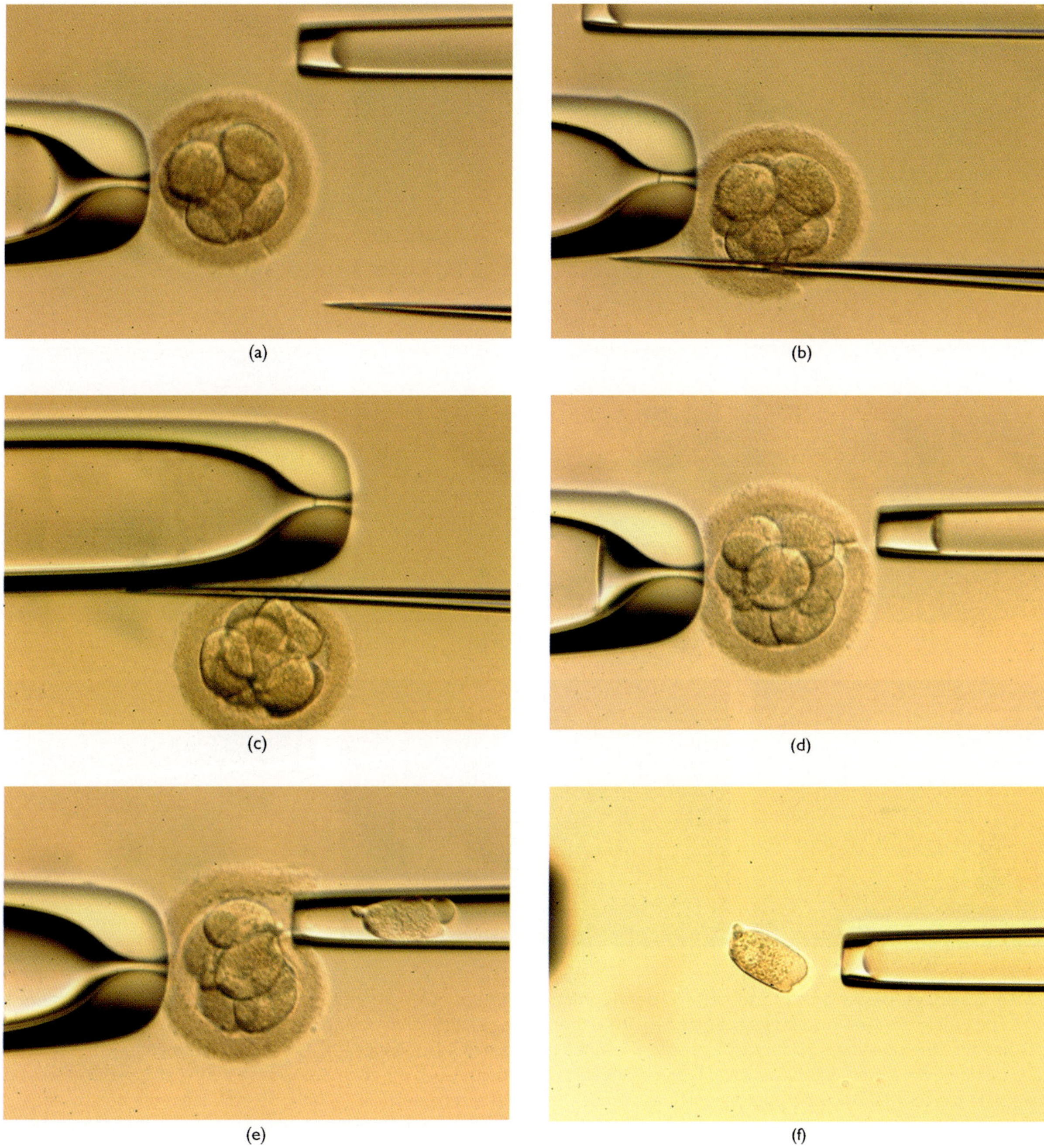

(a) (b) (c) (d) (e) (f)

Figure 2.13 Embryo biopsy following polar body removal and creation of the V-shaped opening in the zona pellucida. (a) To perform the second cut, the embryo is rotated vertically until the first slit created during polar body removal is clearly visible (5 o'clock position). (b) The second intersecting slit is accomplished by entry into the first slit, advancing tangentially through the perivitelline space, and ending at the 7 o'clock position. (c) The embryo is released from the holding pipette and held by the microneedle. The microneedle is brought to the bottom of the holding pipette and pressed to it, pinching a portion of the zona pellucida. By gently rubbing the microneedle against the holding pipette with a sawing motion, partial zona dissection is performed and the embryo is released. (d) The embryo is rotated until the V-shaped opening is at 3 o'clock and then held firmly by suction from the holding pipette. (e) The embryo biopsy micropipette is then brought into focus, and by application of a slight downward pressure freely passes through the opening toward the nearest blastomere. The blastomere is slowly aspirated into the pipette. Aspiration continues slowly until the whole blastomere is inside the micropipette, which is then withdrawn slowly from the perivitelline space. The blastomere is removed with little distortion to the embryo. (f) The embryo is released from the holding pipette, and all the microtools are raised slightly from the bottom of the dish. The microscope stage is moved so that another drop of medium at the 6 o'clock position is visualized. The micropipette containing the blastomere is lowered to the bottom of the dish, and the blastomere is expelled to the middle of the drop of medium.

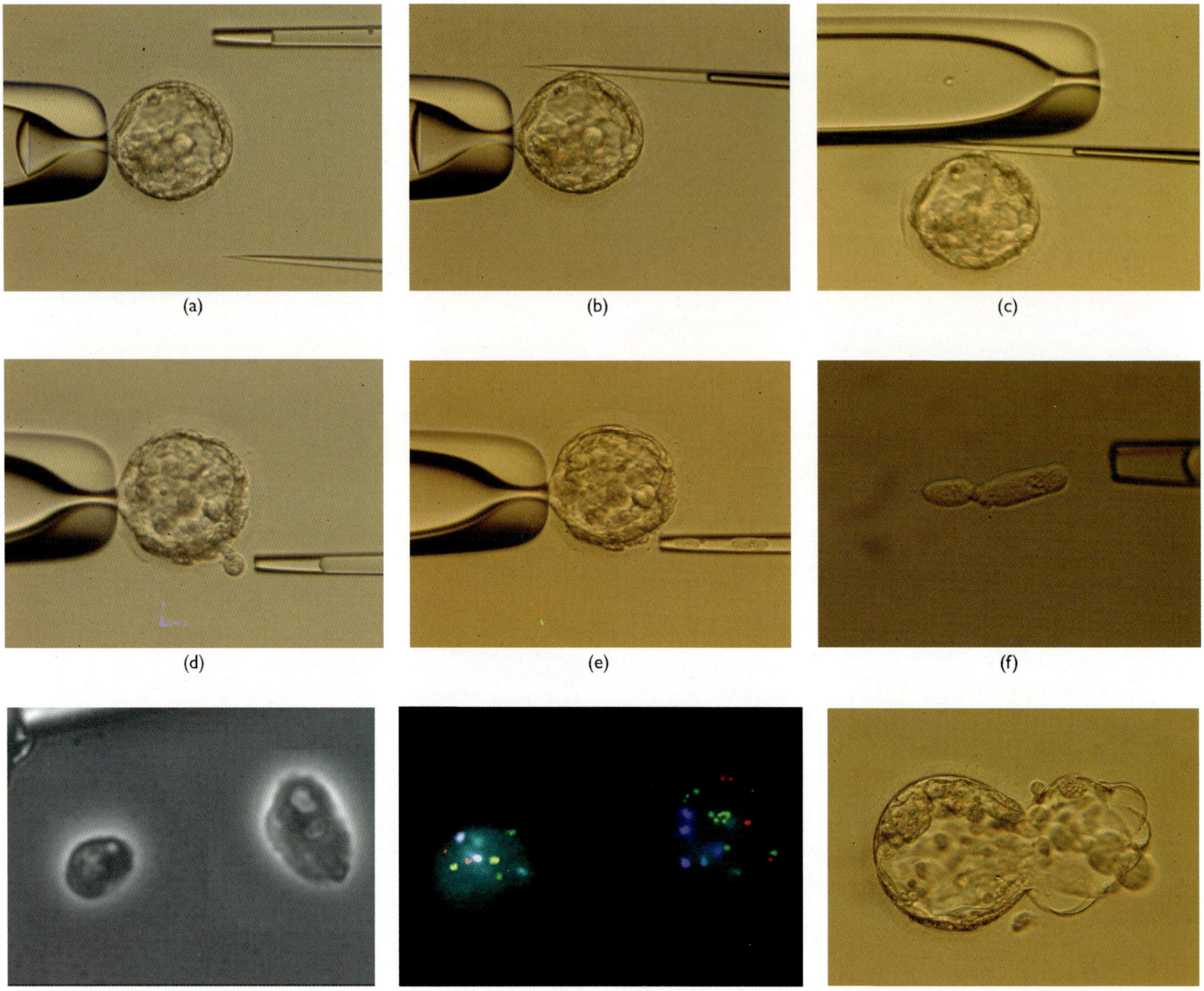

(a) (b) (c) (d) (e) (f) (g) (h) (i)

Figure 2.14 Blastocyst biopsy on day 5 of embryo development. (a) Image of a poor-quality blastocyst prior to beginning the biopsy procedure. The embryo is held loosely by gentle suction from the holding pipette and rotated using the microneedle, in order to position the embryo so that the opening is positioned opposite the inner cell mass (ICM), if visible. (b) The embryo is then held firmly in position using more suction from the holding pipette and the microneedle is passed through the zona pellucida, entering at approximately 1 o'clock and exiting at 11 o'clock. (c) Once the microneedle has passed through the zona pellucida, a slit-type opening is created by releasing the embryo from the holding pipette, bringing the portion of the zona pellucida under which the microneedle has passed to the holding pipette, gently pressing and rubbing against the holding pipette in order to cut the zona pellucida. (d) After an hour or more in culture, trophectoderm cells will begin herniating through the opening. (e) Depending on the cohesiveness of the cells, they may be aspirated into the micropipette, as seen in this example, or may be cut using a microsurgical blade. (f) Image of the two trophectoderm cells that were removed. (g) Phase-contrast image of the nuclei isolated from the corresponding cells (f). (h) Fluorescence *in situ* hybridization (FISH) image after hybridization with MultiVysion polar body (PB) panel probe for chromosomes 13, 16, 18, 21, and 22. One normal diploid and one tetraploid cell are evident by the number of signals present for the five chromosomes tested. (i) Image of the same embryo in which blastocyst biopsy was performed (a) after several hours in culture, hatching through the artificial opening created during biopsy.

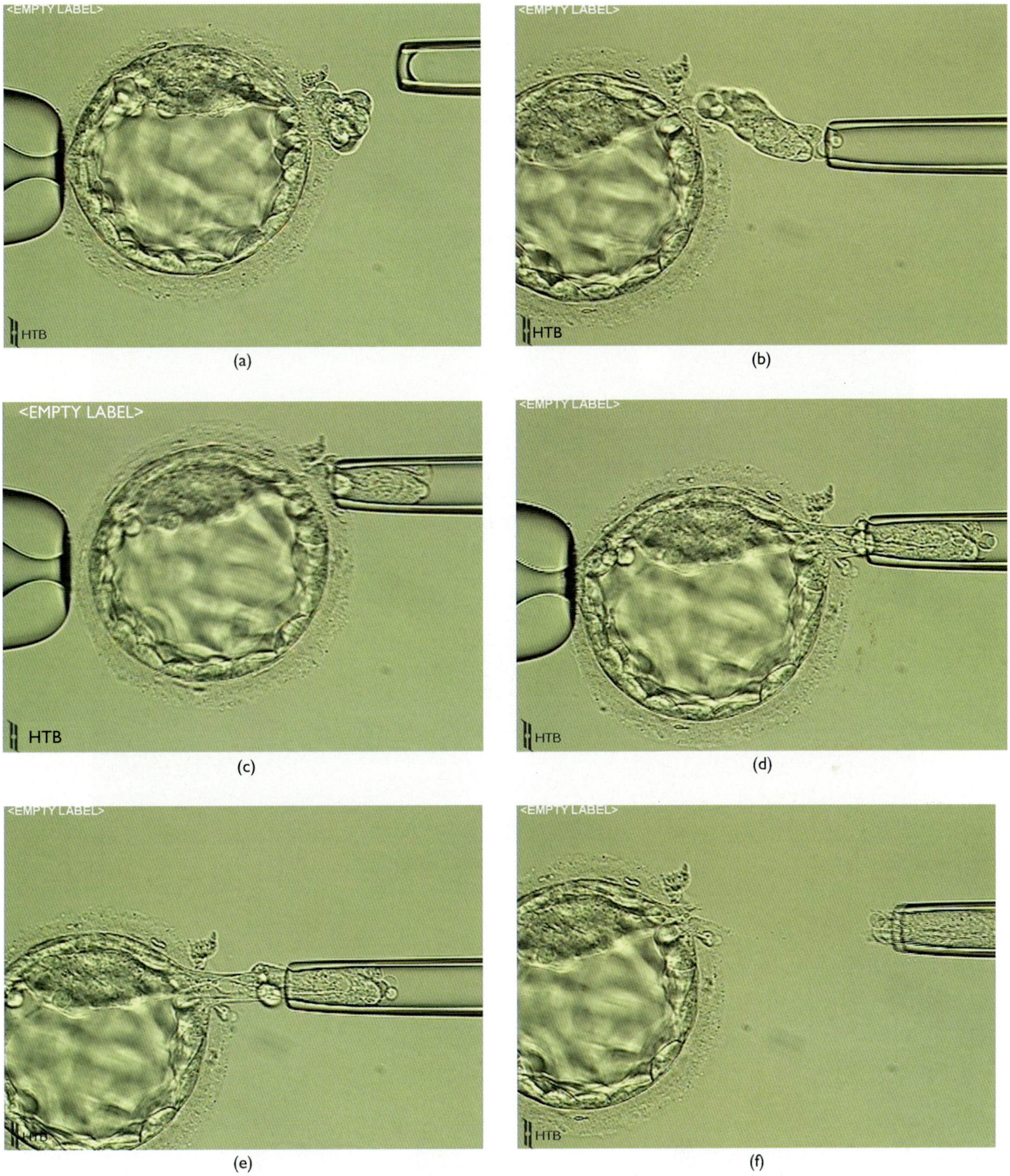

Figure 2.15 Laser-assisted blastocyst biopsy on day 5. (a) Image of a blastocyst prior to beginning the biopsy procedure. The embryo is held loosely by gentle suction from the holding pipette and rotated using the microneedle in order to position the embryo so that the opening is positioned opposite the ICM. (b), (c), and (d) As the trophectoderm is beginning to herniate through the zona pellucida, several trophectoderm cells are smoothly aspirated into the biopsy pipette with internal diameter of 30 μm throughout the zona pellucida. (e) To break down the tight junctions between trophectoderm cells, three laser shots are applied (with a duration of 0.7 msec pulse with each. (f) Biopsied cells transferred for analysis.

3 Nuclear transfer techniques for preimplantation diagnosis and prospect for artificial gamete formation

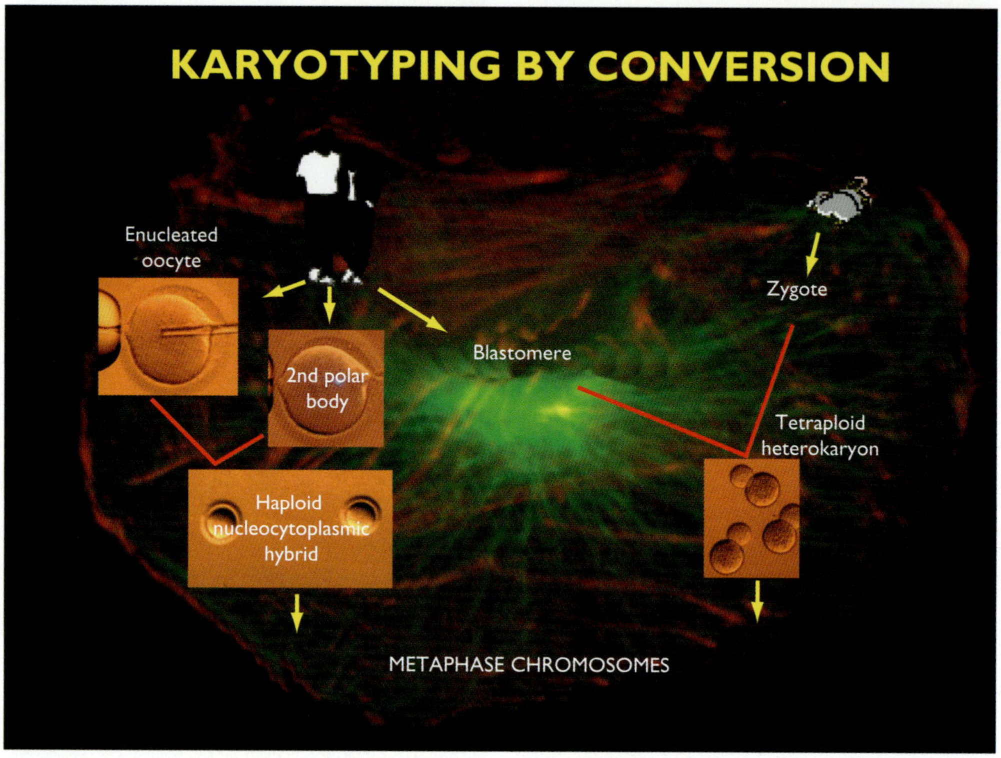

Figure 3.1 Scheme of karyotyping by nuclear transfer technique.

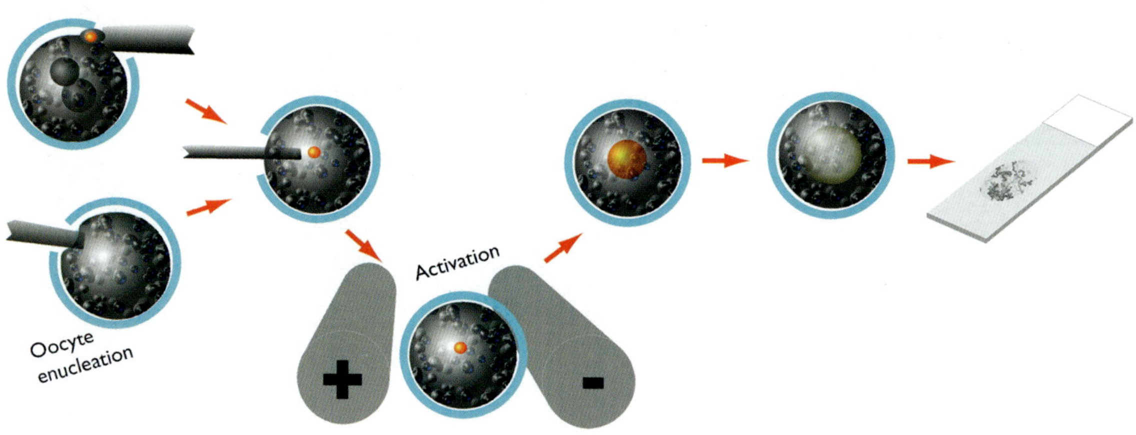

Figure 3.2 Flow chart of second polar body nucleus conversion into metaphase chromosomes.

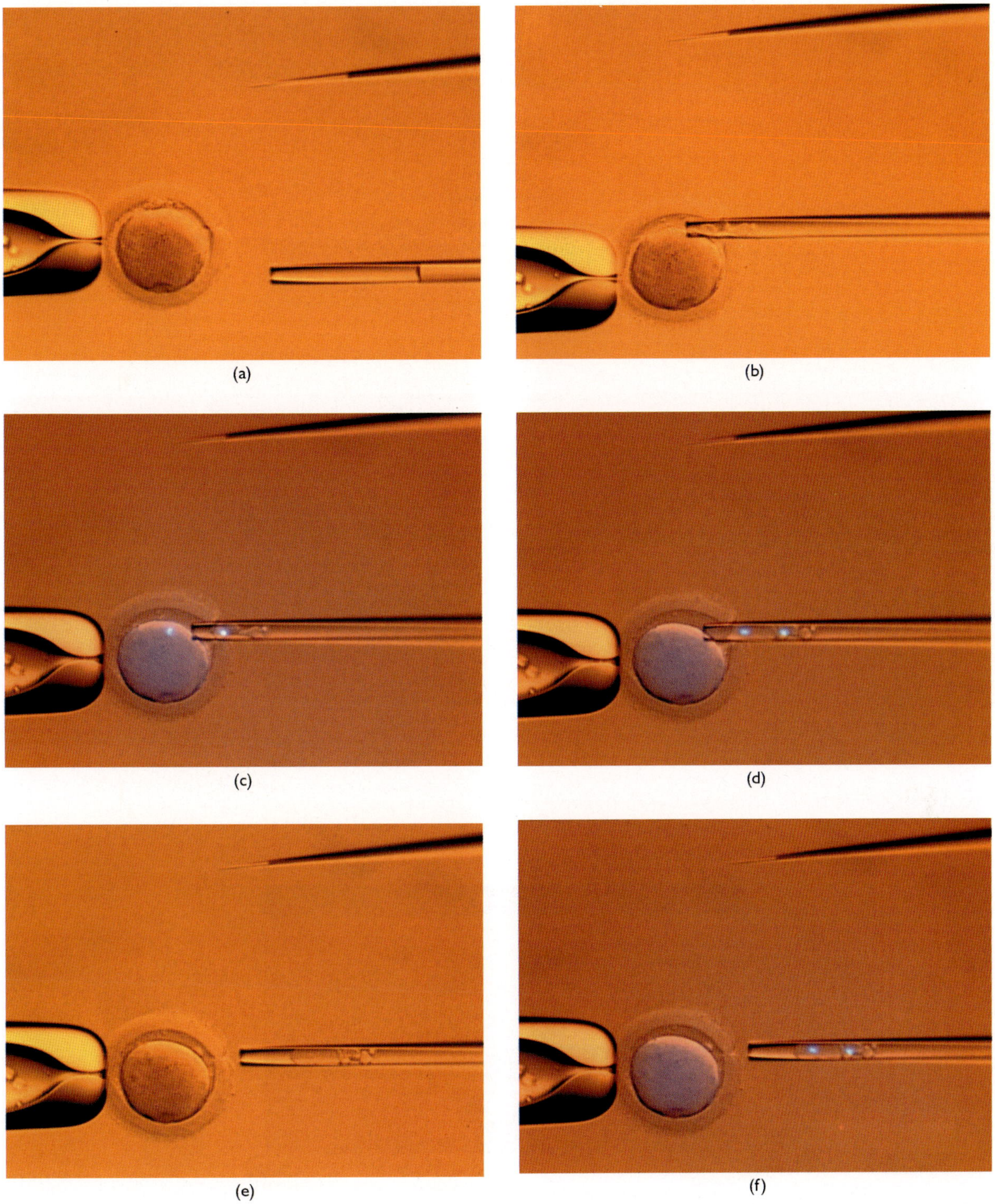

Figure 3.3 Enucleation of human oocytes as a source of cytoplasts for second polar body nucleus conversion into metaphase chromosomes. (a) and (b) After partial zona dissection, a flame-polished biopsy tool is used to remove the first polar body (PB1) from the perivitelline space, as described in Chapter 2. (c) and (d) Chromatin epifluorescence after staining with vital Hoechst stain. (e) and (f) Enucleation is verified by a second brief exposure to epifluorescence, showing that both the PB1 and metaphase II chromosomes are inside the pipette.

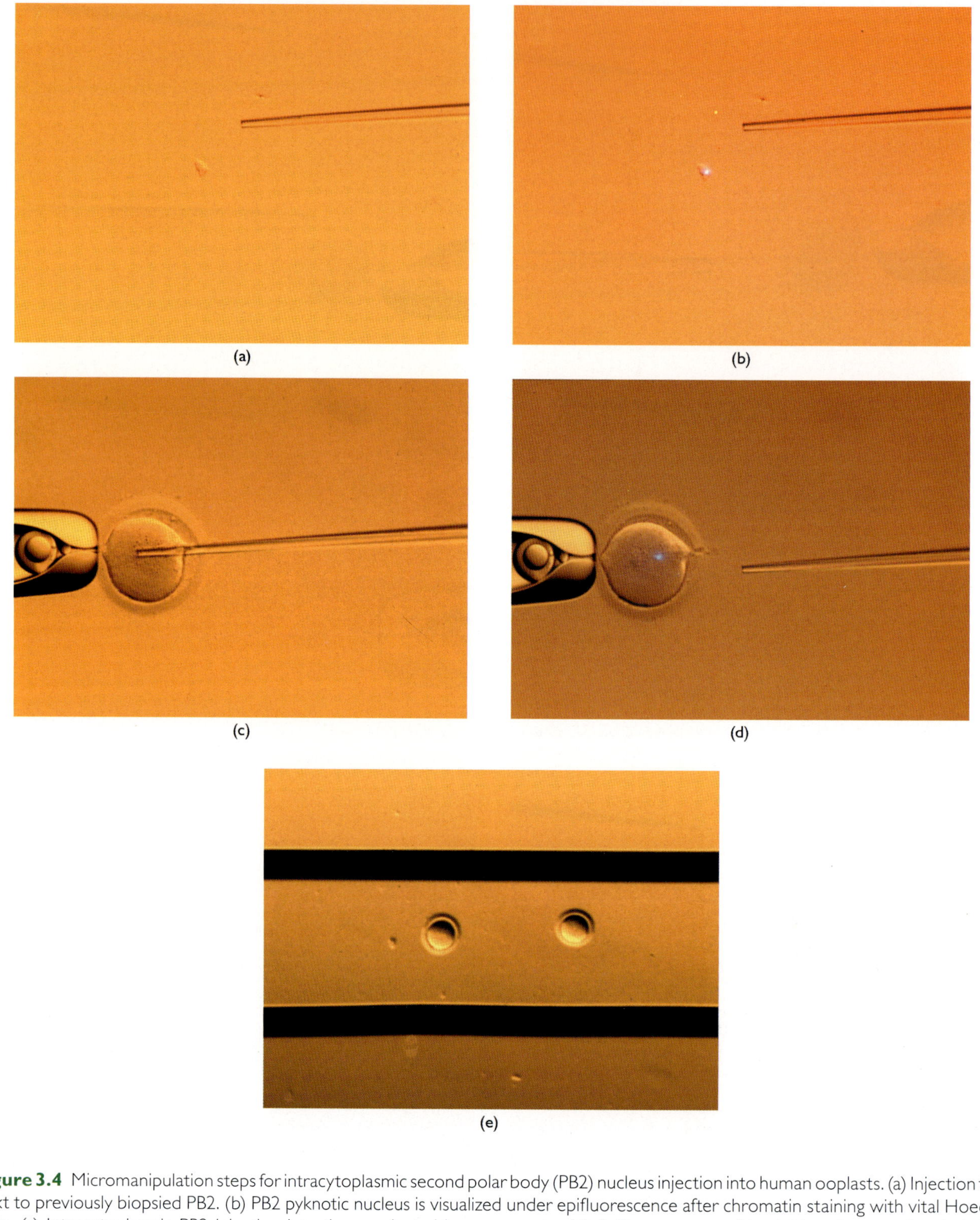

Figure 3.4 Micromanipulation steps for intracytoplasmic second polar body (PB2) nucleus injection into human ooplasts. (a) Injection tool next to previously biopsied PB2. (b) PB2 pyknotic nucleus is visualized under epifluorescence after chromatin staining with vital Hoechst stain. (c) Intracytoplasmic PB2 injection into the enucleated human oocyte. (d) Epifluorescence of haploid nucleocytoplasmic hybrid immediately after polar body injection, confirming the success of the procedure. (e) Activation of the resulting haploid nucleocytoplasmic hybrids by electrostimulation.

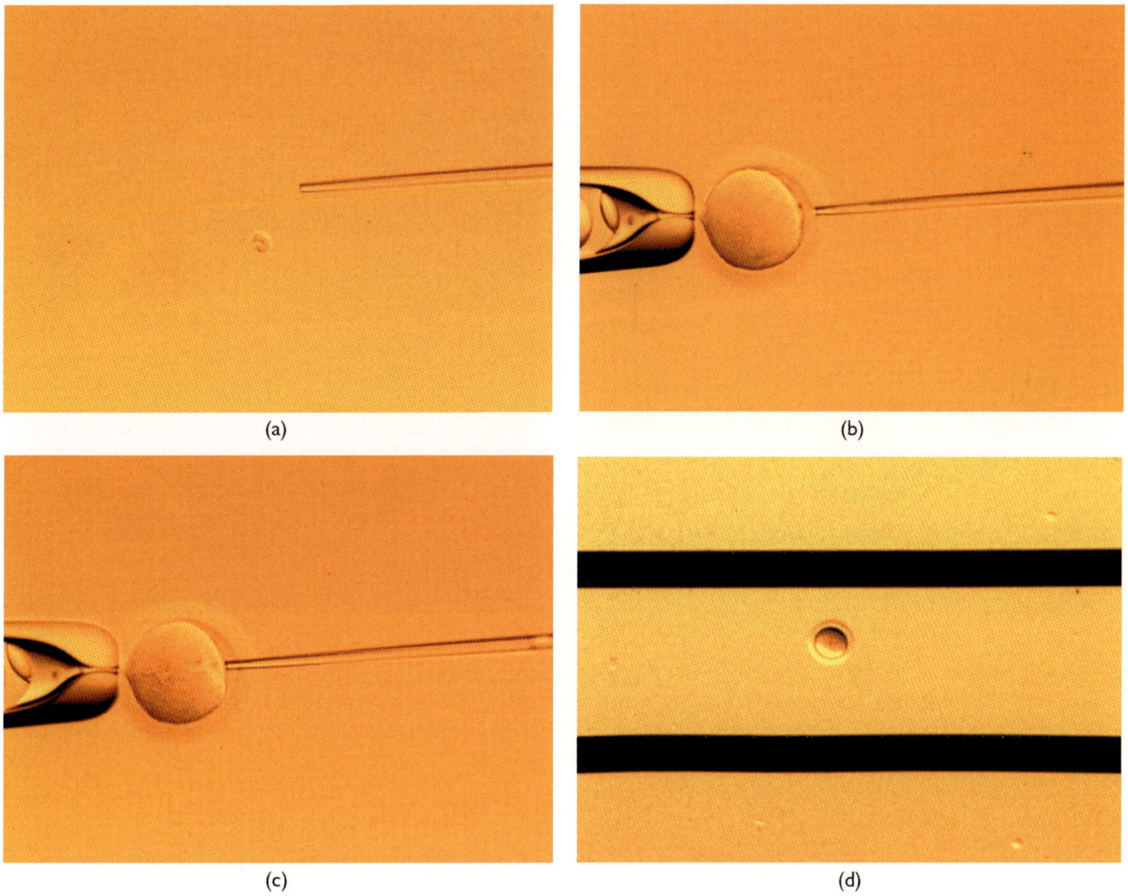

Figure 3.5 Intracytoplasmic second polar body (PB2) nucleus injection into human ooplasts without Hoechst staining and epifluorescence verification. (a) PB2 prior to aspiration into the injection pipette. (b) Human ooplast before intracytoplasmic PB2 injection. (c) Reconstructed haploid nucleocytoplasmic hybrid immediately after PB2 injection into the ooplast. (d) Haploid nucleocytoplasmic hybrid activation, one at a time.

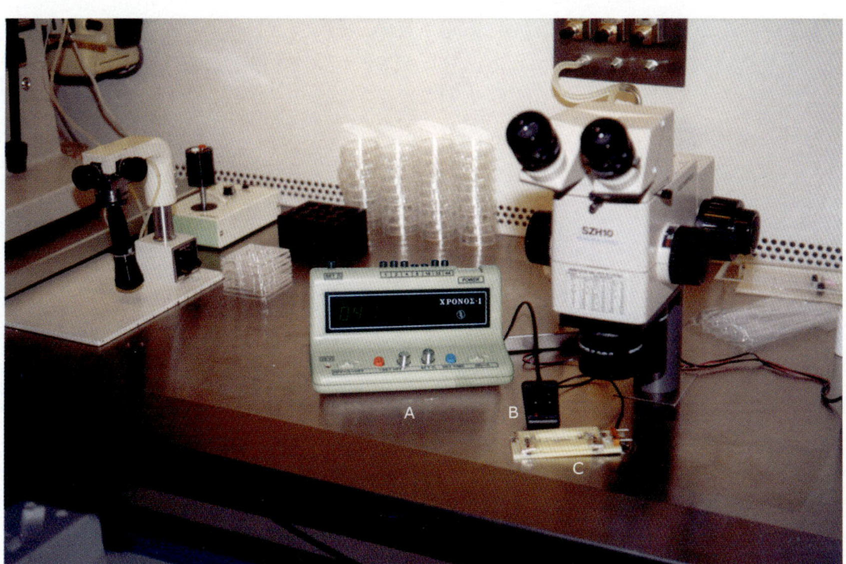

Figure 3.6 Oocyte activation and cell electrofusion device (XRONOS, Chicago, IL). (A) Electrofusion unit, (B) remote control, and (C) chamber for electrofusion.

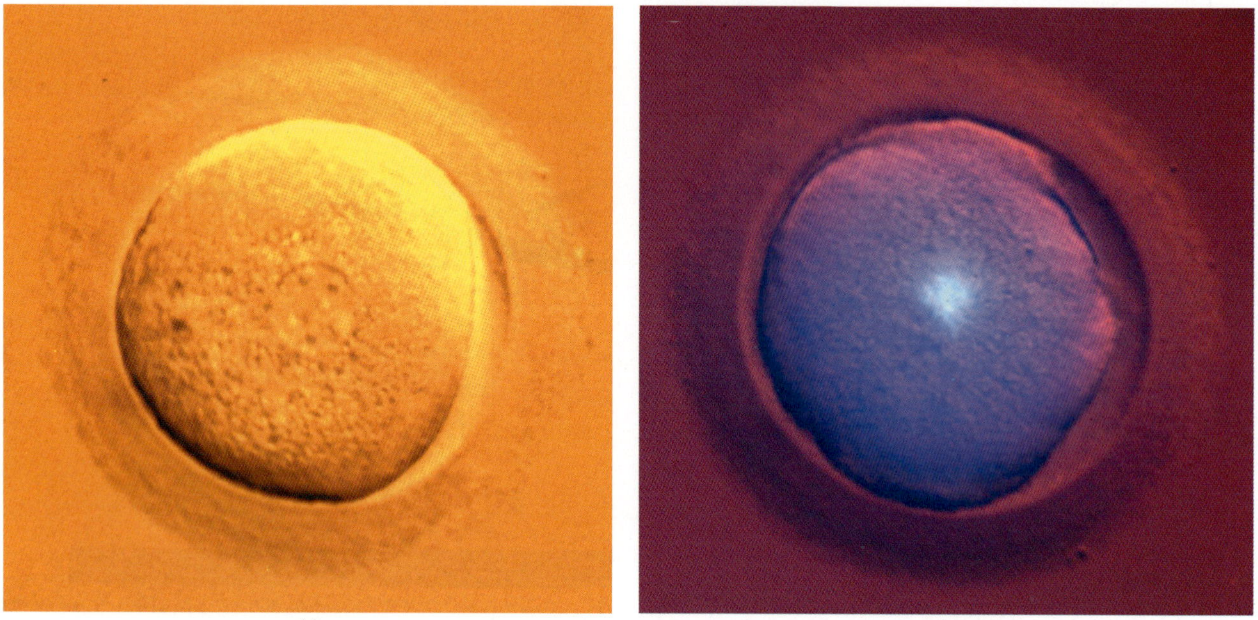

(a) (b)

Figure 3.7 Conversion of the second polar body (PB2) nucleus into metaphase chromosomes. (a) Haploid nucleocytoplasmic hybrid between human PB2 and enucleated oocyte at the pronuclear stage (differential interference contrast using Nomarski optics). (b) The same embryo, at the first metaphase. Chromosomes (blue) are visualized by Hoechst staining; Hoffman modulation contrast optics gives the general view of the embryo.

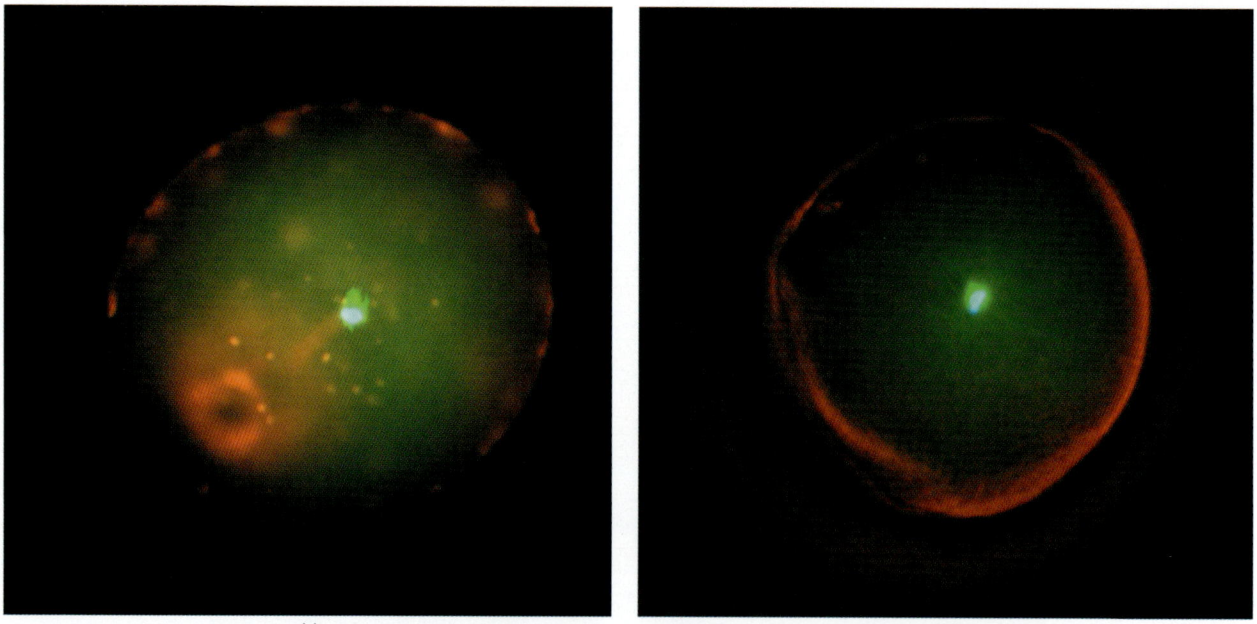

(a) (b)

Figure 3.8 Second polar body (PB2) nucleus transformation following its injection into foreign cytoplasm (immunocytochemical investigation). (a) Haploid nucleocytoplasmic hybrid immediately after intracytoplasmic PB2 injection. Actin stained red, tubulin green, chromatin blue. The PB2 nucleus is inside the cytoplast. Anti-actin antibodies (labeled red) stain the subcortical layer of actin and are used for visualizing membranes. The cavity is still not relaxed after injection. There is no plasma membrane around the PB2 nucleus since it was broken by the injection tool. However, it is surrounded by tubulin microfilaments, abundant in the PB2 (unpublished observations). (b) Two hours after PB2 injection (bright-field view of an embryo is shown in red, tubulin green, chromatin blue). Tubulin microfilaments, initially present only around the nucleus, started to elongate into the cytoplasm.

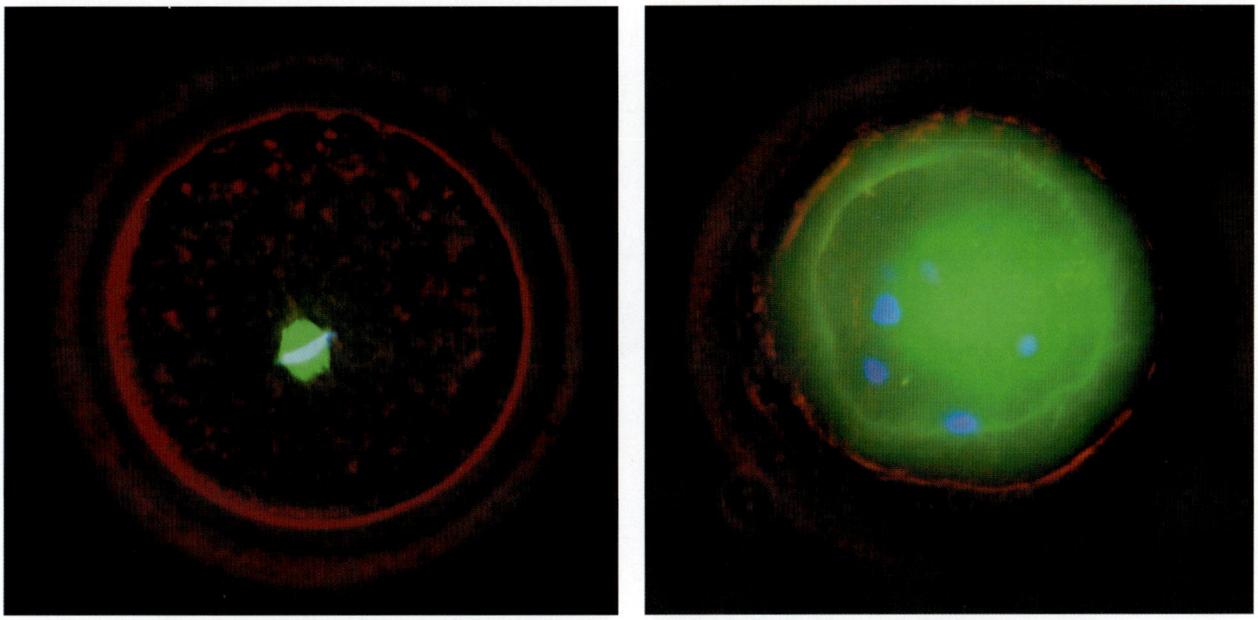

(c) (d)

Figure 3.8 *(Continued)* Second polar body (PB2) nucleus transformation following its injection into foreign cytoplasm (immunocytochemical investigation). (c) First mitotic division of the reconstructed embryo, with metaphase spindle of the PB2 clearly seen. Bright-field view of an embryo is shown in red, tubulin green, chromatin blue. (d) Premature chromosome condensation induced by okadaic acid. PB2 chromosomes (blue) are scattered all over the cytoplasm, with no spindle formed; staining for tubulin (green) also reveals cytoplasm stratification, caused by cytochalasin D.

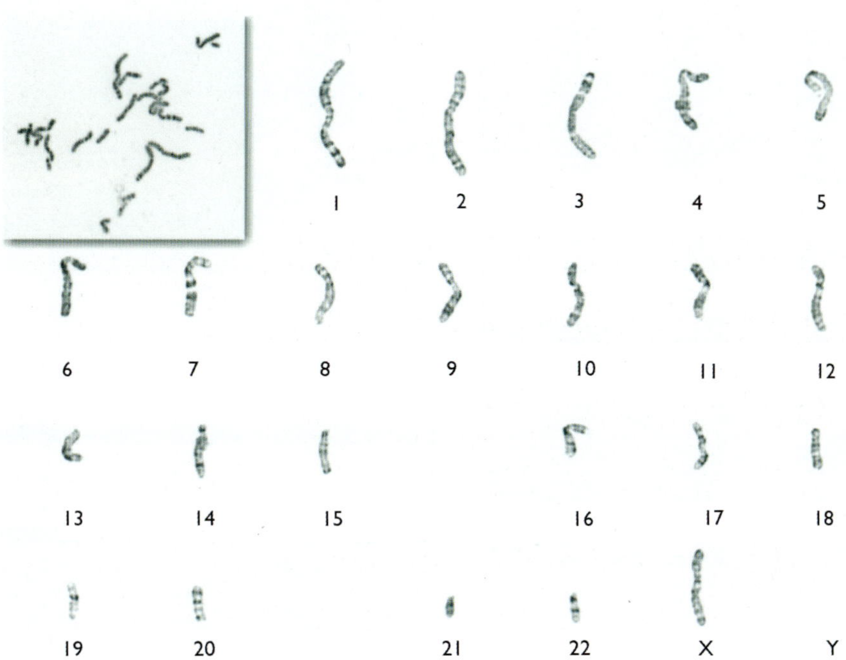

Figure 3.9 Karyotype of a second polar body obtained following its injection into foreign cytoplasm.

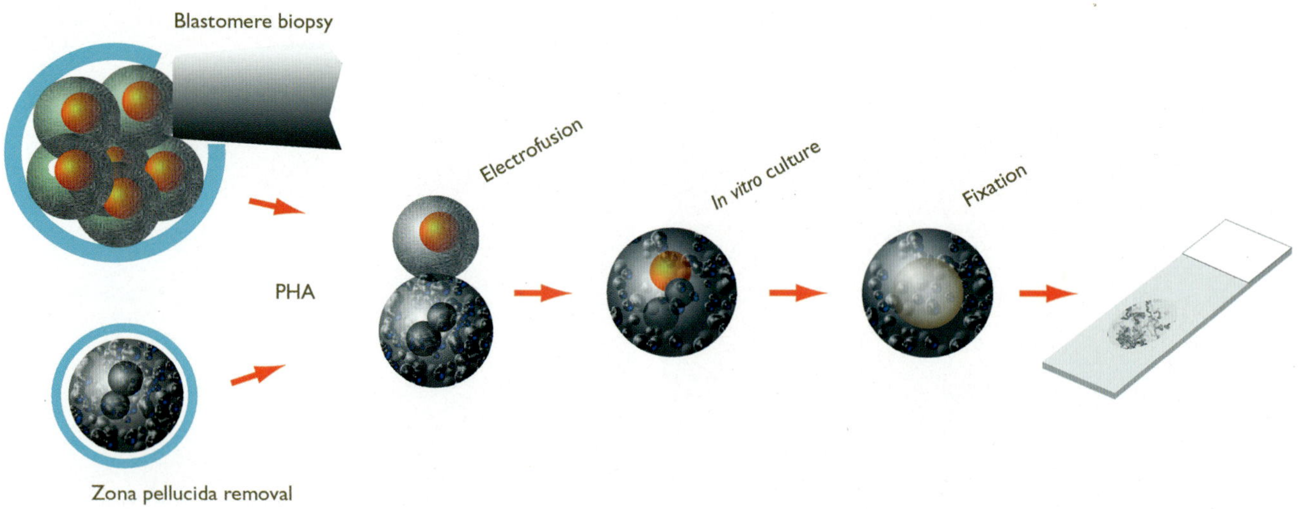

Figure 3.10 Flow chart of blastomere nucleus conversion into metaphase chromosomes. PHA, phytohemagglutinin.

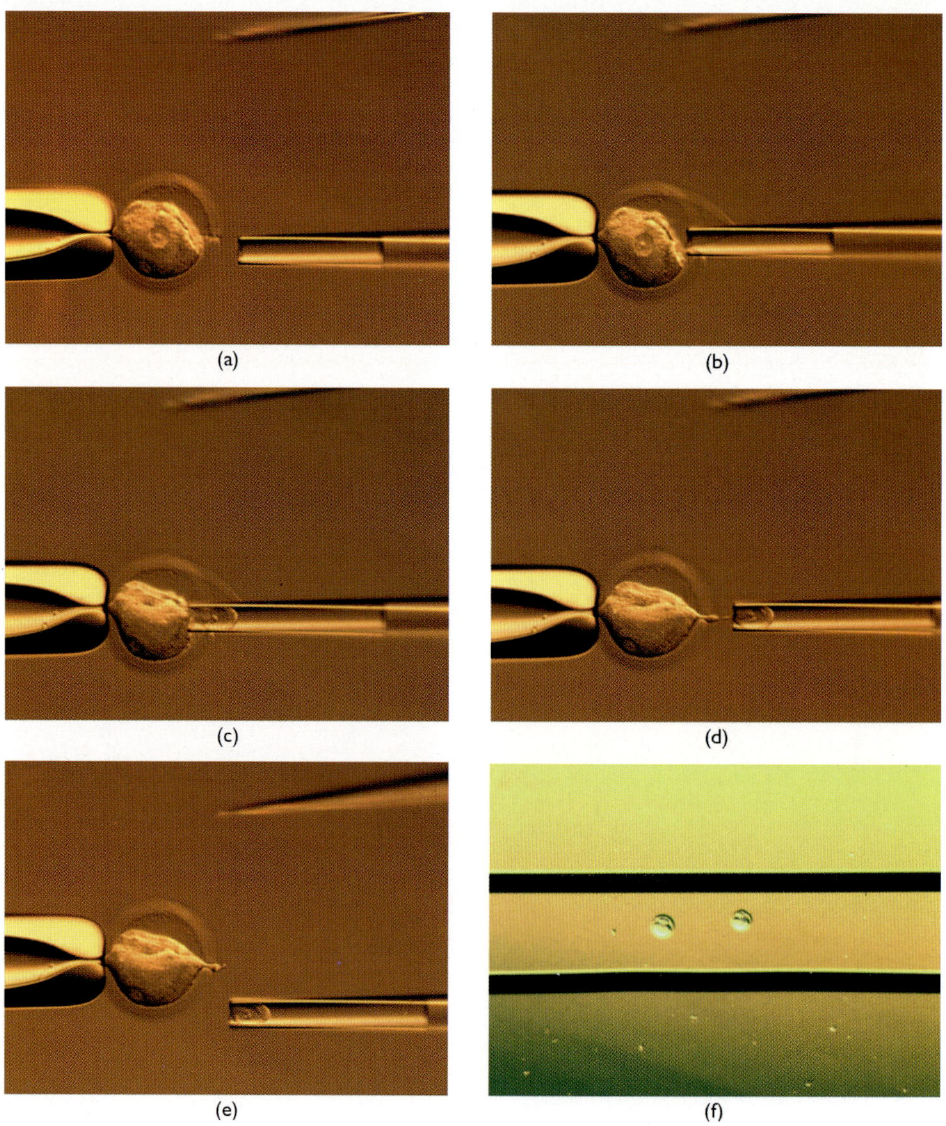

Figure 3.11 Enucleation of haploid human zygote as a source for blastomere nucleus conversion into metaphase chromosomes. (a–e) Steps of human one-pronuclear-zygote enucleation. (f) Blastomere–cytoplast electrofusion .

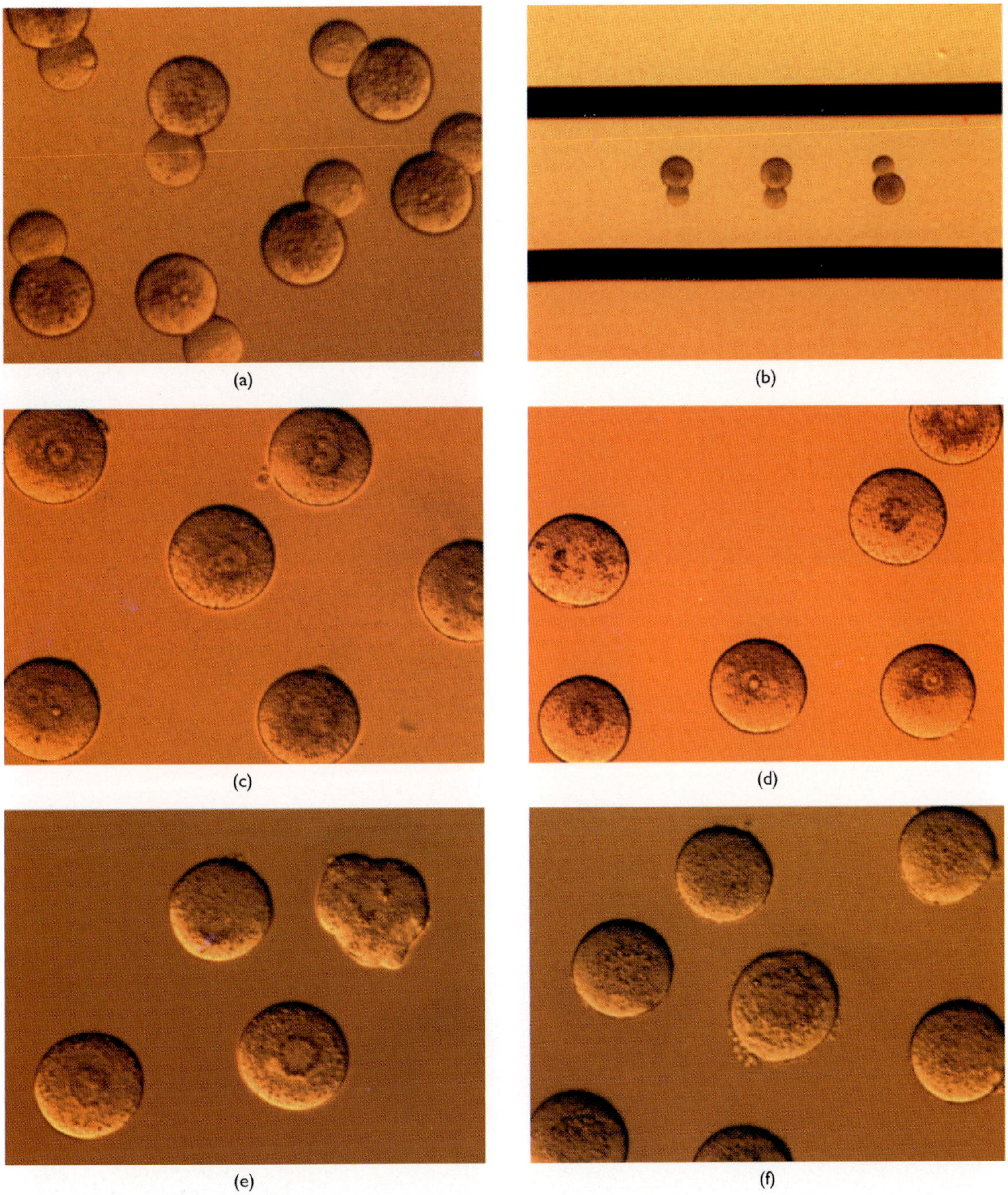

Figure 3.12 Tetraploid heterokaryons between human blastomeres and mouse zygotes. (a) Human blastomere–mouse zygote pairs are kept together by phytohemagglutinin. (b) Blastomere–zygote pairs in the electrofusion chamber, immediately after electric pulse. (c) Tetraploid interspecies hybrids immediately after fusion. Human nuclei and two mouse pronuclei are visible in all heterokaryons. (d) Five hours after fusion. Some embryos start entering metaphase of the first cleavage division. (e) Hybrids 9 h after fusion. Most of the heterokaryons have entered mitosis by this time. An irregular shape of an embryo is an indicator of anaphase or telophase of the first mitosis. (f) Okadaic acid is used to induce premature chromosome condensation. Heterokaryons after 1 h of treatment by okadaic acid. The pronuclei have disappeared. Since okadaic acid disrupts the spindle, no metaphase formation is evident prior to fixation.

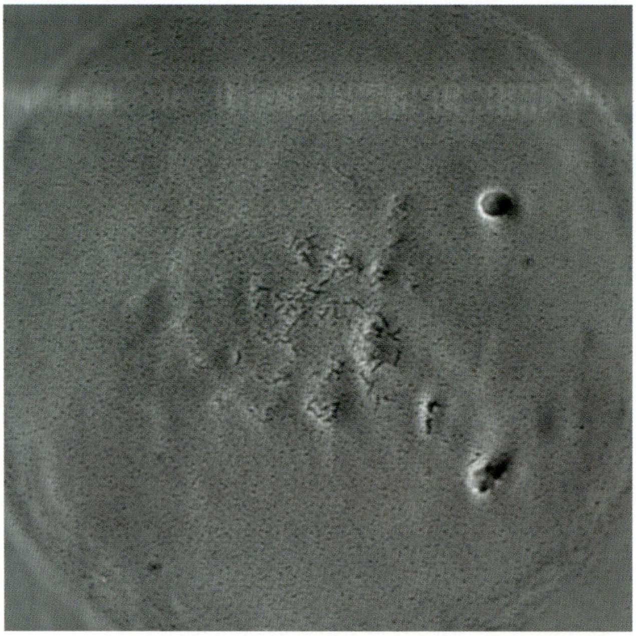

Figure 3.13 Metaphase of an individual human blastomere following conversion. Human–mouse tetraploid hybrid immediately after fixation (phase contrast).

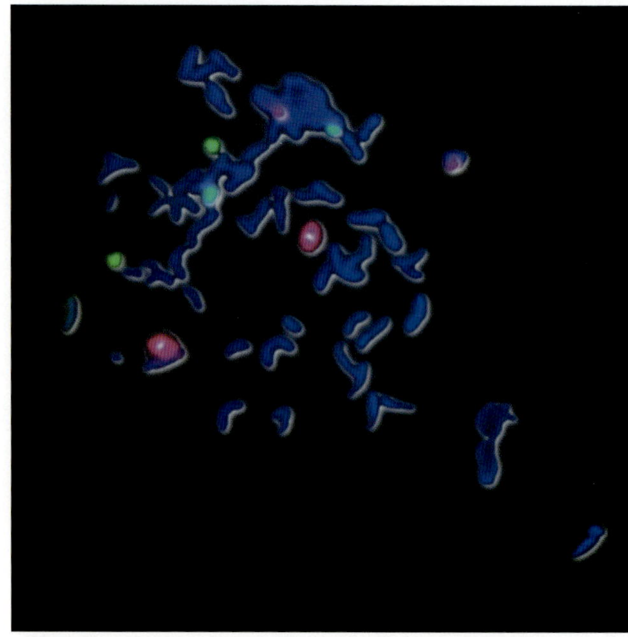

Figure 3.14 The same metaphase as 3.13 hybridized using whole chromosome painting for chromosomes 16, 18, 21, and 22 (Corel Photo-Paint was used during final image processing).

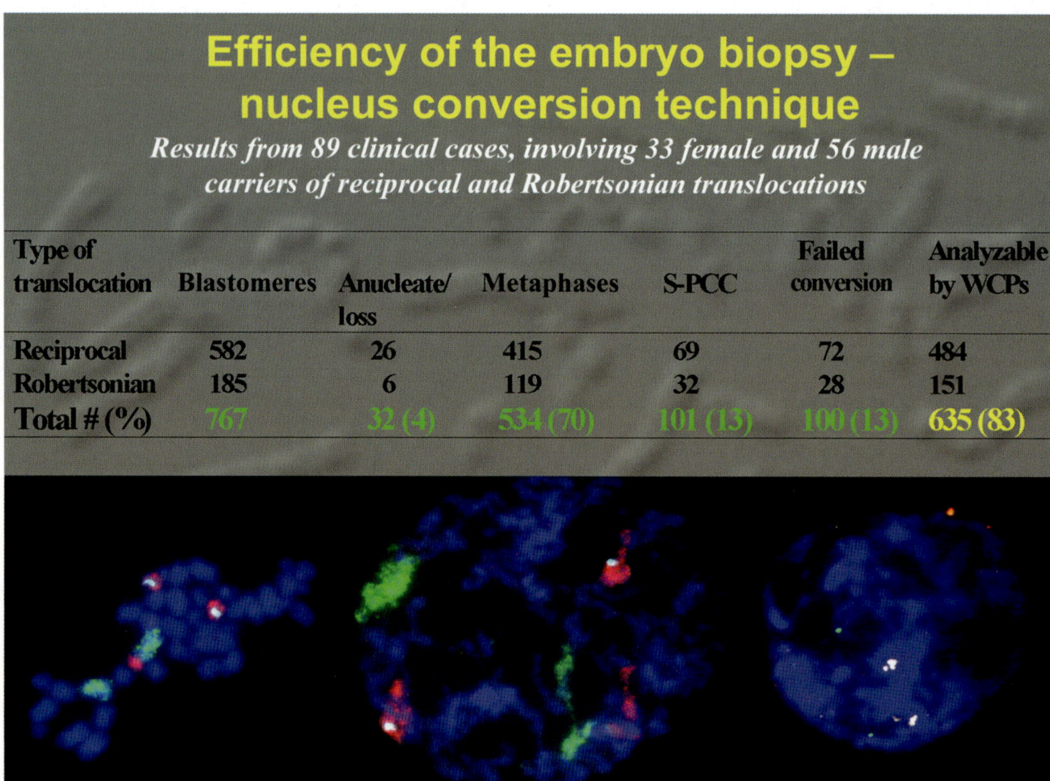

Type of translocation	Blastomeres	Anucleate/ loss	Metaphases	S-PCC	Failed conversion	Analyzable by WCPs
Reciprocal	582	26	415	69	72	484
Robertsonian	185	6	119	32	28	151
Total # (%)	767	32 (4)	534 (70)	101 (13)	100 (13)	635 (83)

Figure 3.15 Efficiency of the blastomere nucleus conversion. Based on a study of 767 embryos from 89 preimplantation genetic diagnosis (PGD) cycles for chromosomal translocations. S-PCC, S-phase premature chromosome condensation; WCP, whole-chromosome paint.

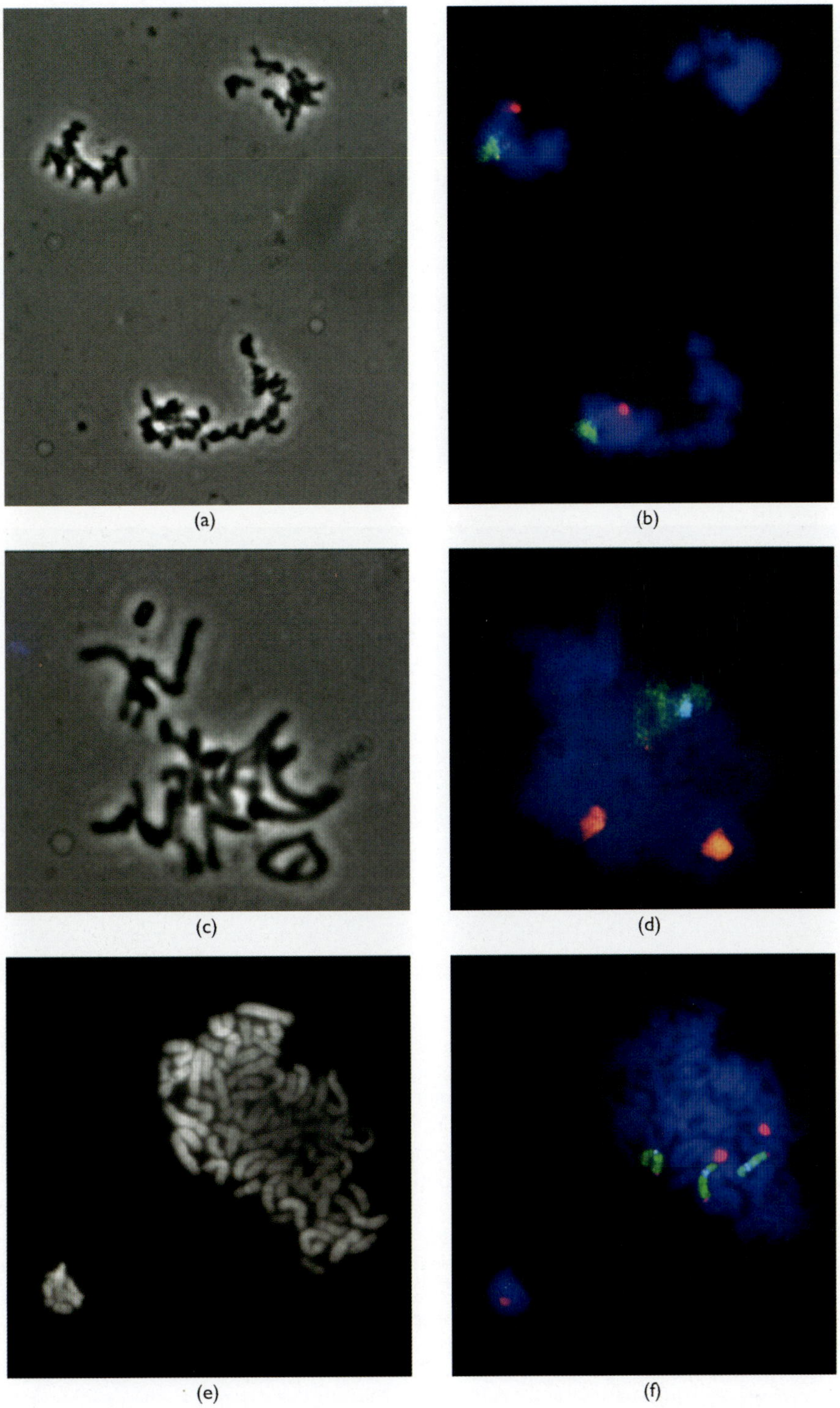

Figure 3.16 Metaphase chromosomes obtained by periodic observation of the natural cell cycle of day-3 embryos without nuclear conversion. (a) Phase-contrast image of chromosomes from a haploid embryo obtained after embryo biopsy and fixation of a blastomere after disappearance of the nucleus. Two distinct chromosome spreads are present. (b) Fluorescence *in situ* hybridization (FISH) image of the corresponding chromosome spreads seen in (a), using a probe cocktail consisting of WCP 10 (green), CEP 10 (aqua), Tel 10q (red), and WCP 22 (orange), showing one chromosome 10 (WCP 10, green) and one chromosome 22 (WCP 22, orange) in each chromosome spread. (c) Phase-contrast image of metaphase chromosomes from a haploid embryo obtained after embryo biopsy and fixation of a blastomere after disappearance of the nucleus. (d) FISH image of the metaphase chromosomes (c) using the probes in (b), showing an extra chromosome 22, and one chromosome 10 in this haploid set. (e) DAPI-stained metaphase chromosomes from a triploid embryo obtained after embryo biopsy and blastomere exposure to an antimitotic agent blocking spindle formation, followed by fixation. (f) FISH image of these metaphase chromosomes using the same probe cocktail previously mentioned (b), in which the expected three chromosomes 10 (green) and three chromosomes 22 (orange) are present.

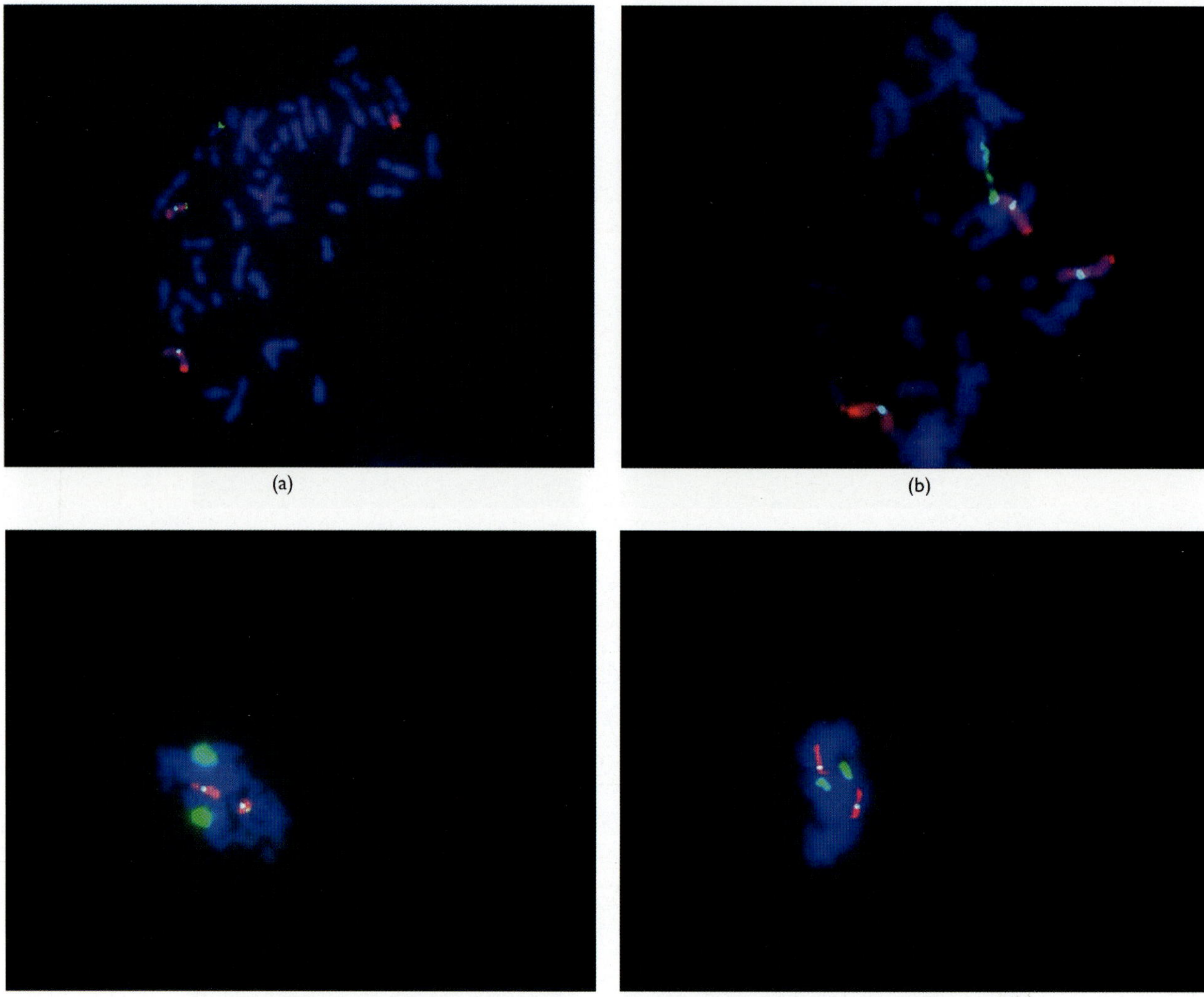

(a) (b) (c) (d)

Figure 3.17 PGD in a family with maternally derived reciprocal translocation 46,XX,t(7;19)(q22,3;p13.3) by chemical conversion method. (a) Fluorescence *in situ* hybridization (FISH) analysis of metaphase chromosomes of a peripheral blood lymphocyte from the mother. Chromosome 7 is identified by whole-chromosome paint (WCP) (red), CEP 7 (aqua), telomeric 7q (red). Chromosome 19 is identified by whole-chromosome paint (WCP) (green) and telomeric 19p (green). The same probes were used for PGD testing for this family. (b) FISH analysis of metaphase cell from an embryo obtained through chemical nuclear conversion. Two normal copies of chromosome 7 as well as an additional derivative –der(7) are present. Only one normal copy of chromosome 19 is present. Karyotype: 46,XX,+der(7)t(7;19)(q22,3;p13.3) mat,-19 representing adjacent-2 segregation pattern. (c) FISH analysis of metaphase cell from an embryo obtained through chemical nuclear conversion. One normal copy and one derivative chromosome 7 are present. Two normal copies of chromosome 19 are present. Karyotype: 46,XX,der(7)t(7;19)(q22,3;p13.3) representing adjacent-1 segregation pattern. (d) FISH analysis of metaphase cell from an embryo obtained through nuclear conversion. Two normal copies for each of the chromosomes are present. Karyotype: 46,XX.

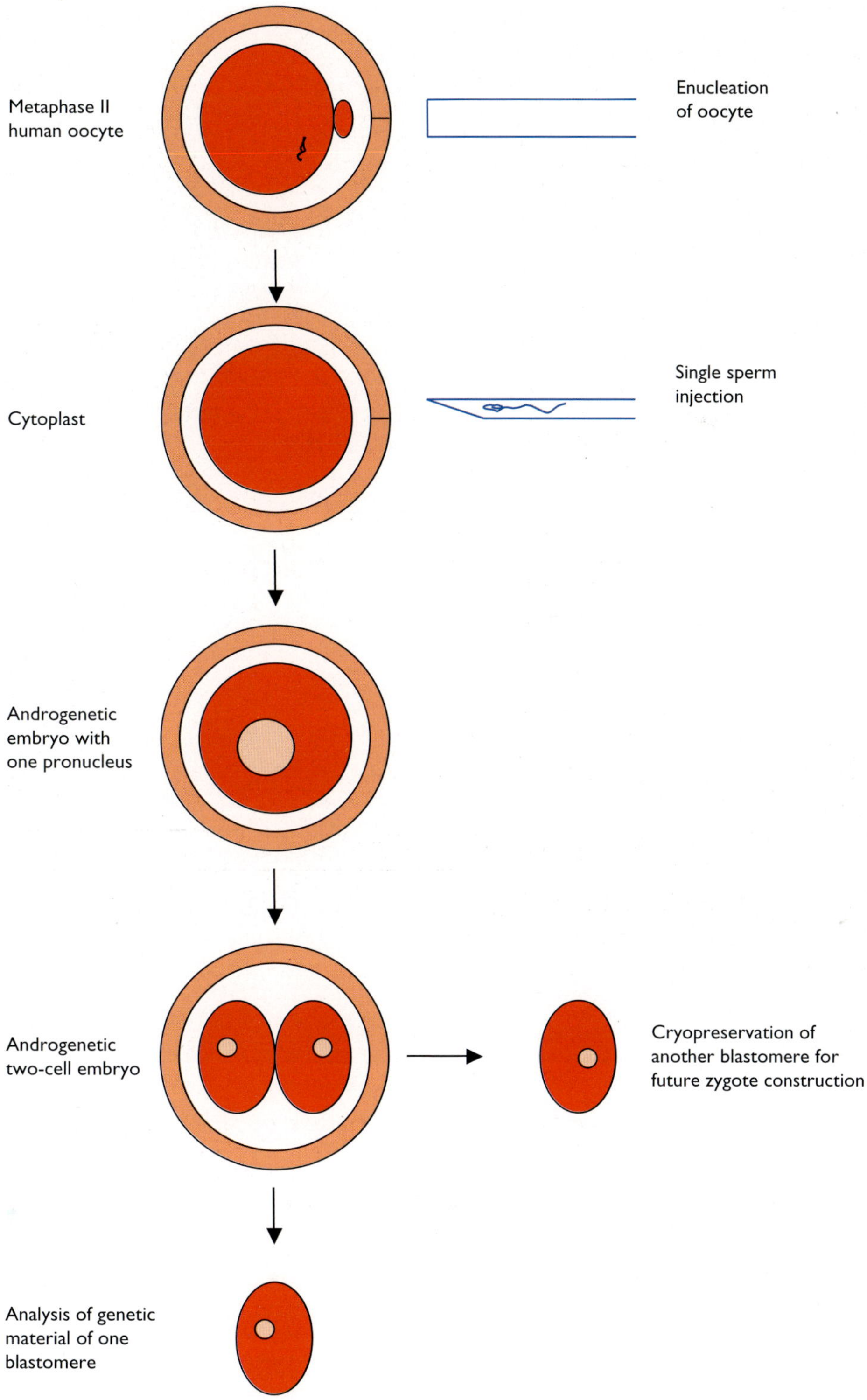

Figure 3.18 Flow chart of sperm duplication in human metaphase II cytoplast. Step 1 – enucleation of human metaphase II oocyte; step 2 – injection of single human sperm into the cytoplast; step 3 – reconstructed haploid androgenic embryo with one pronucleus; step 4 – development of this pronucleus into two-cell embryos; step 5 – testing of one of the cells, with the other one available for further zygote construction of known male contribution.

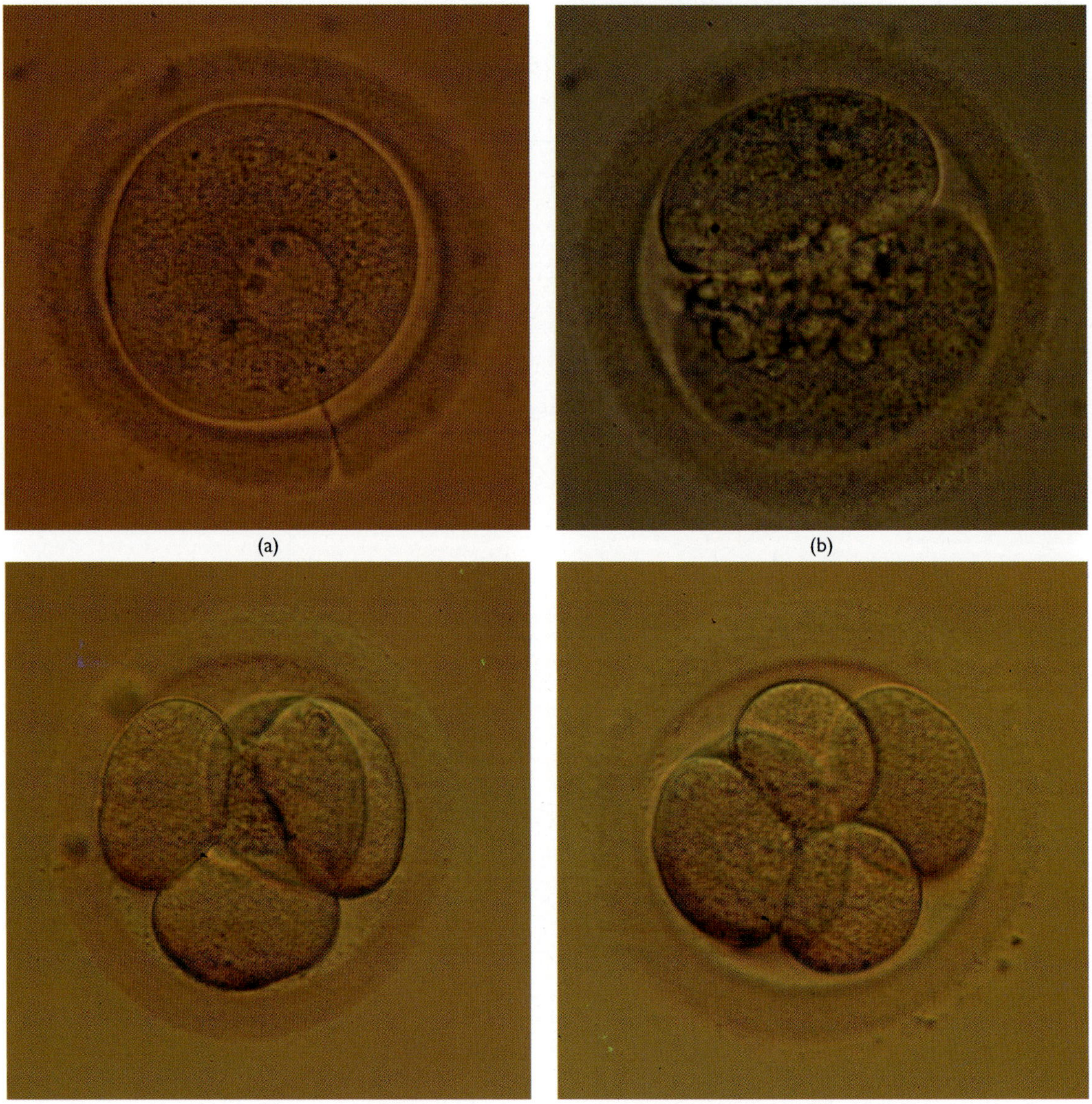

(a) (b) (c) (d)

Figure 3.19 Sperm duplication resulting in an androgenetic five-cell cleaving human embryo. (a) Reconstructed one-cell embryo following enucleation and single sperm injection; (b)–(d) Development of the reconstructed one-cell embryo in cleavage stage five-cell embryo. (a) One-cell embryo with a male pronucleus (20 h after intracytoplasmic sperm injection (ICSI)); (b) two-cell embryo (29 h after ICSI); (c) four-cell embryo (45 h after ICSI); and (d) five-cell embryo (45 h after ICSI).

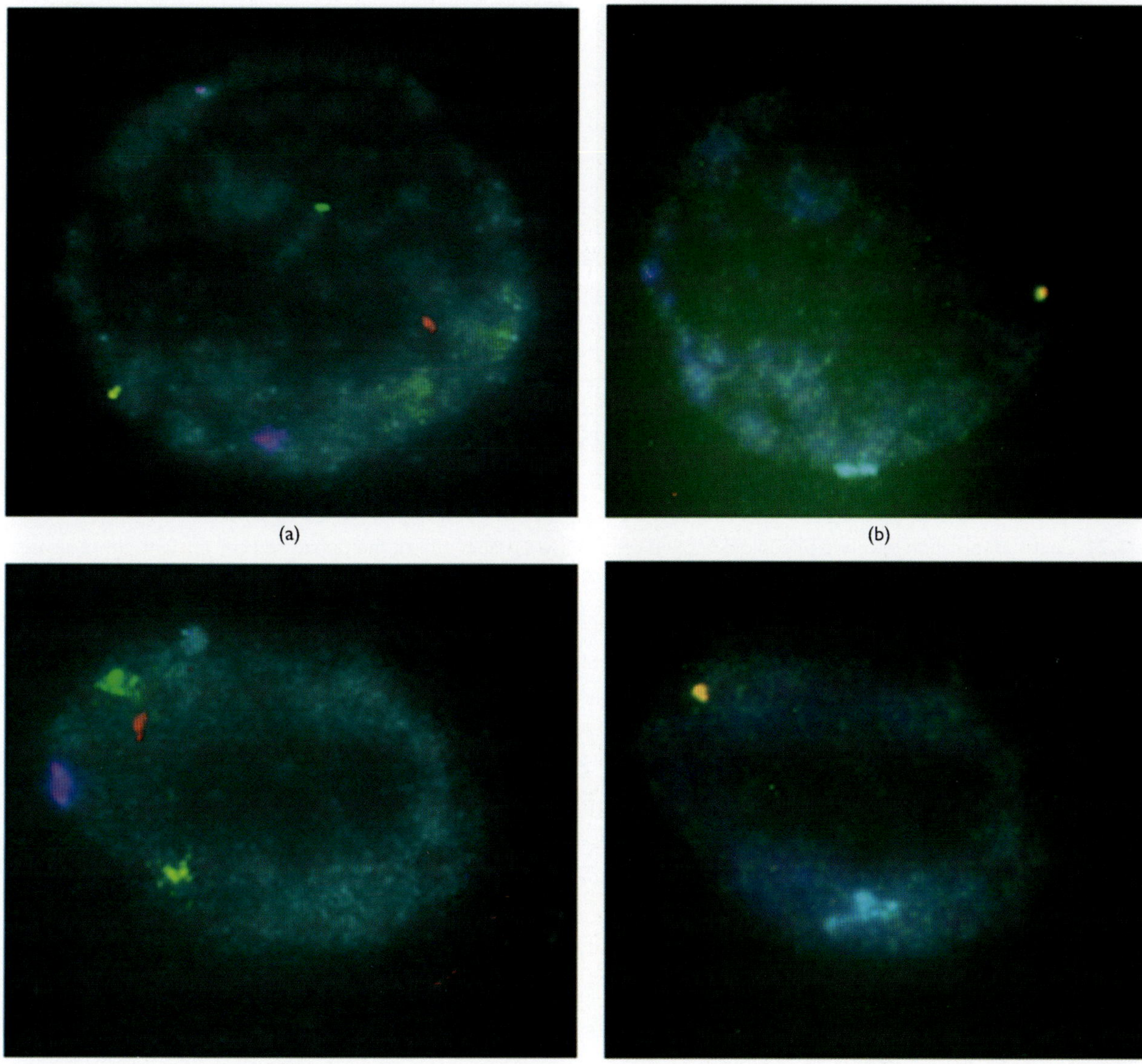

(a) (b) (c) (d)

Figure 3.20 Human sperm duplication into two identical chromosomally normal haploid cells using human metaphase II oocytes. (a) and (c) Two identical cells derived following sperm duplication, shown by fluorescence *in situ* hybridization (FISH) analysis of chromosomes 13, 16, 18, 21, and 22. (b) and (d) Re-hybridization of the same cells with chromosome-specific probes for chromosomes 16 and Y.

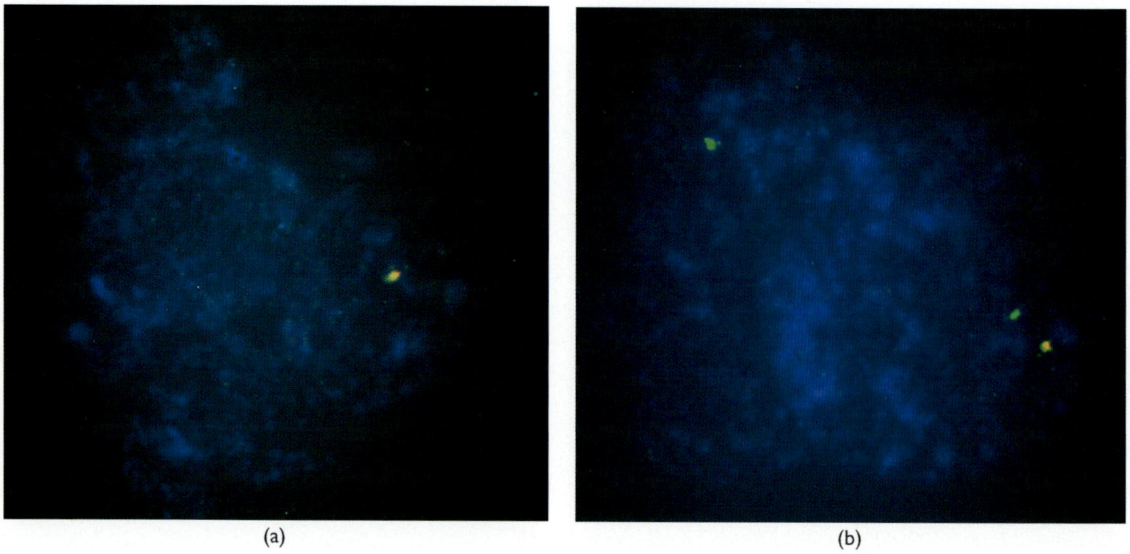

Figure 3.21 Sperm duplication into two aneuploid haploid cells. Single signal in one of the duplicated cell (a), with three signals in the corresponding cell (b), demonstrating non-disjunction of the X chromosome (two green signals).

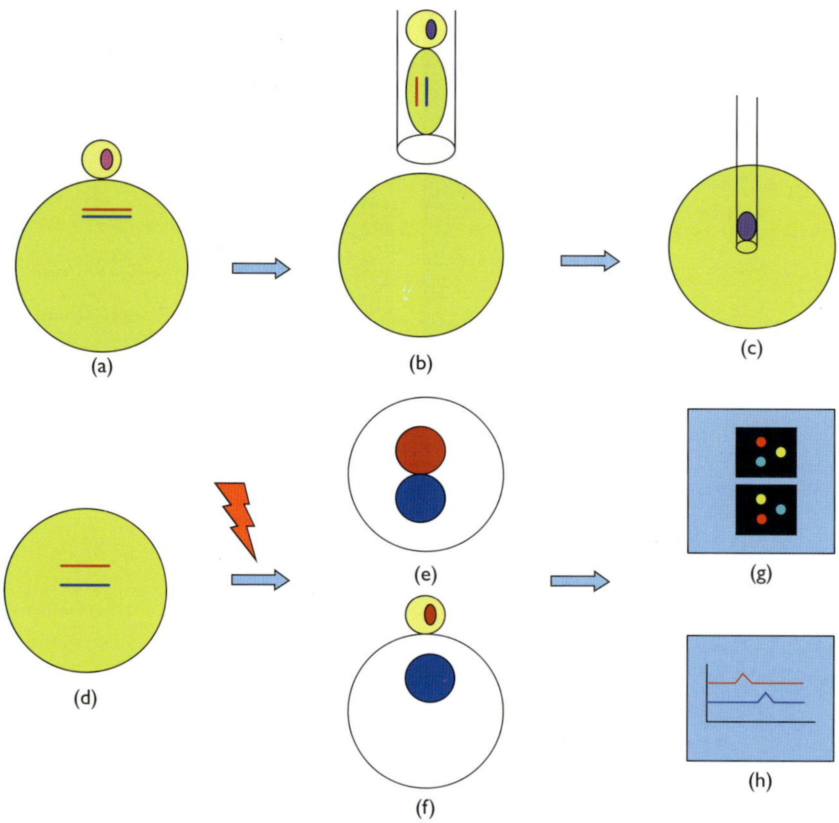

Figure 3.22 Development of artificial human gametes *in vitro*. Flow chart of haploidization procedure for obtaining gametes from somatic cells. (a) *In vitro* matured metaphase II oocyte with extruded first polar body (PB1). (b) Both PB1 and metaphase II chromosomes are removed (shown in pipette), to prepare a recipient enucleated ooplast. (c) Single diploid cumulus cells were prepared as nuclei donors, from which a nucleus was mechanically isolated for the introduction into ooplast. (d) Reconstructed oocyte converting somatic cell nucleus into metaphase chromosomes. (e) Two pronuclei or (f) pronucleus and PB1 obtained after electrostimulation using electrofusion device (Chicago, IL). (g) Fluorescent *in situ* hybridization analysis, or (h) polymerase chain reaction (PCR)-based chromosomal analysis, confirming the formation of two haploid sets of chromosomes in both (e) and (f) scenarios.

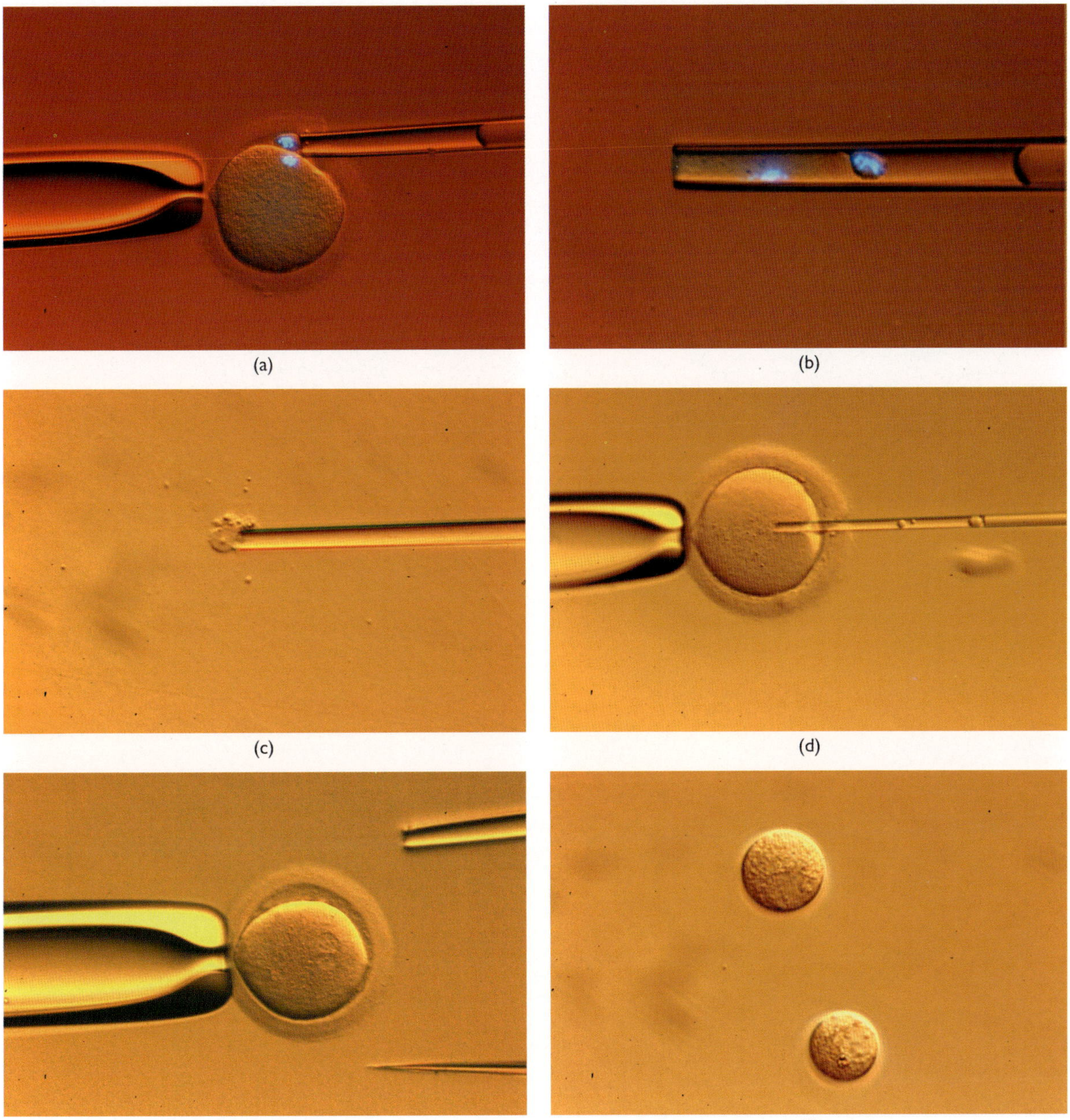

(a) (b) (c) (d) (e) (f)

Figure 3.23 Development of artificial human gametes *in vitro* (continued). Microsurgery procedure for obtaining gametes from somatic cells. (a) Enucleation of recipient matured human oocytes using flame-polished blunt micropipette, following the opening performed by partial dissection of zona pellucida (PZD). (b) The removed first polar body (PB1) and small ooplast with metaphase plate are shown in the micropipette, stained with a vital Hoechst stain. (c) A single nucleus is isolated from an individual donor human cumulus cell. (d) Microinjection of the cumulus nucleus into the recipient enucleated oocyte (ooplast) through the same zona opening. (e) Reconstructed by nuclear transfer oocyte showing two foci, representing metaphase chromosomes, following activation by electrostimulation. (f) Microsurgically removed pronuclei for subsequent analysis.

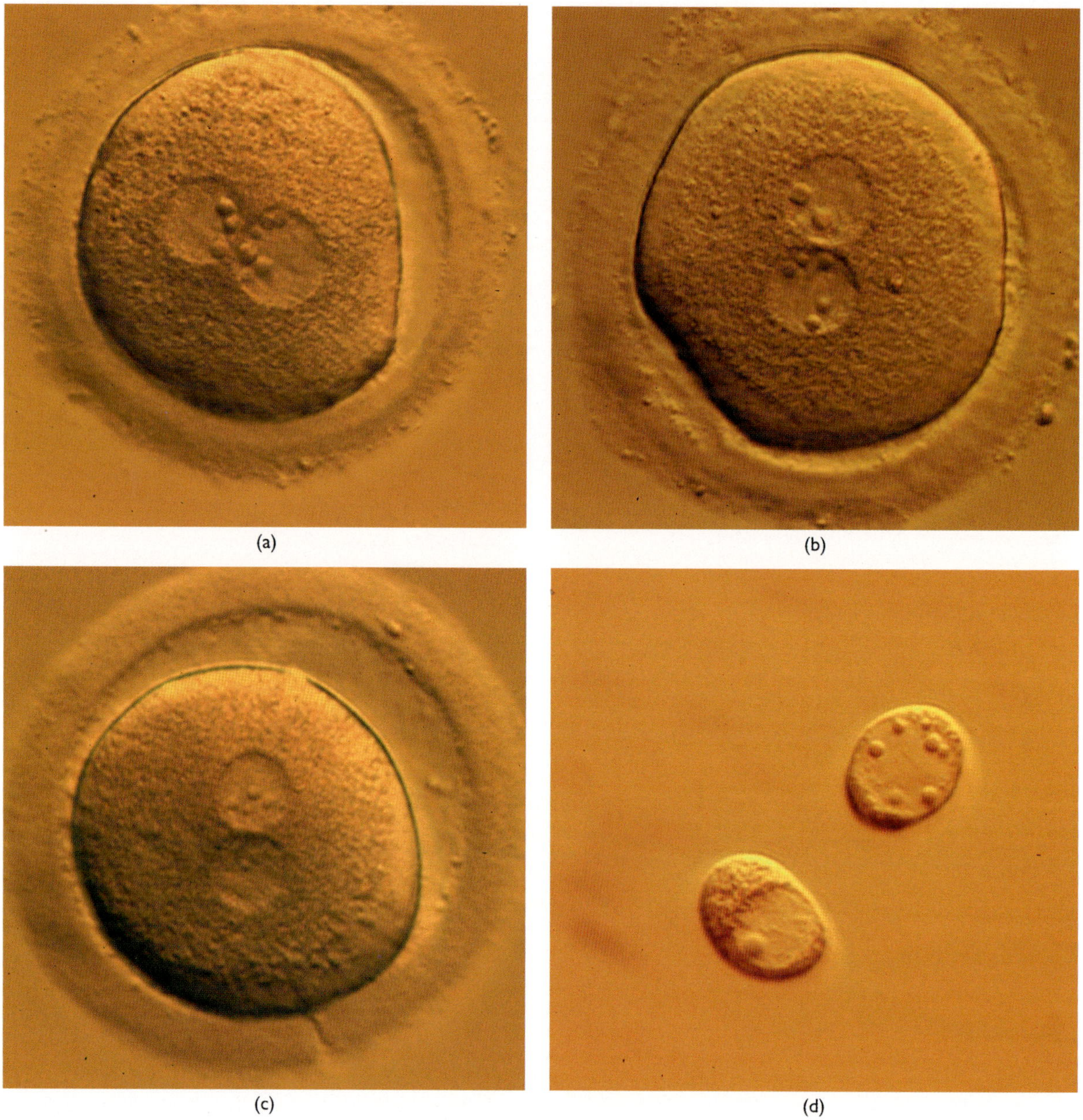

Figure 3.24 Development of artificial human gametes *in vitro* (continued). *In vitro* development of reconstructed oocytes following haploidization. (a), (b), and (c) Reconstructed by somatic cell nucleus injection metaphase II oocytes 10 h after electrostimulation. (d) Isolated pronuclei (×400).

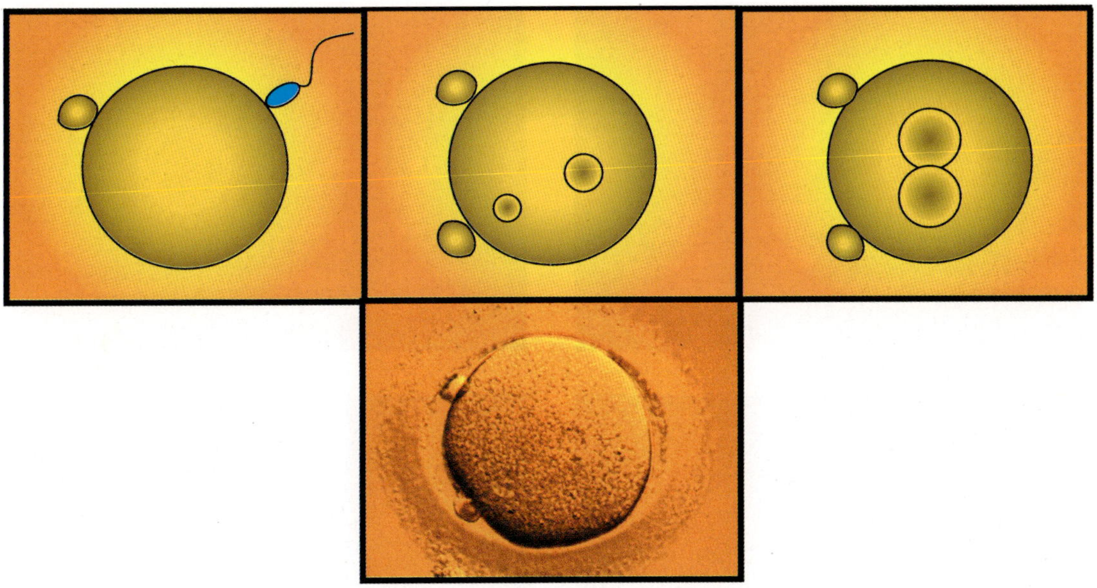

(a)

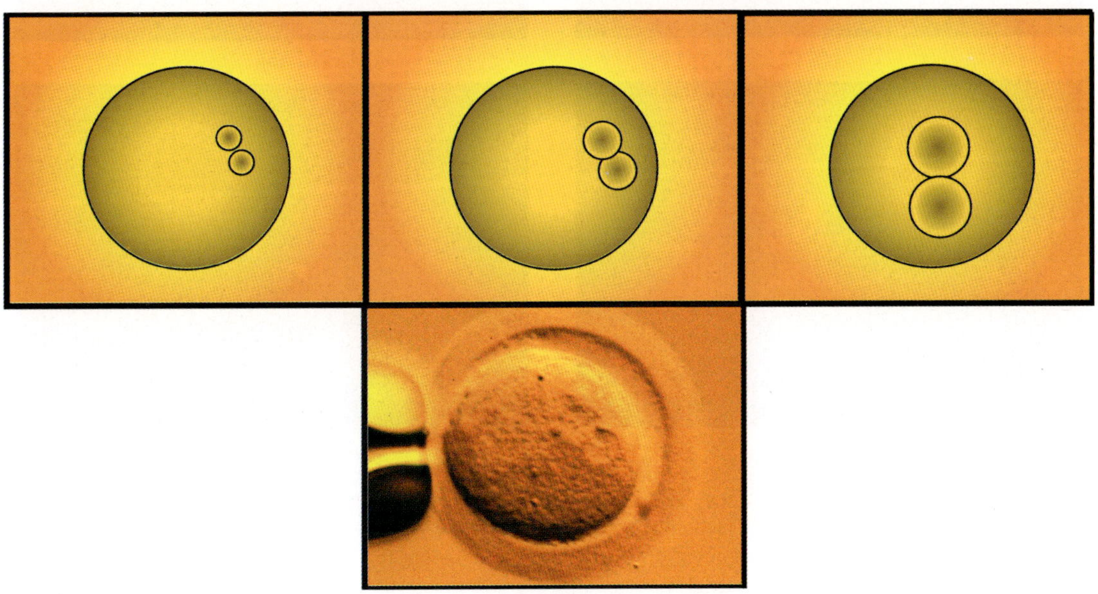

(b)

Figure 3.25 Development of artificial human gametes *in vitro* (continued). Flow chart of pronuclei formation after natural fertilization and somatic cell haploidization. (a) The sequence of events in the matured metaphase II oocyte, following sperm penetration (upper left), resulting in polar body (PB) extrusion and pronuclei formation (upper row middle and second row middle), migrating from the periphery to the middle (upper right). (b) Reconstructed metaphase II oocytes following somatic cell nuclei injection 6 h after electrostimulation, resulting in two haploidization pronuclei positioned close to each other despite the volume growth (shown from upper left to upper right) (×200).

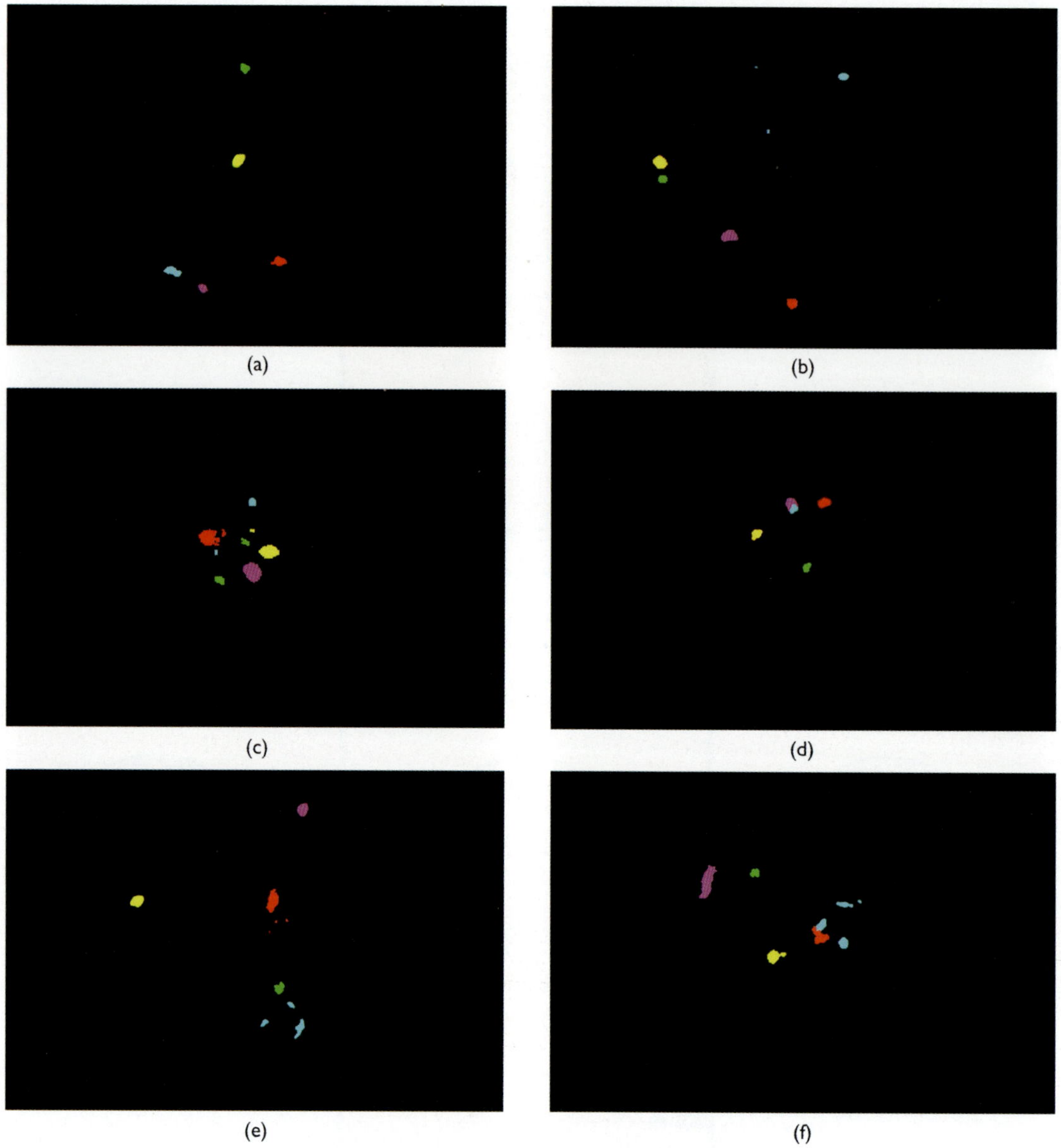

Figure 3.26 Normal segregation of chromosomes 13, 16, 18, 21, and 22 of reconstructed somatic cell nuclei. (a) and (b) Two identical pronuclei obtained from the reconstructed somatic cell injected into an enucleated metaphase II oocyte, showing a single signal for all the chromosomes analyzed by fluorescence *in situ* hybridization (FISH): chromosomes 13 (red), 16 (aqua), 18 (blue), 21 (green), and 22 (yellow) (x600). (c)–(f) Two more examples of normal chromosome segregation in the resulting PB and pronucleus (c) and (d) or haploid pronuclei (e) and (f) obtained through injection into enucleated metaphase II oocytes (chromosomes 16 and 21 in (c) and chromosome 16 in (e) and (f) are pulverized).

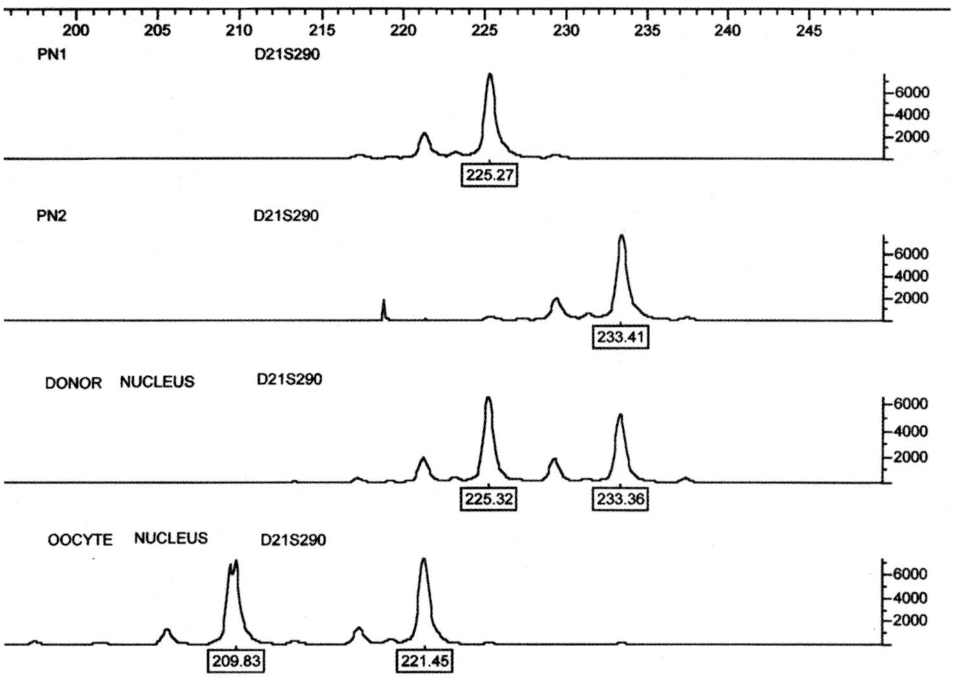

(a)

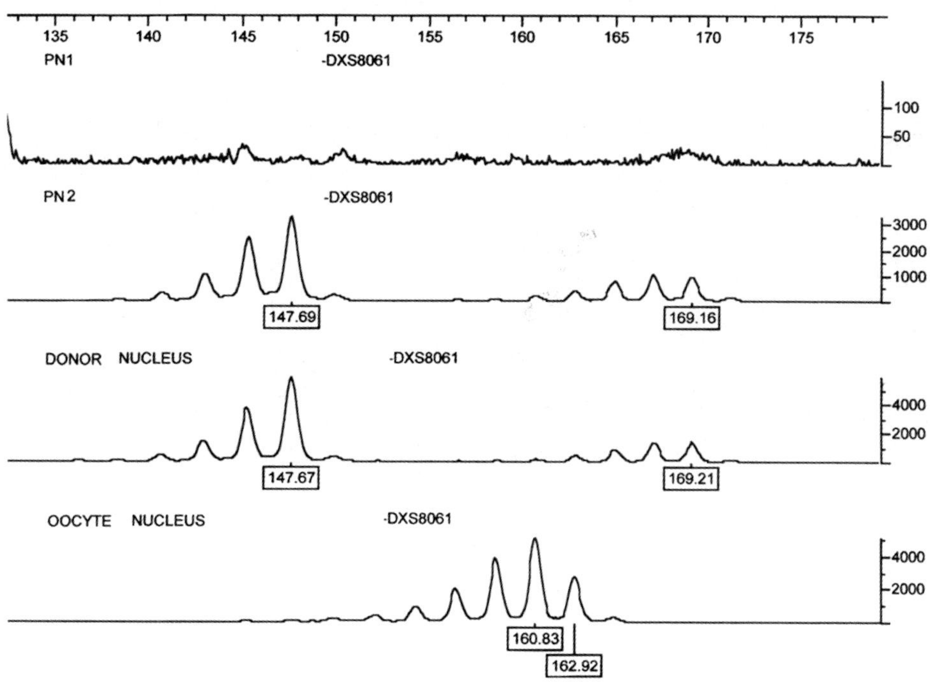

(b)

Figure 3.27 Capillary electrophoresis results of cumulus cell haploidization. (a) Normal segregation of chromosome 21. Each of the pronuclei (PN) obtained from cumulus cells injected into the enucleated recipient metaphase II oocyte has one chromosome 21, based on testing for the STR marker D21S290 located on chromosome 21 (PN1 and PN2), evident from the presence of a single allele 225 or 233 for these markers in each pronucleus. The DNA profiles of donor cumulus cell nucleus (donor nucleus) and recipient oocyte (oocyte nucleus) are presented below, demonstrating that both the resulting pronuclei originated from haploidization. (b) Abnormal segregation of chromosomes X. None of the somatic cell alleles for chromosome X marker are present in one of the resulting pronuclei (PN1), which is in accordance with both of the chromosome X STR marker DXS8061 alleles 160/162 being detected in the corresponding sister pronucleus (PN2). The DNA profiles of donor cumulus cell nucleus (donor nucleus) and recipient oocyte (oocyte nucleus) are presented below, demonstrating the evidence that both of the resulting pronuclei originated from haploidization.

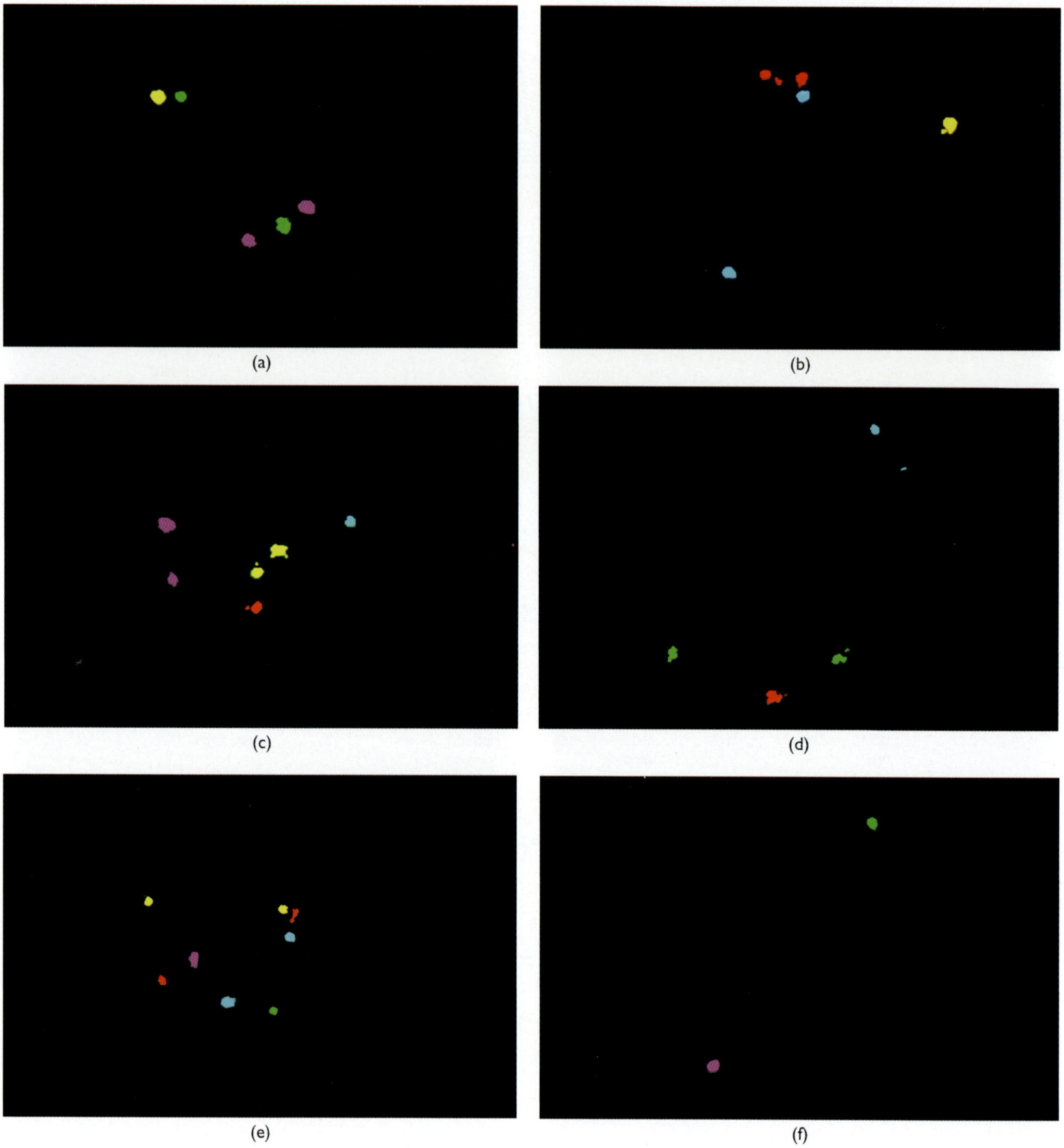

Figure 3.28 Aneuploidies detected in reconstructed somatic cell nuclei. (a) and (b) Abnormal chromosome segregation for chromosomes 13, 16, 18, and 21 found in two pronuclei resulting from haploidization, evident from extra red (chromosome 13) and aqua (chromosome 16) signals (two instead of one) seen in the sister pronucleus (b), while the corresponding signals for these chromosomes were missing in the sister pronucleus (a); and extra blue and green signals in pronucleus (a), in accordance with no blue and green signals for chromosome 18 and 21 in the sister pronucleus (b). (c) and (d) Abnormal chromosome segregation for chromosome 18, 21, and 22 found in two pronuclei resulting from haploidization, as shown by the double signals for chromosome 18 (blue) and chromosome 22 (yellow) (instead of a single signal for each chromosome) in pronucleus (c), in accordance with missing signals for these chromosomes in the corresponding sister pronucleus (d); and an extra green signal for chromosome 21 in pronucleus (d), which is missing in the corresponding sister pronucleus (c). (e) and (f) Abnormal chromosome segregation for chromosomes 13, 16, and 22 found in two pronuclei resulting from haploidization, evident from only two single signals in one of the pronuclei, including one green signal for chromosome 21 and one blue signal for chromosome 18 (f), in accordance with one green, one blue, and two signals for chromosomes 13, 16, and 22 in the corresponding sister pronucleus (e). Magnification ×600.

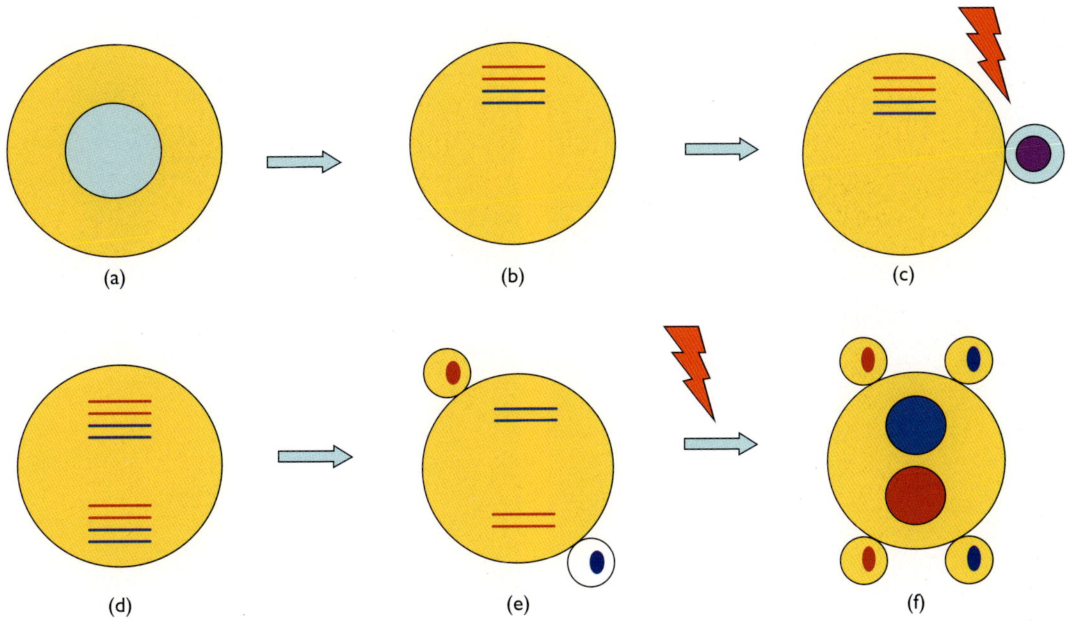

Figure 3.29 Flow chart of somatic cell nucleus haploidization using immature metaphase I oocytes. (a) and (b) *In vitro* matured metaphase I oocyte. (c) The metaphase I oocyte following electrofusion with fibroblasts at G2 (4C) cell cycle stage. (d) Reconstructed metaphase I oocytes forming two metaphases, followed by extrusion of two first polar bodies during maturation into metaphase II stage (e). Fidelity of chromosome segregation was analyzed by five-color fluorescence *in situ* hybridization (FISH) analysis of the resulting polar bodies and oocytes. (f) Reconstructed tetraploid oocytes may potentially develop into diploid embryos.

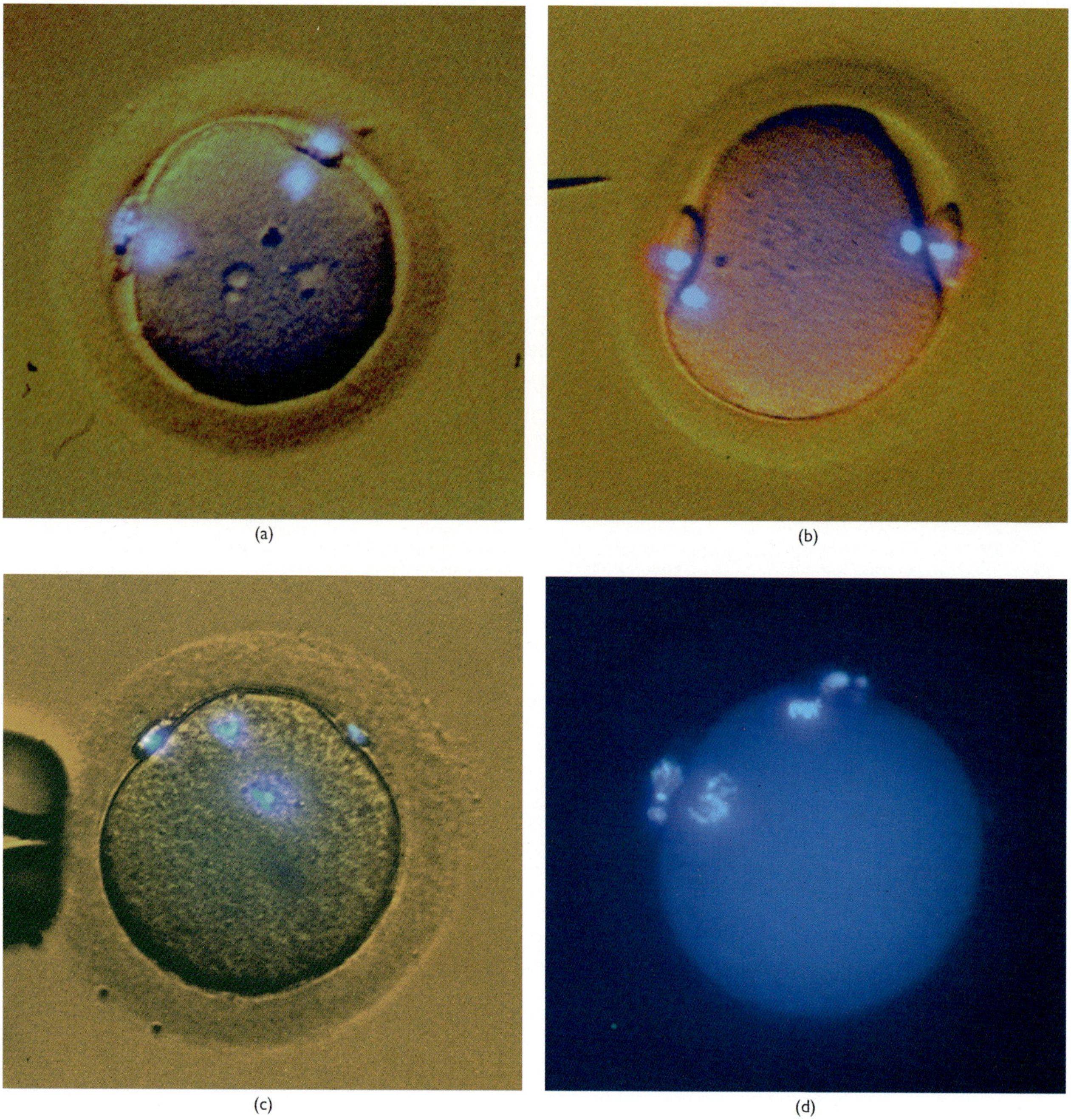

Figure 3.30 Example of somatic cell nucleus haploidization using immature metaphase I oocytes. Fibroblasts at G2 cell cycle stage were fused electrically with metaphase I oocytes. After 12 h of culture and maturation, the oocytes extruded two polar bodies, one originating from the oocyte, the other from somatic metaphase. (a)–(c) Reconstructed metaphase II oocytes with dual set of chromosomes stained with Hoechst 33342. (d) Ultraviolet luminescence of the reconstructed oocyte. Magnification x400.

4 Preimplantation diagnosis for aneuploidies

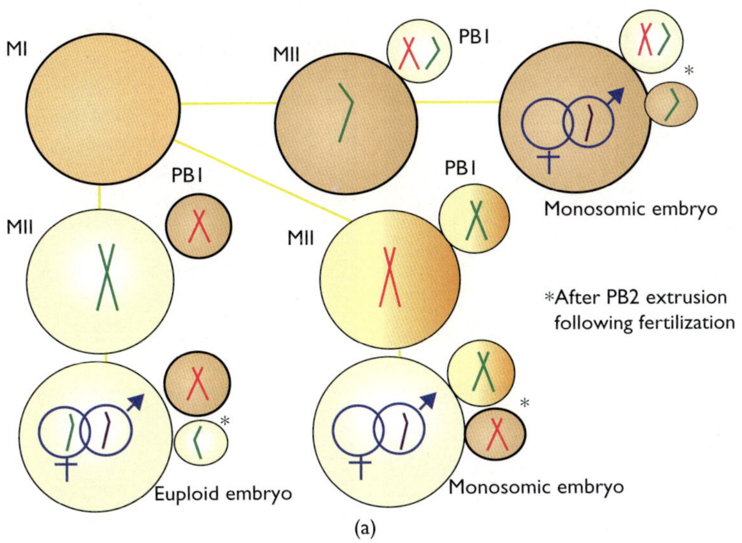

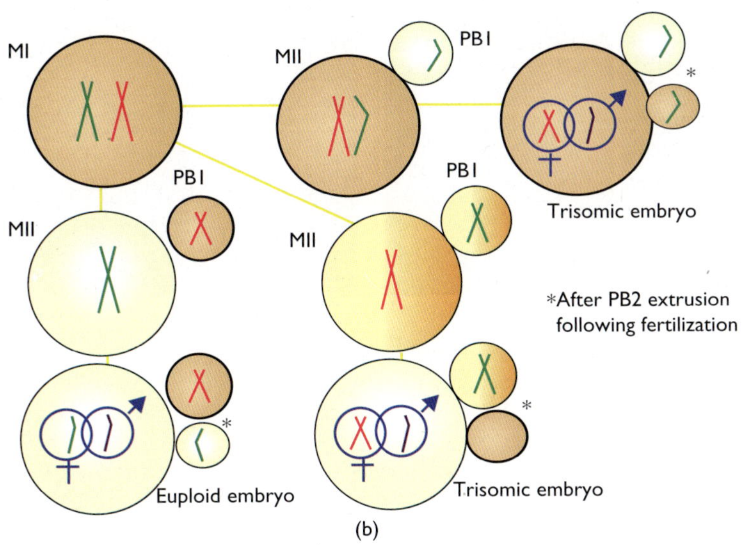

Figure 4.1 Schematic representation of possible chromosome (chromatid) segregation in meiosis I (MI) and II (MII). (a) For simplicity only one pair of homologues (one maternal and one paternal) is shown. Normal chromosome segregation during meiosis I and II is depicted along the vertical pathway, resulting in a euploid embryo. Following the horizontal path, chromatid malsegregation involving one of the homologues has occurred during the first meiotic division in which an additional chromatid has been extruded into the first polar body (PB1), leaving only a single chromatid present in the oocyte. Following meiosis II immediately after fertilization, the remaining chromatid may or may not be extruded in the second polar body (PB2). If extruded during the second meiotic division, the resulting oocyte will be nullisomic for that particular chromosome, resulting in a monosomic embryo following syngamy. Following the diagonal path, normal chromosome segregation has occurred during meiosis I. However, after fertilization chromatid error has occurred in which both chromatids have been extruded in PB2, resulting in a nullisomic oocyte/monosomic embryo. (b) Normal chromosome segregation during meiosis I and II is depicted along the vertical pathway, resulting in a euploid embryo. Following the horizontal path, chromatid malsegregation involving one of the homologues has occurred during the first meiotic division in which an additional chromatid has been retained in the oocyte and only a single chromatid has been extruded in PB1. After fertilization, the extra chromatid may or may not be extruded in PB2. As depicted, if only a single chromatid is extruded in PB2, an additional chromatid is retained in the oocyte, resulting in a trisomic embryo following syngamy. Following the diagonal pathway, normal chromosome segregation has occurred during the first meiotic division; however, after fertilization, chromatid error has occurred during meiosis II in which an extra chromatid has been retained in the oocyte, rendering PB2 nullisomic for that particular chromosome. After syngamy the resulting chromosome complement would be trisomic.

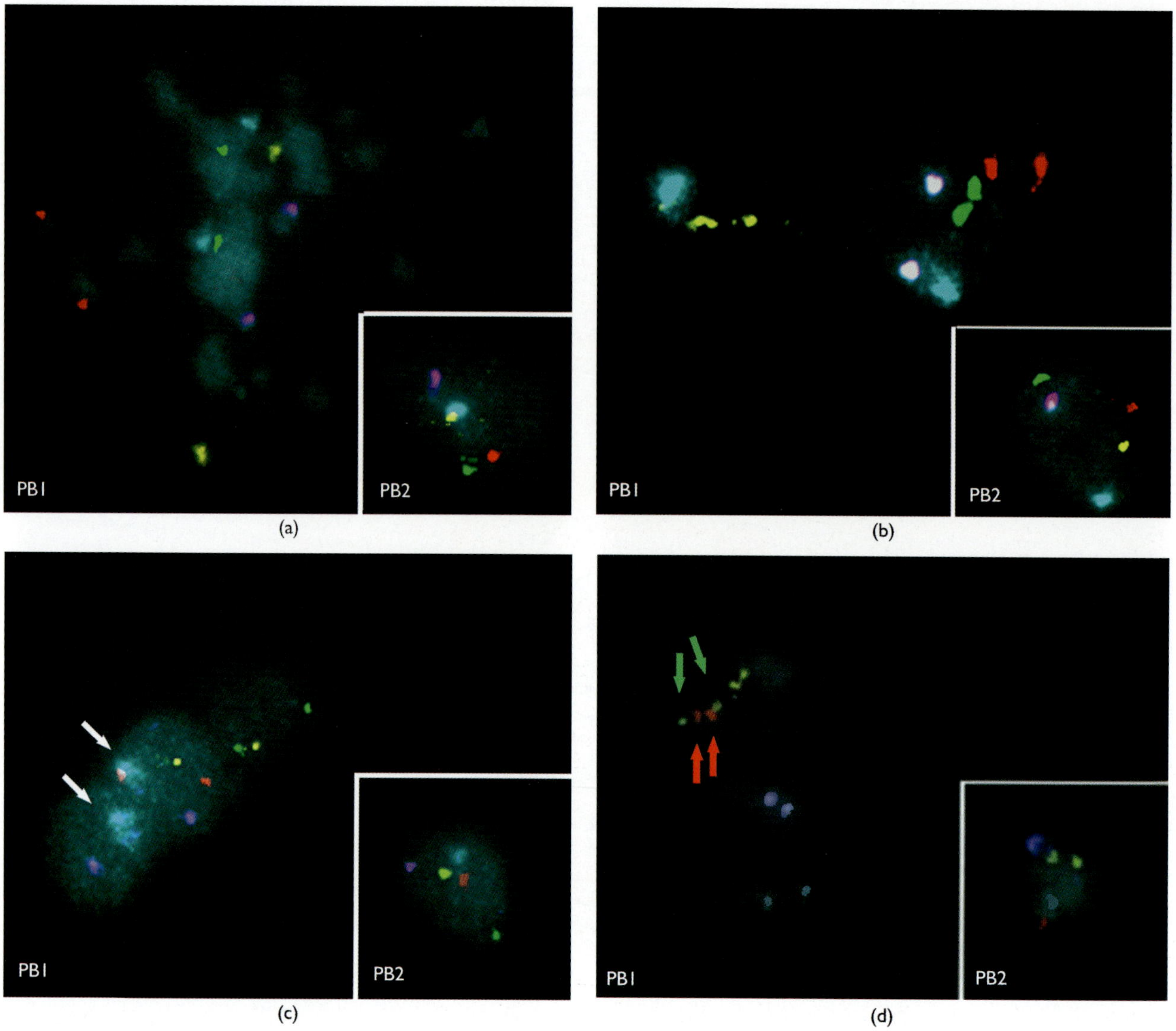

Figure 4.2 Fluorescence *in situ* hybridization (FISH) images of first polar body (PB1) and second polar body (PB2) after a 3-h hybridization with MultiVysion PB panel probe for autosomes 13 (red), 16 (aqua), 18 (violet blue), 21 (green), and 22 (gold). PB1 and PB2 were removed simultaneously on day 1 at the pronuclear stage of development following fertilization assessment. (a) PB1 chromosomes showing a normal number of single dot signals (two per chromosome, representing each chromatid) in which all chromatids are separate. This chromatid separation allows for easy enumeration of chromatids, enabling identification of not only chromosome non-disjunction, but also chromatid errors found to be more prevalent. A normal number of signals (one per chromosome (chromatid)) are present in the PB2 interphase nucleus (lower right), implying a normal chromosome complement in the oocyte and resulting embryo. (b) FISH image of PB1 in which a normal number of signals are seen. Some chromatids are in closer proximity to one another (e.g. chromatids for chromosome 21 in green). Centromeric enumeration signals for chromosome 16 (16q11.2) in aqua appear equally large and diffuse and can vary depending upon the degree of chromatin condensation, since the probe targets a region of highly repetitive satellite DNA sequences. The PB2 nucleus contains a normal number of signals for the five autosomes tested. (c) FISH image of PB1 in which a normal number of signals are seen, with all chromatids being separate and easily counted, except signals for chromosome 16 (white arrows), which once again are diffuse, with one in particular being split, necessitating re-hybridization using a probe that targets the same chromosome but at a different locus. The PB2 nucleus contains a normal number of signals for each of the autosomes tested. (d) FISH image of PB1 in which a normal number of signals are seen. The chromatids are seen paired with a slight overlap for chromosomes 13 (red arrows) and 21 (green arrows). The PB2 nucleus contains a normal number of signals for each of the autosomes tested.

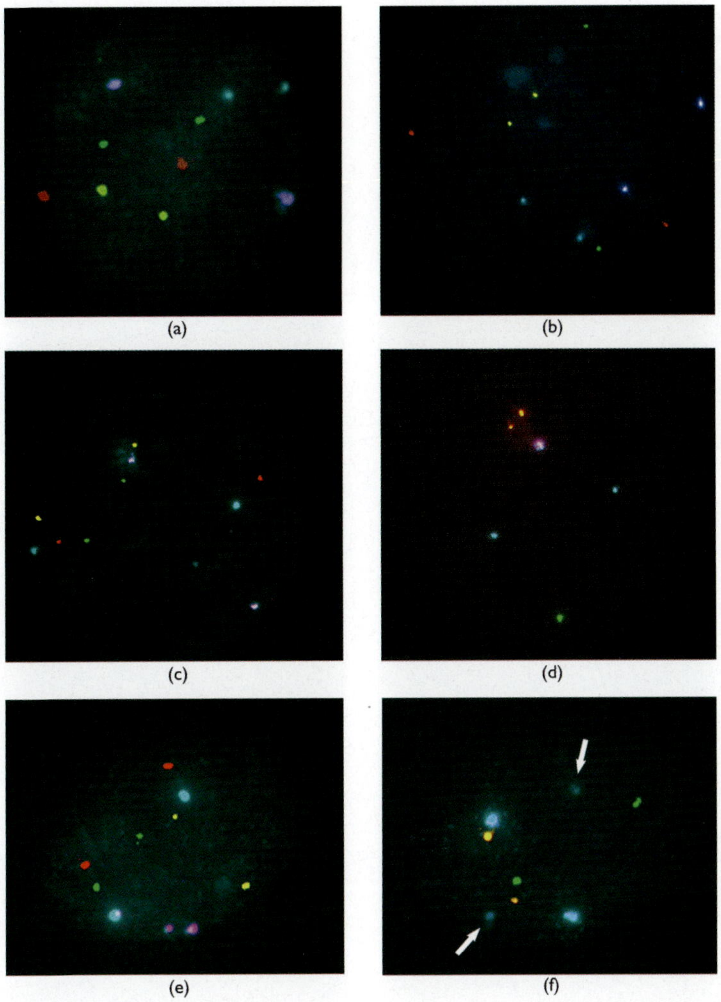

Figure 4.3 Normal fluorescence *in situ* hybridization (FISH) images of interphase nuclei isolated from blastomeres after embryo biopsy on day 3 of embryo development. (a) FISH image of an interphase nucleus from a blastomere removed from an embryo in a 39-year-old female. A normal number of signals are present (two for each of the autosomes tested) following hybridization with MultiVysion PB panel for autosomes 13 (red), 16 (aqua), 18 (violet blue), 21 (green), and 22 (gold). (b) FISH image of an interphase nucleus obtained after embryo biopsy and blastomere fixation from a 43-year-old female. A normal number of signals are present for the five autosomes tested after 3 h of hybridization with the MultiVysion PB panel probe. (c) FISH image of an interphase nucleus obtained after embryo biopsy and blastomere fixation in a 33-year-old female suffering from primary infertility. A normal number of signals are present for the five autosomes tested after 3 h of hybridization with the MultiVysion PB panel probe. (d) FISH image of re-hybridization of the same interphase nucleus shown in (c) using a four-color custom probe (Vysis) for chromosomes X (green), Y (blue), 15 (orange), and 17 (aqua). Since all the probes in this cocktail target the centromeric region consisting of highly repetitive satellite DNA sequences, analysis can be accomplished after a short hybridization time of 4 h. A normal number of signals are present for the autosomes and sex chromosomes, in which one signal for both chromosomes X and Y is present, indicating a male embryo. (e) FISH image of an interphase nucleus obtained after blastomere biopsy from a second embryo from the same 33-year-old patient. A normal number of signals are present for the five autosomes tested. (f) FISH image of re-hybridization of the same interphase nucleus, shown in (e), using the four-color custom probe (Vysis). A normal number of signals are present for the autosomes and X chromosome (two green signals), indicating a female embryo. Also seen are faint residual signals left over from the first hybridization for chromosome 16 (aqua) appearing as flat non-fluorescing spots (white arrows) that were not eliminated entirely with the second round of denaturation and reannealing of DNA.

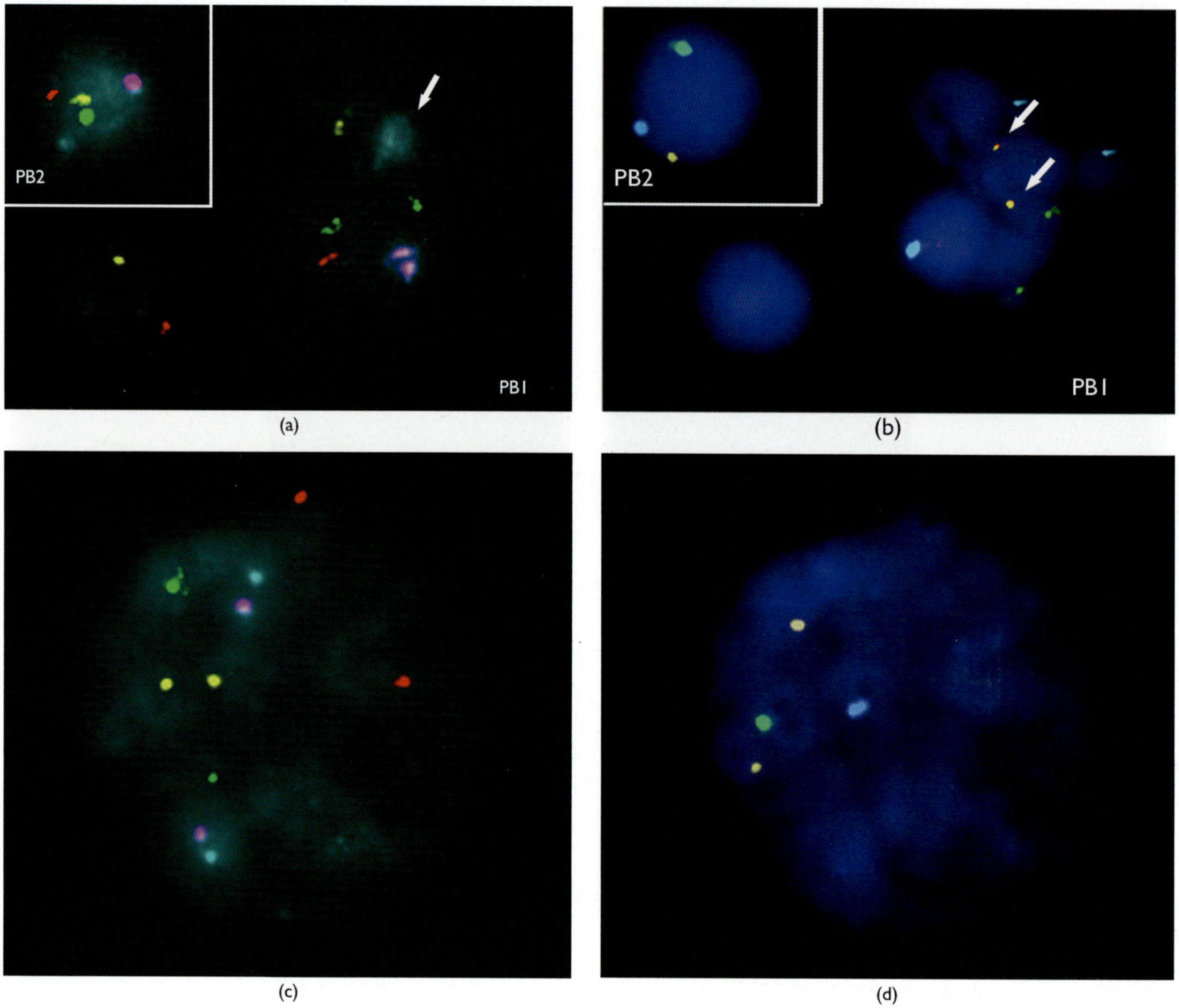

Figure 4.4 First polar body (PB1) and second polar body (PB2) testing followed by blastomere analysis of the resulting embryo by fluorescence *in situ* hybridization (FISH) for eight chromosomes. (a) FISH images of PB1 and PB2 after a 3-h hybridization with MultiVysion PB panel probe for chromosomes 13 (red), 16 (aqua), 18 (violet blue), 21 (green), and 22 (gold). PB1 and PB2 were removed simultaneously on day 1 at the pronuclear stage of development following fertilization assessment of an oocyte retrieved from a 36-year-old woman. A normal number of signals are present for four of the five autosomes tested in PB1, the exception being chromosome 16, which appears as a single large and diffuse signal (white arrow), requiring further investigation by re-hybridization. Also seen are split signals for one of the two signals present for chromosomes 13 (red) and 21 (green) that are often seen with the locus-specific probes, depending on the condition of chromatin with respect to degradation and degree of condensation. (b) Re-hybridization of the same PB1 and PB2 with a probe cocktail for chromosomes 15 (CEP 15; green), 17 (CEP 17; aqua), and 16 (sub-telomeric 16q; orange), showing a normal number of signals present for both PB1 and PB2, including chromosome 16. (c) FISH image of an interphase nucleus after blastomere removal from the embryo derived from the oocyte tested by PB1 and PB2 in (a) and (b). A normal number of signals are present for chromosomes 13, 16, 18, 21, and 22. (d) FISH image of re-hybridization of the same interphase nucleus shown in (c) for chromosomes 15 (CEP 15; orange), X (CEP X; green), and Y (CEP Y; aqua). Two signals for chromosome X are present as well as two signals for chromosome 15 (appearing yellow when seen through a yellow single-bandpass filter). Upon completion of the testing, this embryo was deemed suitable for embryo transfer.

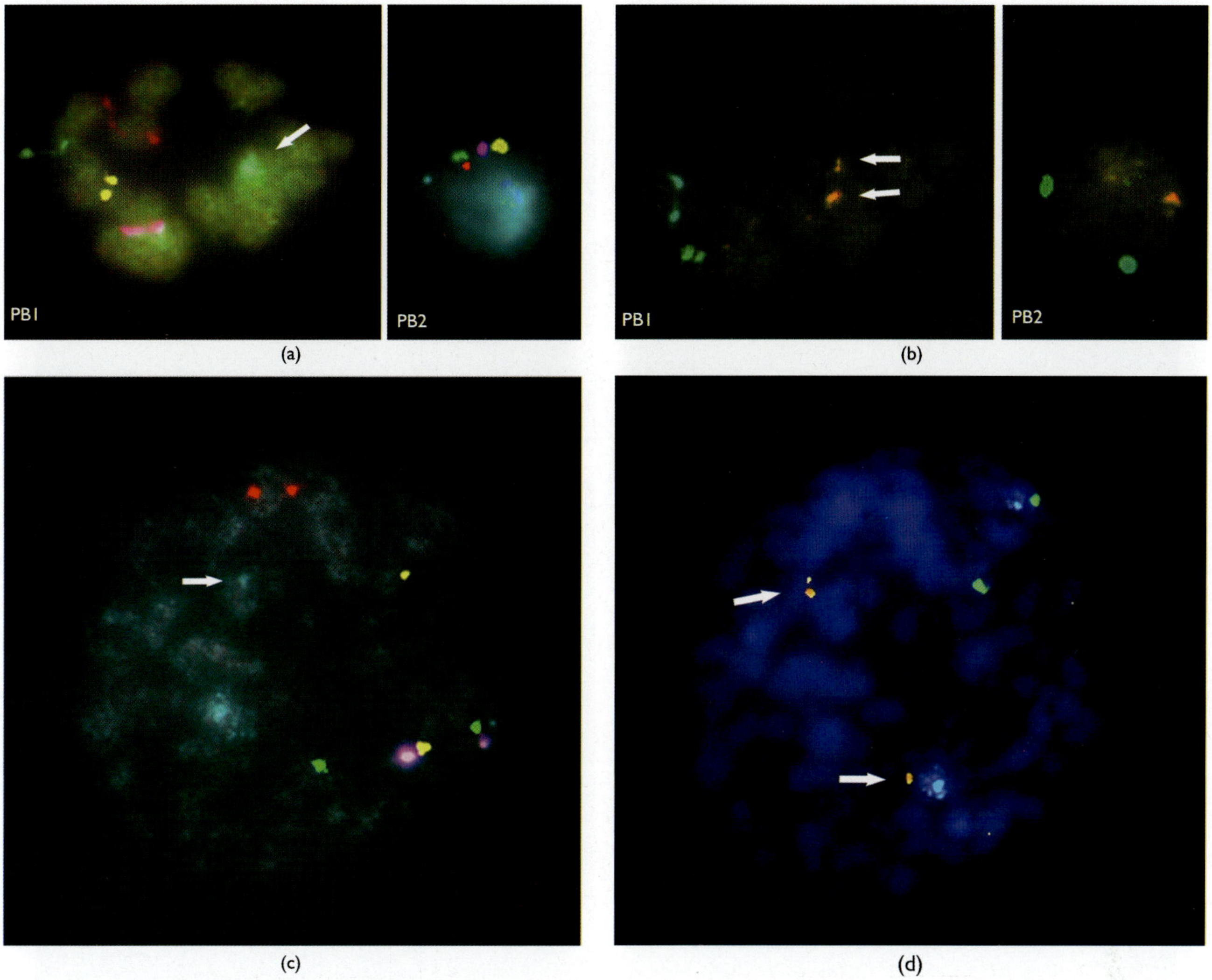

Figure 4.5 First polar body (PB1) and second polar body (PB2) testing followed by blastomere analysis of the resulting embryo by fluorescence *in situ* hybridization (FISH) for seven chromosomes. (a) FISH images of PB1 and PB2 after a 3-h hybridization with MultiVysion PB panel probe for autosomes 13 (red), 16 (aqua), 18 (violet blue), 21 (green), and 22 (gold). PB1 and PB2 were removed simultaneously on day 1 at the pronuclear stage of development following fertilization assessment of an oocyte retrieved from a 29-year-old oocyte donor. A normal number of signals are present for four of the five autosomes tested in PB1, the exception being chromosome 16, which appears as a single large and diffuse signal (white arrow), requiring further investigation by re-hybridization. PB2 contains a normal number of signals present for the chromosomes tested. (b) FISH image of the re-hybridization of the same PB1 and PB2 in (a) for chromosomes 15 (CEP 15; green), 17 (CEP 17; aqua), and 16 (sub-telomeric 16q; orange). Normal numbers of signals (two for each chromatid present in PB1 and one for each in PB2) are seen. (c) FISH image of an interphase nucleus after blastomere removal from the embryo derived from the oocyte corresponding to PB1 and PB2 in (a) and (b). Two signals for each of the chromosomes tested can be seen; however, one signal for chromosome 16 appears faint (white arrow) so that in the second round of hybridization for chromosomes 15 and 17, chromosome 16 was retested using a probe that targeted a different locus (sub-telomeric 16q; orange). (d) FISH image of the second round of hybridization for the same interphase nucleus shown in (c), showing a normal number of signals, including chromosome 16, and therefore considered to be suitable for transfer to the oocyte recipient.

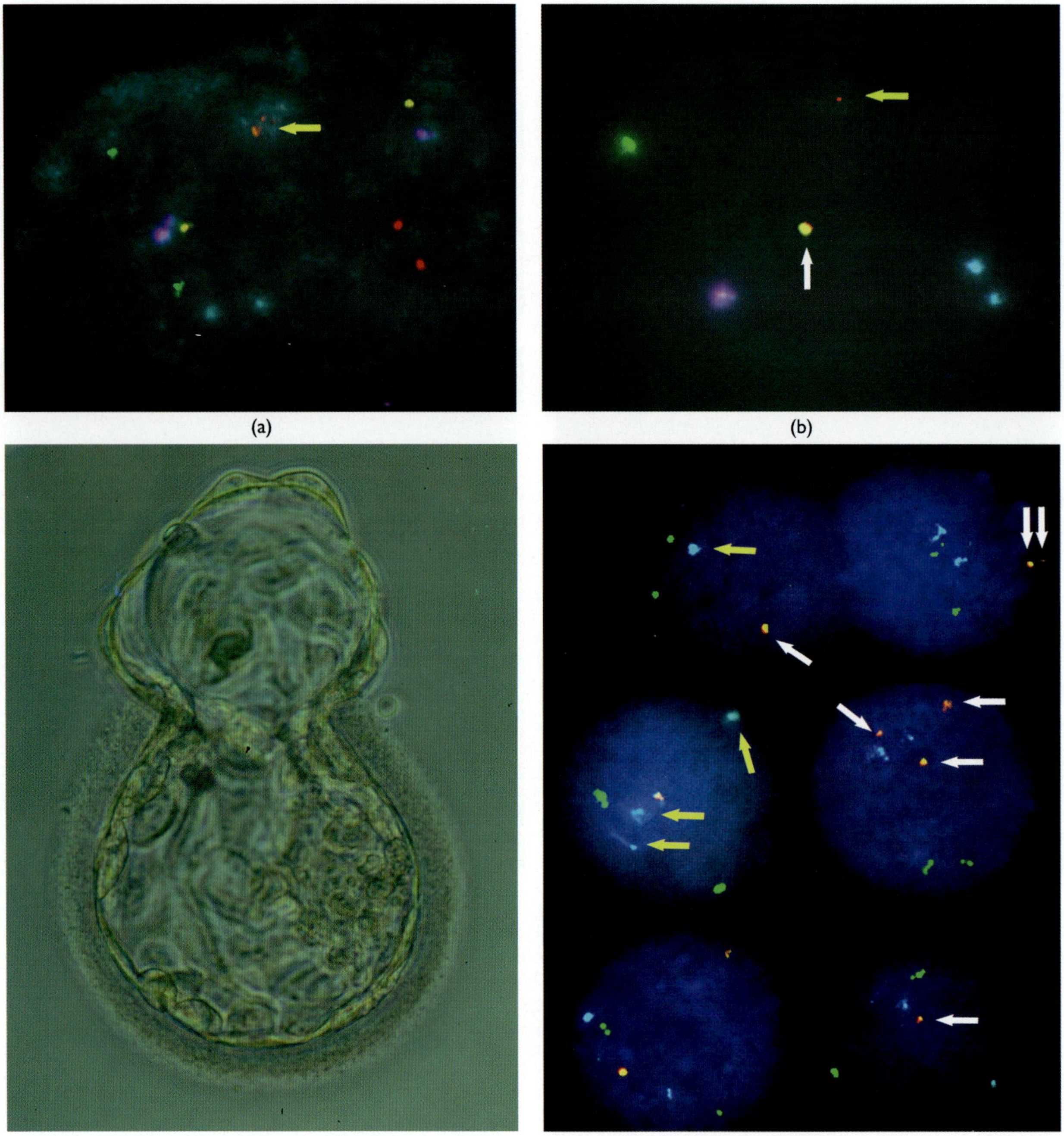

(a) (b) (c) (d)

Figure 4.6 Aneuploidy testing by embryo biopsy and interphase nucleus fluorescence *in situ* hybridization (FISH) analysis for nine chromosomes. (a) FISH image of an interphase nucleus obtained after embryo biopsy of an eight-cell embryo (grade 1, no fragmentation present) on day 3 following fertilization of an oocyte retrieved from a 40-year-old patient. FISH was performed using the MultiVysion polar body (PB) panel probe as previously described in Figure 4.4. A normal number of signals can be seen, including an artifact showing non-specific hybridization (yellow arrow) seen as a dull spot during observation with different single-bandpass filters. (b) FISH image after re-hybridization using the four-color custom probe for chromosomes 15 (orange), 17 (aqua), X (green), and Y (violet blue). Two aqua signals for chromosome 17 and one signal for each sex chromosome X and Y, identifying a male embryo, were visualized along with only one signal for chromosome 15 (white arrow) and the same non-specific artifact seen with the first round of hybridization (yellow arrow). The embryo was identified as having an abnormal chromosome complement (monosomy 15) and was omitted from embryo transfer. (c) Image of the corresponding embryo (a) and (b) on day 5 of embryo development using Hoffman modulation contrast optics and a magnification of ×200. As seen from this image, this embryo reached the blastocyst stage and began hatching through the artificial opening created during embryo biopsy, despite the abnormal chromosome complement monosomy 15 (b). (d) Follow-up FISH analysis, performed by a probe cocktail consisting of CEP 15 (orange), CEP 17 (aqua), and sub-telomeric 22q (green), which revealed an embryo (approximately 50 cells) mosaic for chromosome 15. Nuclei with trisomy, disomy, and monosomy 15 (white arrows) were present, as well as two nuclei with errors for chromosome 17, one trisomic and one monosomic (yellow arrows).

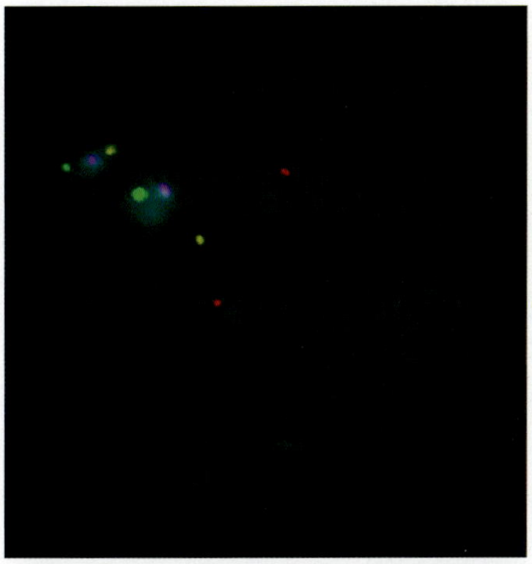

(a)

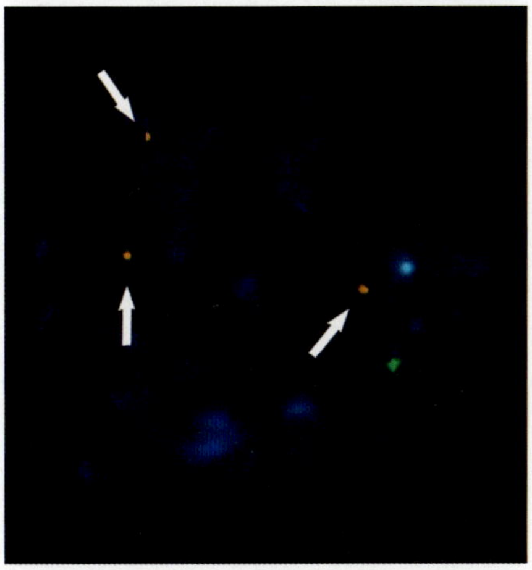

(b)

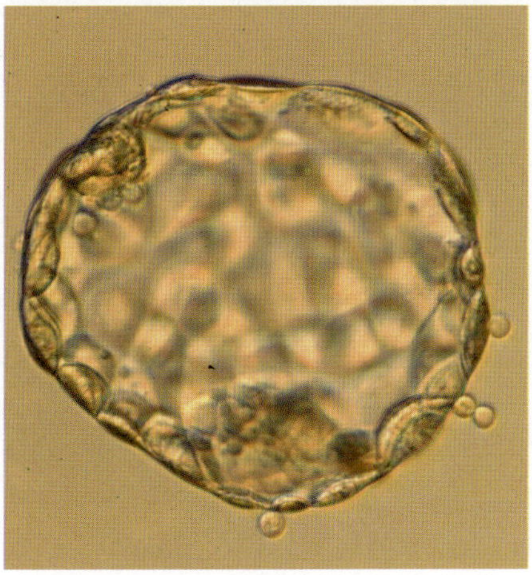

(c)

Figure 4.7 Trisomy 16 detected by embryo biopsy and interphase fluorescence *in situ* hybridization (FISH) analysis. Embryo biopsy was performed on day 3 of embryo development on an eight-cell embryo (grade 1; no fragmentation). The embryo was derived from a cycle in a 35-year-old patient. (a) FISH image of an interphase nucleus after hybridization with the MultiVysion PB panel probe (see Figure 4.4). Two signals for each of the chromosomes are present except for chromosome 16. Considering the possibility of hybridization failure, the nucleus was subjected to a second round of overnight hybridization for chromosomes X (CEP X; green), Y (CEP Y; aqua), and 16 (subtelomeric 16q). (b) FISH image after re-hybridization revealing trisomy 16, evident by the presence of three signals for chromosome 16 (white arrows). (c) Image of the same embryo with trisomy 16 on day 5, which reached a fully expanded blastocyst, that had completely hatched from the zona pellucida through the artificial opening created during embryo biopsy. Inner cell mass (ICM) is present at 6 o'clock.

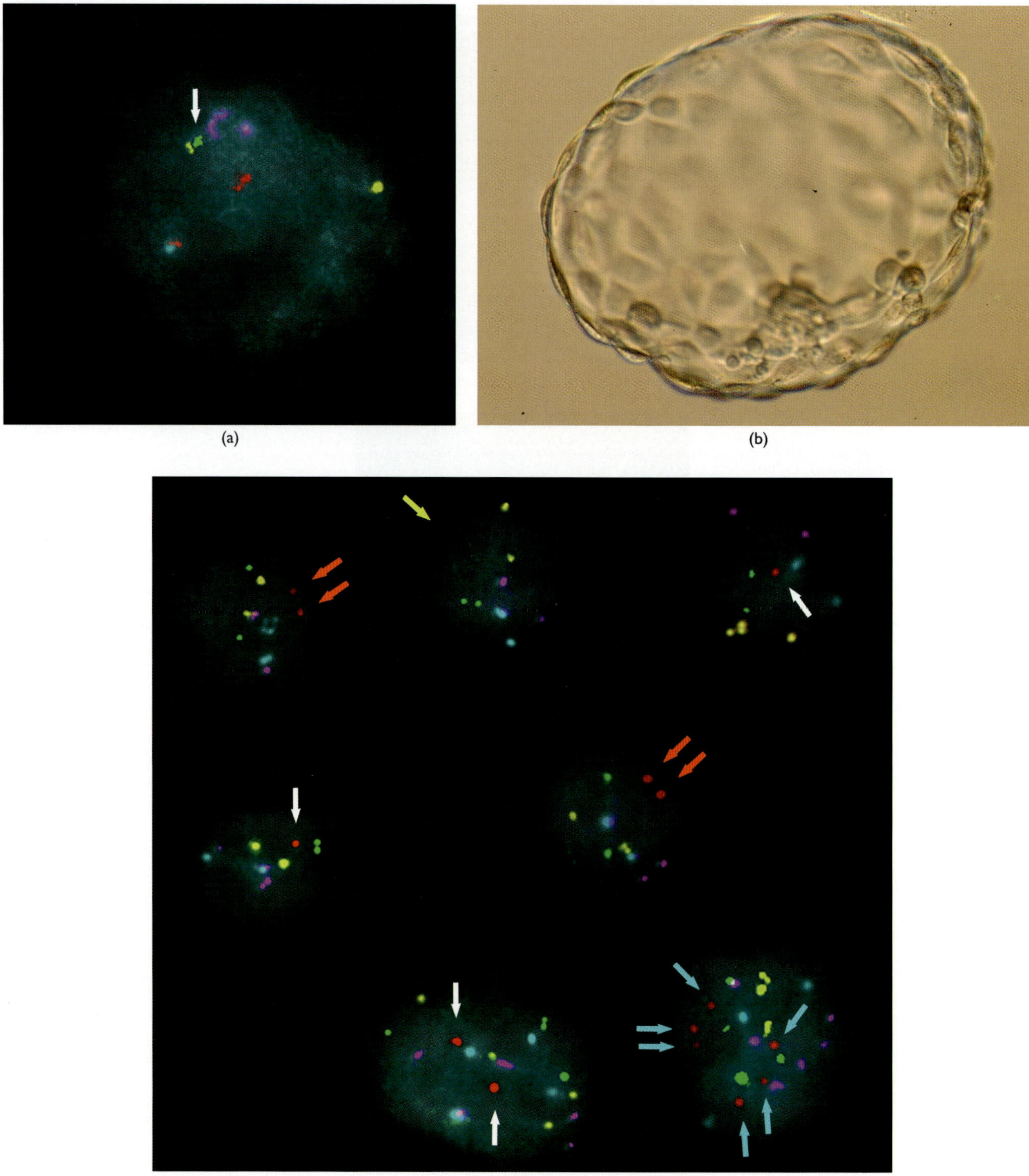

(a) (b)

(c)

Figure 4.8 Monosomy 21 detected by aneuploidy testing at cleavage stage resulting in a mosaic blastocyst. Embryo biopsy was performed on day 3 of embryo development on a six-cell embryo (grade 2, with approximately 15% fragmentation), derived from a 29-year-old oocyte donor. (a) Fluorescence *in situ* hybridization (FISH) image of an interphase nucleus after hybridization with the MultiVysion PB panel probe, which revealed two signals for each of the chromosomes except for a single signal for chromosome 21 in green (white arrow). This embryo was omitted from transfer and cultured to fully hatched blastocyst, the image of which is shown in (b), with a small inner cell mass (ICM) at 6 o'clock. (c) Follow-up FISH analysis of this blastocyst using a custom probe cocktail (research use only), consisting of LSI 21 (21q22 to 21q22.2) (red); LSI BCR (22q11.2) (gold); sub-telomeric 16p (green); LSI 13 (13q14) (aqua); and LSI BCL2 (18q21) (violet blue). FISH image of nuclei obtained after whole embryo fixation revealed mosaicism for chromosome 21 (red), evidenced by nullisomic (yellow arrow), monosomic (white arrows), disomic (red arrows), and polyploid (aqua arrows) nuclei.

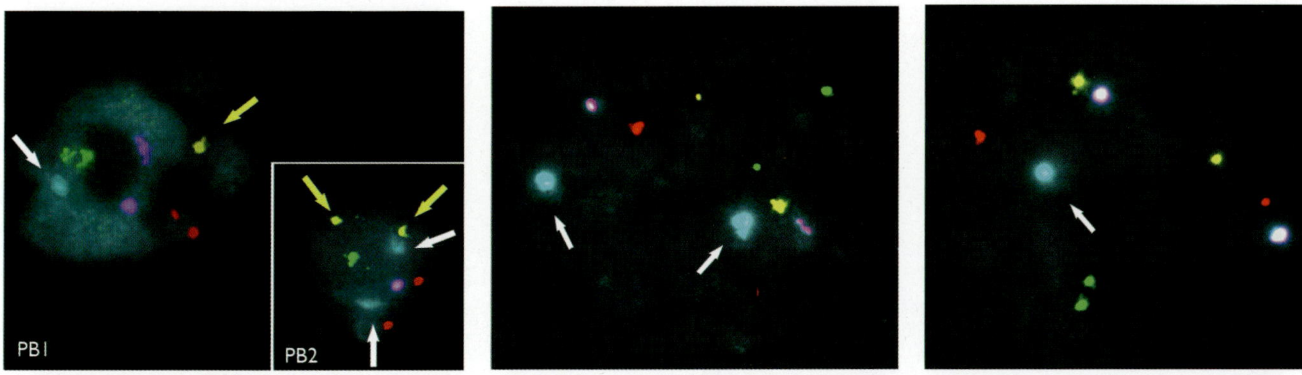

(a) (b) (c)

Figure 4.9 Complex error of chromosomes 16 and 22 deriving from meiosis I and II. First polar body (PB1) and second polar body (PB2) were removed simultaneously on day 1 at the pronuclear stage of development following fertilization assessment. (a) Fluorescence *in situ* hybridization (FISH) images of PB1 and PB2 after a 3-h hybridization with MultiVysion PB panel probe for chromosomes 13 (red), 16 (aqua), 18 (violet blue), 21 (green), and 22 (gold). Chromatid errors are evident by the presence of a single signal for chromosomes 16 (white arrow) and 22 (yellow arrow) in PB1, and additional signals for chromosomes 16 and 22 in the PB2 nucleus, which should have resulted in a balanced embryo with a normal number for the chromosomes tested. However, follow-up embryo testing revealed mosaicism for chromosome 16, evidenced by a normal number of signals present for each of the chromosomes tested, including chromosome 16, in one cell (b), but with only one signal present for chromosome 16 (white arrow) in the other (c).

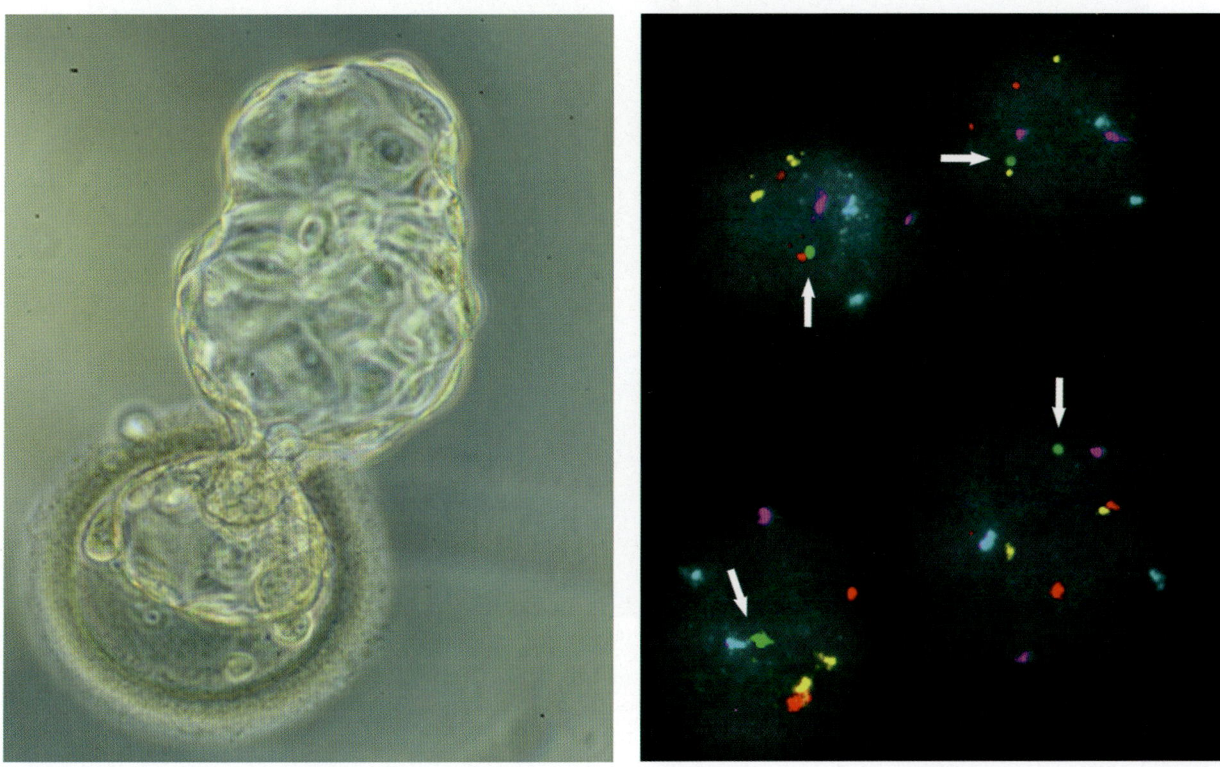

(a) (b)

Figure 4.10 Monosomy 16 blastocyst originating from meiosis II error. (a) Image of a blastocyst hatching through the artificial opening created during biopsy procedures with a compact inner cell mass (ICM) located near the opening in the zona pellucida. The embryo, obtained from a 33-year-old woman with primary infertility, was omitted from transfer because of chromosome 16 meiosis II error (two signals for chromosome 16 in PB2 instead of one), indicating the absence of chromosome 16 in the resulting oocyte. (b) Fluorescence *in situ* hybridization (FISH) image of nuclei isolated from the embryo in (a) hybridized using a custom probe cocktail (research use only) consisting of LSI 21 (21q22 to 21q22.2) (red); LSI BCR (22q11.2) (gold); sub-telomeric 16p (green); LSI 13 (13q14) (aqua); and LSI BCL2 (18q21) (violet blue). Follow-up analysis of the embryo confirmed the polar body diagnosis, showing a single chromosome 16 (white arrows) present in all 80 nuclei isolated after whole embryo fixation.

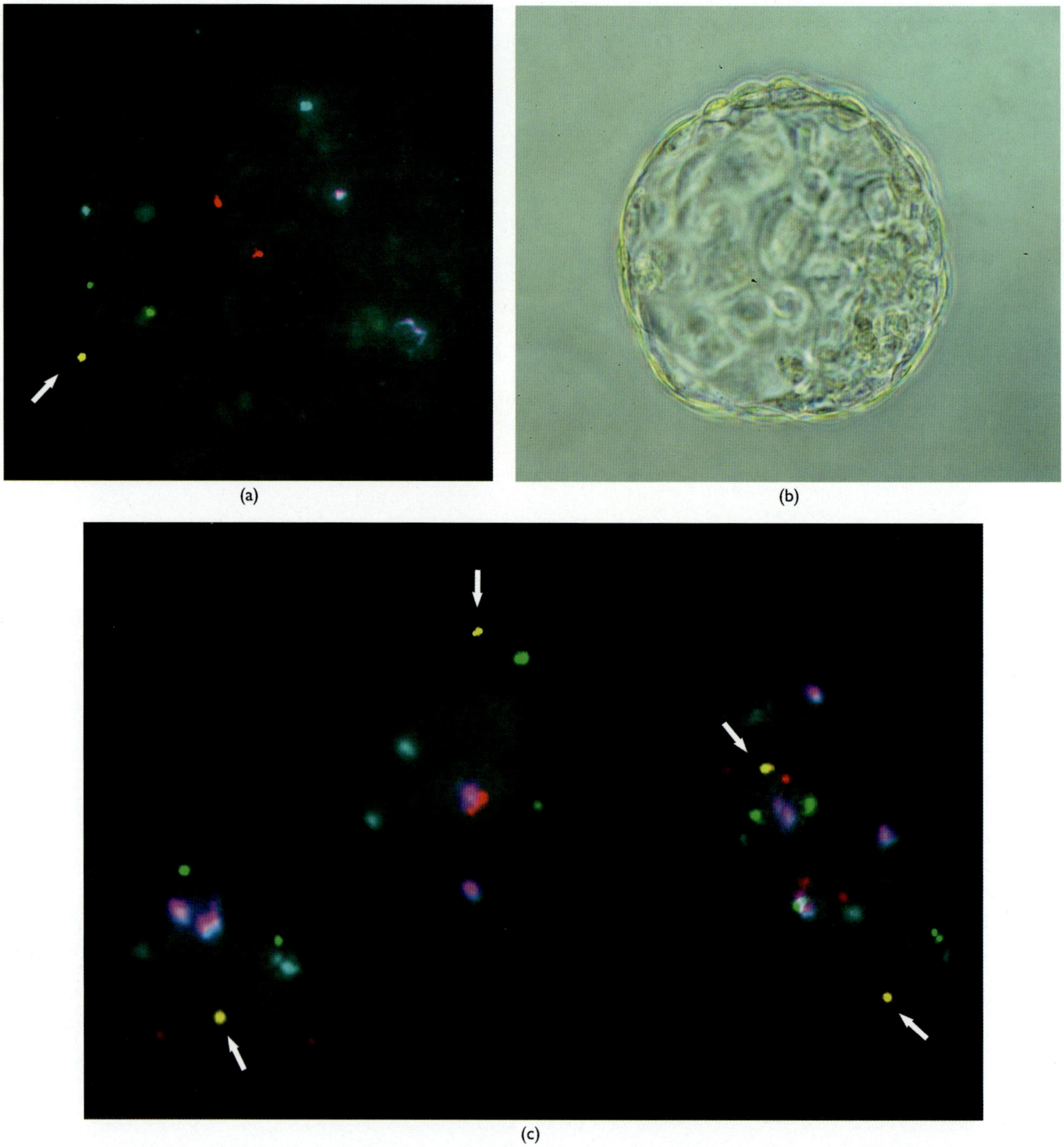

Figure 4.11 Monosomy 22 detected at day-3 cleavage stage confirmed in hatched blastocyst. (a) Fluorescence *in situ* hybridization (FISH) image of an interphase nucleus obtained after embryo biopsy of an eight-cell, grade 1 (no fragmentation) embryo derived from a couple in which the maternal age was 38 years. FISH was performed with the MultiVysion PB panel probe, showing two signals for each of the chromosomes except for a single signal for chromosome 22 in gold (white arrow). (b) Image of a fully hatched blastocyst, 144 h post-ICSI, deriving from the embryo corresponding to (a). Complete hatching is observed more often because of the artificial opening created during biopsy procedures. Although there appears to be a substantial number of trophectoderm cells, no inner cell mass (ICM) is distinguishable. (c) FISH image of nuclei isolated from the embryo in (b), performed with MultiVysion PB panel probe for autosomes 13, 16, 18, 21, and 22 (in gold, white arrows), confirming monosomy 22 in all 40 nuclei isolated after whole embryo fixation.

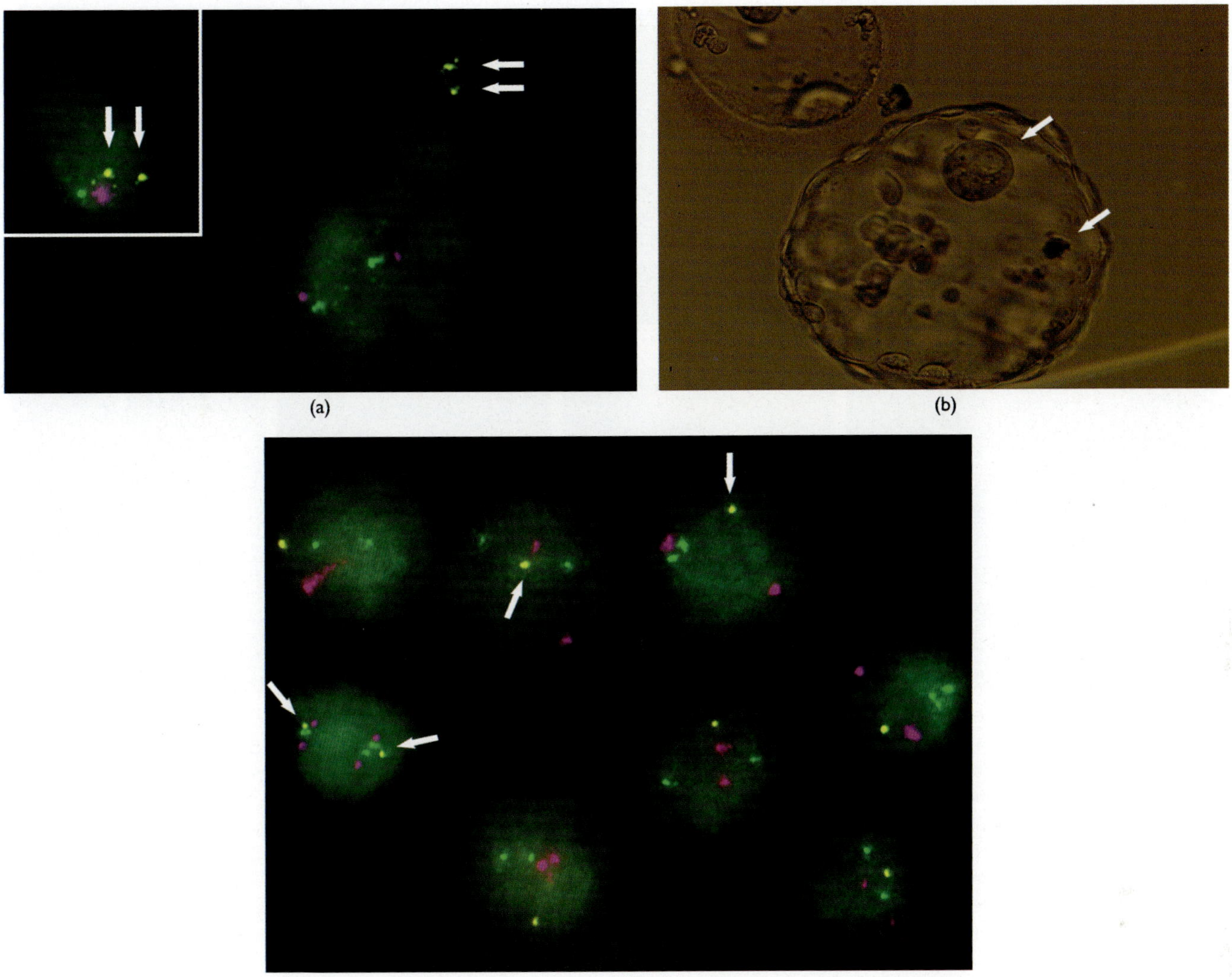

Figure 4.12 Polar-body-based detection of monosomy 22 confirmed at the hatched blastocyst stage. (a) Fluorescence *in situ* hybridization (FISH) image of first polar body (PB1) and second polar body (PB2) following hybridization with the MultiVysion PB panel probe. PB1 and PB2 were removed simultaneously following fertilization of an oocyte derived from a 40-year-old woman. Three of the five fluorophores are shown in which a normal number of signals are seen for chromosomes 18, 21, and 22 (white arrows) in PB1; however, an additional signal for chromosome 22 is seen in PB2 (white arrows), indicating a monosomic embryo. (b) Image of a fully hatched blastocyst from the corresponding embryo, which was omitted from transfer because of chromosome 22 meiosis II error. Some degenerating cells, including a blastomere with a clearly visible interphase nucleus (white arrows), which did not participate in the formation of this blastocyst, are seen in the blastocele. (c) FISH image of nuclei isolated from this embryo (b), performed with MultiVysion PB panel probe (only three of the five chromosomes tested, seen in the green, violet blue, and yellow fluorophores, are shown), including the signals for chromosome 22 in gold (white arrows). Follow-up analysis of the embryo confirmed the polar-body-based diagnosis of monosomy 22, which was seen in all 45 nuclei isolated after whole embryo fixation.

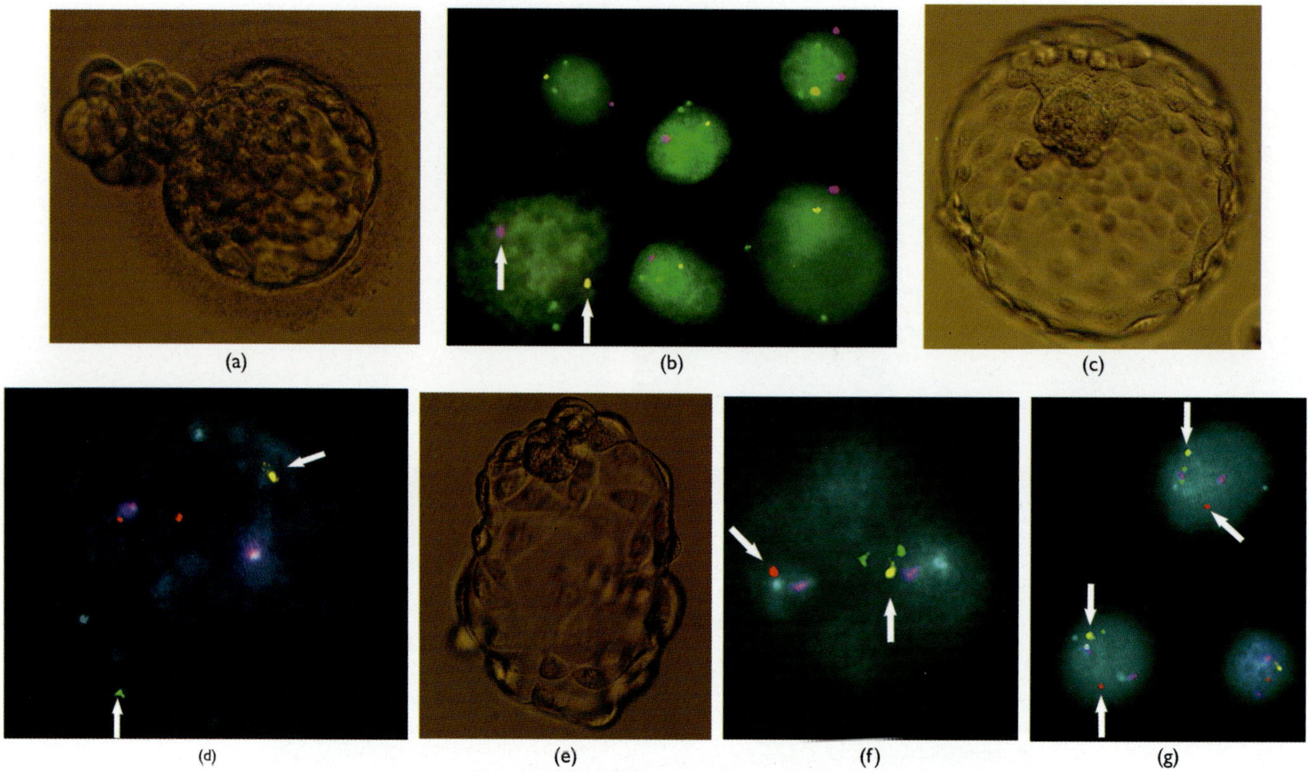

Figure 4.13 Development of double monosomic embryos to blastocyst stage. (a) Image of a contracted blastocyst that had begun hatching through the artificial opening in the thick zona pellucida. Some cells have begun to show signs of degeneration. This embryo was omitted from transfer based on polar body detection of meiosis II errors of chromosomes 18 and 22 predicting a double monosomy in the resulting embryo, obtained from a couple in which the maternal age was 45 years. (b) Fluorescence *in situ* hybridization (FISH) image of nuclei isolated from the blastocyst shown in (a), performed with MultiVysion PB panel probe, confirming monosomy 18, visualized in violet blue, and monosomy 22 in gold (white arrows); only three of the five chromosomes tested, 18, 21, and 22 (seen in the green, violet blue, and yellow fluorophores), are shown. However, only 30 of 38 nuclei isolated by whole embryo fixation contained double monosomy, with the remaining eight cells showing either monosomy 22 (five cells) or monosomy 18 (three cells), indicating mosaicism as a result of later mitotic division errors. (c) Image of a fully hatched blastocyst with a visible inner cell mass (ICM) derived from a couple suffering from primary infertility in which the maternal age was 29 years. Despite the young age of the female patient, 13 of 19 embryos were determined to be abnormal after testing by both polar body and blastomere analysis. (d) FISH image of an interphase nucleus obtained after embryo biopsy of an eight-cell, grade 1 (no fragmentation) embryo, corresponding to (c). FISH performed with the MultiVysion PB panel probe for chromosomes 13, 16, 18, 21, and 22, showing two signals for each of the chromosomes tested except for a single signal for chromosome 21 in green and 22 in gold (white arrows). (e) Image of a fully hatched blastocyst with a visible ICM at 12 o'clock, derived from a couple in which the maternal age was 42 years, which was predicted to have a double monosomy (f) and (g) based on embryo biopsy on day 3, at which time the embryo was 7–8 cells, grade 1 (no fragmentation). (f) FISH image of the interphase nucleus isolated on day 3 from the embryo corresponding to (e), performed with the MultiVysion PB panel probe, showing two signals present for three of the five autosomes tested and only one signal present for chromosomes 13 and 22 (white arrows). (g) Follow-up FISH analysis of nuclei isolated from the embryo in (e), confirming double monosomies 13 and 22 in all nuclei (approximately 50 cells isolated after whole embryo fixation), predicted by blastomere analysis (f).

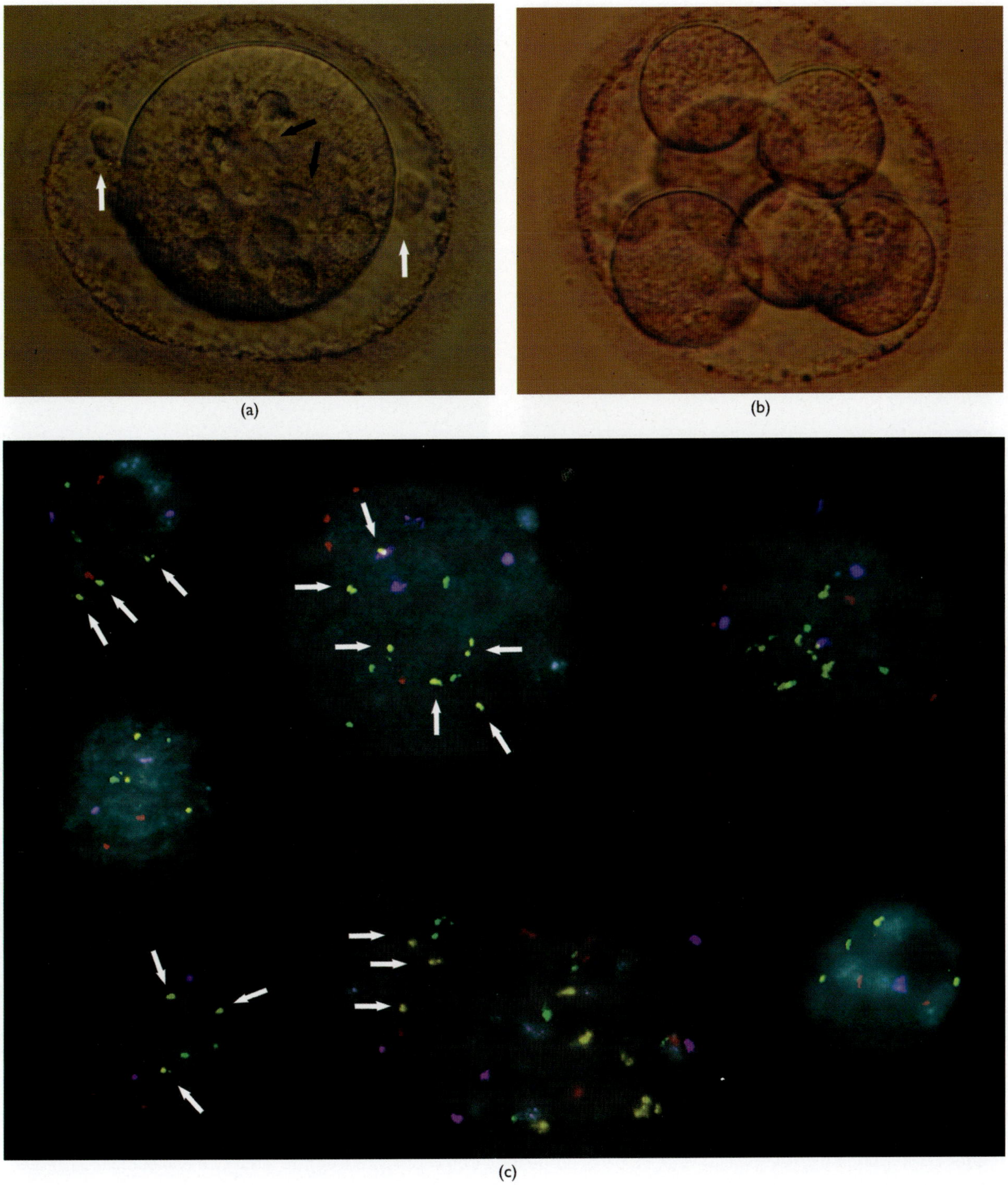

(a) (b) (c)

Figure 4.14 Development of embryo with trisomy 22 of meiosis II origin up to the hatched blastocyst stage. (a) Image of a highly vacuolized zygote with two pronuclei (black arrows) derived from a couple in which the maternal age was 39 years. First polar body (PB1) and second polar body (PB2) are present (white arrows); both are round and located on opposite sides of the oocyte. Following PB testing, the embryo was omitted from transfer because of a trisomy 22 prediction based on a missing LSI 22 signal in PB2. (b) Image of a 7–8-cell embryo with an irregular cell configuration, in which little cell-to-cell contact is seen on day 3; however, this embryo did reach the early blastocyst stage on day 5. (b) Follow-up fluorescence *in situ* hybridization (FISH) analysis of the embryo (corresponding to (a) and (b)), after hybridization with MultiVysion PB panel probe for chromosomes 13, 16, 18, 21, and 22 (gold), showing trisomy 22 in approximately 40 nuclei isolated following whole embryo fixation, with six gold signals present in tetraploid nuclei (white arrows).

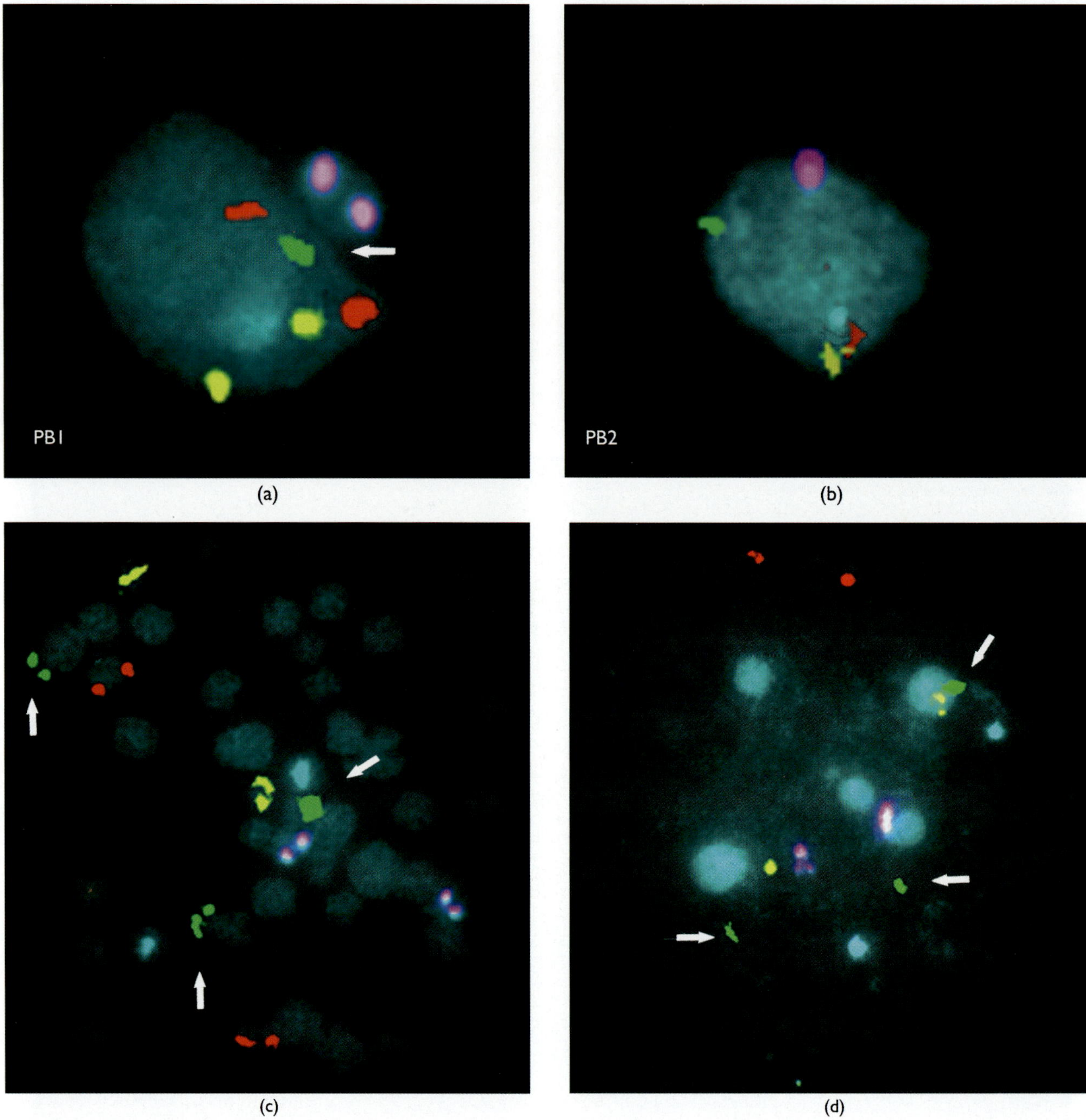

Figure 4.15 Meiosis I error resulting in trisomy 21. First polar body (PB1) and second polar body (PB2) were simultaneously removed on day 1 at the pronuclear stage of development following fertilization assessment. (a) Fluorescence *in situ* hybridization (FISH) image of PB1 after a 3-h hybridization with MultiVysion PB panel probe for chromosomes 13 (red), 16 (aqua), 18 (violet blue), 21 (green), and 22 (gold), showing one chromosome 21 signal (white arrow) instead of two, indicating an extra chromatid 21 retained in the oocyte. (b) FISH image of PB2 showing a normal number of signals for each of the chromosomes tested. Information obtained by the PB testing indicated trisomy 21 to be present in the embryo attributable to the chromatid error in meiosis I. (c) FISH image of metaphase chromosomes obtained after embryo biopsy and fixation on day 3, confirming the presence of three chromosomes 21 (white arrows). Some double dot (paired) signals are seen representing each chromatid of these metaphase stage chromosomes. (d) FISH image of an interphase nucleus isolated from a second cell from the corresponding embryo in (a), (b), and (c), also showing three signals for chromosome 21 (white arrows).

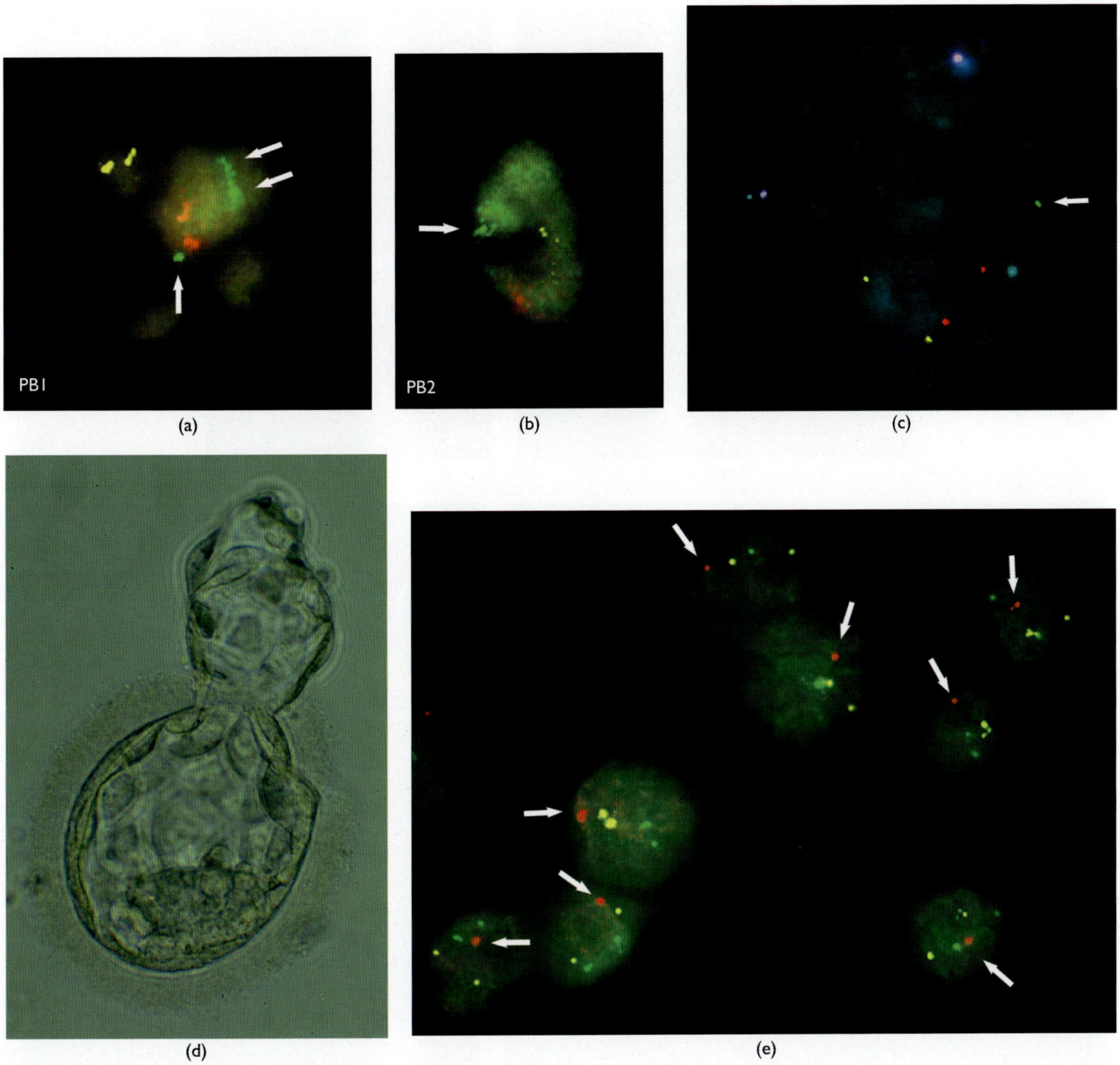

Figure 4.16 Meiosis I error resulting in monosomy 21. (a) Fluorescence *in situ* hybridization (FISH) image of first polar body (PB1) chromatin after hybridization with MultiVysion PB panel probe (only three of the five autosomes are shown: chromosome 13 in red, 21 in green, and 22 in gold), showing three signals for chromosome 21 instead of two, predicting the missing chromatid 21 in the oocyte; the oocyte was derived from an IVF couple suffering from primary infertility, with the maternal age of 33 years. (b) FISH image of second polar body (PB2) shows a normal number of signals for the same three chromosomes, suggesting no maternally derived chromosome 21 in the resulting embryo. (c) FISH image of an interphase nucleus obtained after biopsy of the corresponding embryo in (a) and (b) showing two signals for each of the chromosomes tested with the exception of chromosome 21 (white arrow), in which only one signal is present, confirming the PB findings. (d) Day 5 image of the developing embryo corresponding to (a), (b), and (c); hatching is seen through the opening created during biopsy procedures, although expansion is minimal. (e) FISH image of nuclei isolated from the embryo in (d) hybridized using a custom probe cocktail (research use only) consisting of LSI 21 (21q22 to 21q22.2) (red); LSI BCR (22q11.2) (gold); subtelomeric 16p (green); LSI 13 (13q14) (aqua); and LSI BCL2 (18q21) (violet blue) (only chromosomes labeled in the red, green, and gold fluorophores are shown), confirming monosomy 21 (white arrows) in all 65 nuclei isolated after whole embryo fixation.

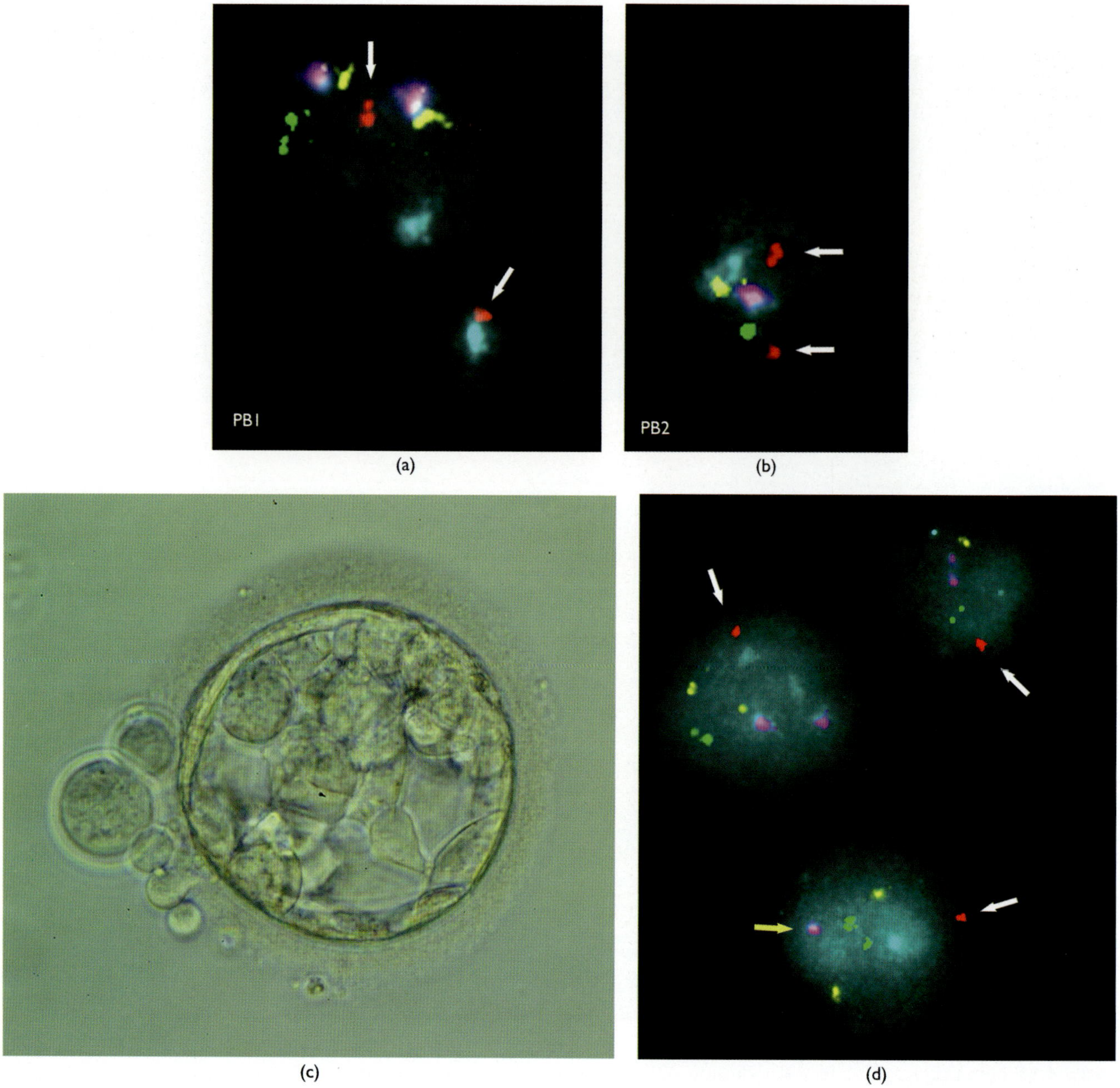

Figure 4.17 Meiosis II error resulting in monosomy 13. (a) Fluorescence *in situ* hybridization (FISH) image of isolated chromatin from first polar body (PB1) removed from an oocyte retrieved from a 44-year-old patient, showing a normal number of signals after hybridization with MultiVysion PB panel probe. Two signals, one of which is split, are present for chromatid 13 (white arrows). (b) FISH image of second polar body (PB2) nucleus in which two signals (instead of one) for chromosome 13 are present, indicating the lack of chromosome 13 in the oocyte. Following syngamy this embryo was predicted to be monosomic for chromosome 13. (c) Image of a poor-quality cavitating morula resulting from this oocyte (a) and (b), in which few cells make up the trophectoderm as evidenced by the stretched out cells along the periphery. A few cytoplasmic fragments have escaped through the artificial opening created during biopsy. (d) Follow-up FISH analysis after hybridization with MultiVysion PB panel probe for chromosomes 13 (red), 16, 18, 21, and 22, confirming monosomy 13 (one red signal shown by white arrows) in each of 45 nuclei isolated after whole embryo fixation.

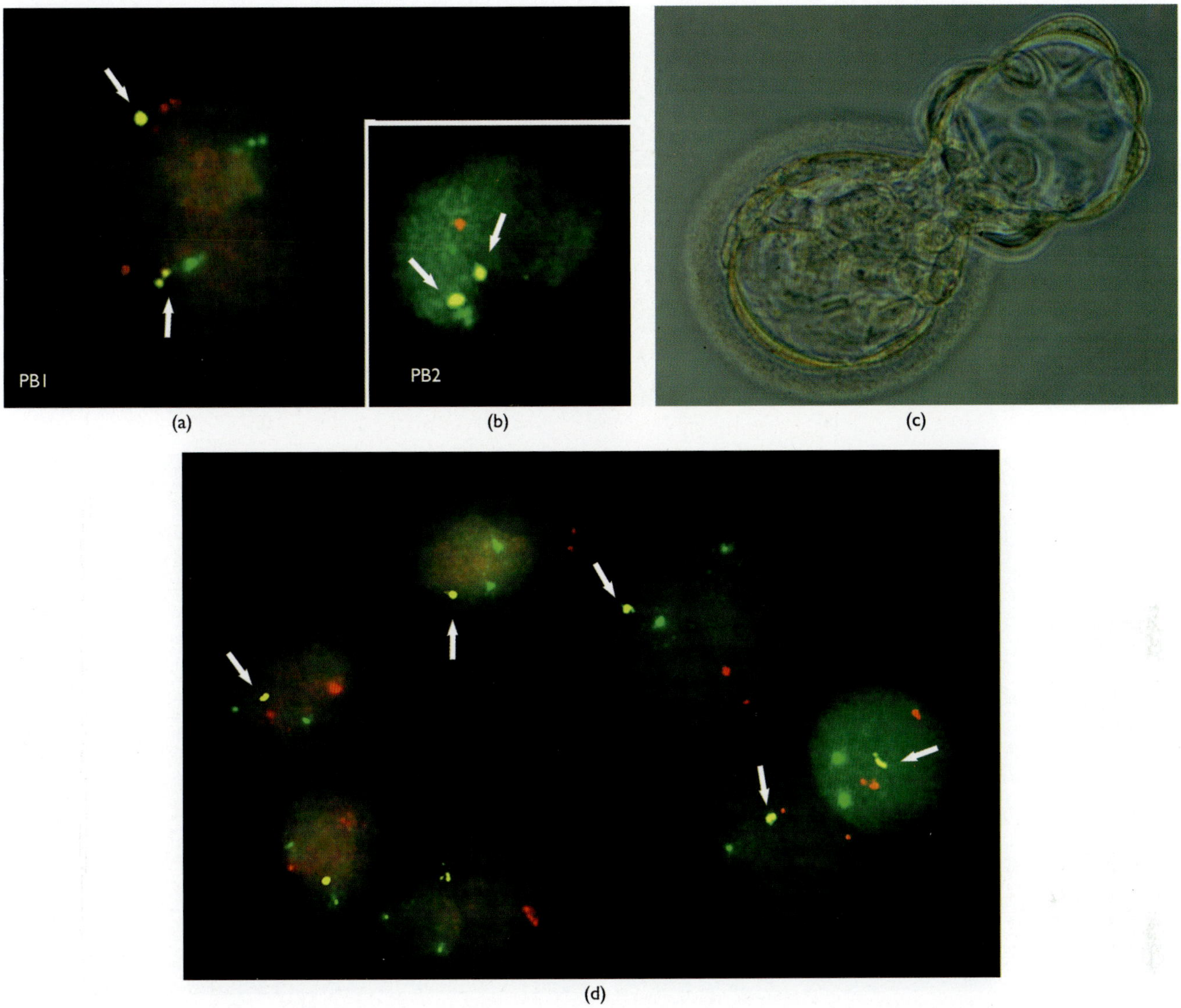

Figure 4.18 Meiosis II error resulting in monosomy 22. (a) Fluorescence *in situ* hybridization (FISH) image of isolated chromatin from first polar body (PB1) removed from an oocyte retrieved from a 42-year-old patient, showing a normal number of signals after hybridization with MultiVysion PB panel probe (only three of the five chromosomes are shown in fluorophores red, green, and gold). Two signals, one of which is split, are present for chromatid 22 (white arrows). (b) FISH image of second polar body (PB2) nucleus in which two signals for chromosome 22 are present, indicating nullisomy 22 in the resulting oocyte and monosomy 22 in the developing embryo. (c) Image of a non-expanded blastocyst herniating through the opening created during biopsy resulting from this monosomy 22 embryo. (d) Follow-up FISH analysis of this embryo after hybridization with MultiVysion PB panel probe (three of the five chromosomes are shown in fluorophores red, green, and gold), confirming monosomy 22 (one gold signal shown by white arrows) in each of 60 nuclei isolated after whole embryo fixation.

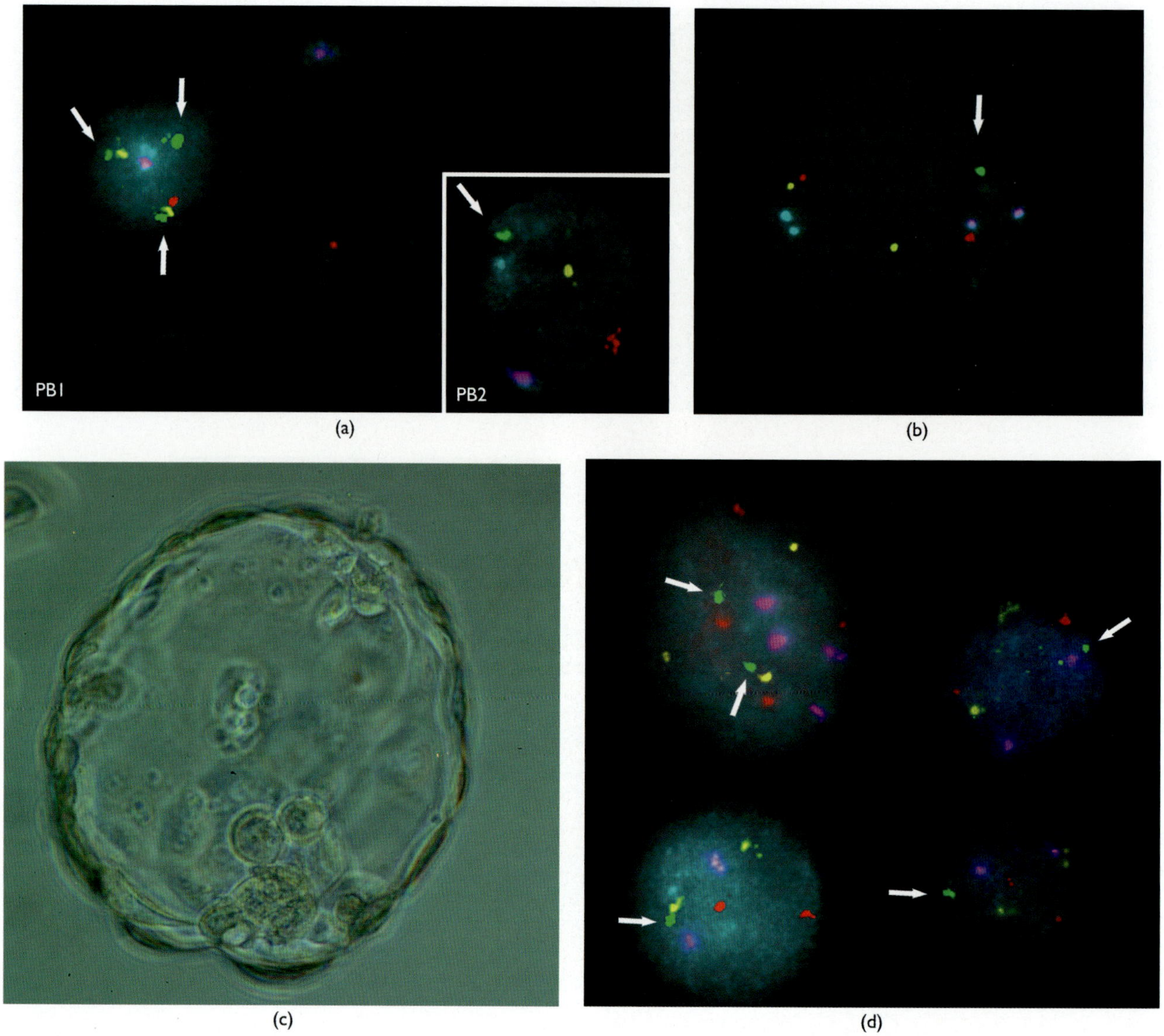

Figure 4.19 Meiosis I error resulting in monosomy 21. (a) Fluorescence *in situ* hybridization (FISH) image of first polar body (PB1) and second polar body (PB2) chromatin after hybridization with MultiVysion PB panel probe, showing three signals (instead of two) for chromosome 21 (white arrows) in PB1, and a normal number of signals present in the PB2 nucleus, including one chromosome 21 signal (white arrow), suggesting nullisomy 21 in the oocyte retrieved from a 40-year-old woman. (b) Follow-up testing of the resulting embryo by blastomere interphase analysis confirmed the predicted monosomy 21, evidenced by a single signal for chromosome 21 from the paternal contribution (white arrow). (c) Day 5 fully hatched blastocyst derived from this monosomy 21 embryo shown in (a) and (b). (d) Follow-up FISH analysis of the embryo confirming monosomy 21 (white arrows) in all 50 nuclei isolated after whole embryo fixation.

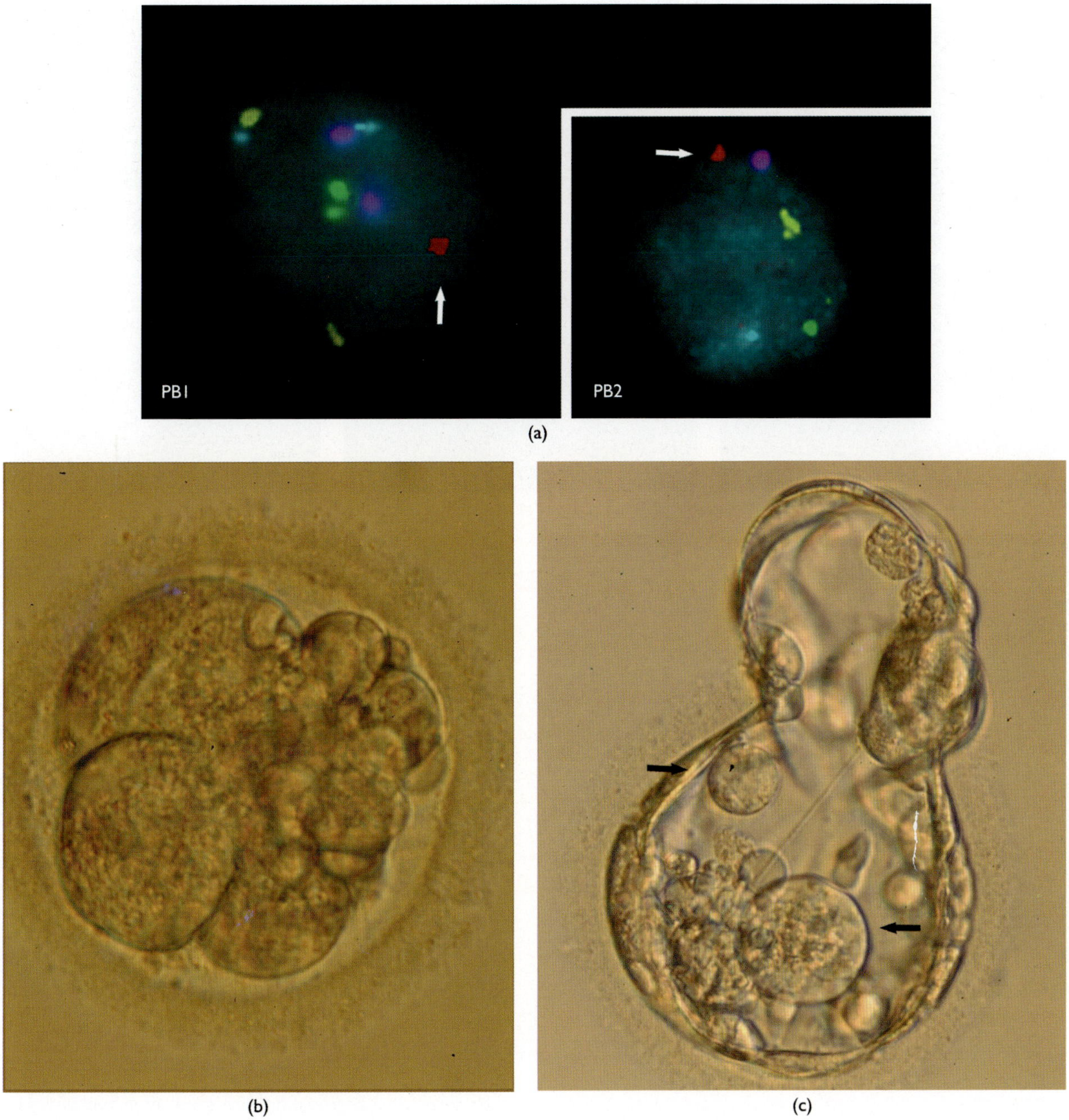

Figure 4.20 Meiosis I error resulting in trisomy 13. First polar body (PB1) and second polar body (PB2) were simultaneously removed on day 1 at the pronuclear stage of development following fertilization of an oocyte retrieved from a 35-year-old patient. (a) Fluorescence *in situ* hybridization (FISH) image of PB1 and PB2 after a 3-h hybridization with MultiVysion PB panel probe for autosomes 13 (red), 16 (aqua), 18 (violet blue), 21 (green), and 22 (gold), showing a single (instead of double) signal for chromosome 13 (white arrow) in PB1 and a normal number of signals for each chromosome in PB2, indicating trisomy 13 in the resulting embryo. (b) Image of the corresponding aneuploid embryo on day 3, showing that only a few uneven blastomeres are present, with greater than a quarter of the embryo being fragmented. (c) Despite chromosome abnormality and poor morphologic quality, this embryo developed further, forming a poor-quality early blastocyst, with a few cytoplasmic fragments (black arrows), originally seen at the cleavage stage and which did not participate in formation of this abnormal blastocyst, remaining within the blastocele.

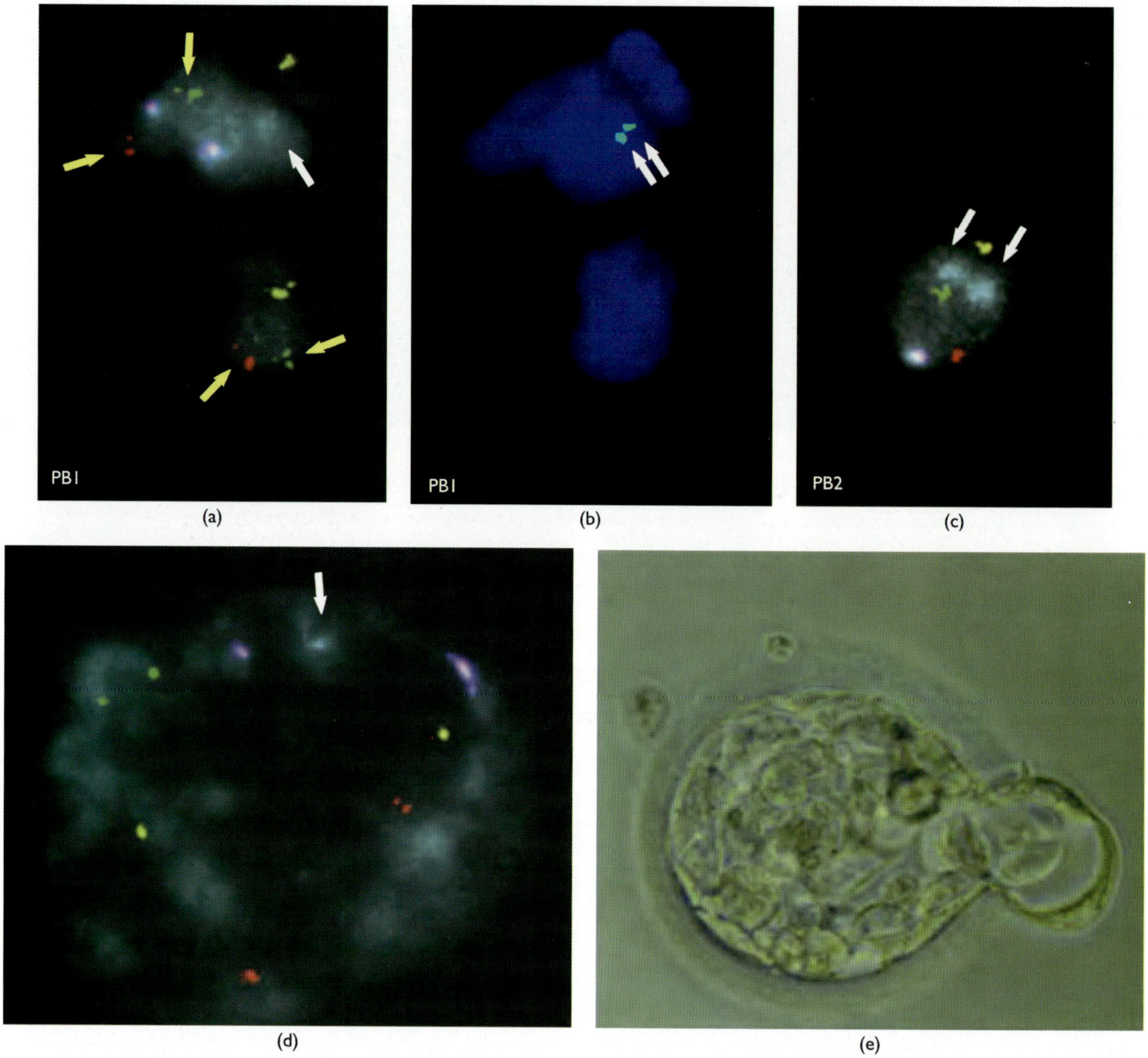

Figure 4.21 Meiosis II errors resulting in monosomy 16. (a) Fluorescence *in situ* hybridization (FISH) image of isolated chromatin from first polar body (PB1) removed from an oocyte retrieved from a 39-year-old patient. A normal number of signals (LSI signals for chromosomes 13 and 21 (yellow arrows) appear equally split due to chromatin degradation) are seen after hybridization with MultiVysion PB panel probe, with the exception of chromosome 16, in which a large diffuse CEP signal is present. Enumeration was impossible, requiring further testing to be conducted for chromosome 16. (b) FISH image after re-hybridization of PB1 chromatin for chromosome 16 targeting a different locus using a sub-telomeric 16p probe in green. Two signals are present, albeit in close proximity. (c) FISH image of PB2 nucleus, showing two signals (instead of one) for chromosome 16 (white arrows), indicating that the oocyte is nullisomic for chromosome 16, which will result in a monosomy 16 embryo. (d) FISH image of an interphase nucleus obtained after embryo biopsy showing two signals for each of the chromosomes tested, with the exception of chromosome 16, for which a single signal (white arrow) is seen, confirming the PB diagnosis of monosomy 16. (e) Image of the corresponding embryo on day 5 of development, presenting as an early hatching blastocyst, in which follow-up FISH analysis confirmed monosomy 16 in all (approximately 50) nuclei isolated after whole embryo fixation.

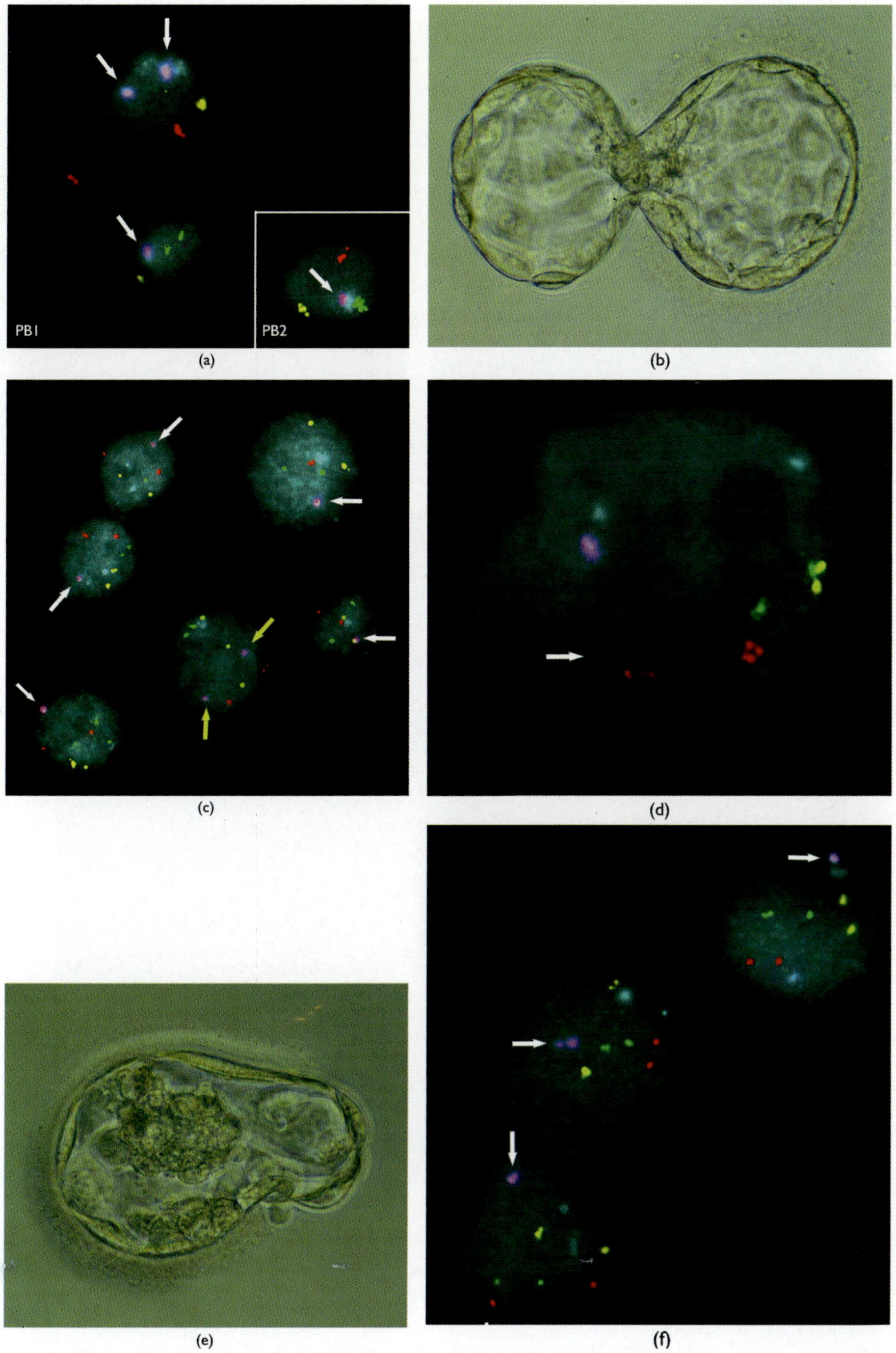

Figure 4.22 Meiosis I error resulting in monosomy 18. First polar body (PB1) and second polar body (PB2) were simultaneously removed on day 1 at the pronuclear stage of development following fertilization of an oocyte retrieved from a 40-year-old patient. (a) Fluorescence *in situ* hybridization (FISH) image of PB1 and PB2 after a 3-h hybridization with MultiVysion PB panel probe for autosomes 13 (red), 16 (aqua), 18 (violet blue), 21 (green), and 22 (gold), showing three (instead of two) signals for chromosome 18 (white arrows) in PB1. A normal number of signals in the PB2 nucleus, including chromosome 18 (white arrow), suggests nullisomy 18 in the corresponding oocyte, which will result in an embryo with monosomy 18. (b) Image of a hatching expanded blastocyst derived from this monosomy 18 embryo, consisting of over 80 cells. (c) FISH image of nuclei isolated after whole embryo fixation of this blastocyst confirming monosomy 18 (a single signal for chromosome 18 in violet blue is present (white arrows) in the majority of the nuclei). The embryo is mosaic, as cells with two signals for chromosome 18 are also present (yellow arrows) along with three signals for chromosome 22 (gold) in one nucleus. (d) FISH image of an interphase nucleus isolated after embryo biopsy of an eight-cell, grade-1 embryo derived from a couple in which the maternal age was 31 years. A single signal is present for chromosome 18 (white arrow) after hybridization with the MultiVysion PB panel probe (signals for chromosome 13 in red are both equally split). (e) Image of a poor-quality blastocyst derived from this embryo (d), consisting of approximately 35 cells on day 5. (f) FISH image of nuclei isolated after whole embryo fixation, in which a single signal for chromosome 18 is present (white arrows) in each of the nuclei, confirming the initial diagnosis.

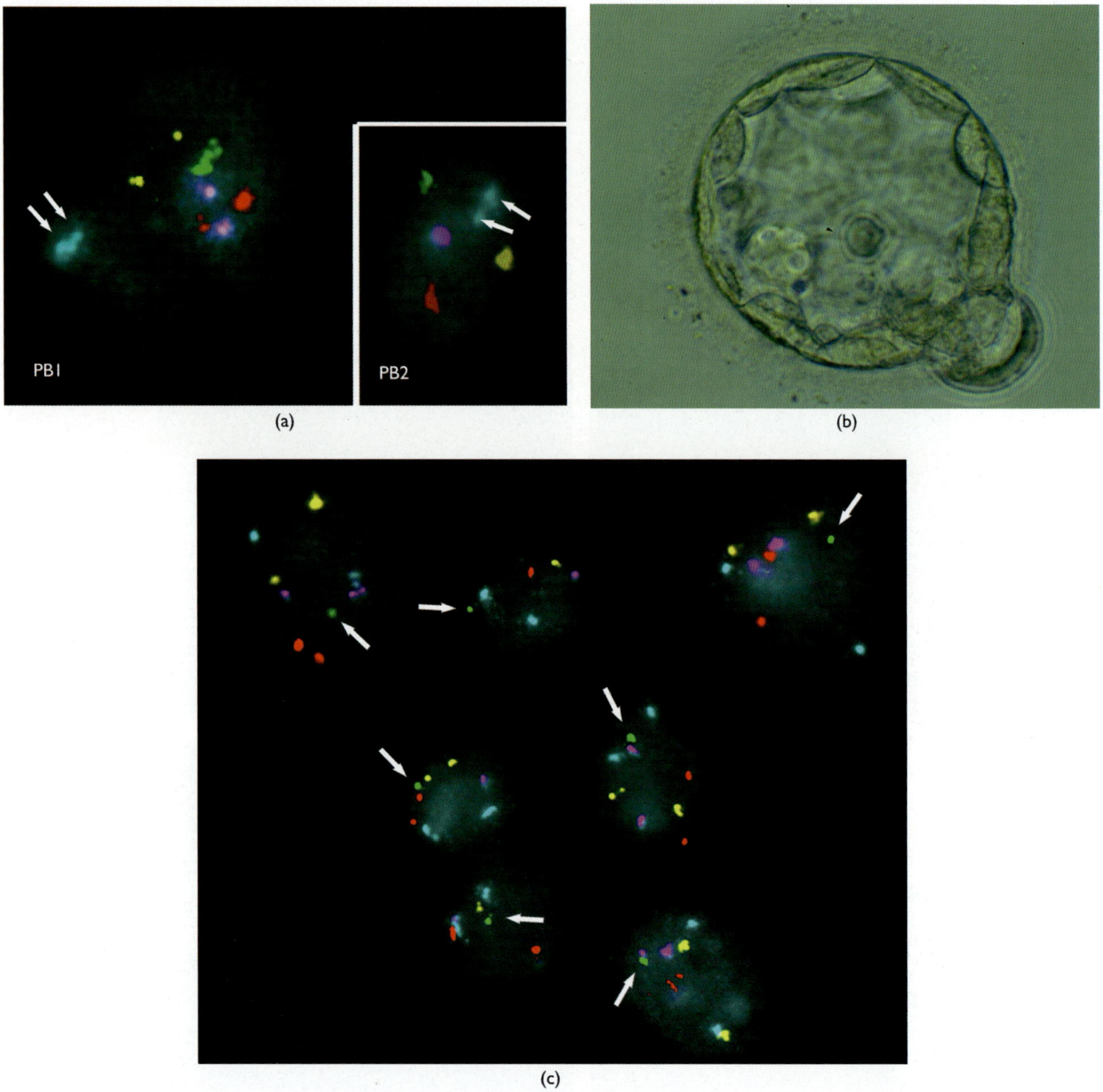

Figure 4.23 Meiosis II error resulting in monosomy 16. (a) Fluorescence *in situ* hybridization (FISH) image of isolated chromatin from first polar body (PB1) and second polar body (PB2) removed simultaneously following fertilization of an oocyte retrieved from a 31-year-old woman, who had previously experienced a first-trimester loss due to trisomy 14. A normal number of signals are seen in PB1 after hybridization with MultiVysion PB panel probe. Chromatids for chromosomes 16 and 21 are in close proximity, creating a strip-like signal. Two signals for chromosome 16 are present in the PB2 nucleus, indicating nullisomy 16 in the oocyte. (b) Image of the day-6 expanding blastocyst derived from this embryo (a), consisting of approximately 60 cells. (c) FISH image of nuclei isolated from the embryo in (b) hybridized using a custom probe cocktail (research use only) consisting of LSI 21 (21q22 to 21q22.2) (red); LSI BCR (22q11.2) (gold); sub-telomeric 16p (green); LSI 13 (13q14) (aqua); and LSI BCL2 (18q21) (violet blue), which confirms monosomy 16 (white arrows) in each of the nuclei tested.

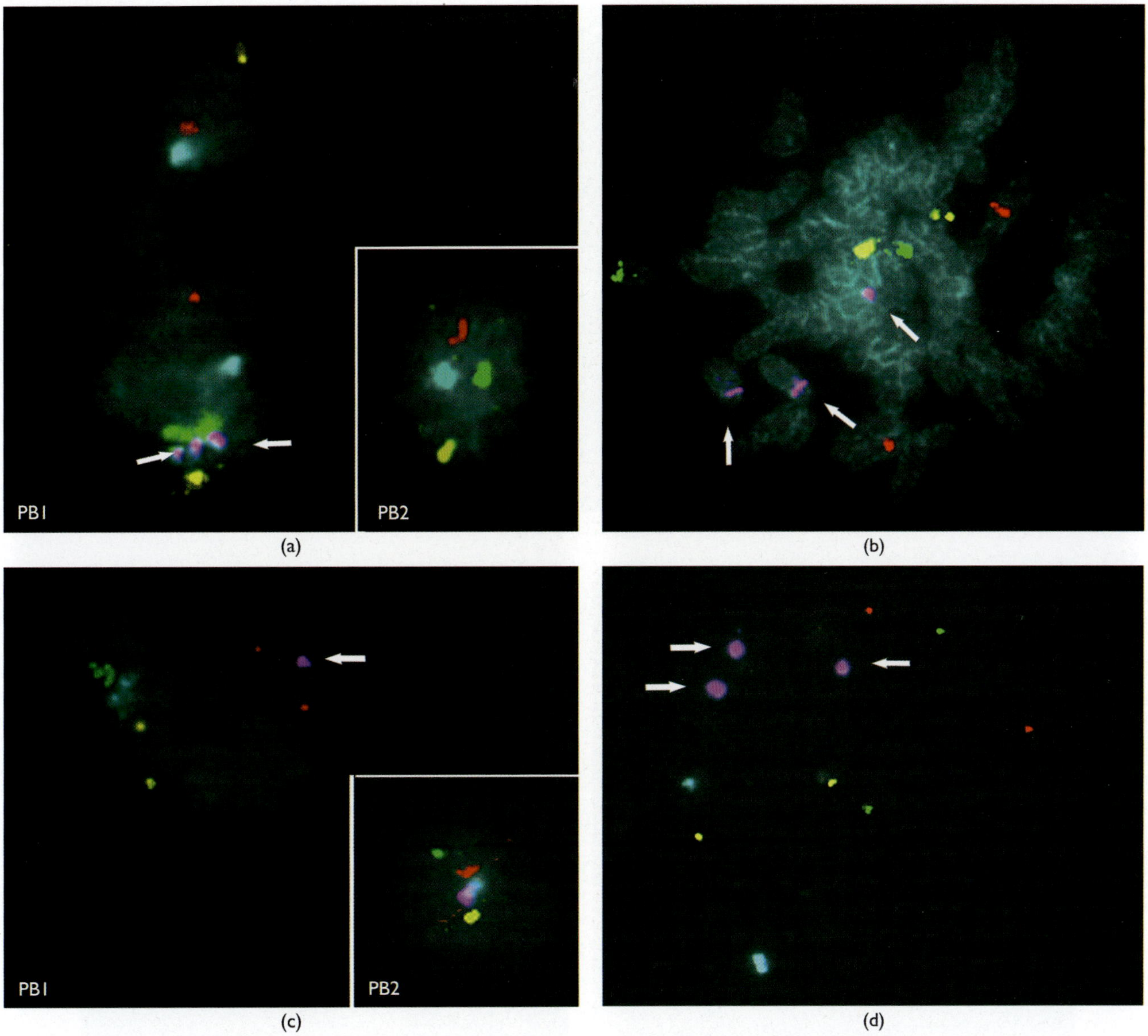

Figure 4.24 Meiosis I (c) and meiosis II (a) errors both resulting in trisomy 18. (a) Fluorescence *in situ* hybridization (FISH) image of first polar body (PB1) and second polar body (PB2) after hybridization with the five-color MultiVysion PB panel probe, showing normal number of signals in PB1 for all the chromosomes tested, including signals for chromosome 21 (green), which are in close proximity to one another, and for chromosome 18 (violet blue) (white arrows). However, only four of five signals are present in PB2 (shown in the right lower corner), the missing signal being for chromosome 18, indicating an extra chromatid 18 in the oocyte, which will lead to trisomy 18 in the resulting embryo. (b) Follow-up FISH analysis of the resulting embryo after blastomere removal and nucleus conversion (see Chapter 3), confirming the predicted trisomy 18, evident from the three signals for chromosome 18 present (white arrows). (c) and meiosis II (a) errors both resulting in trisomy 18. (c) FISH image of PB1 and PB2 after hybridization with the five-color MultiVysion PB panel probe, showing two signals for each chromosome tested in PB1, some in close proximity, such as chromosome 21 in green, except for chromosome 18, in which only one signal is present (white arrow). Since a normal number of signals are present in PB2 from this oocyte (one signal for each of the chromosomes tested), the missing chromosome 18 signal in PB1 indicates that an additional chromatid was retained in the oocyte, leading to a trisomy 18 embryo. (d) FISH image of an interphase nucleus from the resulting embryo, in which trisomy 18 is evident by the presence of three signals in the violet blue fluorophore (white arrows), confirming the PB diagnosis.

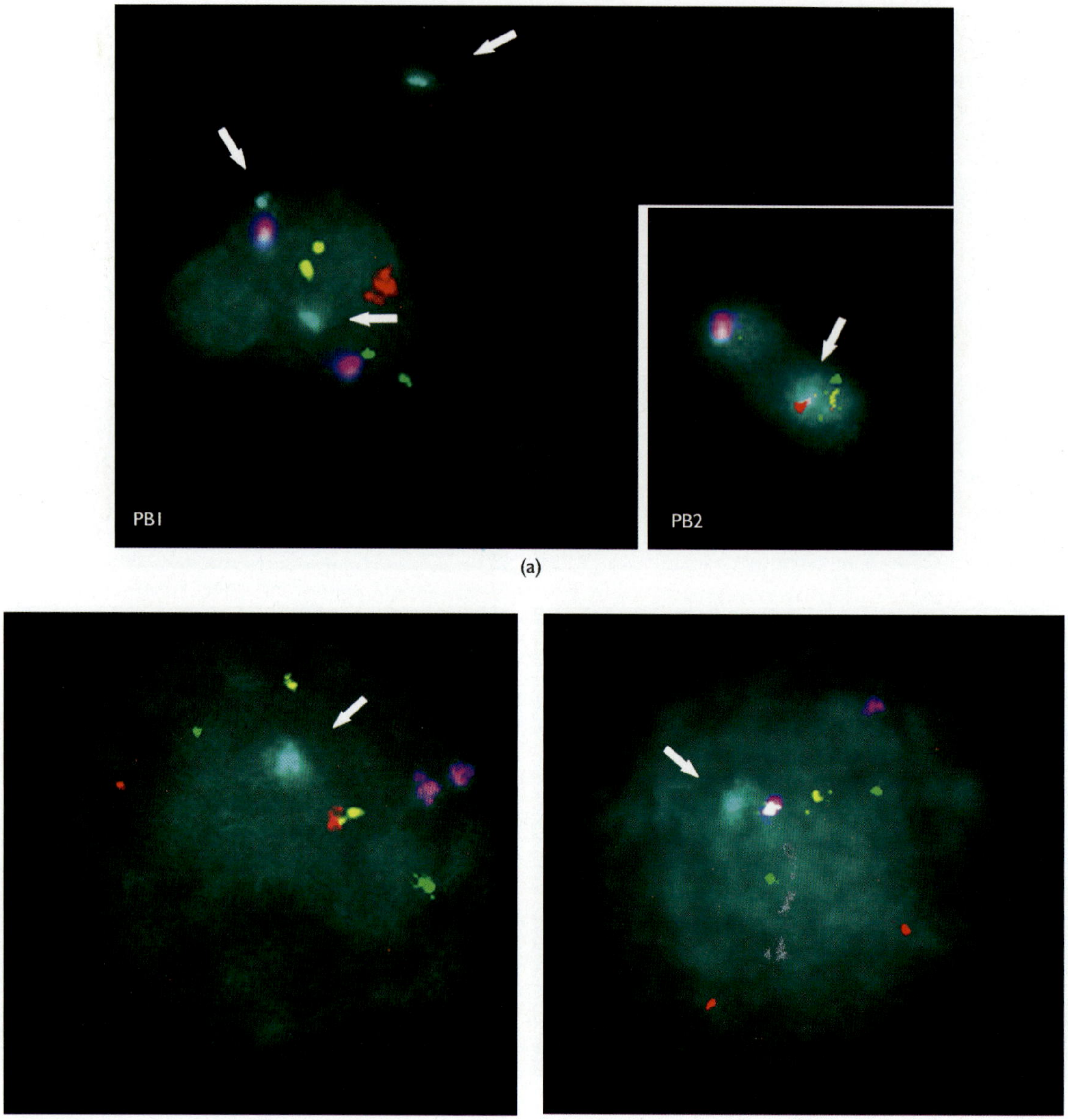

(a)

(b) (c)

Figure 4.25 Monosomy 16 originating from meiosis I error detected by polar body analysis. (a) Fluorescence *in situ* hybridization (FISH) image of first polar body (PB1) and second polar body (PB2) chromatin after hybridization for autosomes 13 (red), 16 (aqua), 18 (violet blue), 21 (green), and 22 (gold), showing an extra chromosome 16 signal (three instead of two, indicated by white arrows). A normal pattern of signals is present in PB2, including a very diffuse signal for chromosome 16 (white arrow) overlapping with the LSI 13 signal (red), indicating a corresponding nullisomic 16 oocyte, which will develop into a monosomy 16 embryo; (b) and (c) FISH images of interphase nuclei from the embryo derived from this oocyte, confirming predicted monosomy 16, evident from only a single signal for chromosome 16 (white arrows) in both cells.

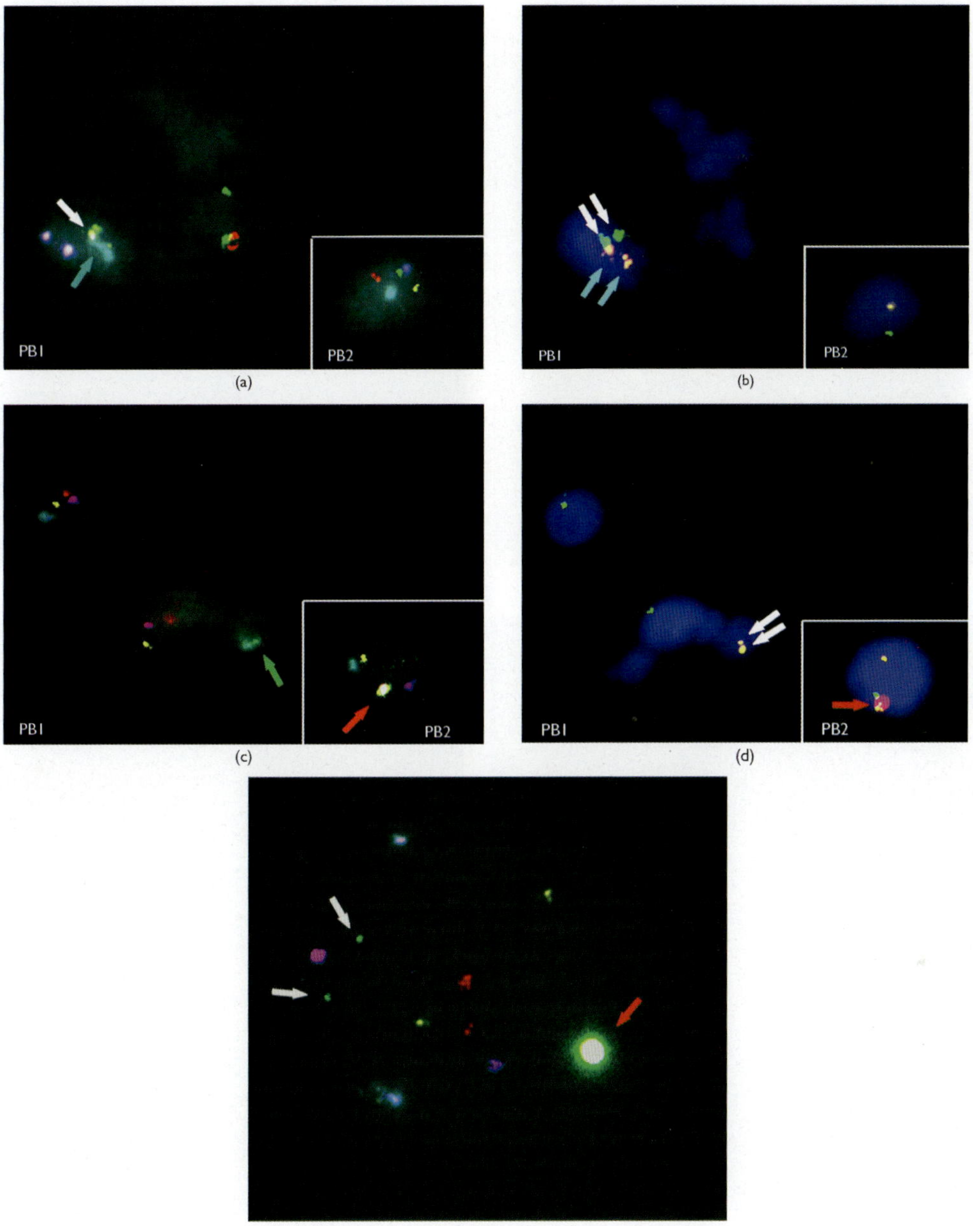

Figure 4.26 First polar body (PB1) and second polar body (PB2) fluorescence *in situ* hybridization (FISH) analysis of highly condensed chromatin, requiring re-hybridization. (a) FISH image of PB1 and PB2 after hybridization with a five-color chromosome cocktail for chromosomes 13 (red), 16 (aqua), 18 (violet blue), 21 (green), and 22 (gold) removed from an oocyte obtained from a 36-year-old woman. A normal number of signals are present in PB1 for chromosomes 13, 18, and 21, but close proximity and overlapping of signals for chromosome 22 (white arrow) and chromosome 16 (strip-like signal indicated by aqua arrow) render an inconclusive result. PB2 contains a normal number of signals. Interpretation of results in this PB1 cannot be undertaken without a second round of hybridization targeting the terminal region of each chromosome. (b) FISH image following re-hybridization of PB1 and PB2 chromatin with a sub-telomeric 16q probe in orange (aqua arrows) and a sub-telomeric 22q in green (white arrows), showing two signals for each of these chromosomes tested in PB1 along with one signal for each chromosome in PB2 (representing a control in this system), suggesting the resulting zygote is normal and can be transferred. (c) FISH image of highly condensed PB1 and PB2 chromatin from the same patient as (a) and (b). Two separate signals are seen for each of the chromatids present in PB1 with the exception of chromosome 21, which appears as a single signal (green arrow); however, it is located near or overlapping with the aqua signal for chromosome 16. Additionally, signal overlap and artifact interference (red arrow) are seen in the PB2 nucleus, about which no conclusion can be made regarding chromosomes 13 and 21. (d) Re-hybridization performed for chromosomes 13 and 21 using sub-telomeric 13q (green) and 21q (orange), showing two signals for chromosome 13 (representing an internal control) and chromosome 21 (located in close proximity to one another) in PB1; one signal each for chromosome 13 and chromosome 21 are now evident in PB2 following the second round of hybridization, along with the same artifactual interference seen with the first hybridization. (e) FISH image of an interphase nucleus from the resulting embryo, confirming a normal number of signals for each of the chromosomes tested, including chromosome 21 (white arrows). Also present is a large, bright artifact (red arrow) causing a dimming effect for the chromosome signals owing to its intensity when attempting to capture the image.

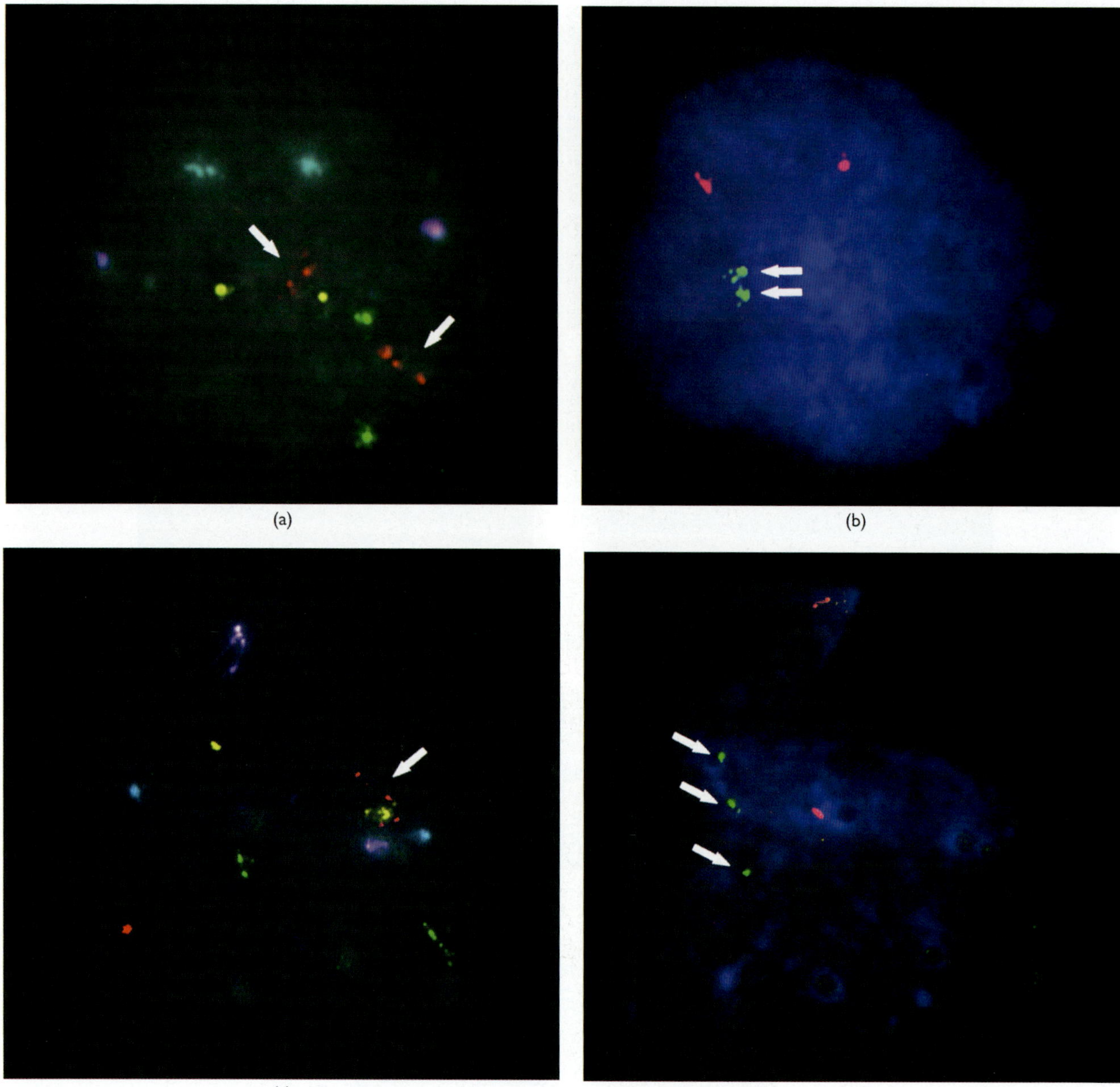

(a) (b) (c) (d)

Figure 4.27 Split fluorescence *in situ* hybridization (FISH) signals requiring an additional round of hybridization. (a) FISH image of an interphase nucleus after hybridization with MultiVysion PB panel probe, showing two signals for each of the chromosomes tested with the exception of chromosome 13 (white arrows), in which both signals are split, consisting of two and three dots. (b) FISH image after a second round of hybridization, using a probe cocktail targeting the sub-telomeric region of chromosomes 13 (green) and 16 (orange, which appears red through a red single-bandpass filter), showing two signals for both of the chromosomes re-investigated, indicating that the embryo is normal for the five autosomes tested. (c) FISH image of an interphase nucleus after hybridization with MultiVysion PB panel probe, showing split signals for chromosomes 13, 18, and 21, caused by overspreading during fixation. Because of the decondensed state of the chromatin and the fact that signal dots are less than one domain apart, split signals are counted as one. However, in this particular nucleus a single signal for chromosome 13 (red) is seen in the lower left area, while the second, located on the right, appears pulverized (white arrow), making it difficult to draw any conclusion regarding chromosome 13 without further testing. (d) FISH image after a second round of hybridization, using a probe cocktail targeting the sub-telomeric region of chromosomes 13 (green) and 18 (orange), showing two signals present for chromosome 18 (internal control), but three signals for chromosome 13 (white arrows), all of which are more than two domains apart, indicating a trisomy 13 in the embryo.

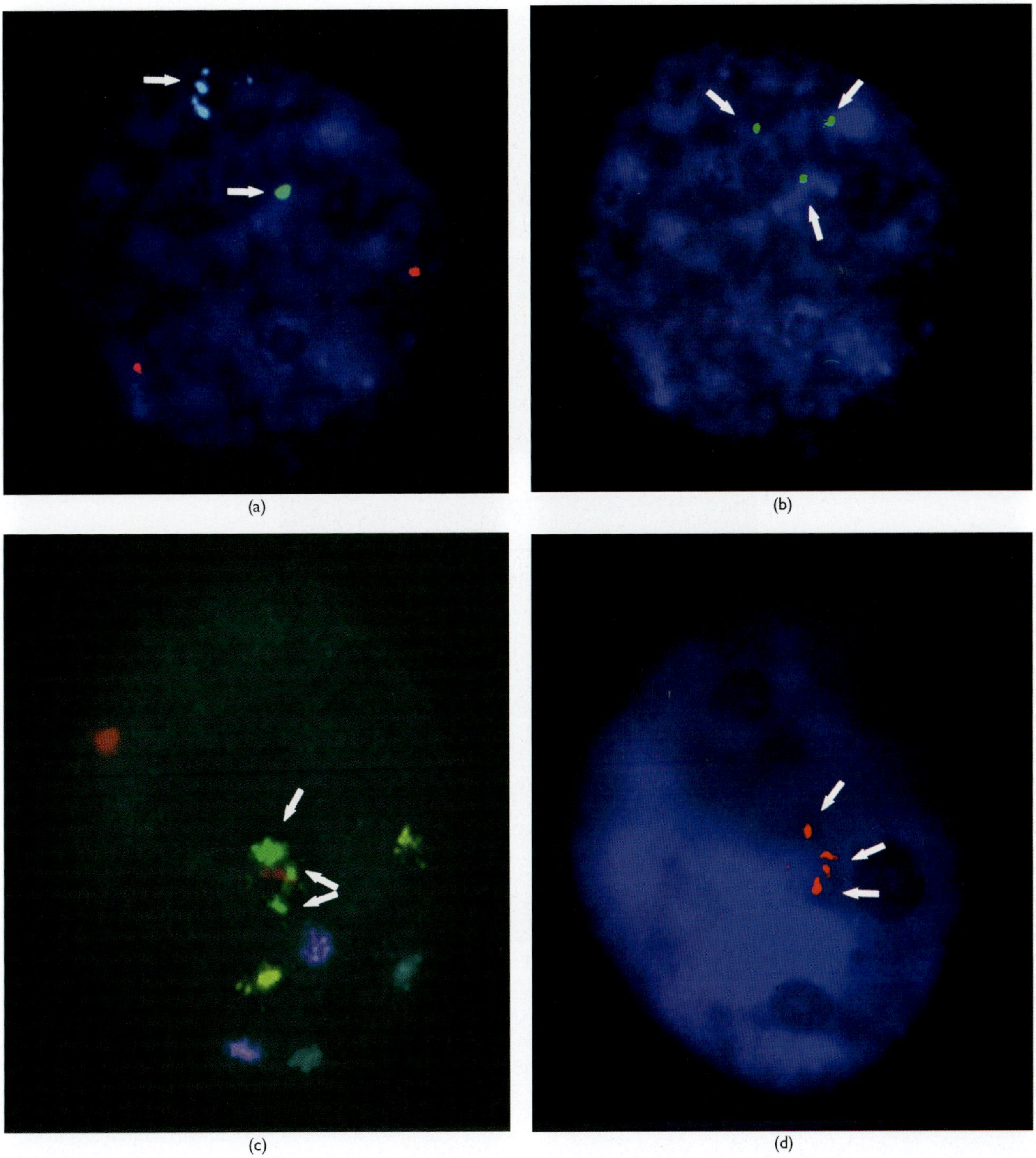

Figure 4.28 Value of re-hybridization in split signals. (a) Fluorescence *in situ* hybridization (FISH) image of an interphase nucleus after a second round of hybridization for chromosomes X (CEP X; green), Y (CEP Y; aqua), and 16 (sub-telomeric 16q; orange), revealing a single signal for chromosome X (yellow arrow), two signals for chromosome 16, and a double dot signal for chromosome Y (white arrow), requiring further testing of chromosome Y to avoid a misdiagnosis. (b) FISH image after a third round of hybridization with a sub-telomeric Xp/Yp in green, which hybridizes to common sequences of the sub-telomeric region of the p-arm for both chromosomes X and Y, showing three signals (white arrows), which indicates an embryo abnormal for the sex chromosomes by the presence of an extra Y chromosome. (c) FISH image of an interphase nucleus after hybridization with MultiVysion PB panel probe, showing two signals for each of the chromosomes tested with the exception of chromosome 21 (white arrows), for which one signal is large, and the other is split, consisting of two separate smaller dots, preventing a conclusion from being made regarding chromosome 21. (d) FISH image following re-hybridization of the same nucleus (c) for chromosome 21 with a sub-telomeric 21q in orange, showing at least three small signals, indicating a possible trisomy 21, despite the close proximity of signals.

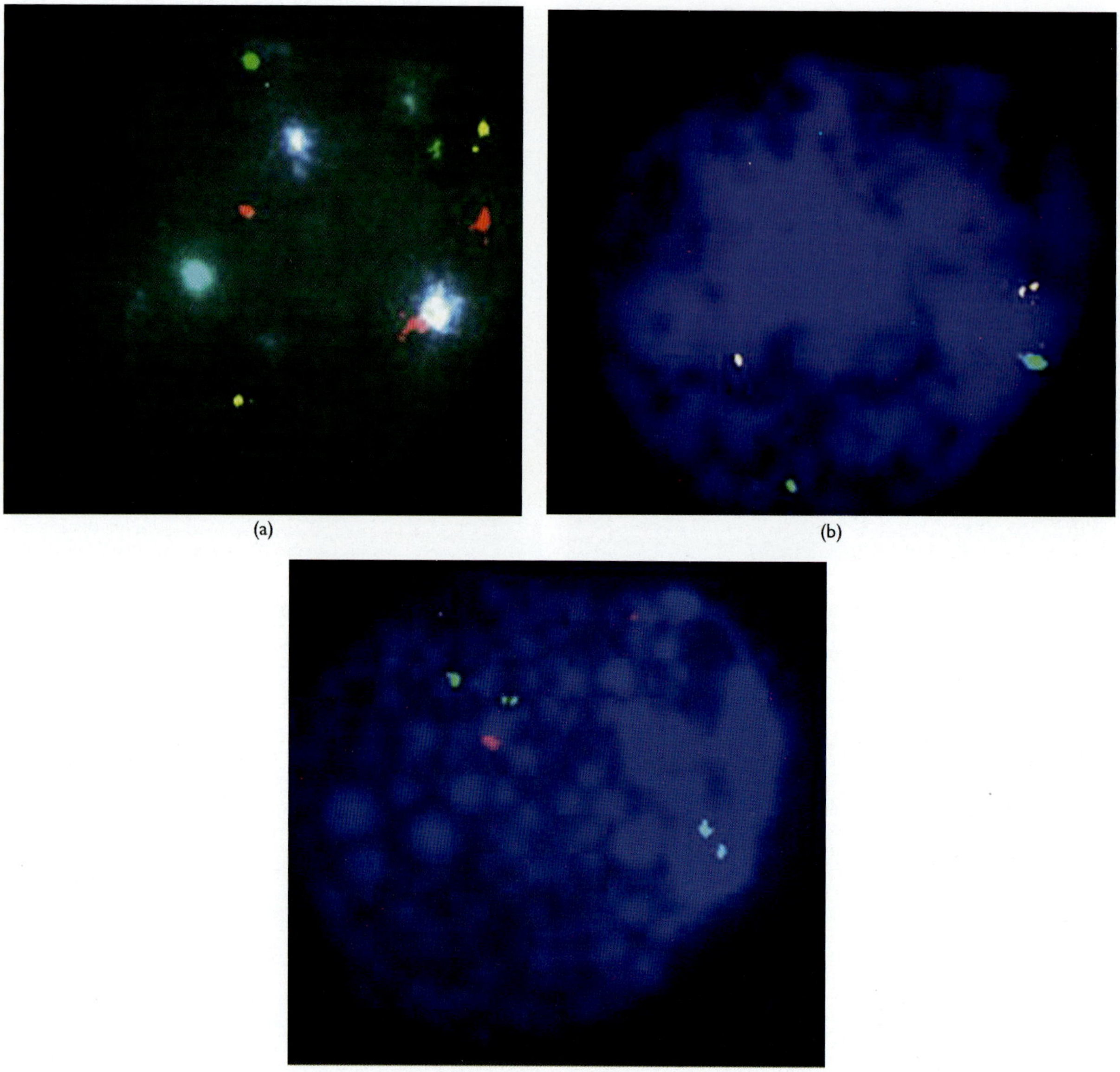

(a) (b) (c)

Figure 4.29 Re-hybridization with different probes in uncertain results on fluorescence *in situ* hybridization (FISH) signals requiring an additional round of hybridization. (a) FISH image of an interphase nucleus after hybridization with MultiVysion PB panel probe, showing two signals for each of the chromosomes tested, with the exception of chromosomes 13 (red) and 16 (aqua). Chromosome 13 looks to have an extra signal, which appears as an artifact under the visual microscopic examination. Results for chromosome 16 are not clear. (b) FISH image after a second round of hybridization, using a probe cocktail targeting the sub-telomeric region of chromosomes 13 (green) and 16 (gold), showing two signals for both of the chromosomes re-investigated, indicating that the embryo is normal for the five autosomes tested. (c) FISH image of re-hybridization of the same interphase nucleus tested with a custom-made mixture of probes that includes chromosomes X (green), 8 (aqua), and 15 (red). A normal number of signals are present for the autosomes and sex chromosomes, indicating a normal female embryo.

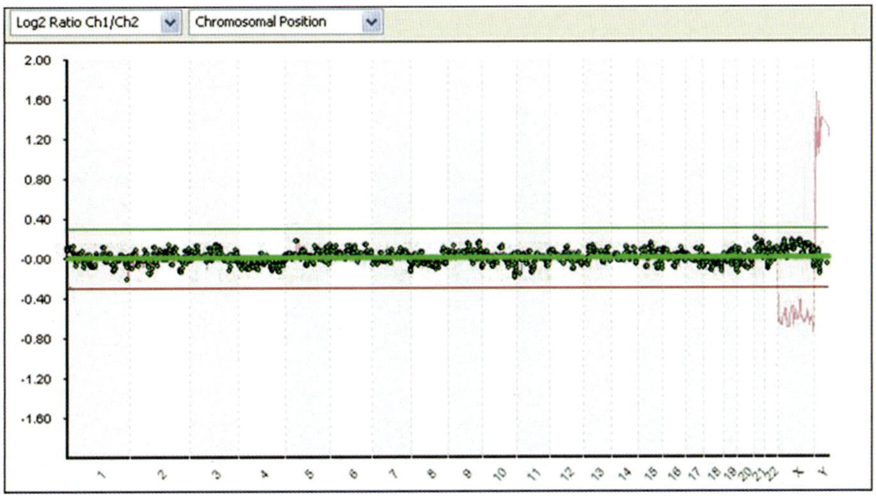

Figure 4.30 Normal results of array-CGH analysis for 24-chromosome aneuploidy testing in blastocyst biopsy sample.

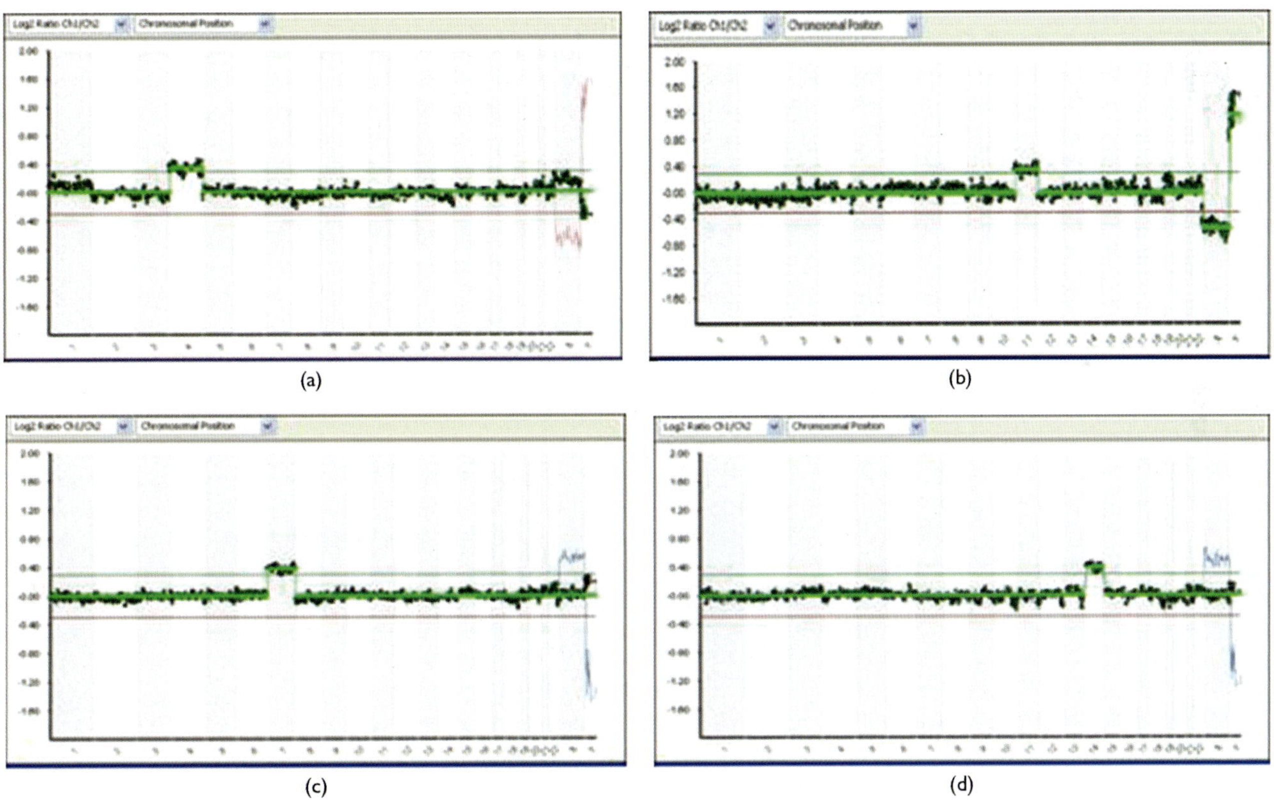

Figure 4.31 Aneuploidies detected by array-CGH testing for 24 chromosomes using an aCGH testing platform on trophectoderm biopsy on day 5. Trisomies 4, 7, 11, and 14 presented, which would not have been diagnosed using standard FISH testing, and thus would have led to transfers of abnormal embryos. Upper left chart represents 47, XY,+4 karyotype. Upper right shows chart shows karyotype 46, Y,–X,+11. Bottom left chart represents 47, XX,+7. Bottom right chart represents 47, XX,+14.

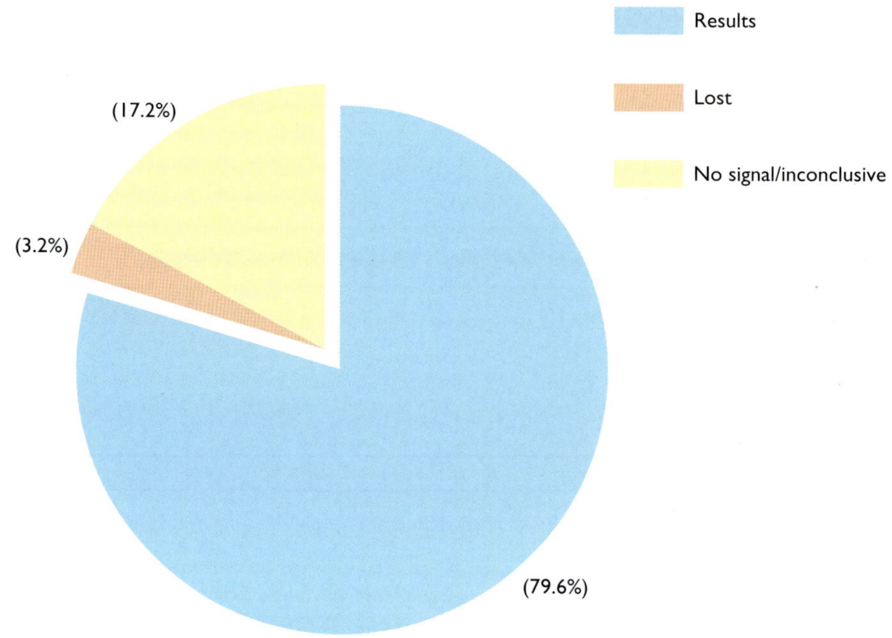

Figure 4.32 Pie chart of polar body fluorescence *in situ* hybridization (FISH) analysis efficiency in prediction of oocyte chromosomal constitution. Results were obtained in approximately 80% of oocytes tested. No or inconclusive results were the result of either the loss of polar bodies during micromanipulation procedures (3.2%), or failure of adequate hybridization (17.2%).

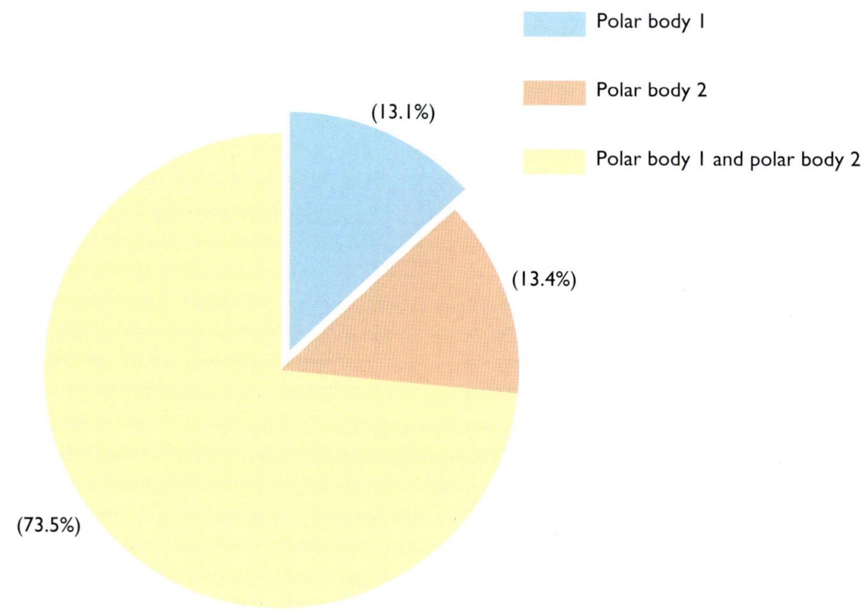

Figure 4.33 Pie chart demonstrating the proportion of oocytes in which results were obtained by one or both polar bodies. Results were obtained by first polar body (PBI) only in 13.1%, second polar body (PB2) only in 13.4%, and by both PBI and PB2 in 73.5%. While the detection of abnormalities by only one polar body (PBI or PB2) may avoid transfer of the corresponding embryo, no decision can be made if information is available for only one polar body with a normal pattern, since errors may occur during meiosis I and/or meiosis II. Embryos may be transferred only if both PBI and PB2 are found to have normal fluorescence *in situ* hybridization (FISH) patterns.

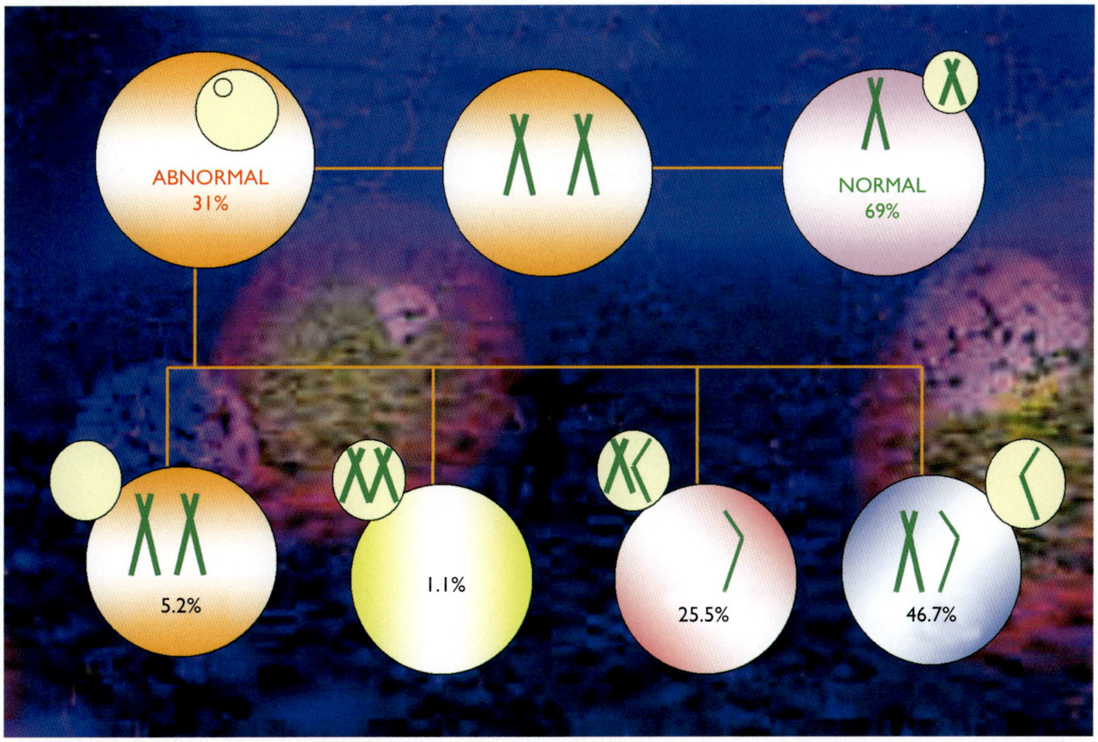

Figure 4.34 Schematic representation of segregation patterns and relative proportions of each type of error occurring in meiosis I. Upper panel shows an overall proportion of the resulting normal and abnormal metaphase II oocytes. Lower panel shows the types and proportion of each error, providing evidence of non-random distribution, with the majority representing missing chromatids in the first polar body (PB1). In addition 21.5% of PB1 were with complex errors (not shown).

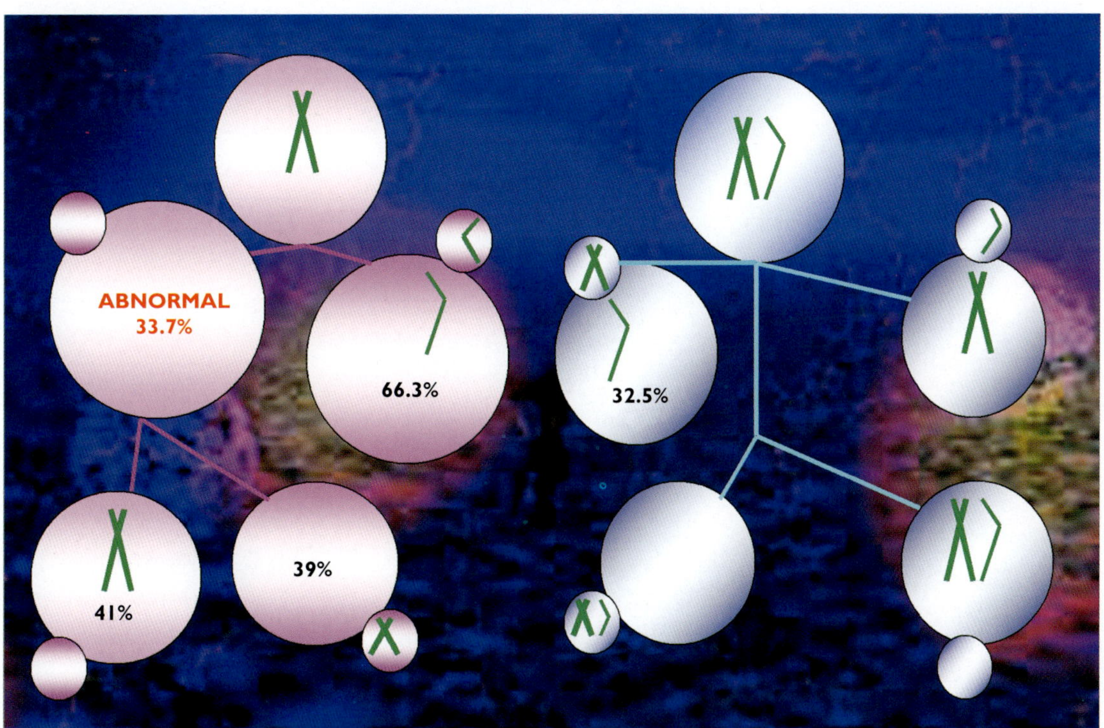

Figure 4.35 Schematic representation of segregation patterns and relative proportions of each type of error occurring in meiosis II. Left panel shows the types and proportions of errors resulting from normal metaphase II oocytes (20% of PB2 were with complex errors; not shown). Right panel shows the expected outcome of second meiotic division from a metaphase II oocyte with an extra chromatid resulting from meiosis I error. Of the resulting normal oocytes, 32.5% have a single chromatid, including all the types of sequential errors that result in a balanced oocyte.

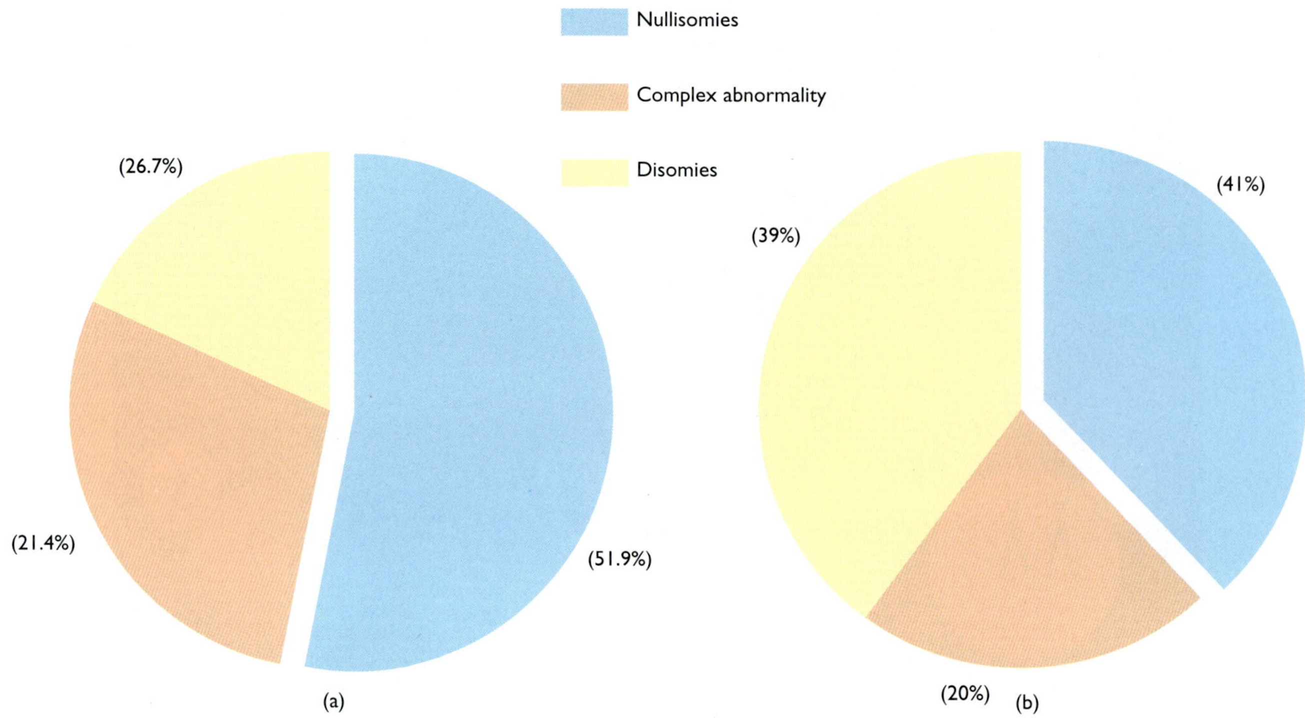

Figure 4.36 Pie charts demonstrating the distribution of the types of chromosomal abnormalities observed in first polar body (PB1) (a) and second polar body (PB2) (b). Nullisomies (missing chromosomes or chromatids) in PB1 (a) were more prevalent compared to other types of abnormalities, while there was no such difference in PB2 (b). Complex errors are comparable in both PB1 and PB2.

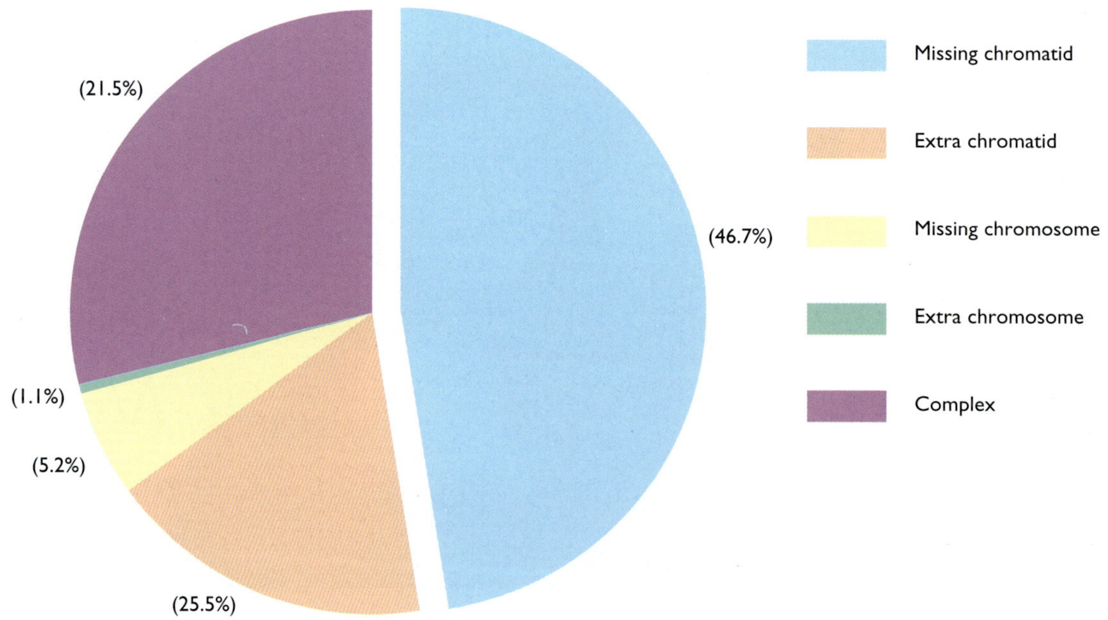

Figure 4.37 Pie chart demonstrating the distribution of types of errors in first polar body (PB1). Missing chromatids (47.4%) were far the most prevalent, followed by complex abnormalities (28.8%) involving more than one chromosome, compared to other types of errors. Chromosomal non-disjunction (yellow and green) was almost ten-fold less frequent than chromatid malsegregation (blue and orange).

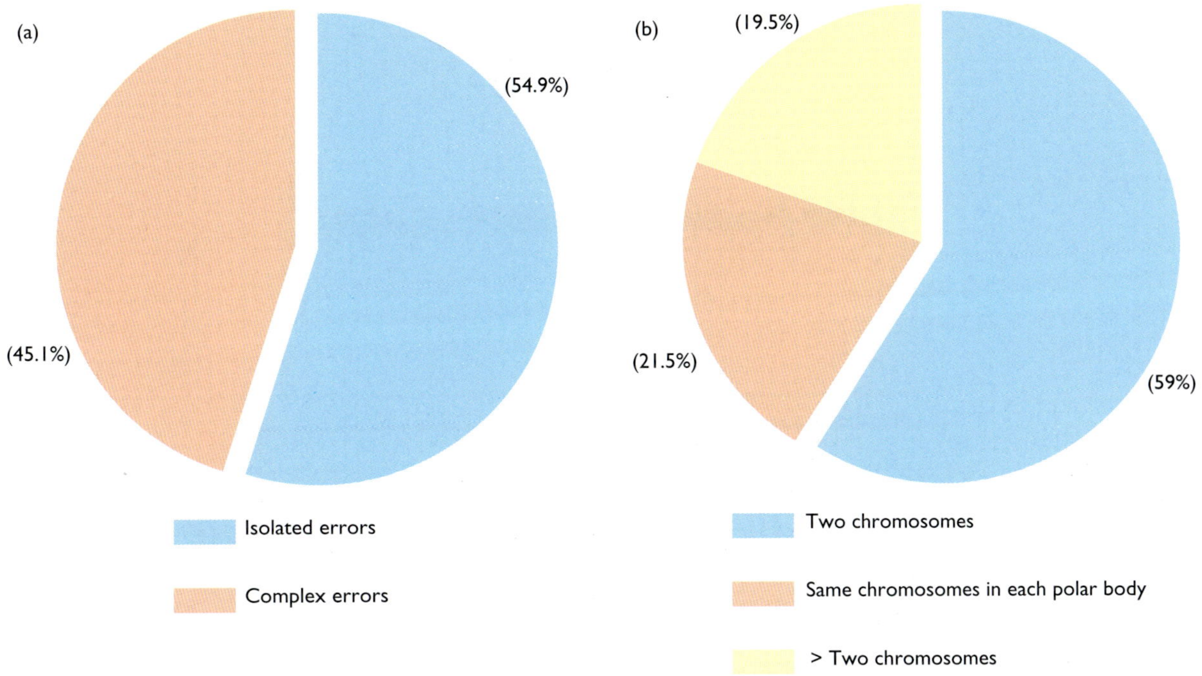

Figure 4.38 Pie charts showing proportions and types of complex aneuploidies. (a) Overall prevalence of complex errors involving either errors of the same chromosome in both meiotic divisions or involvement of two or more chromosomes; (b) relative distribution of various types of complex errors.

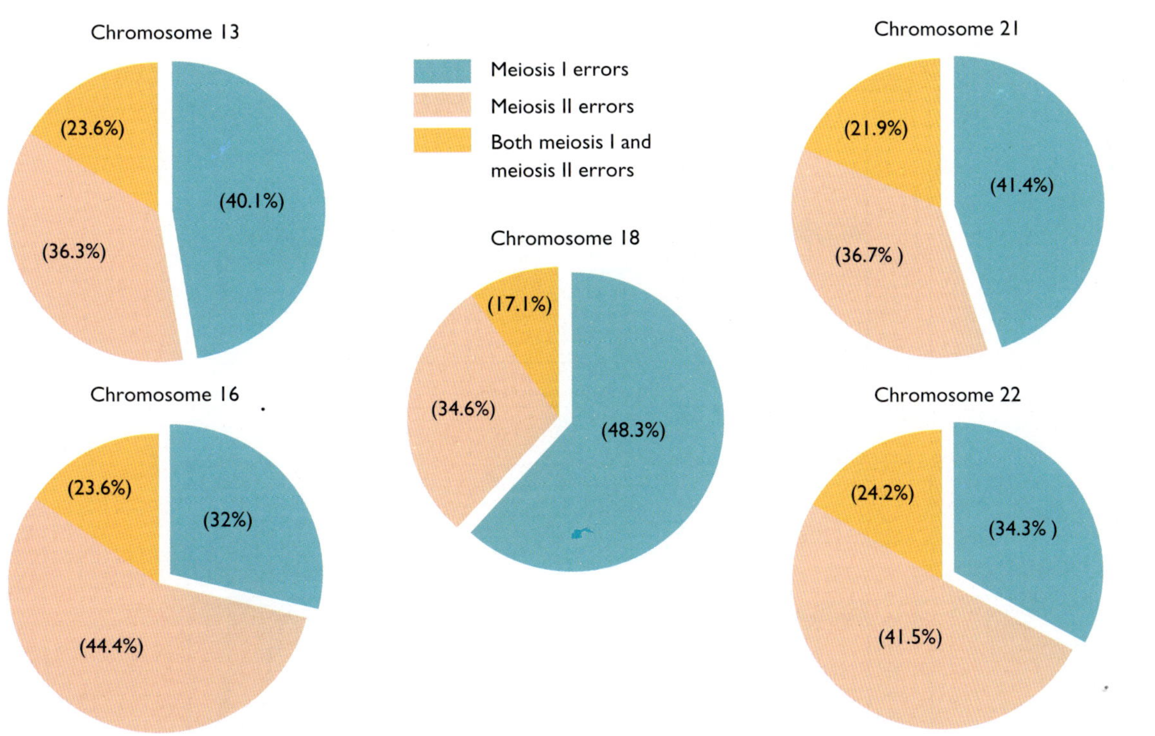

Figure 4.39 Pie charts of meiotic origin of chromosome 13, 16, 18, 21, and 22 aneuploidies detected by first polar body (PB1) and second polar body (PB2) and fluorescence *in situ* hybridization (FISH) analysis. Meiosis I errors shown in aqua, meiosis II in pink, and both meiotic divisions in orange. Chromosome 16 and 22 errors originate predominantly from meiosis II (bottom left and bottom right), chromosome 18 errors originate predominantly from meiosis I, and chromosome 13 and 21 errors comparably in meiosis I and meiosis II.

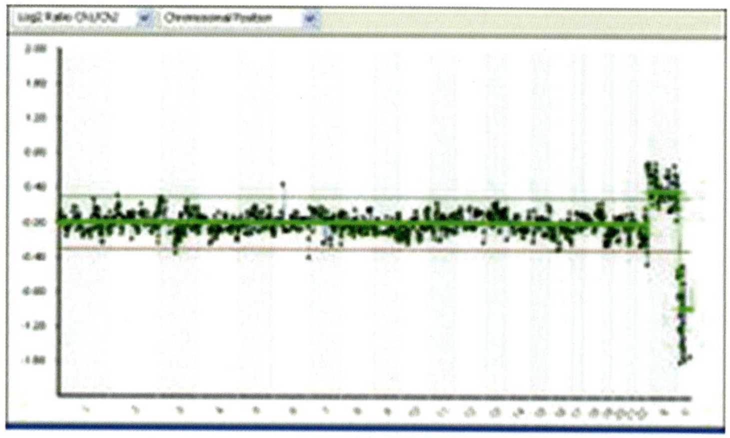

(a)

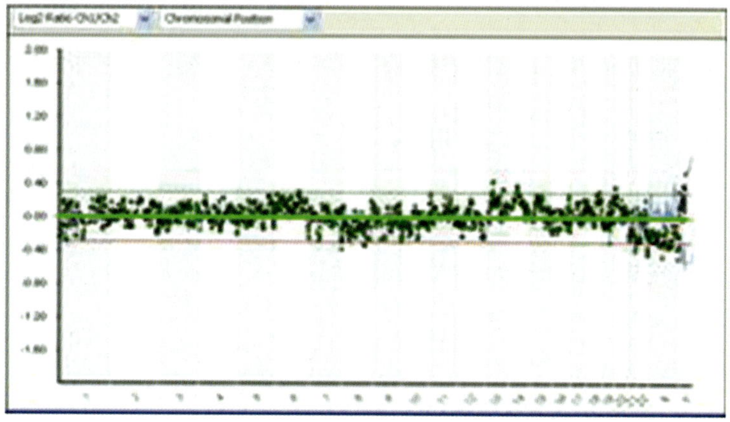

(b)

Figure 4.40 Normal pattern of 24-chromosome aneuploidy testing of PB1 (top) and PB2 (bottom) by array-CGH analysis.

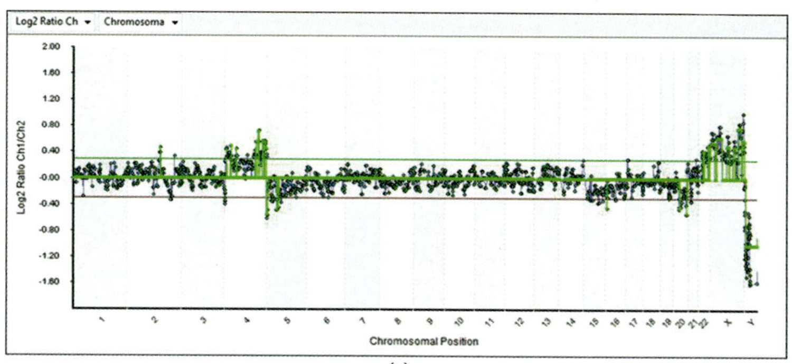

(a)

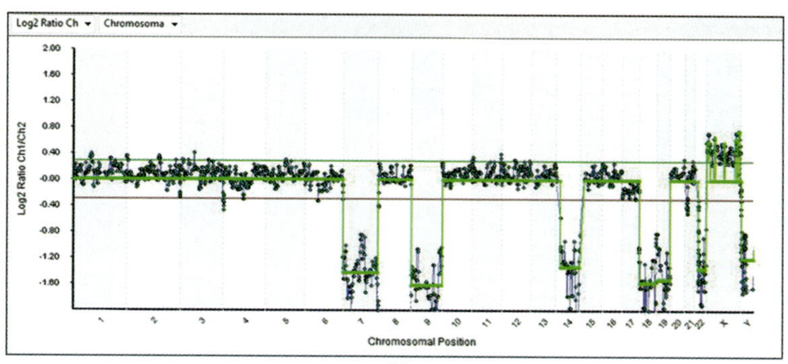

(b)

Figure 4.41 Aneuploidies detected by array-CGH in PB1 and PB2. (a) Aneuploidies detected by array-CGH in PB1: extra chromatid 4 and missing chromatids 5 and 21. (b) Aneuploidies detected by array-CGH in PB2: missing chromatids 7, 9, 14, 18, 19, and 22.

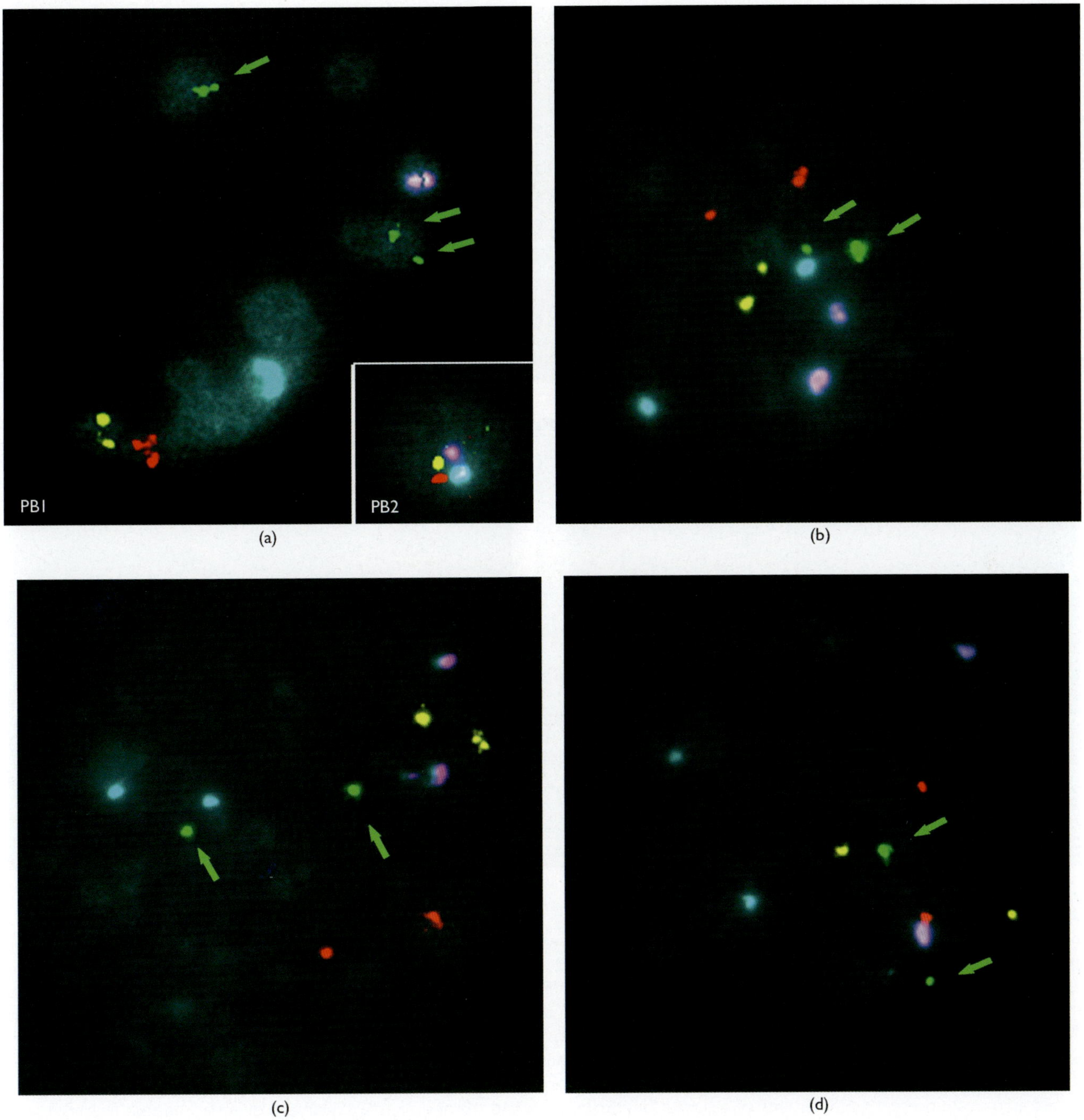

Figure 4.42 Sequential chromosome 21 errors in meiosis I and II resulting in a chromosomally normal embryo. (a) Fluorescence *in situ* hybridization (FISH) image of first polar body (PB1) and second polar body (PB2) after hybridization with the MultiVysion PB panel probe, showing a normal number of signals (two per chromosome) in PB1 with the exception of three signals for chromosome 21 (green arrows), indicating chromatid error in meiosis I. The same four of five chromosomes show a normal number of signals present in PB2, again with the exception of the chromosome 21 signal, which was missing, indicating a possible normal chromosome complement, including chromosome 21. (b) – (d) Follow-up FISH analysis of the resulting embryo, confirming a normal pattern of chromosomes in all three nuclei, including chromosome 21 (green arrows), obtained after whole embryo fixation.

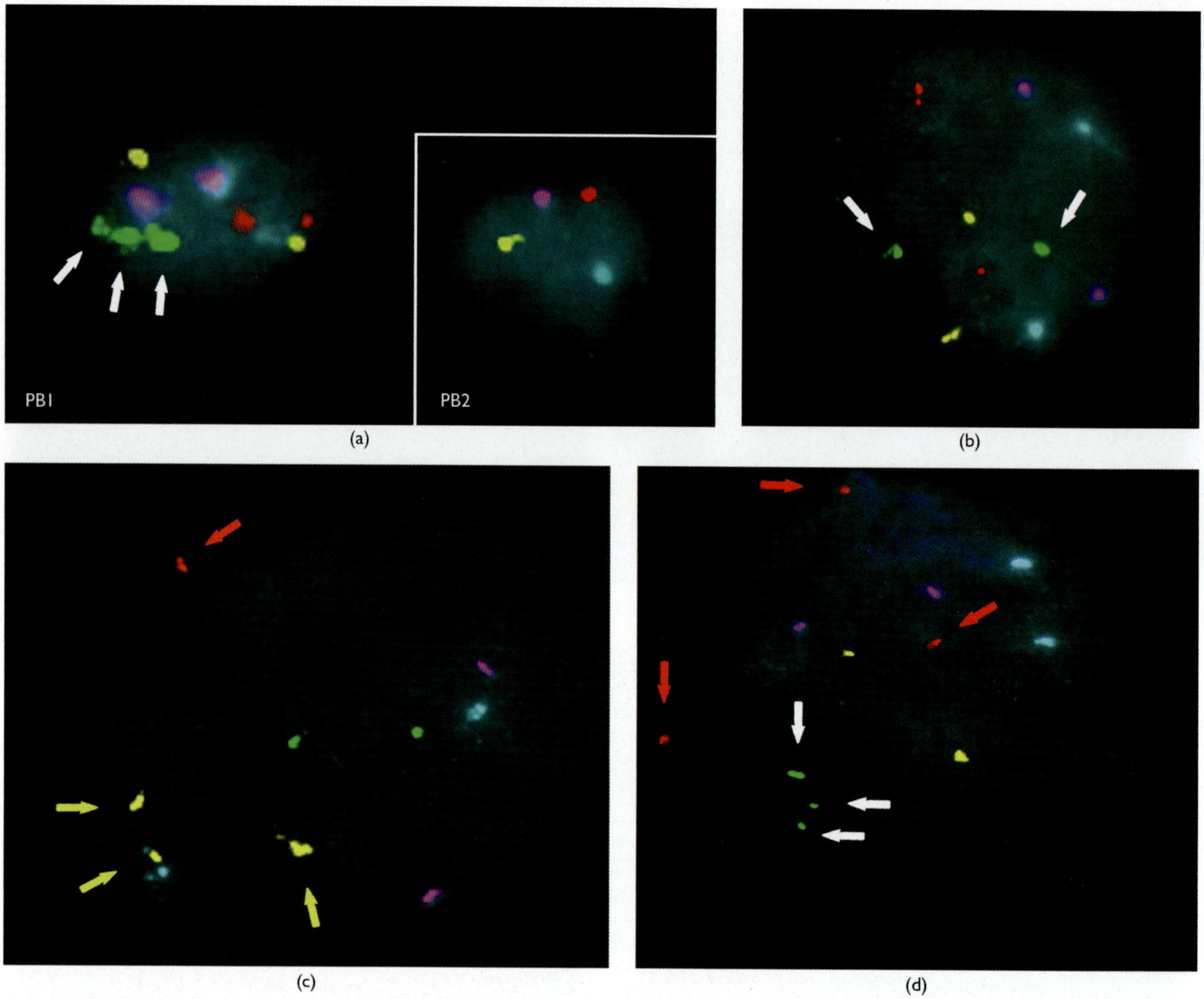

Figure 4.43 Sequential chromosome 21 errors in meiosis I and II resulting in an abnormal mosaic embryo. First polar body (PB1) and second polar body (PB2) were removed simultaneously following fertilization of an oocyte retrieved from a 39-year-old woman. (a) Fluorescence *in situ* hybridization (FISH) image of PB1 and PB2 after hybridization with the MultiVysion PB panel probe, showing a normal number of signals for each chromosome (double dots) in PB1 with the exception of three signals for chromosome 21 (white arrows). Four instead of five signals are detected in PB2 (shown in the right lower corner), with a missing green signal for chromosome 21, suggesting the normal number for all five chromosomes in the resulting oocyte. (b) FISH image of an interphase nucleus from the resulting embryo with normal number of signals, including chromosome 21 (white arrows). (c) FISH image of a second interphase nucleus from the same embryo as (a) and (b), in which three signals for chromosome 22 (yellow arrows) and only one signal for chromosome 13 (red arrow) are present, together with two signals for chromosomes 16, 18, and 21. (d) FISH image of a third nucleus from the same embryo as (a), (b), and (c), in which three signals for chromosome 13 (red arrows) and chromosome 21 (white arrows) are present with a normal number of signals for chromosomes 16, 18, and 22. The observed mosaicism may be associated with the sequential errors of chromosome 21 in meiosis I and meiosis II.

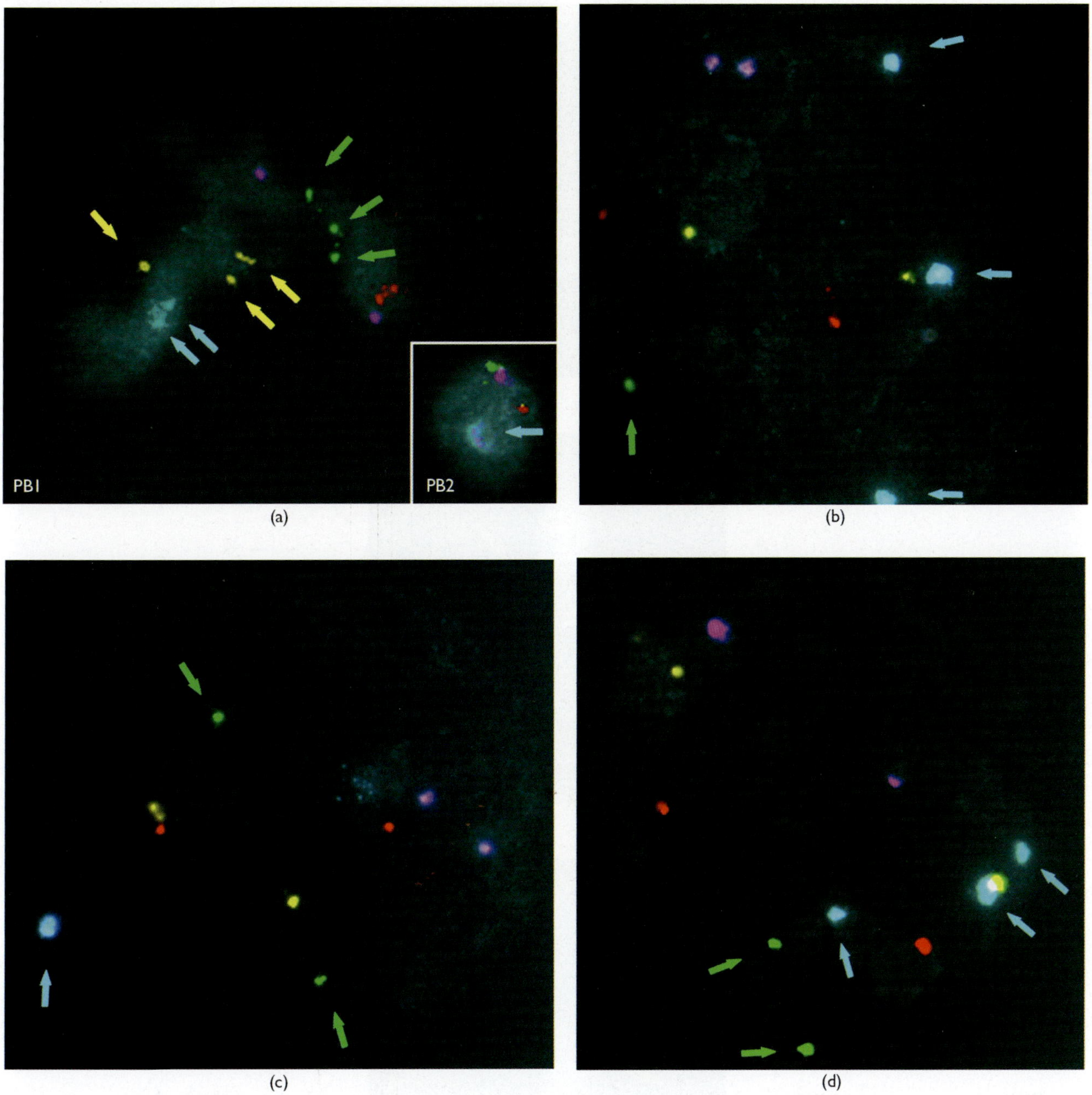

Figure 4.44 Complex errors involving more than one chromosome resulting in mosaicism. First polar body (PB1) and second polar body (PB2) were removed simultaneously following fertilization of an oocyte retrieved from a 36-year-old woman. (a) Fluorescence *in situ* hybridization (FISH) image of PB1 and PB2 after hybridization with the MultiVysion PB panel probe, revealing an abnormal number of signals (three) in PB1 for chromosome 21 (green arrows) and chromosome 22 (yellow arrows), with a normal pattern of signals (two) for each of the remaining chromosomes tested, 13, 16, and 18. A normal number of signals are present for four of the five chromosomes tested in PB2 (lower right corner), with evident absence of a gold signal for chromosome 22. (b) FISH image of an interphase nucleus from the resulting embryo, showing only one signal present for chromosome 21 (green arrow) as predicted by the number of chromatids extruded during meiosis. There are a normal number of signals for chromosome 22 also expected, together with an unexpected three signals for chromosome 16 (aqua arrows). (c) FISH image of a second interphase nucleus from the same embryo as shown in (a) and (b). Two signals for each chromosome tested, including chromosome 21 (green arrows), are present, with the exception of chromosome 16 (aqua arrows), represented by only one signal. (d) FISH image of a third interphase nucleus from this embryo, in which two signals for each of the chromosomes tested are present, including chromosome 21, but three instead of the expected two signals are present for chromosome 16, indicating mosaicism in the embryo.

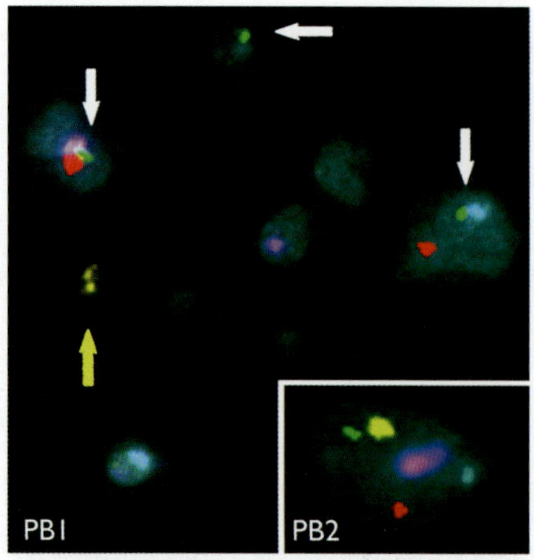

(a)

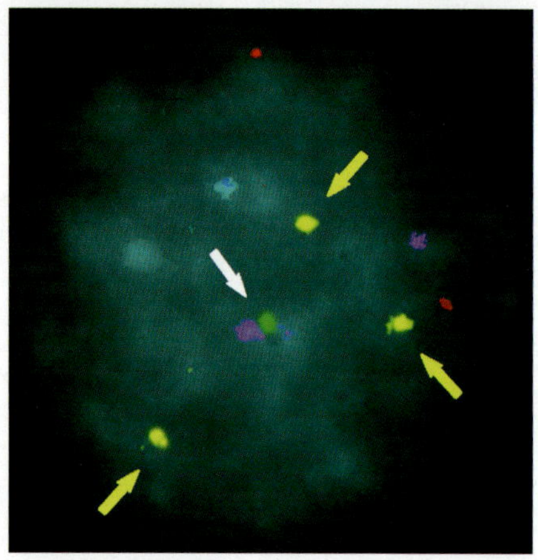

(b)

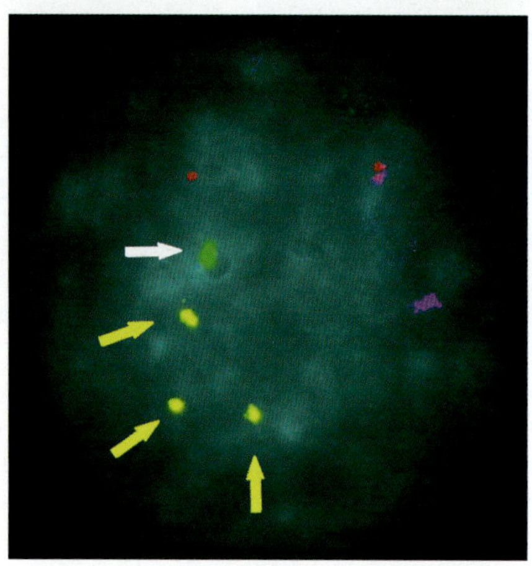

(c)

Figure 4.45 Complex errors in meiosis I resulting in monosomy 21 and trisomy 22. (a) Fluorescence *in situ* hybridization (FISH) image of first polar body (PB1) and second polar body (PB2) after hybridization with the MultiVysion PB panel probe, revealing a double error in PB1, represented by three (instead of two) chromosome 21 signals (white arrows) and only one split chromosome 22 signal (yellow arrow). A normal number of signals (one each) are present in PB2 (right lower corner). (b) and (c) FISH images of nuclei obtained from the resulting embryo, showing three chromosome 22 signals and one chromosome 21 signal, confirming the predicted double aneuploidy. (Note that chromosome 16 is not seen owing to strong aqua background from the nuclear staining as a result of fluorophore-labeled (aqua) human placental DNA incorporated into this probe cocktail.)

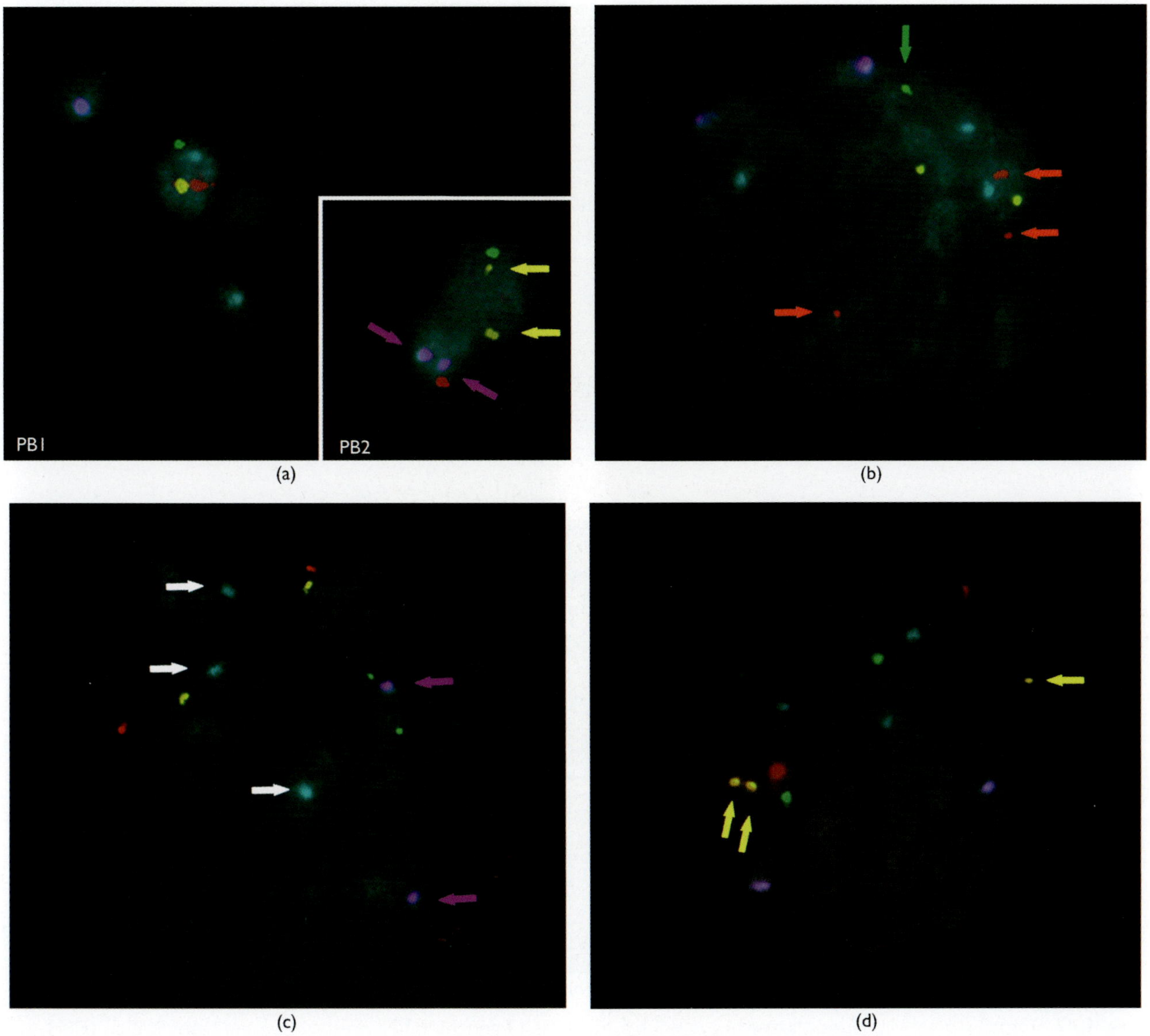

Figure 4.46 Complex errors in meiosis I and II resulting in a mosaic embryo. First polar body (PB1) and second polar body (PB2) were removed simultaneously following fertilization of an oocyte retrieved from a 35-year-old woman suffering from secondary infertility with a reproductive history that included four previous spontaneous abortions. (a) Fluorescence *in situ* hybridization (FISH) image of PB1 and PB2 following hybridization with the MultiVysion PB panel probe, showing only one signal (instead of two) for chromosomes 18, 21, and 22 in PB1. Additional errors are seen in PB2, evident from two signals present for chromosomes 18 (red arrows) and 22 (yellow arrows) and the absence of a signal for chromosome 16. (b) FISH image of an interphase nucleus from the resulting embryo, showing only one chromosome 21 signal (green arrow) and three signals for chromosome 13 (three red arrows) and 16 (not indicated by arrows). (c) FISH image of a second interphase nucleus from the same embryo, corresponding to (a) and (b), showing two signals for each of the chromosomes tested, including chromosome 18 (purple arrows), with the exception of chromosome 16 (white arrows), in which three signals are seen. (d) FISH image of a third interphase nucleus from the same embryo, in which two signals for each of the chromosomes tested are present, with the exception of three signals for chromosome 16 and 22 (gold arrows), revealing extensive mosaicism in the embryo, which may be caused by complex errors in meiosis I.

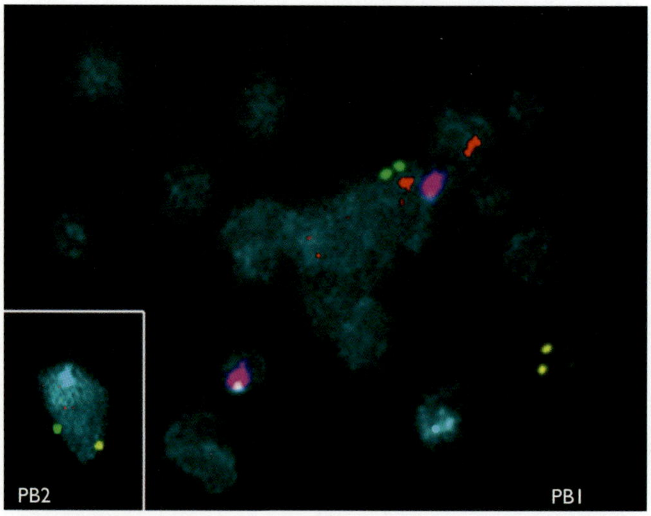

(a)

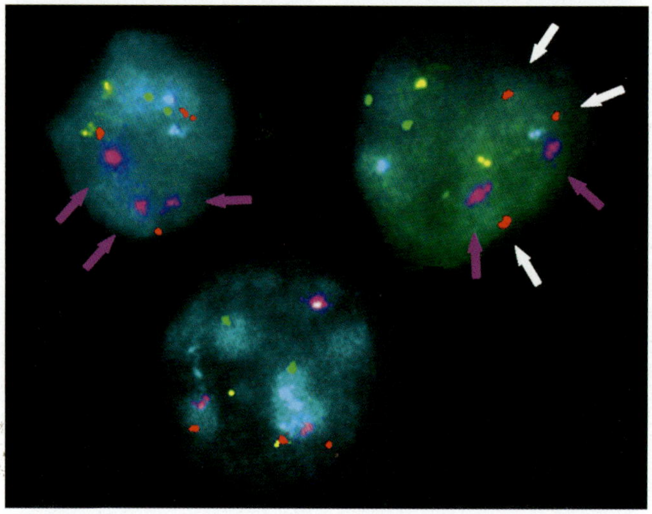

(b)

Figure 4.47 Complex errors in meiosis II resulting in double trisomies 13 and 18. (a) Fluorescence *in situ* hybridization (FISH) image of first polar body (PB1) and second polar body (PB2) following hybridization with the MultiVysion PB panel probe, showing a normal number of signals (two) for each of the chromosomes tested in PB1. However, double errors in meiosis II are evident from missing signals for chromosomes 13 and 18 in PB2. (b) Follow-up FISH analysis of the embryo by whole embryo fixation confirms the predicted double trisomy 13 and 18, evident from the presence of three signals for chromosome 13 (white arrows) and chromosome 18 (purple arrows) in two of the three cells shown (upper left and lower middle nuclei). However, three chromosome 13 signals with a normal number of signals (two) for the other chromosomes, including chromosome 18, are present, suggesting mosaicism for chromosome 18 (upper right).

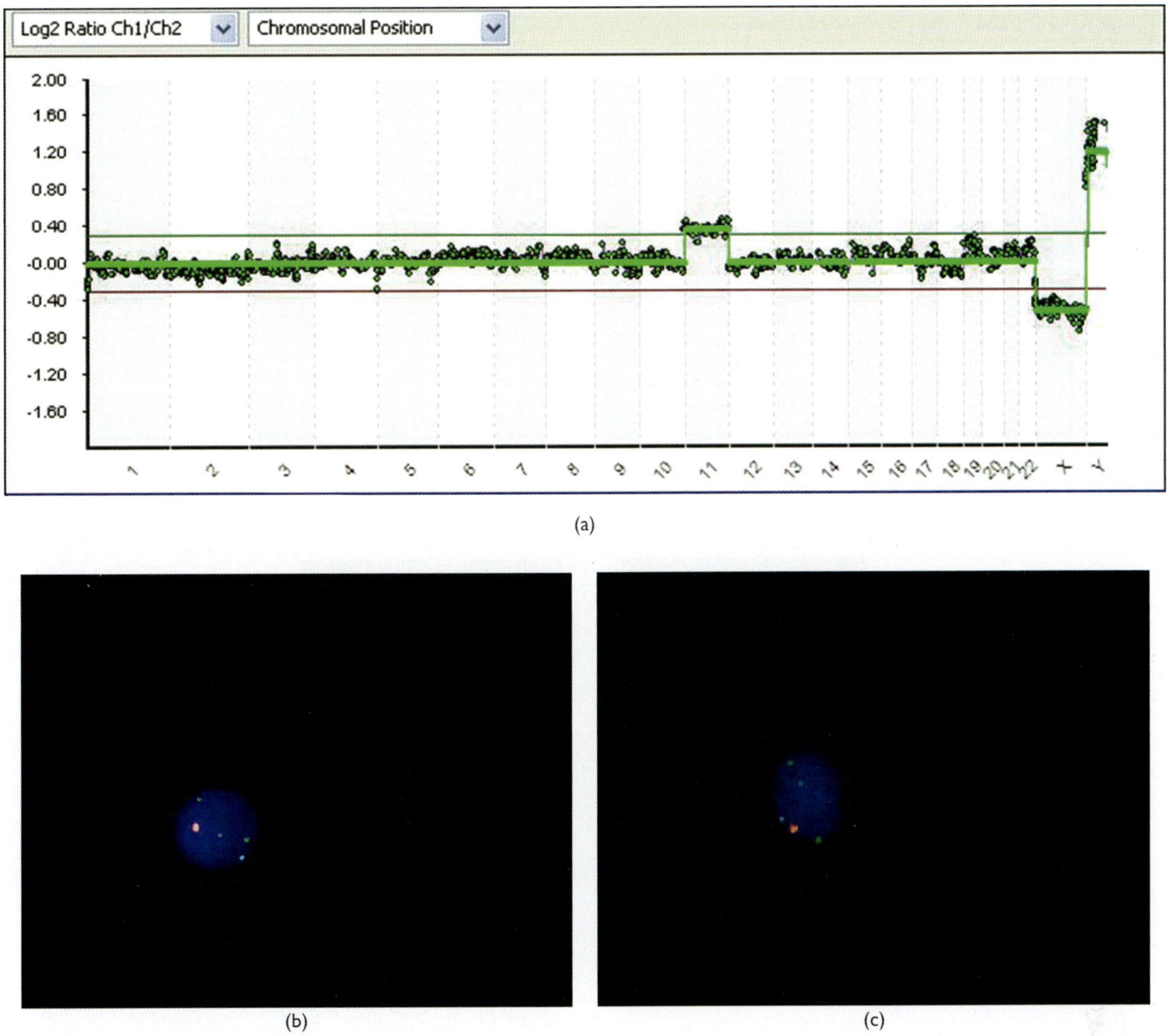

Figure 4.48 Confirmation of trisomy 11 detected by array-CGH and FISH analysis. (a) Trisomy 11 detected by array-CGH, and (b) and (c) confirmed by FISH analysis.

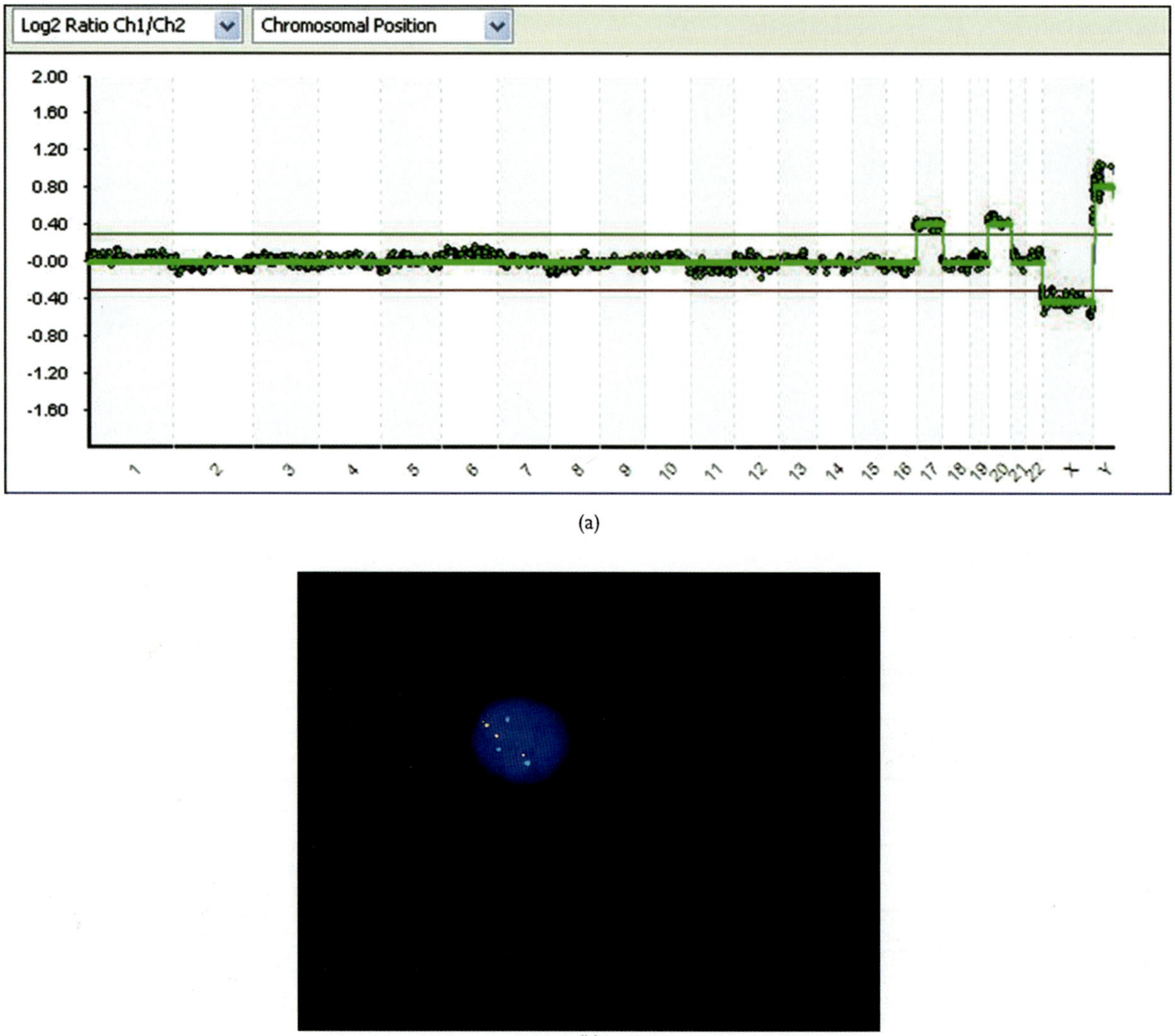

(a)

(b)

Figure 4.49 FISH confirmation of double trisomy 17 and 19 detected by array-CGH in blastocyst. (a) Double trisomy 17 and 19 detected by array-CGH in blastocyst. (b) Confirmation of the finding by FISH analysis, showing three signals for chromosomes 17 and 19.

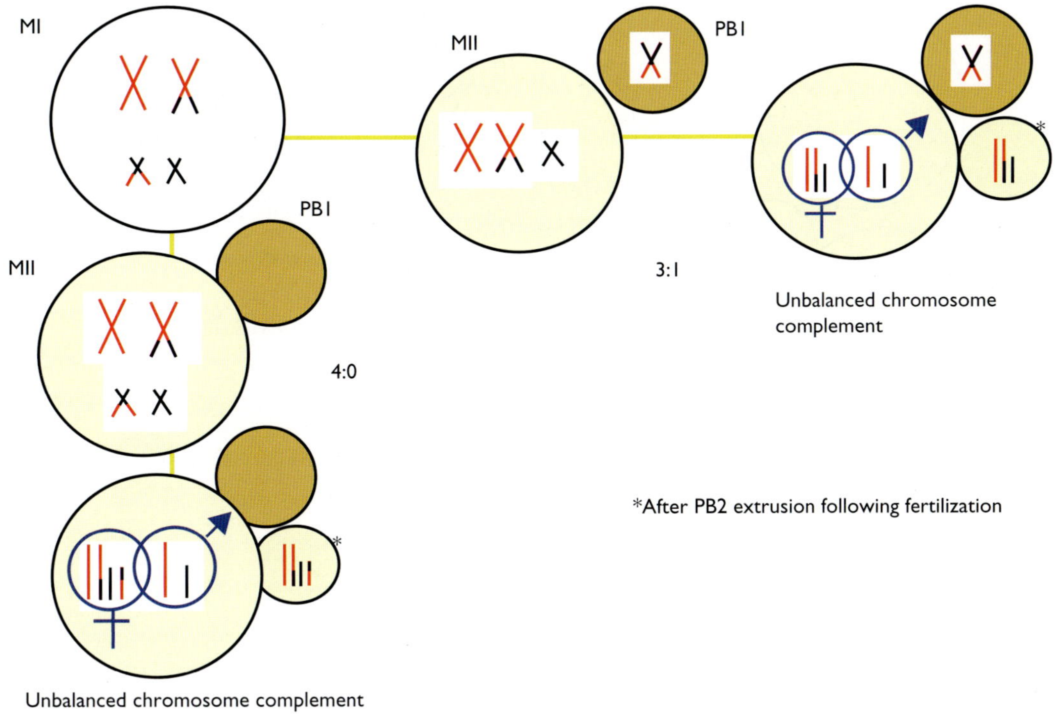

Figure 5.5 Schematic representation of 3:1 and 4:0 chromosome segregation during meiosis I and II for a maternal carrier of a reciprocal translocation. The vertical path depicts a 4:0 segregation pattern in which both normal and derivative chromosomes are extruded from or retained in the oocyte during meiosis I, resulting in a more lethal chromosome imbalance. After fertilization and barring anaphase II non-disjunction, the resulting unbalanced embryo would consist of a double trisomy or double monosomy. Along the horizontal path, 3:1 segregation is depicted in which only one normal or derivative chromosome is retained in the oocyte or extruded in the first polar body (PB1), resulting in an unbalanced oocyte. After fertilization, the chromosome complement of the embryo could consist of a tertiary trisomy/monosomy or an interchange trisomy/monosomy, as depicted in this example of interchange trisomy in which extra genetic material from both chromosomes is present. Neither outcome of these types of segregation patterns is suitable for transfer. Depending on the chromosomes involved, a 3:1 segregation pattern may result in a viable unbalanced conceptus.

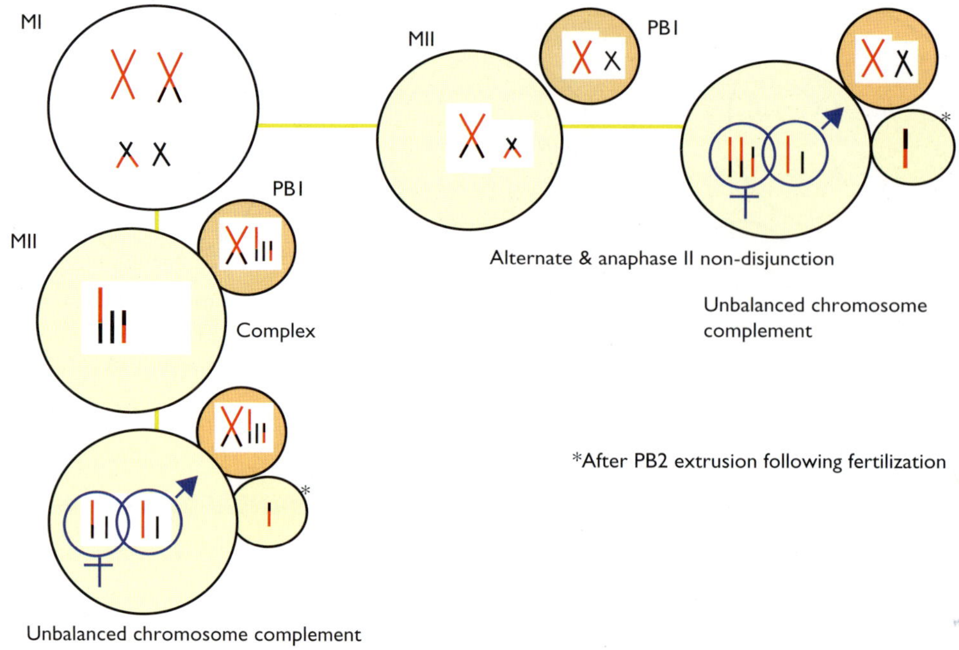

Figure 5.6 Schematic representation of complex chromosome segregation during meiosis I and II and an alternate chromosome segregation during meiosis I with anaphase II non-disjunction for a maternal carrier of a reciprocal translocation. Along the vertical path, complex segregation is depicted in which chromatid exchange and chromatid non-disjunction during meiosis I are identified, resulting in an unbalanced oocyte. As a result, a textbook segregation pattern cannot be identified. Second polar body (PB2) analysis is required to predict accurately the chromosome complement of the oocyte and resulting embryo, in which, if this example were studied by blastomere analysis alone, it may appear as if adjacent-1 segregation had occurred. More often this type of abnormal segregation leads to an unbalanced oocyte and would not be considered for embryo transfer. Along the horizontal path, alternate segregation is depicted in which both normal chromosomes have been extruded during meiosis I; however, by analysis of PB2, anaphase II non-disjunction has been identified in which extra chromosome material has been retained in the oocyte, resulting in an unbalanced oocyte. This illustrates the necessity for analysis of both first polar body (PB1) and PB2 when performing PGD for maternal translocation carriers.

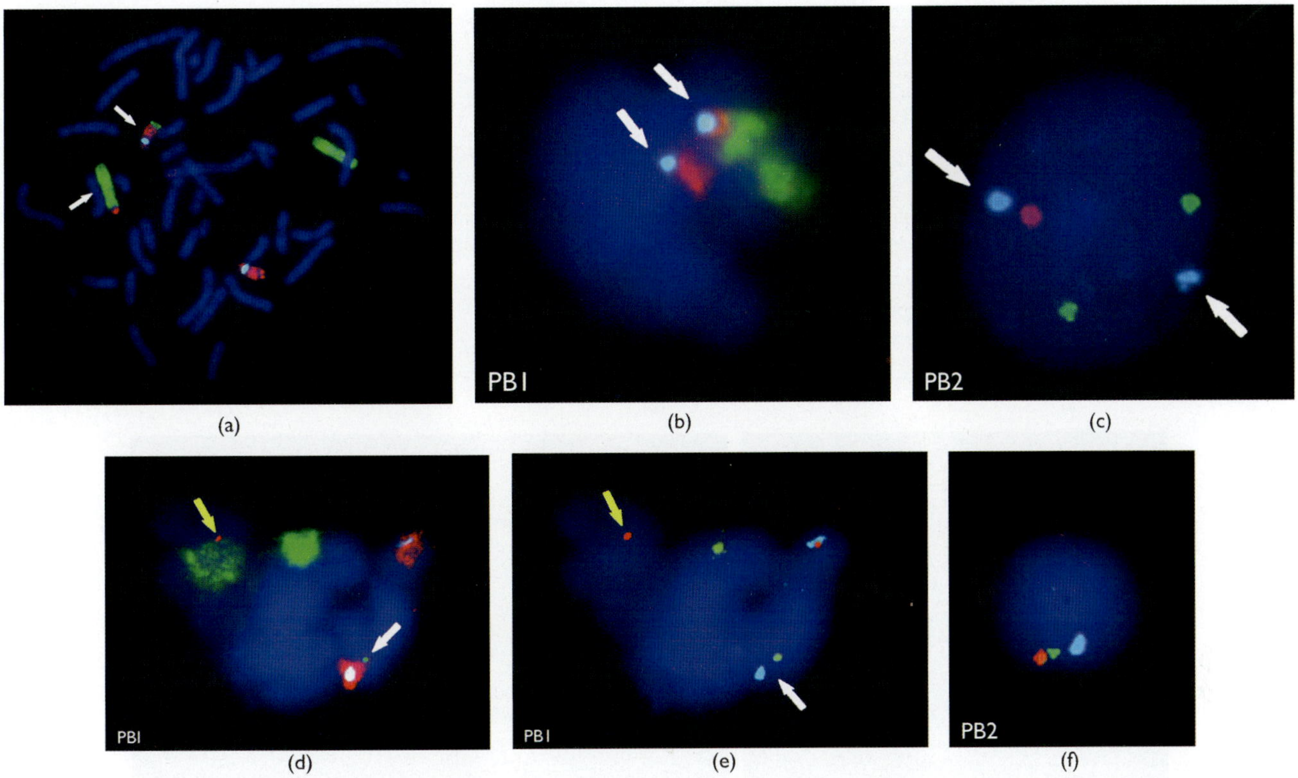

Figure 5.7 PGD for a maternally derived reciprocal translocation (46,XX,t(12;18)(p13.31;q21.32)) by polar body (PB) analysis. (a) Fluorescence *in situ* hybridization (FISH) analysis of metaphase chromosomes of a peripheral blood lymphocyte from the carrier. Chromosome 12 is identified with whole-chromosome paint (WCP) in green in conjunction with the sub-telomeric (Tel) probe 12p in green for easy visualization of the small translocated portion of chromosome 12 located on derivative 18. Chromosome 18 is identified with WCP in orange, which appears red due to visualization through a red single-bandpass filter in conjunction with the centromeric-enumeration probe (CEP) 18 in aqua and a Tel 18q in orange added to the probe cocktail for easy visualization of the terminal segment of chromosome 18 located on derivative 12. Derivative chromosomes are identified by a combination of both red and green fluorescence (white arrows). Derivative 18 is distinguished from derivative 12 not only by size, but also by the presence of the CEP 18 in aqua. (b) Clumped metaphase chromosomes of a first polar body (PB1) removed on the day of oocyte recovery. Two chromatids for chromosome 18 are present, evidenced by two CEP aqua signals (white arrows). Two chromatids for chromosome 12 are present, identified by the two areas of WCP in green. Further testing through re-hybridization with sub-telomeric probes would be required to distinguish derivative chromatids from normal chromatids because the translocated segments are small and difficult to see when chromosomes are poorly spread. (c) Additionally, investigation of the second polar body (PB2) by FISH with CEP 18 (aqua), Tel 12p (green), and Tel 18q (orange) is essential for accurate prediction of the chromosome status of the oocyte. An unbalanced oocyte is easily recognized by the presence of an additional CEP 18 signal (white arrows), indicating that anaphase II non-disjunction had occurred, which resulted in the extrusion of both normal and derivative chromatids for chromosome 18 so that after fertilization the resulting embryo is monosomic for chromosome 18. (d) Another PB1 removed from an oocyte from the same carrier (a). Individual normal and derivative (der) chromatids are seen by visualization of the sub-telomeric signals (yellow and white arrows). (e) Re-hybridization using only CEP 18 and sub-telomeric probes confirms the findings from the first round of hybridization, which was shown in (d); there is one chromatid present for each of the chromosomes of interest (12, der(12), 18, der(18)). Normal chromatid 12 is identified by a single Tel 12p signal in green, der(12) is identified by a single Tel 18q signal in orange (yellow arrow), normal chromatid 18 is identified by a single aqua CEP 18 signal and a single orange Tel 18q signal, and der(18) is identified by a single signal for both CEP 18 and Tel 12p (white arrow). Based on these findings, the PB2 must be studied in order to rule out anaphase II non-disjunction and to predict accurately the chromosome complement of the oocyte. (f) FISH of the PB2 nucleus. Three signals (expected normal number of signals representing 12, 18 or der(12), and der(18)) are present in PB2, suggesting a normal or balanced chromosome complement in the oocyte.

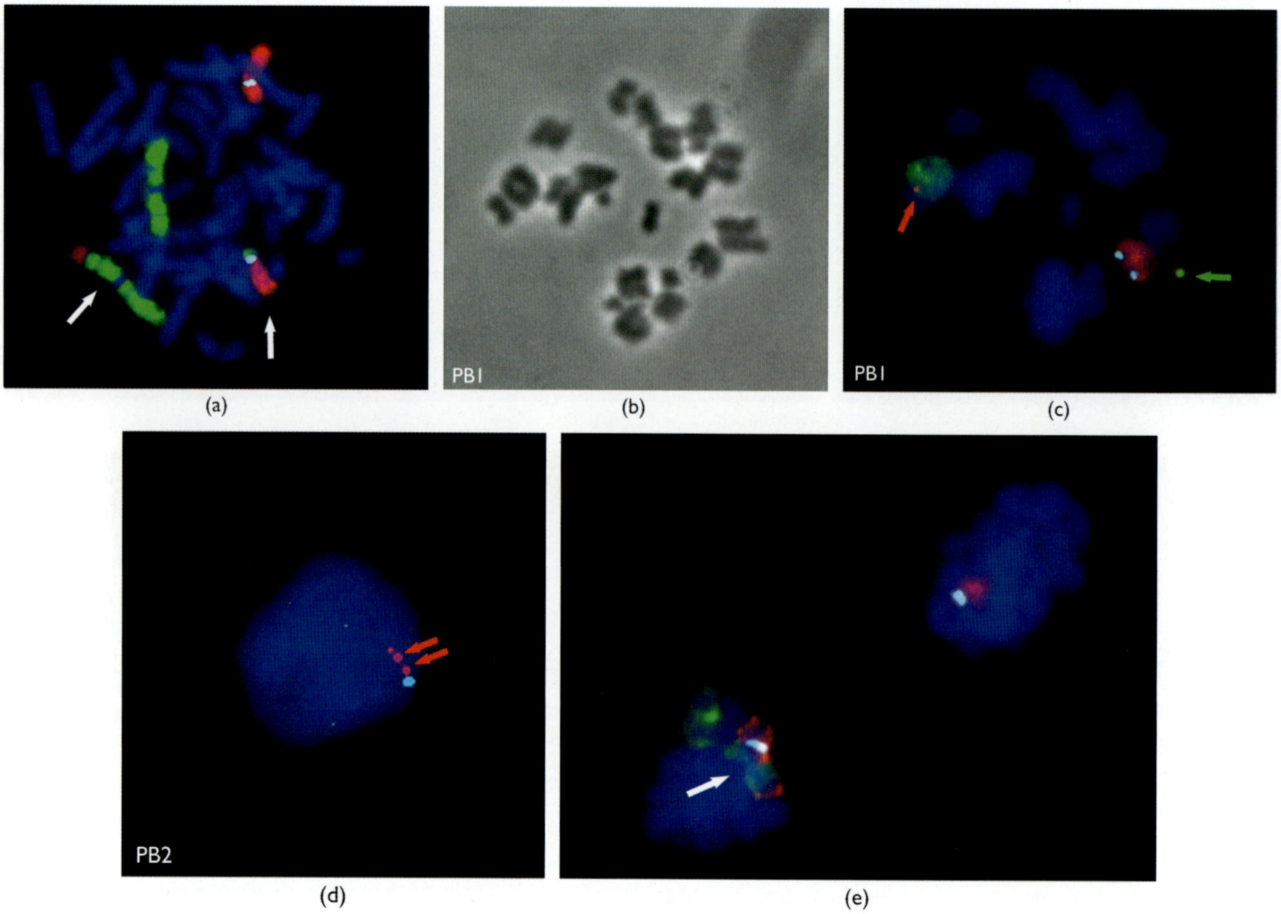

Figure 5.8 PGD for a maternally derived reciprocal translocation (46,XX,t(1;8)(q42;p11.2)) by polar body analysis. (a) Fluorescence *in situ* hybridization (FISH) analysis of metaphase chromosomes of a peripheral blood lymphocyte from the carrier. Chromosome 1 is identified with whole-chromosome paint (WCP) in green. Chromosome 8 is identified with WCP in orange, which appears red due to visualization through a red single-bandpass filter, in conjunction with a centromeric enumeration probe (CEP) 8 in aqua. Derivative chromosomes are identified by a combination of both red and green fluorescence (white arrows). Since the translocated segments are small, Tel 1q (orange) and Tel 8p (green) were added to the initial probe cocktail to ensure identification of chromatid exchange (CE). (b) Phase-contrast image of metaphase chromosomes from first polar body (PB1). (c) FISH image of PB1 shown in (b) in which CE of both is observed showing two CEP signals for chromosome 8, indicating two chromatids are present; however, only one chromatid carries the signal for Tel 8p (green arrow), indicating that the other chromatid contains the translocated segment from chromosome 1. Chromosome 1 is identified by WCP in green; however, only a single signal for the Tel 1q probe (red arrow) is seen, indicating that the sister chromatid carries the translocated segment for chromosome 8. (d) FISH image of second polar body (PB2) after hybridization with Tel 1q (orange), Tel 8p (green), and CEP 8 (aqua). A single signal for CEP 8 and two signals for Tel 1q (red arrows) are present, indicating that the normal chromosome 1 and the der(8) are present. Based on PB2 findings, it was predicted that this oocyte carried an unbalanced chromosome complement by the presence of der(1), and the developing embryo was omitted from embryo transfer. (e) Follow-up FISH analysis of metaphase chromosomes obtained after embryo biopsy and blastomere nucleus conversion of the corresponding unbalanced embryo identified by PB analysis (c) and (d). PGD by polar body analysis is confirmed by the presence of der(1) (white arrow).

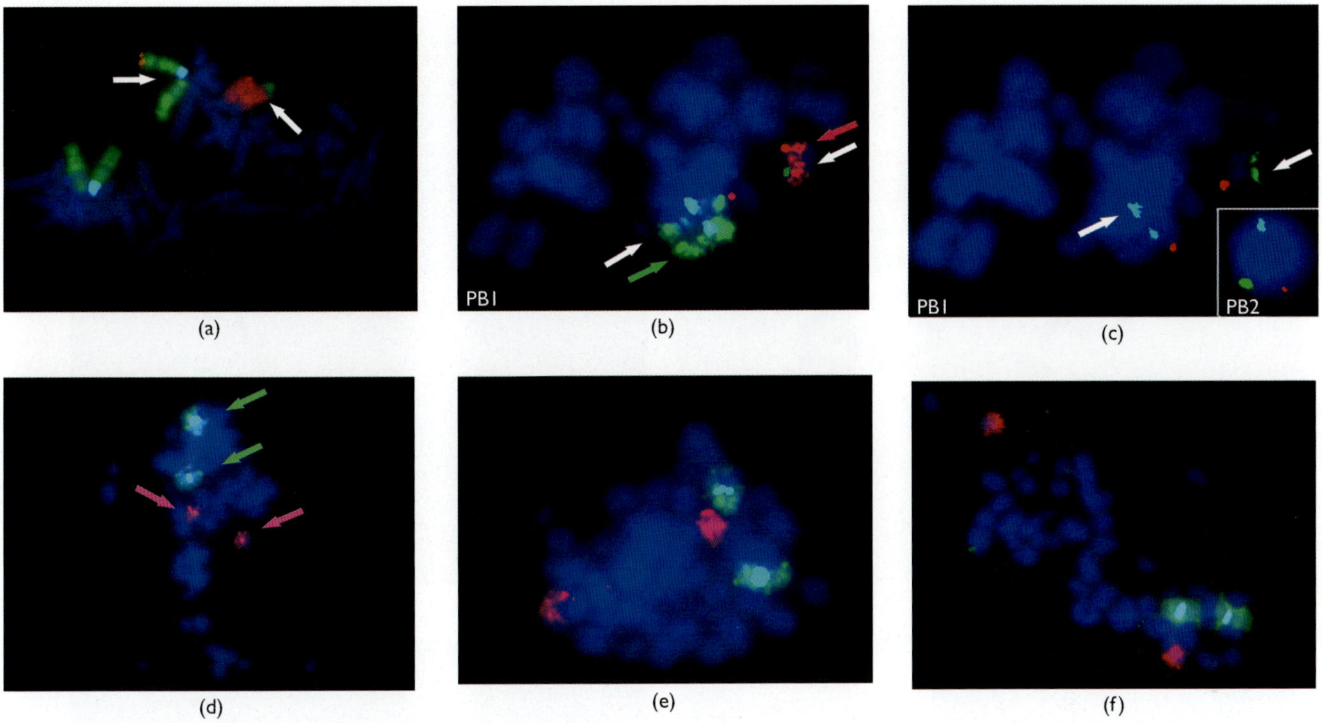

Figure 5.9 PGD for a maternally derived reciprocal translocation (46,XX,t(1;15)(q32;q26)) by polar body analysis. (a) Fluorescence *in situ* hybridization (FISH) analysis of metaphase chromosomes of a peripheral blood lymphocyte from the carrier. Chromosome 1 is identified with whole-chromosome paint (WCP) in green in conjunction with a centromeric-enumeration probe (CEP) 1 in aqua. Chromosome 15 is identified with WCP in orange (visualization through a red single-bandpass filter), in conjunction with Tel 15q in orange since the translocated segment of chromosome 15 onto chromosome 1 is small. Derivative chromosomes are identified by a combination of both red and green fluorescence (white arrows). (b) FISH image of metaphase chromosomes from first polar body (PB1), in which chromatid exchange (CE) of both is observed. Chromosome 1 is identified by WCP in green showing two CEP signals in aqua, indicating both chromatids are present; however, only one chromatid carries the signal for Tel 15q (derivative chromatid, white arrow), while the other chromatid does not (normal chromatid, green arrow). Chromosome 15 (orange) is visualized in red, with one chromatid seen as only red (normal chromatid, red arrow) and one chromatid seen as red and green (der(15), white arrow). (c) Re-hybridization of PB1 metaphase chromosomes shown in (b) with CEP 1 (aqua), Tel 1q (orange), and CEP 15 (green). Centromeric probes confirm the number of chromatids present, while Tel 1q confirms the presence of one normal and one derivative chromatid for each of the chromosomes of interest. Hybridization of second polar body (PB2) with the same probe cocktail is seen (lower right) showing a balanced/normal number of signals, indicating that the oocyte carries either a normal or balanced chromosome complement. (d), (e), and (f) Embryo follow-up analysis by embryo biopsy and blastomere nucleus conversion to metaphase chromosomes confirms the prediction by PB analysis, showing a normal chromosome complement. Normal chromosomes 1 (green arrows) and chromosomes 15 (red arrows) are present.

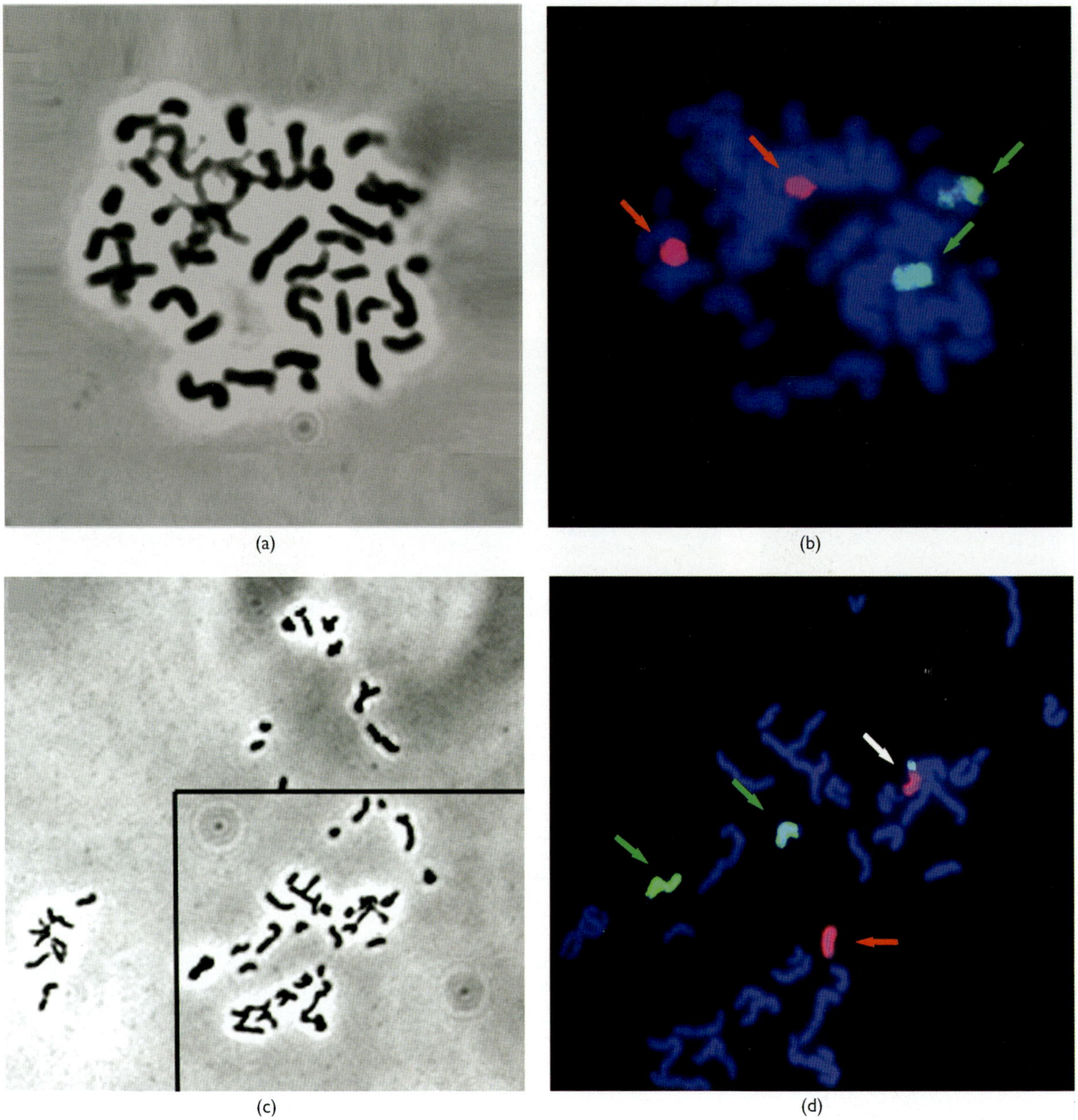

Figure 5.10 PGD for paternally derived reciprocal translocation (46,XY,t(13;20)(q22;p11.2)) by embryo biopsy and blastomere nucleus conversion to obtain metaphase chromosomes. (a) Phase-contrast image of metaphase chromosomes obtained after fixation and pretreatment of the human–mouse heterokaryon (see Chapter 3). (b) Fluorescence *in situ* hybridization (FISH) image of the same metaphase chromosomes in (a) showing a normal chromosome complement consisting of two chromosomes 13 in green (green arrows) and two chromosomes 20 in orange (red arrows), indicating that the corresponding embryo is suitable for transfer. (c) Phase-contrast image of metaphase chromosomes from a second embryo from the same couple obtained after fixation and pretreatment of the human–mouse heterokaryon. (d) FISH image of the metaphase chromosomes in (c) showing an unbalanced chromosome complement consisting of two chromosomes 13 in green (green arrows), one chromosome 20 in orange (red arrow), and one der(20) in red and green (white arrow), indicating that the corresponding embryo is not suitable for transfer.

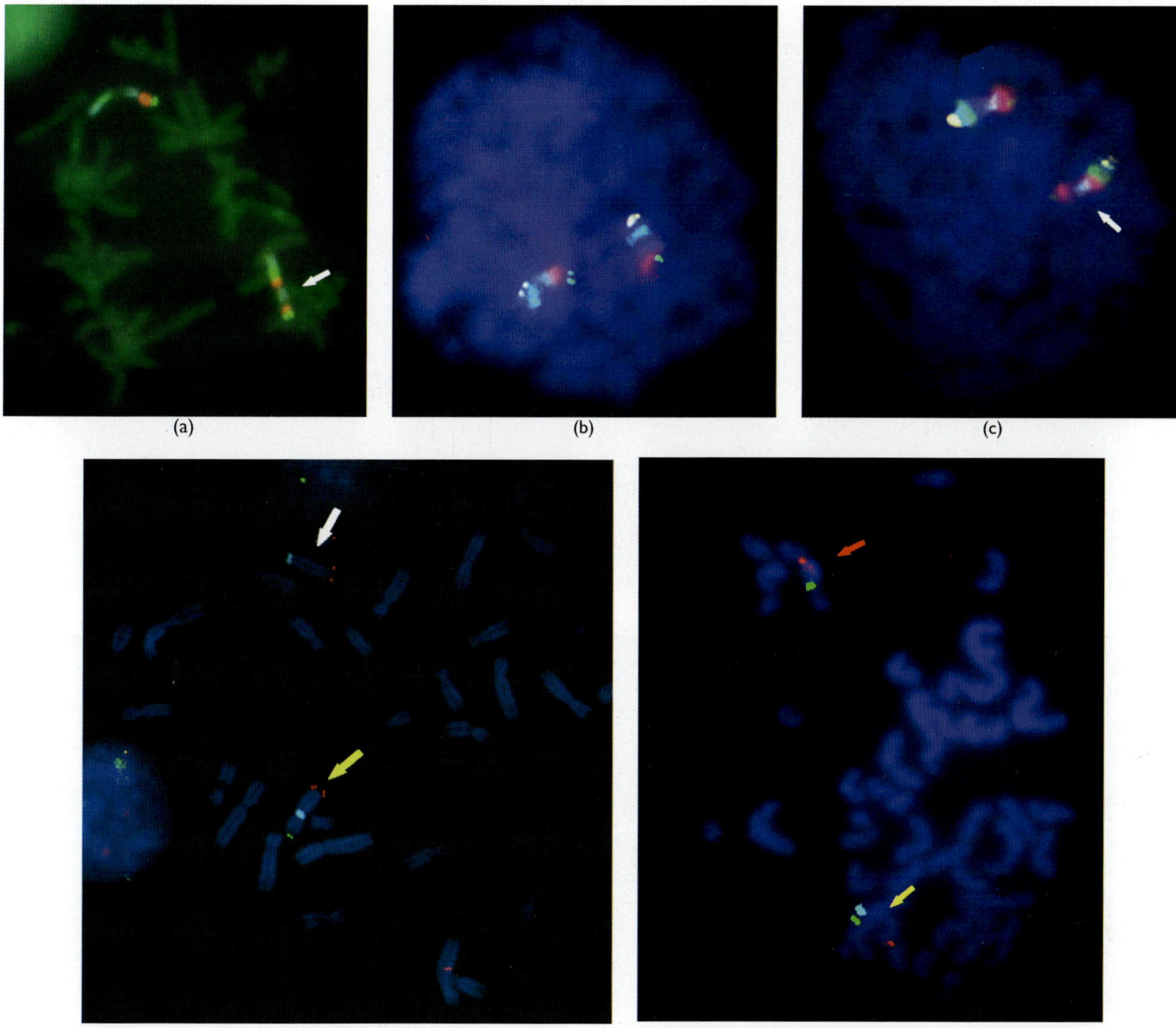

(a) (b) (c) (d) (e)

Figure 5.11 PGD for a paternally derived pericentric inversion of chromosome 5 (46,XY,inv(5)(p13q13)) by embryo biopsy and blastomere nucleus conversion to obtain metaphase chromosomes. (a) Fluorescence *in situ* hybridization (FISH) analysis of metaphase chromosomes of a peripheral blood lymphocyte from the carrier. MetaSystems Xcyte 5 mBand whole-chromosome painting, which identifies chromosome regions for a particular chromosome by labeling with different fluorophores, was used to distinguish the normal chromosome 5 from the chromosome carrying the pericentric inversion (white arrow). The chromosome carrying the inversion was identified by two areas of red paint along the chromosome in contrast to one large area seen on the normal chromosome. (b) FISH image of metaphase chromosomes obtained after embryo biopsy and blastomere nucleus conversion from same patient in (a), in which a probe cocktail consisting of MetaSystems XCyte 5 mBAND with Tel 5p in green and Tel 5q in orange was used to distinguish the normal chromosome from the chromosome carrying the inversion. Both normal chromosomes 5 are present, indicating that the corresponding embryo is suitable for transfer. (c) FISH image of clumped metaphase chromosomes obtained from a second embryo after blastomere nucleus conversion from same patient in (a), in which both the normal chromosome 5 and inv(5) (white arrow) are present. Telomeric signals 5p and 5q are present and terminally located on both chromosomes, indicating a balanced chromosome complement. (d) PGD for a maternally derived pericentric inversion of chromosome X (46,X,inv(X)(p22.3q13)) by embryo biopsy and blastomere nucleus conversion to obtain metaphase chromosomes. FISH analysis of metaphase chromosomes of a peripheral blood lymphocyte from the carrier. Chromosome X was investigated using CEP X (aqua), Tel Xp/Yp (green), and Tel Xq/Yq (orange). The inv(X) chromosome (white arrow) is distinguished from the normal (yellow arrow) by the terminal location of CEP X, making visualization of the Tel Xp signal difficult owing to overlap. (e) FISH image of metaphase chromosomes obtained after embryo biopsy and blastomere nucleus conversion from same patient in (d). This chromosome complement consists of a normal chromosome X (yellow arrow) and chromosome Y (red arrow) identified by Tel Xp/Yp (green) signal and Tel Xq/Yq (orange) signal and the absence of CEP X (aqua). Embryo transfer of the corresponding embryo resulted in the delivery of a healthy male.

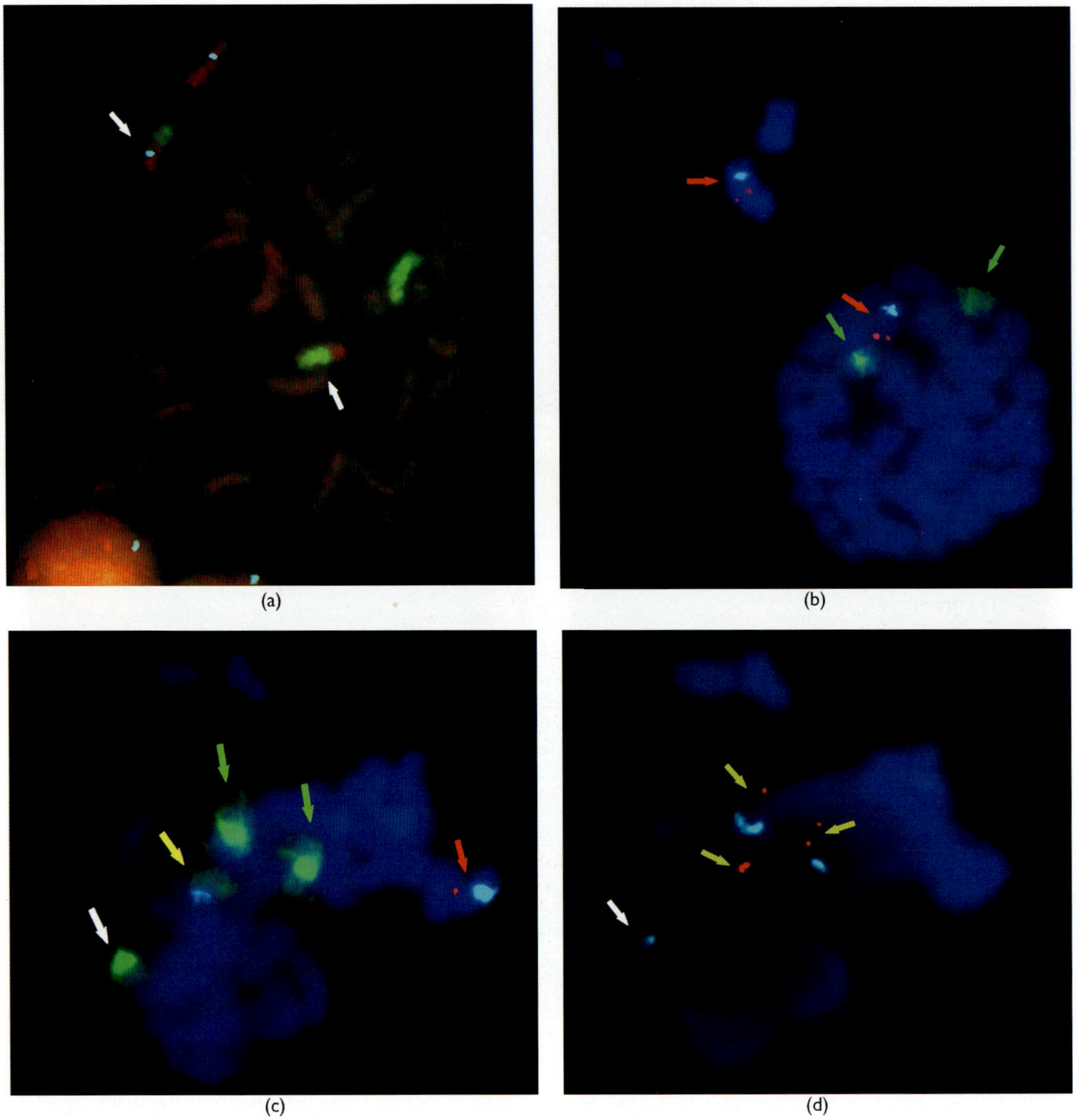

Figure 5.12 PGD for a maternally derived reciprocal translocation (46,XX,t(9;11)(q13;q13.5)) by embryo biopsy and blastomere nucleus conversion. (a) Fluorescence *in situ* hybridization (FISH) analysis of metaphase chromosomes of a peripheral blood lymphocyte from the carrier. Chromosome 9 is identified with whole-chromosome paint (WCP) (green). Chromosome 11 is identified with WCP (orange) in conjunction with CEP 11 (aqua). Derivative chromosomes are identified by a combination of both red and green fluorescence (white arrows). (b) FISH image of metaphase chromosomes obtained after embryo biopsy and blastomere nucleus conversion. Tel 11q (orange) was added to the probe cocktail in case of the WCP 11 failure occasionally seen with paints using Spectrum Orange™ (Vysis). This was done to ensure identification of the translocated segment of chromosome 11 onto chromosome 9. A normal chromosome complement is evidenced by the presence of both normal chromosomes 9 (WCP, green) and chromosomes 11 (CEP 11, aqua; Tel 11q, orange). (c) FISH image of metaphase chromosomes obtained after embryo biopsy and blastomere nucleus conversion from another embryo. An unbalanced chromosome complement is immediately evidenced by the presence of five chromosomes in which only one normal chromosome 11 (red arrow) is present. Derivative (11) is identified by CEP 11 and WCP 9 (green) (yellow arrow), and three chromosomes 9 (WCP, green) (white and green arrows) are seen. (d) Re-hybridization of (c) with a probe cocktail consisting of CEP 9 (aqua) and Tel 9q (orange). Three signals for the Tel 9q (yellow arrows) are seen, one of which is split, representative of both chromatids for a single chromosome. One Tel 9q correlates with the first round of hybridization in which der(11) was identified (yellow arrow in (c)). Additionally, one der(9) is identified by CEP 9 and by the absence of the Tel 9q (white arrow) that was not readily seen with the first hybridization. Upon completion of the testing, this unbalanced chromosome complement consisted of (9, 9, der(9), 11, der(11)), a possible product of 3:1 interchange trisomy or alternate segregation combined with anaphase II non-disjunction.

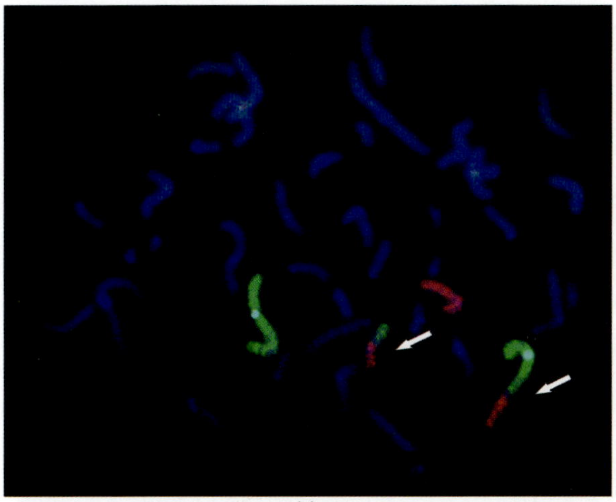

(a)

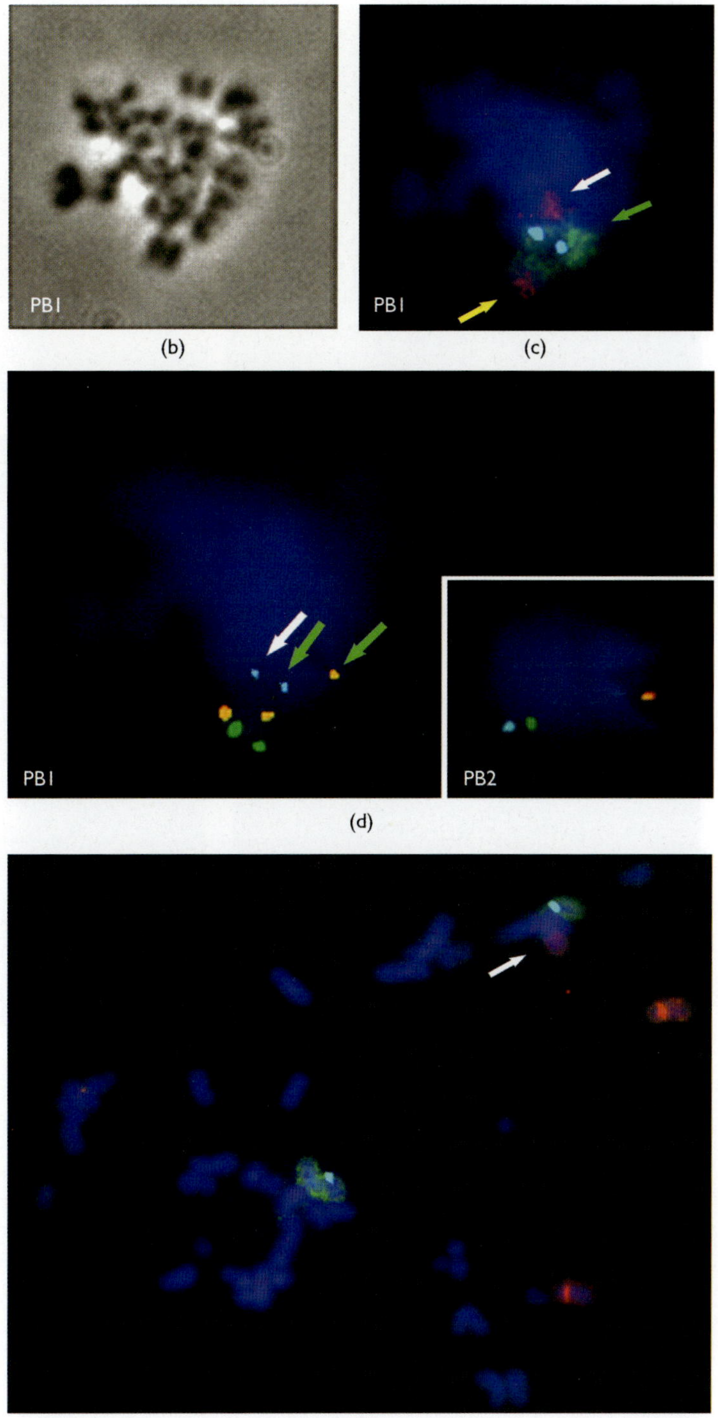

(b) (c) (d) (e)

Figure 5.13 PGD for a maternally derived reciprocal translocation (46,XX,t(2;10)(q31;q11.2)) by polar body analysis. (a) Fluorescence *in situ* hybridization (FISH) analysis of metaphase chromosomes of a peripheral blood lymphocyte from the carrier. Chromosome 2 is identified with whole-chromosome paint (WCP) in green in conjunction with CEP 2 in aqua. Chromosome 10 is identified with WCP in orange seen through a red single-bandpass filter. (b) Phase-contrast image of metaphase chromosomes from first polar body (PB1). (c) FISH image of PB1 in (b) in which chromatid exchange (CE) of one chromosome is observed showing two CEP signals for chromosome 2, indicating two chromatids are present; however, only one chromatid is seen in both red and green (white arrow), indicating that it carries the translocated segment for chromosome 10 while the other chromatid does not (normal chromatid, green arrow). Derivative (10) is present (yellow arrow), identified by the combination of red and green fluorescence and the absence of an aqua signal. Further hybridization is required since the chromosomes of interest are in close proximity and also to enumerate the number of chromatids for der(10). (d) Re-hybridization of PB1 (in (b) and (c)) metaphase chromosomes using a probe cocktail consisting of CEP 2 (aqua), CEP 10 (green), and Tel 2q (orange). Both derivative chromatids for chromosome 10 are present, identified by two CEP 10 (green) and two Tel 2q (orange) signals; one normal chromatid for chromosome 2 is present, identified by one CEP 2 (aqua) and one Tel 2q (orange) (green arrows); and one derivative chromatid for chromosome 2, previously identified in the first hybridization, is confirmed by the CEP 2 (aqua) and the absence of a signal for Tel 2q (white arrow). Hybridization of the second polar body (PB2) nucleus using the same probe cocktail (lower right) showed a balanced number of signals that can only represent a normal chromosome 10 (CEP 10, green) since both derivative chromatids were extruded during meiosis I, and the normal chromosome 2 (CEP 2, aqua, Tel 2q, orange) indicates that the oocyte contains an unbalanced chromosome complement by the presence of der(2). This embryo was omitted from transfer. (e) Follow-up analysis of the corresponding embryo by biopsy and blastomere nucleus conversion confirms the polar body investigation, showing an unbalanced chromosome complement by the presence of der(2) (white arrow).

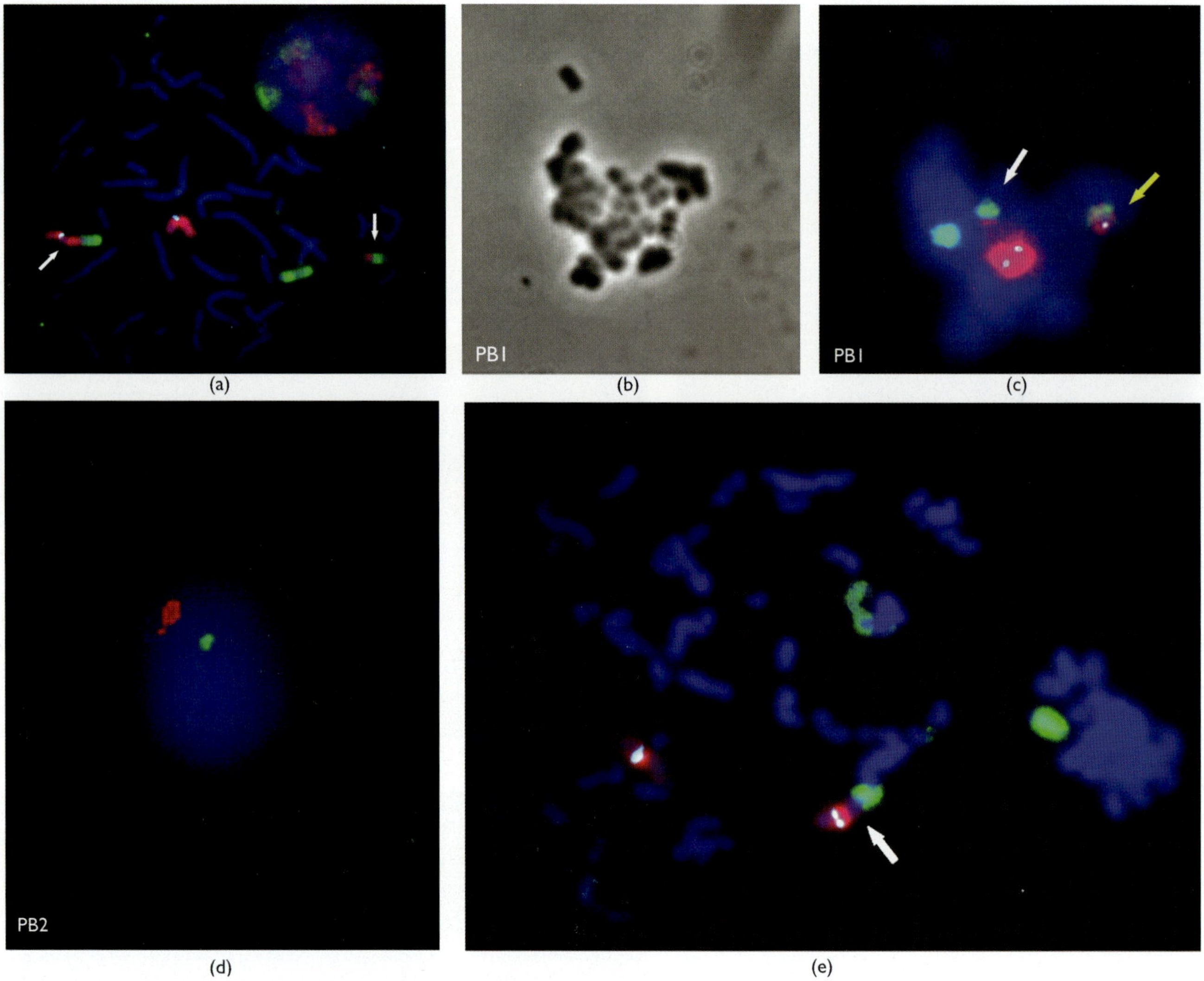

Figure 5.14 PGD for a maternally derived reciprocal translocation (46,XX,t(9;13)(q22;q14)) by polar body analysis. (a) Fluorescence *in situ* hybridization (FISH) analysis of metaphase chromosomes of a peripheral blood lymphocyte from the carrier. Chromosome 9 is identified with whole-chromosome paint (WCP) in orange in conjunction with centromeric-enumeration probe (CEP) 9 in aqua. Chromosome 13 is identified with WCP in green. (b) Phase-contrast image of metaphase chromosomes from first polar body (PB1). (c) FISH image of first polar body (PB1) in (b) in which complex chromosome segregation most likely involved chromatid exchange (CE) of one chromosome along with chromatid non-disjunction. Both chromatids for normal chromosome 9 are identified by CEP 9 (aqua) and WCP (orange), a single chromatid for chromosome 13 (green), a single chromatid for der(13) (orange and green) (white arrow); and a single chromatid for der(9) is identified by CEP 9 (aqua) with red and green fluorescence (yellow arrow). (d) Hybridization of second polar body (PB2) nucleus with a probe cocktail consisting of CEP 9 (aqua); LSI 13 (13q14) (green), used for enumeration of chromosome 13 since hybridization is just above the breakpoint; and Tel 9q (orange). Only one signal for Tel 9q and LSI 13 is seen representing der(13), indicating that the oocyte contains an unbalanced chromosome complement due to the presence of der(9). (e) FISH image of follow-up analysis of the corresponding embryo by biopsy and blastomere nucleus conversion confirms the polar body analysis by the presence of der(9) (white arrow).

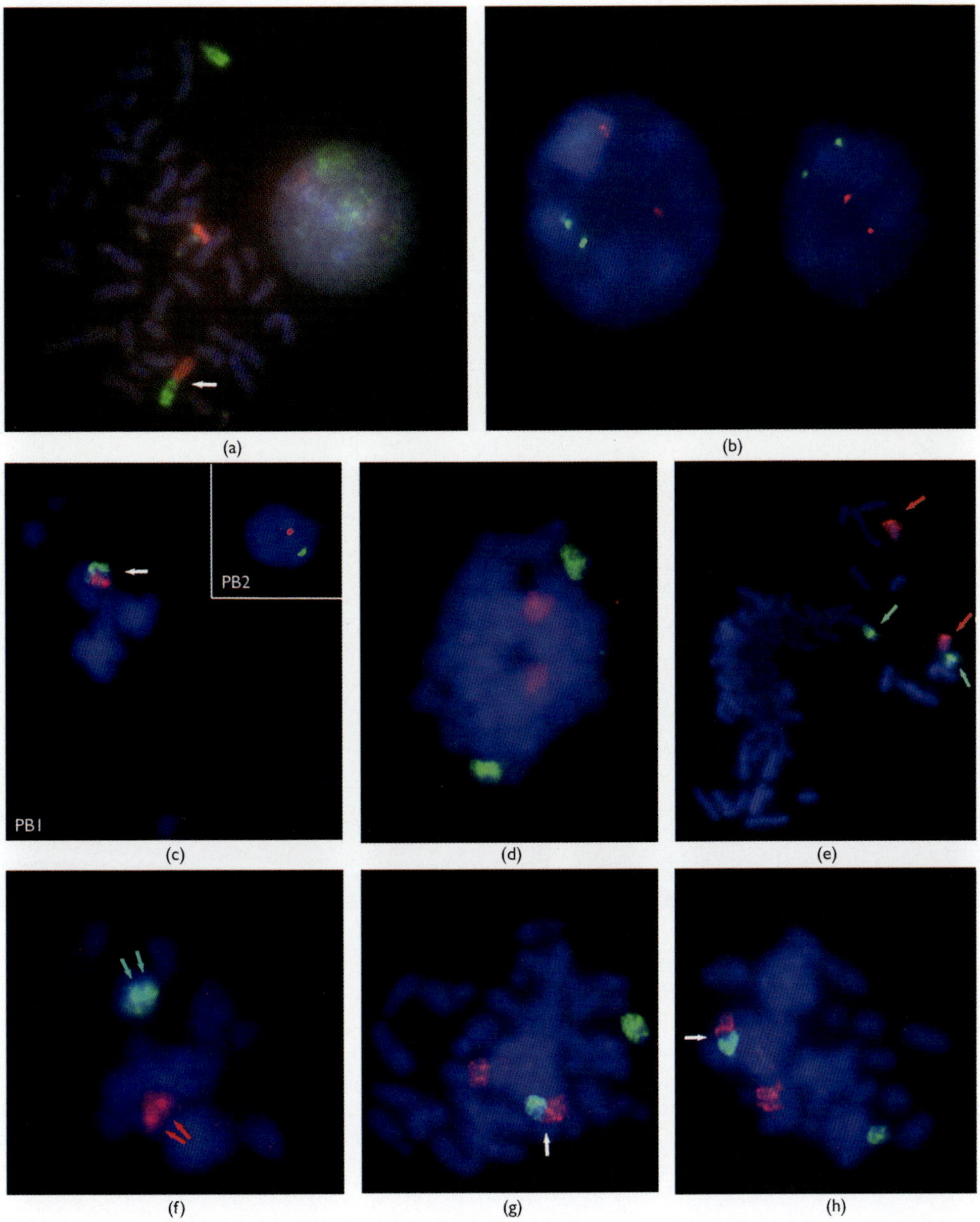

Figure 5.21 PGD of maternally derived Robertsonian translocation (45,XX,der(13;14)(q10;q10)), identification of balanced and normal chromosome complements. Robertsonian translocations originate through centric fusion of the long arms of two acrocentric chromosomes, usually with simultaneous loss of both short arms, resulting in a total chromosome number of 45. (a) Fluorescence *in situ* hybridization (FISH) analysis of metaphase chromosomes of a peripheral blood lymphocyte from the carrier. Chromosome 13 is identified by WCP 13 (green) and chromosome 14 by WCP 14 (orange). The derivative (13;14) is identified by fluorescence of both WCP in orange (appears red through a red single-bandpass filter) and green (white arrow). (b) FISH image of interphase nuclei after hybridization with a probe cocktail consisting of sub-telomeric probes Tel 13q (orange) and Tel 14q (green) showing a balanced/normal number of signals. PGD can be performed using interphase nuclei by enumerating the chromosomes present; however, as with all chromosome rearrangements, one cannot distinguish a balanced complement carrying the derivative(s) from one in which normal chromosomes are present. (c) FISH image of first polar body (PB1) metaphase chromosomes using WCP. Derivative (13;14) (white arrow) appears to be present based on the close proximity of the orange and green fluorescence. Hybridization of second polar body (PB2) using sub-telomeric probes as previously mentioned shows a balanced/normal number of signals, indicating that the corresponding oocyte carries the normal chromosomes 13 and 14. (d) and (e) Follow-up analysis of the corresponding embryo to (c) after embryo biopsy and blastomere nucleus conversion showing a normal chromosome complement (13, 13, 14, 14) easily identified by the physical separation of the chromosomes of interest. (f) FISH image of PB1 metaphase chromosomes using WCP. Normal chromosomes 13 (green arrows) and 14 (red arrows) are identified by their distant location from one another. Based on this information, barring anaphase II non-disjunction, the embryo is predicted to carry a balanced chromosome complement. (g) and (h) Follow-up analysis of the corresponding embryo to (f) after embryo biopsy and blastomere nucleus conversion. Derivative (13;14) (white arrow) is present, seen by the hybridization of both WCP 13 and WCP 14 to one large chromosome, confirming the diagnosis originally made by PB1 testing.

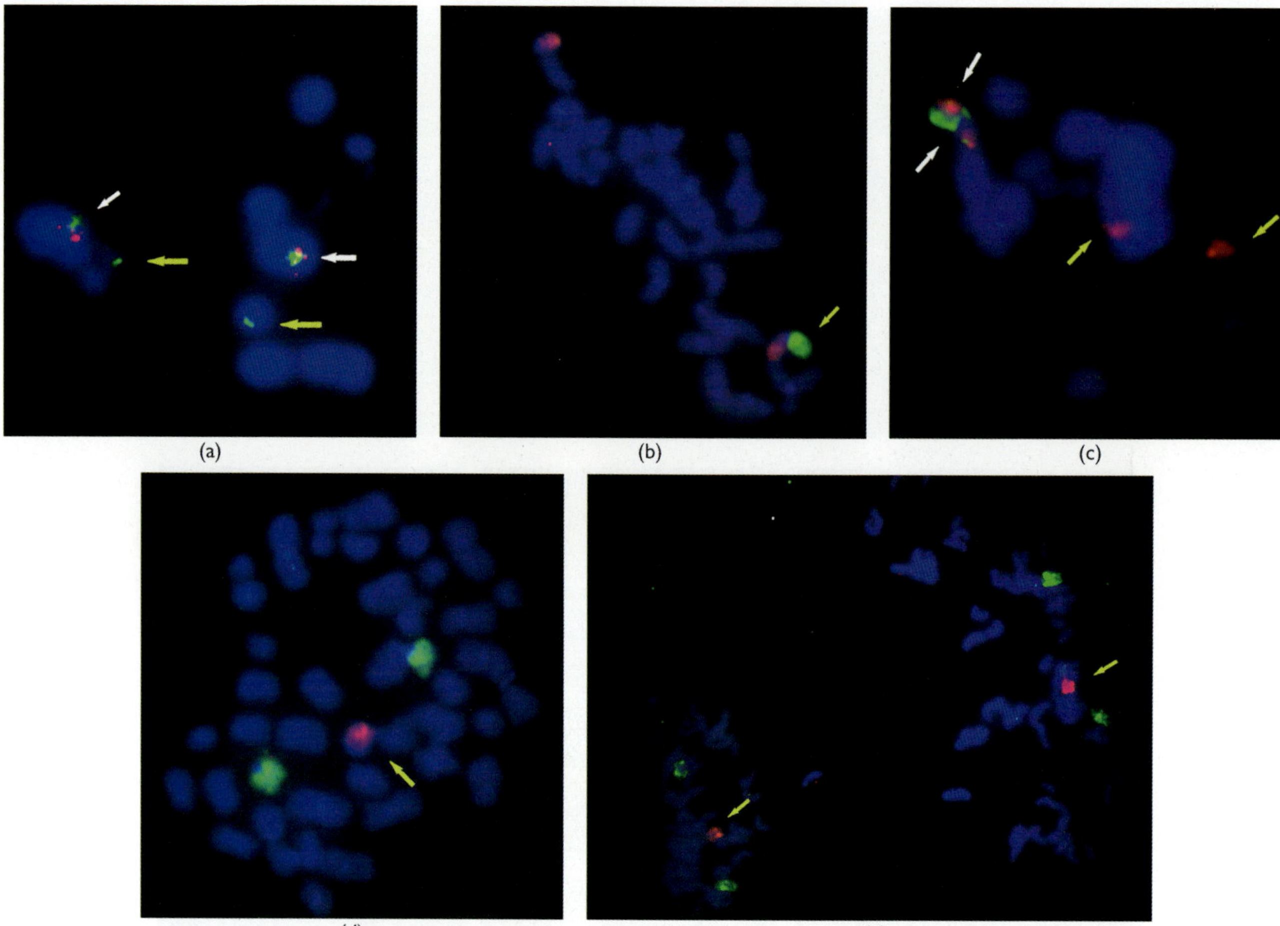

(a) (b) (c) (d) (e)

Figure 5.22 PGD of maternally derived Robertsonian translocation (45,XX,der(13;14)(q10;q10)), identification of unbalanced chromosome complements. (a) Fluorescence *in situ* hybridization (FISH) image of first polar body (PB1) chromosomes after hybridization with a probe cocktail containing locus-specific identifier (LSI) 13 (13q14) (green) and Tel 14q (orange). Separate chromatids for chromosome 13 (yellow arrows) identified by two LSI 13 signals and separate chromatids for der(13;14) identified by LSI 13 and Tel 14q signals (white arrows) are present, suggesting that the oocyte is unbalanced and after fertilization would result in a monosomy 13 embryo. (b) FISH image of metaphase chromosomes following embryo biopsy, blastomere nucleus conversion, and hybridization with whole-chromosome paint (WCP) 13 (green) and WCP 14 (orange). Only one chromosome 13 (yellow arrow) is present, confirming the diagnosis made by PB analysis. (c) FISH image after hybridization of PB1 metaphase chromosomes using WCP 13 (green) and WCP 14 (orange). Two separate chromatids for chromosome 14 (yellow arrows) are present along with two chromatids for der(13;14) (white arrows), indicating that the corresponding oocyte is unbalanced and following fertilization would result in a monosomy 14 embryo. (d) FISH image of metaphase chromosomes following embryo biopsy, blastomere nucleus conversion, and hybridization with WCP13 (green) and WCP 14 (orange). Only one chromosome 14 (yellow arrow) is present, confirming the diagnosis made by PB analysis. (e) Two metaphase plates obtained after fixation of the human–mouse heterokaryon in which a binucleate blastomere from the same embryo was fused. After hybridization with the previously mentioned WCP cocktail, monosomy 14 is present in both metaphase spreads, in agreement with the first cell shown in (d).

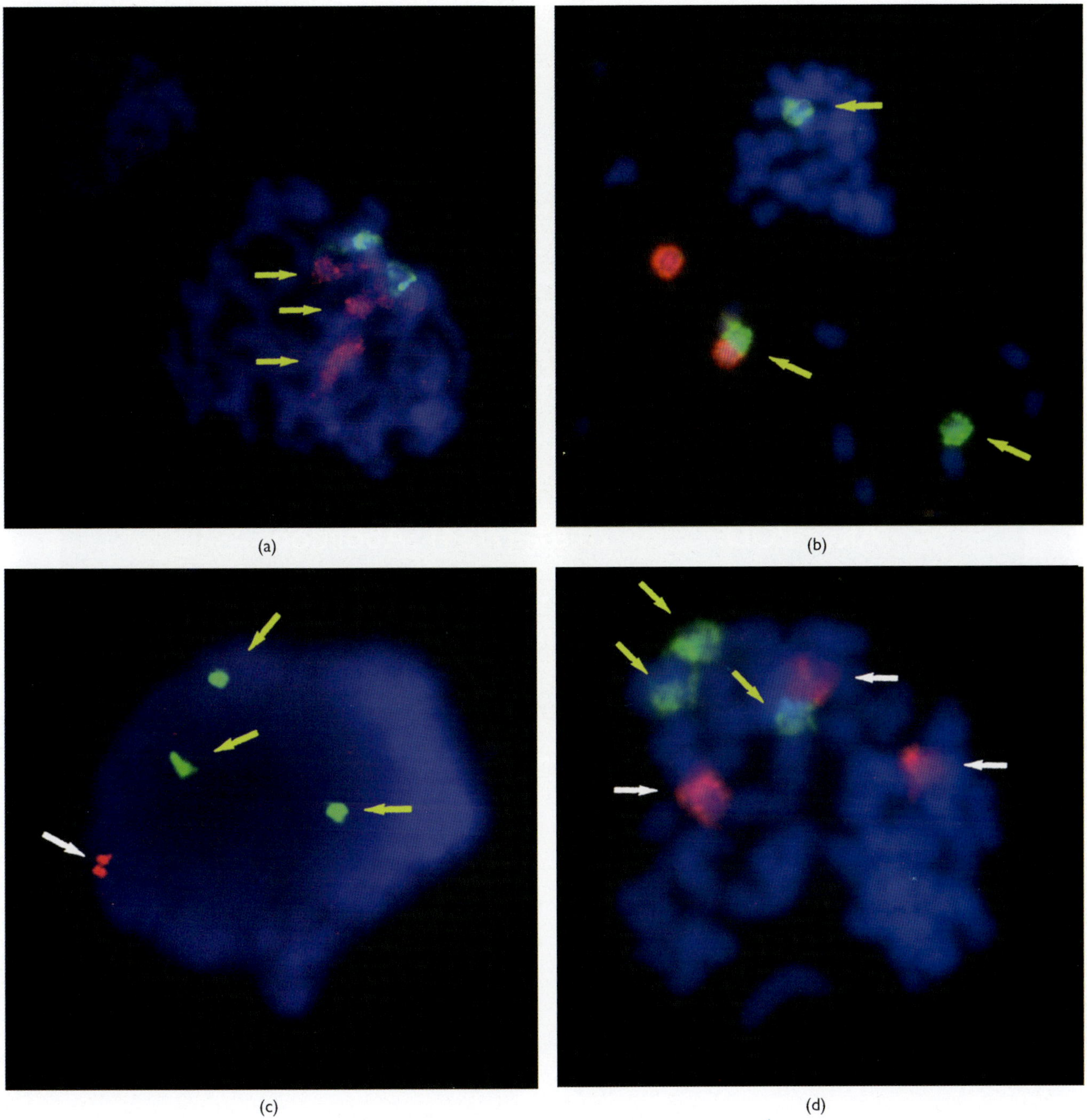

Figure 5.23 PGD of paternally or maternally derived Robertsonian translocation der(13;14)(q10;q10) by blastomere analysis. (a) Fluorescence *in situ* hybridization (FISH) image of partially condensed chromatin obtained after embryo biopsy and blastomere nucleus conversion. Although chromatin is only partially condensed, a whole-chromosome paint (WCP) cocktail was used and successfully revealed trisomy 14 (yellow arrows), indicating that the corresponding embryo was unsuitable for transfer. (b) FISH image in which an unbalanced embryo was identified by the presence of der(13;14) resulting in trisomy 13 (green) (yellow arrows). (c) FISH image of an interphase nucleus that failed to convert after embryo biopsy and blastomere fusion with a mouse zygote. Failure to convert seems to be a reflection of embryo quality since the corresponding embryos more often arrest in their development. FISH was performed using LSI 13 (green) and Tel 14q (orange) showing an unbalanced chromosome complement evidenced by three LSI 13 signals (yellow arrows). Signals for Tel 14q are in close proximity to one another (white arrow). (d) FISH image of metaphase chromosome after embryo biopsy and blastomere nucleus conversion. After hybridization with the WCP cocktail, an unbalanced chromosome complement is seen, consisting of trisomies 13 (yellow arrows) and 14 (white arrows) due to the presence of der(13;14).

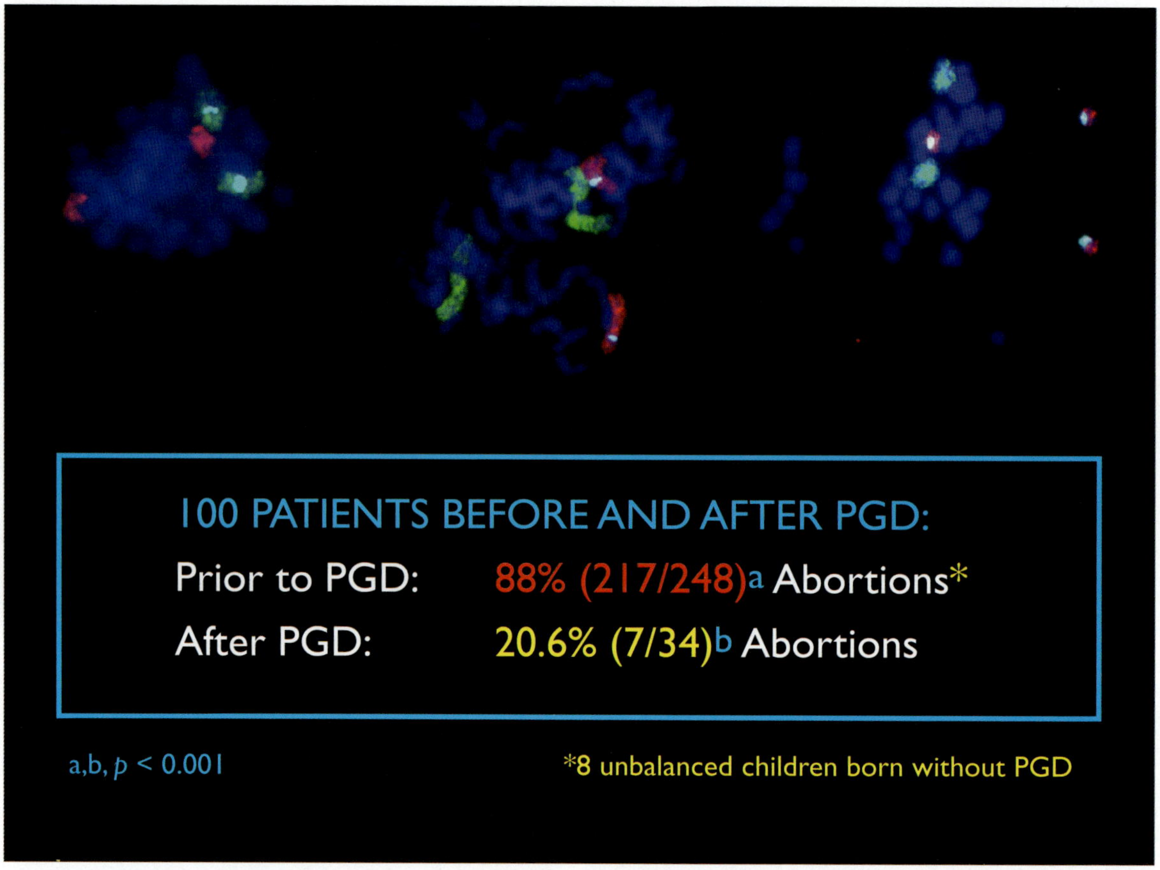

Figure 5.24 Comparison of the incidence of abortion before and after PGD for chromosomal rearrangements. The significant reduction in the abortion rate seen after PGD demonstrates the beneficial effect of PGD testing.

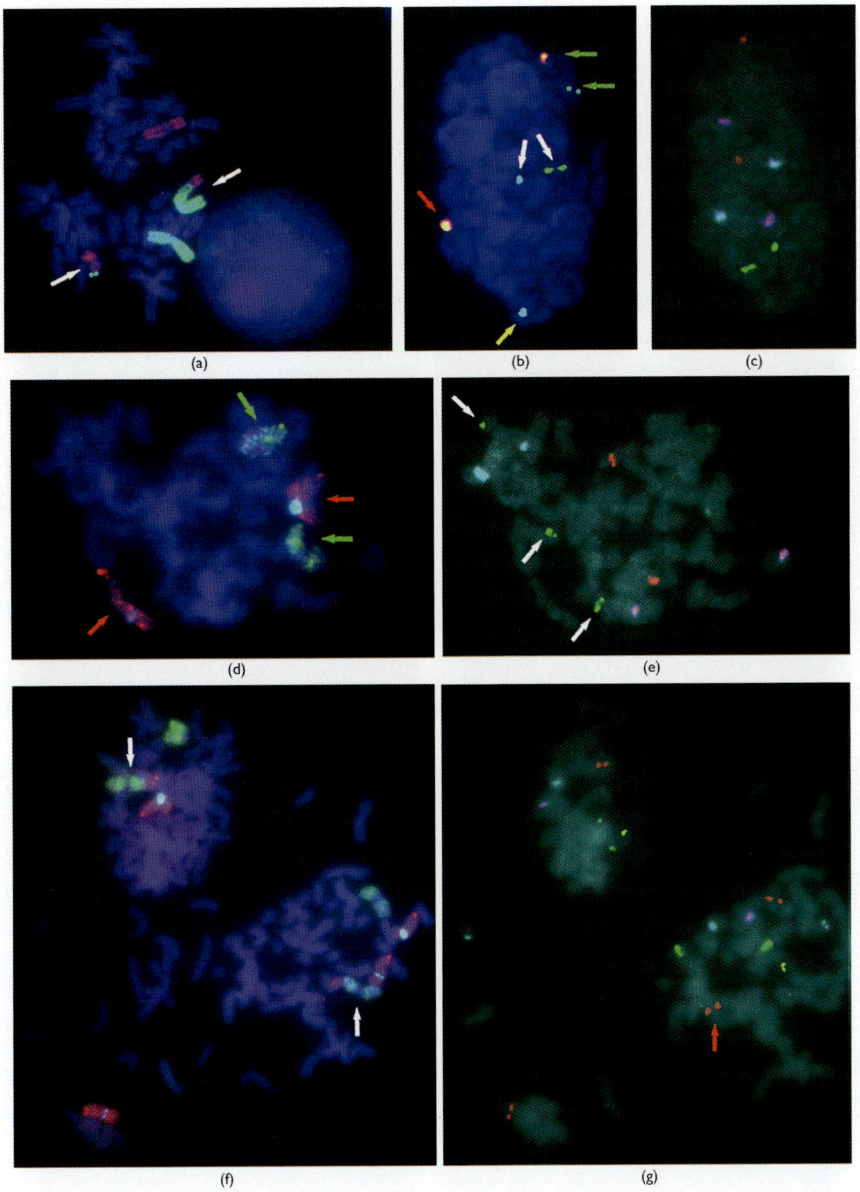

Figure 5.25 PGD for a maternally derived reciprocal translocation (46,XX,t(3;6)(p26.2;q21)) and for common aneuploidies involving chromosomes X, Y, 13, 18, and 21 by embryo biopsy and blastomere nucleus conversion. (a) Fluorescence *in situ* hybridization (FISH) analysis of metaphase chromosomes of a peripheral blood lymphocyte from the carrier. Chromosomes 3 and 6 are identified by whole-chromosome paint (WCP) 3 (orange) and WCP 6 (green). Derivatives are identified by a combination of orange (seen as red through a red single-bandpass filter) and green fluorescence (white arrows). (b) Poorly spread metaphase chromosomes after embryo biopsy and blastomere nucleus conversion. FISH image after hybridization with a probe cocktail of centromeric-enumeration probe (CEP) 3 (orange), CEP 6 (aqua), and Tel 3p (green) showing a balanced chromosome complement. Chromosome 3 is identified by CEP 3 and Tel 3p (green arrows), and der(3) is identified by CEP 3 and the absence of Tel 3p (red arrow). Chromosome 6 is identified by CEP 6 (yellow arrow), and der(6) is identified by CEP 6 and Tel 3p (white arrows). (c) Re-hybridization of the same chromosomes in (b) with the MultiVysion PGT probe (Vysis) for chromosomes 13 (red), 18 (aqua), 21 (green), X (blue), and Y (gold). Two signals are present for each of the autosomes tested and for chromosome X. The corresponding embryo was the only embryo found to be suitable for transfer out of the eight embryos tested, resulting in the delivery of a healthy girl. (d) Metaphase chromosomes obtained after embryo biopsy and blastomere nucleus conversion. A probe cocktail consisting of WCP 3 (green), WCP 6 (orange), CEP 6 (aqua), and Tel 6q (orange) was used and revealed normal chromosomes 3 (green arrows) and 6 (red arrows) present. (e) Re-hybridization of the same metaphase spread in (d) with the MultiVysion PGT probe revealed trisomy 21 (three green signals, white arrows), and therefore the corresponding embryo was omitted from transfer. (f) FISH image of two metaphase spreads obtained after embryo biopsy of a binucleate blastomere and blastomere nucleus conversion. Both consist of an unbalanced chromosome complement by the presence of der(3) (white arrows), and therefore the corresponding embryo was omitted from transfer. (g) For academic reasons, re-hybridization with MultiVysion PGT probe of the same metaphase spreads in (f) revealed a male embryo by the presence of one blue and one gold signal with two signals for each of the autosomes tested, some of which were seen as double dot signals corresponding to each chromatid (e.g. LSI 13, red arrow), as often seen when studying metaphase chromosomes.

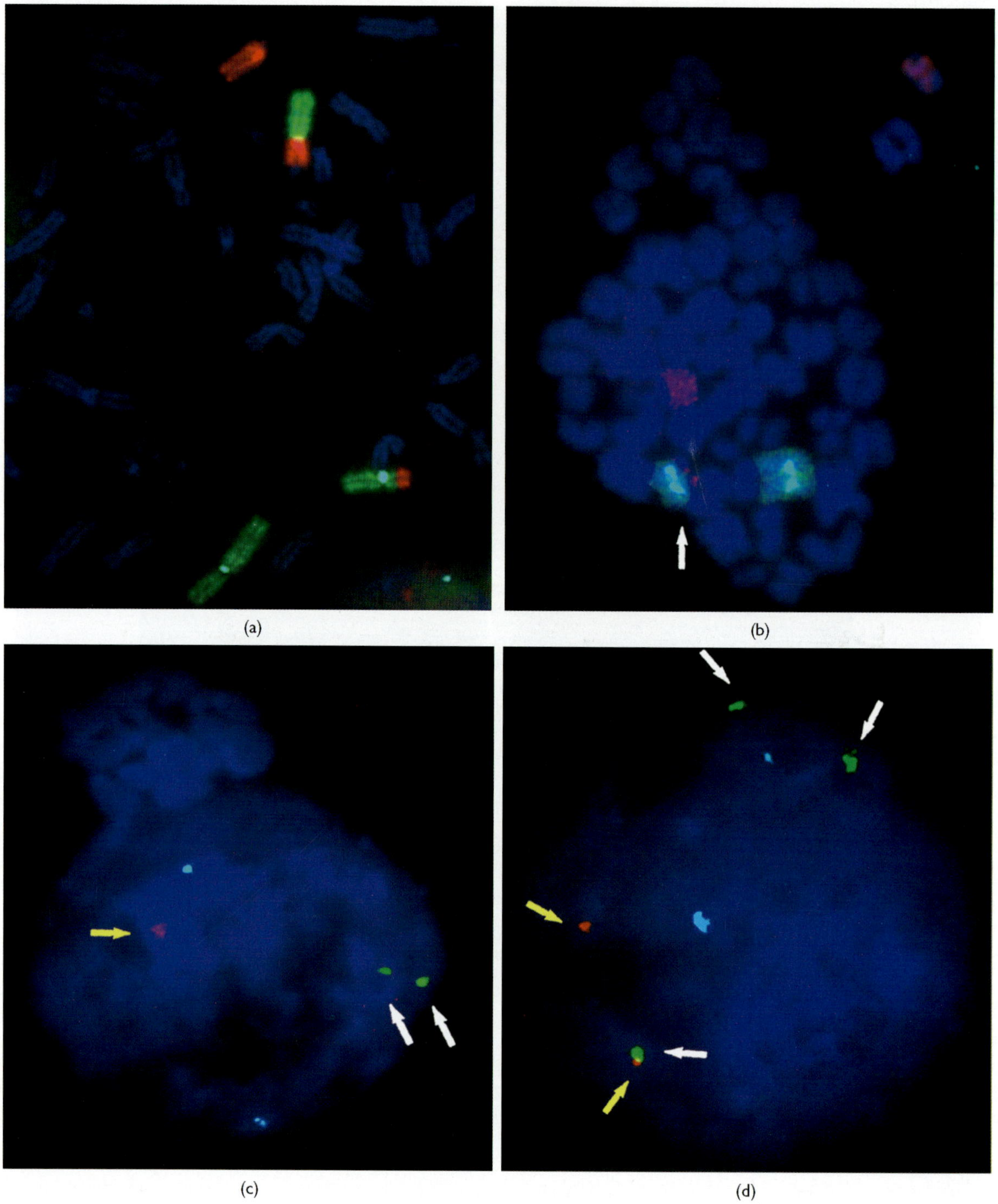

Figure 5.26 PGD for a maternally derived reciprocal translocation (46,XX,t(2;13)(q22;q33)). (a) Fluorescence *in situ* hybridization (FISH) analysis of metaphase chromosomes of a peripheral blood lymphocyte from the carrier. Chromosome 2 is identified by whole-chromosome paint (WCP) 2 (green) in conjunction with centromeric-enumeration probe (CEP) 2 (aqua). Chromosome 13 is identified by WCP 13 (orange) (seen as red through a single bandpass filter). (b) FISH image of metaphase chromosomes after embryo biopsy and blastomere nucleus conversion. An unbalanced chromosome complement is identified by the presence of der(2) (white arrow). (c) FISH image of an interphase nucleus from the same embryo in (b) from follow-up studies. FISH was performed using a probe cocktail consisting of CEP 2 (aqua), Tel 2q (orange), and LSI 13 (13q14) (green), which hybridizes above the breakpoint on der(13). Based on the findings shown in (b), the chromosome complement of the other interphase cells being investigated should result in two CEP 2 aqua signals, one Tel 2q orange signal (yellow arrow), and two LSI 13 green signals (white arrows), as seen. (d) Embryo mosaicism becomes apparent by the presence of additional signals Tel 2q (yellow arrows) and LSI 13 (white arrows), indicating that der(13) is also present (identified by an additional Tel 2q and LSI 13 signal) and that the analysis of the first cell in (b), though indicating an unbalanced chromosome complement, did not reveal the complete set of chromosomes being studied, because of mosaicism.

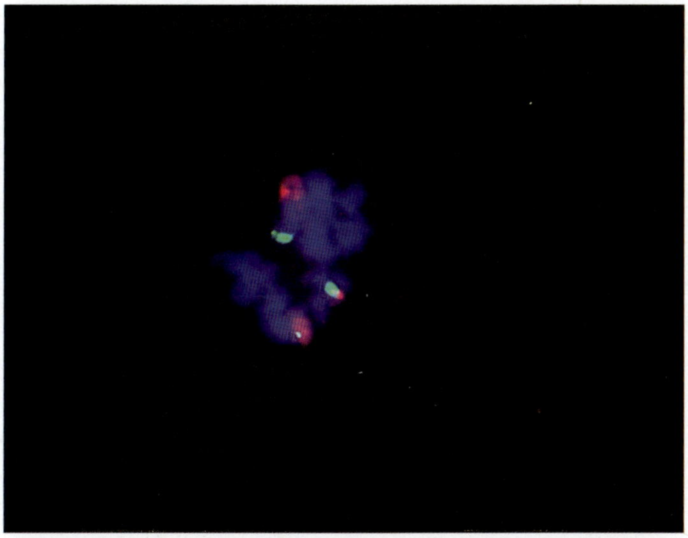

(a)

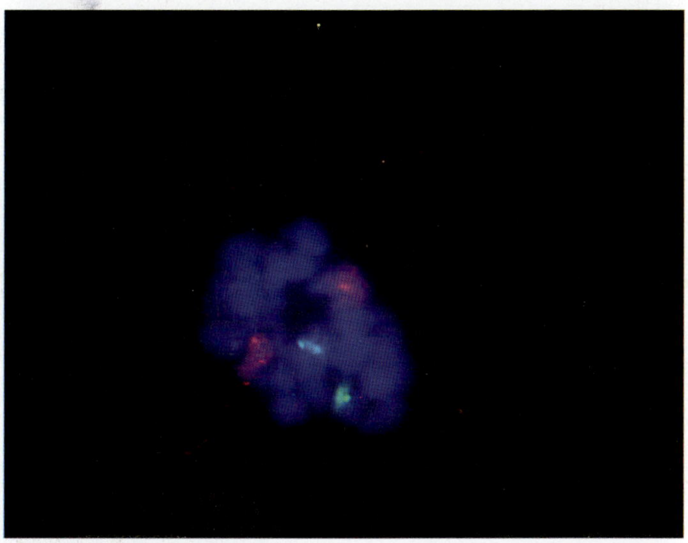

(b)

Figure 5.27 PGD for translocation using the chemical conversion method: (a) FISH analysis of metaphase cell from an embryo obtained through chemical nuclear conversion. Chromosome 5 is identified by whole-chromosome paint (WCP) (red) and telomeric 5p (red). Chromosome 13 is identified by whole-chromosome paint (WCP) (green) and telomeric 13q (green). One normal copy of chromosome 5 and a derivative –der(5) as well as one normal copy of chromosome 13 and a derivative –der(13) are present. The resulting karyotype is 46,XX,t(5;13)(p15.3;q34), indicating a balanced embryo fit for transfer. (b) FISH analysis of metaphase cell from an embryo obtained through chemical nuclear conversion. Two normal copies for each of the chromosomes are present. The resulting karyotype is 46,XX, indicating a normal, translocation-free embryo fit for transfer.

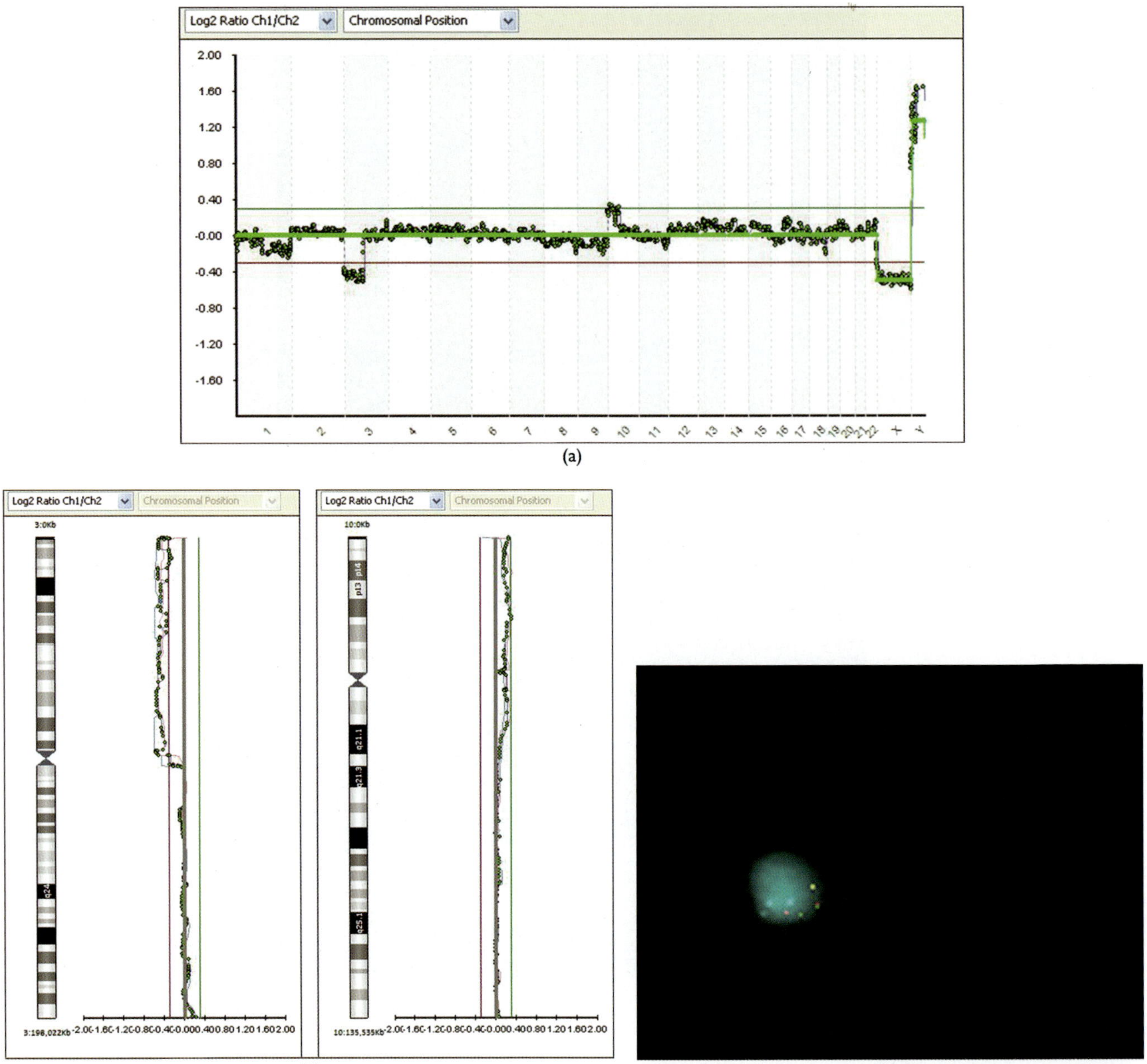

(b) (c)

Figure 5.28 (a) Combined aneuploidy and translocation study of a family with a known carrier of 46,XY,t(3;10)(q11.2;q11.2) detected by array-CGH and confirmed by FISH analysis. (b) CGH chart depicting chromosomes 3 and 10 with respective deletion in the p area and duplication in the q area. (c) FISH image obtained after a whole embryo fixation of the same embryo, confirming array-CGH findings.

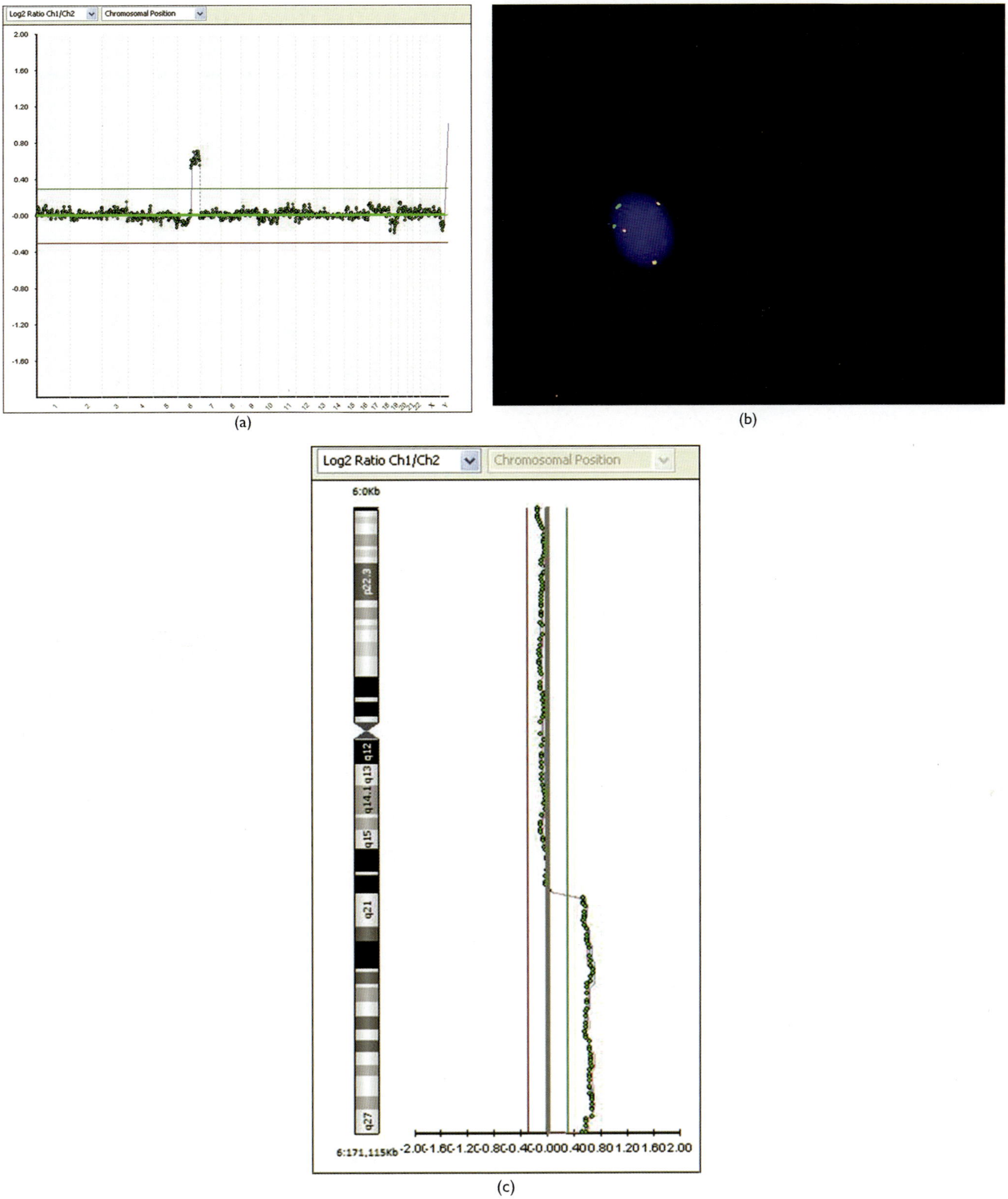

Figure 5.29 PGD for duplication of q arm of chromosome 6 (dup(6)(q21q27)) by array-CGH testing after a trophectoderm biopsy of a day-5 embryo. (a) Duplication of the q arm of chromosome 6. (b) A separate array-CGH chart depicting chromosome 6 with duplication in the q area. (c) FISH image obtained after a whole embryo fixation (WEF) of the same embryo, confirming the above array-CGH findings. Interphase nucleus shows two signals for the p-CEP area of chromosome 6 identified by telomeric 6p (green), while three signals are present for the 6q area identified by telomeric 6q (gold). The karyotype is 46,XY,dup(6)(q21q27).

6 Preimplantation diagnosis for single-gene disorders

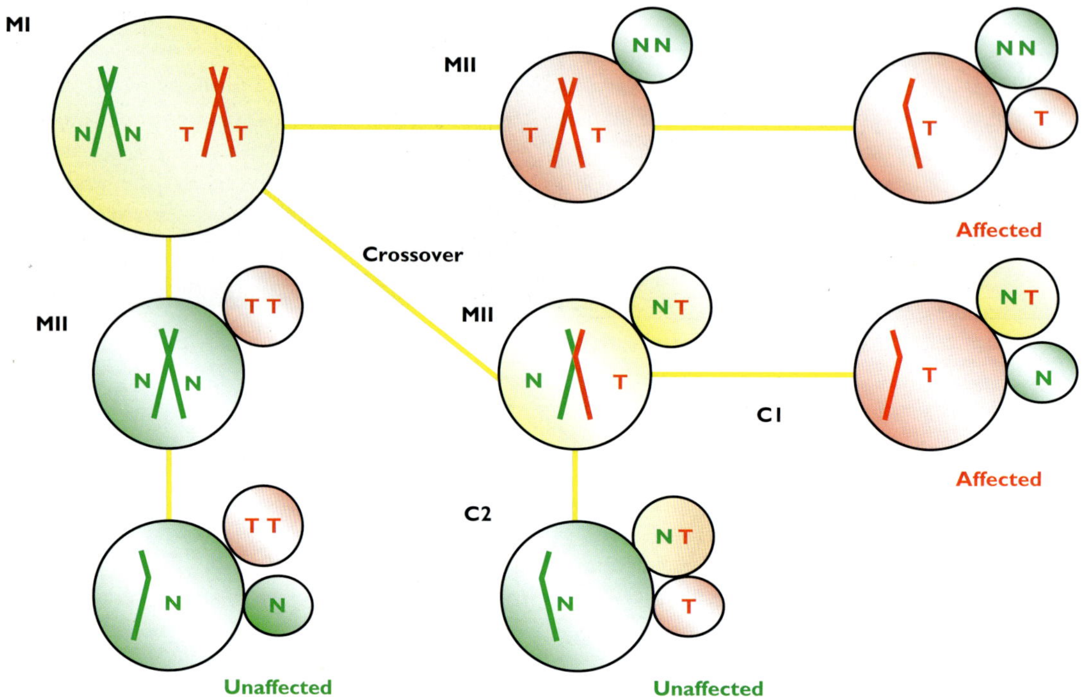

Figure 6.1 Principles of PGD for single-gene disorders by two-step sequential analysis of first and second polar bodies (PB1 and PB2) shown for thalassemia mutations. The large circle represents the genotype of an oocyte obtained from a heterozygous carrier of a mutant gene prior to PB1 extrusion (metaphase I, MI). The other seven large circles show oocytes resulting from the first (metaphase II, MII) and second meiotic divisions. The seven medium-sized circles show extruded PB1s, and the five smallest circles show PB2s. The upper portion of the figure shows extrusion of a homozygous normal PB1, resulting in an affected oocyte. This is confirmed by a mutant PB2 (shaded small circle). The left portion presents the opposite sequence of events. The crossover situation (evidenced by heterozygous PB1) is shown in the middle portion, resulting in either an affected (C1) (evidenced by normal PB2 extrusion) or normal (C2) oocyte (evidenced by abnormal PB2 extrusion). N, normal allele; T, affected (thalassemia) allele; C1 and C2, possible outcomes from heterozygous MII oocyte after the second meiotic division.

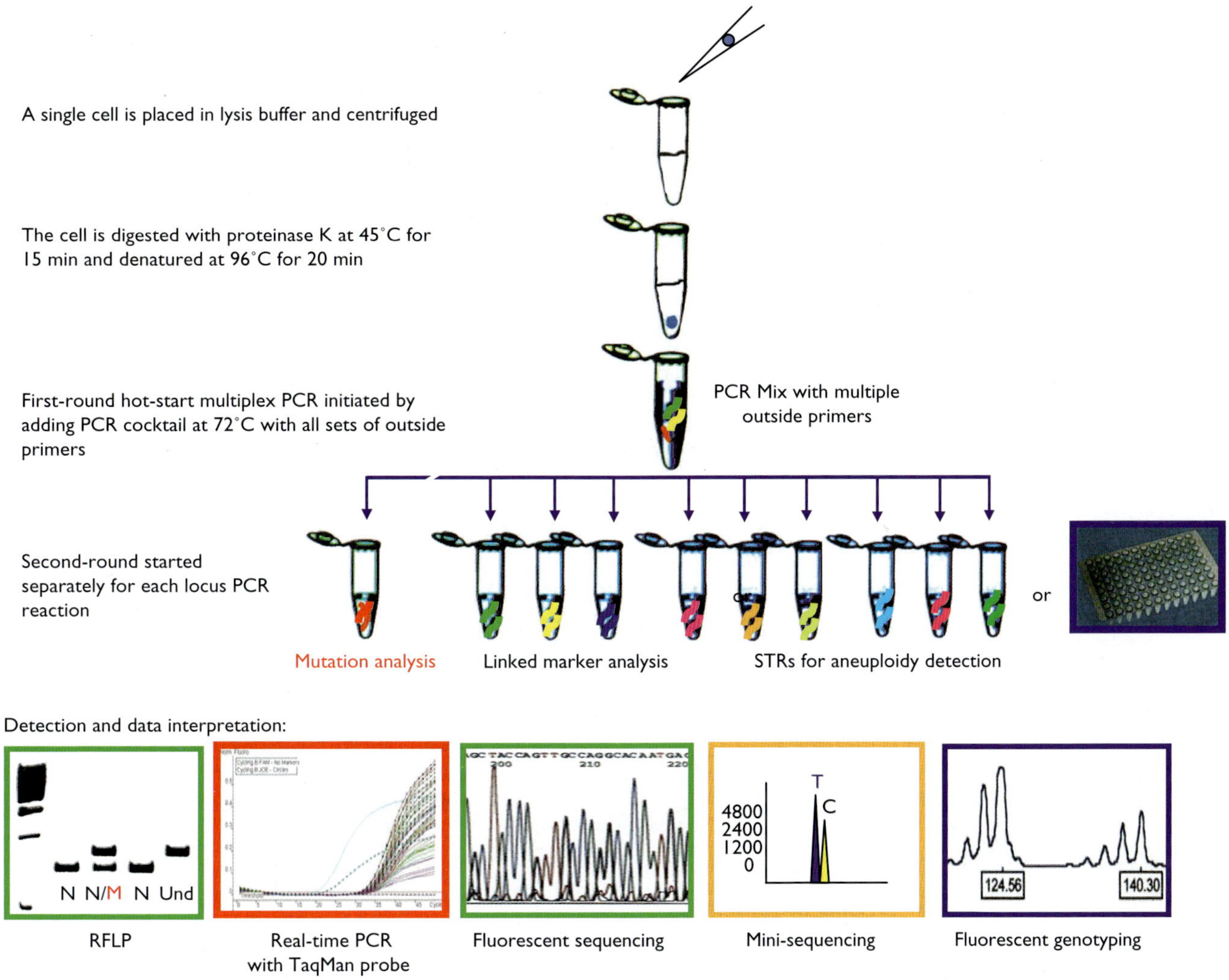

Figure 6.2 Flow chart for multiplex nested PCR applied for PGD. (Top) Scheme showing first-round PCR, with addition of all ten sets of outside primers, followed by aliquoting into ten separate tubes for second-round PCR, with addition of specific inside primers to each tube. (Bottom) Examples of various detection techniques applied for PGD cases, including restriction fragment length polymorphism (RFLP), real-time PCR with TaqMan probes for normal sequence and ΔF508 mutation in *CFTR* gene, fluorescent DNA sequencing reaction for HLA typing, minisequencing for T/C polymorphism, and fluorescent fragment-size analysis of STRs on chromosome 21.

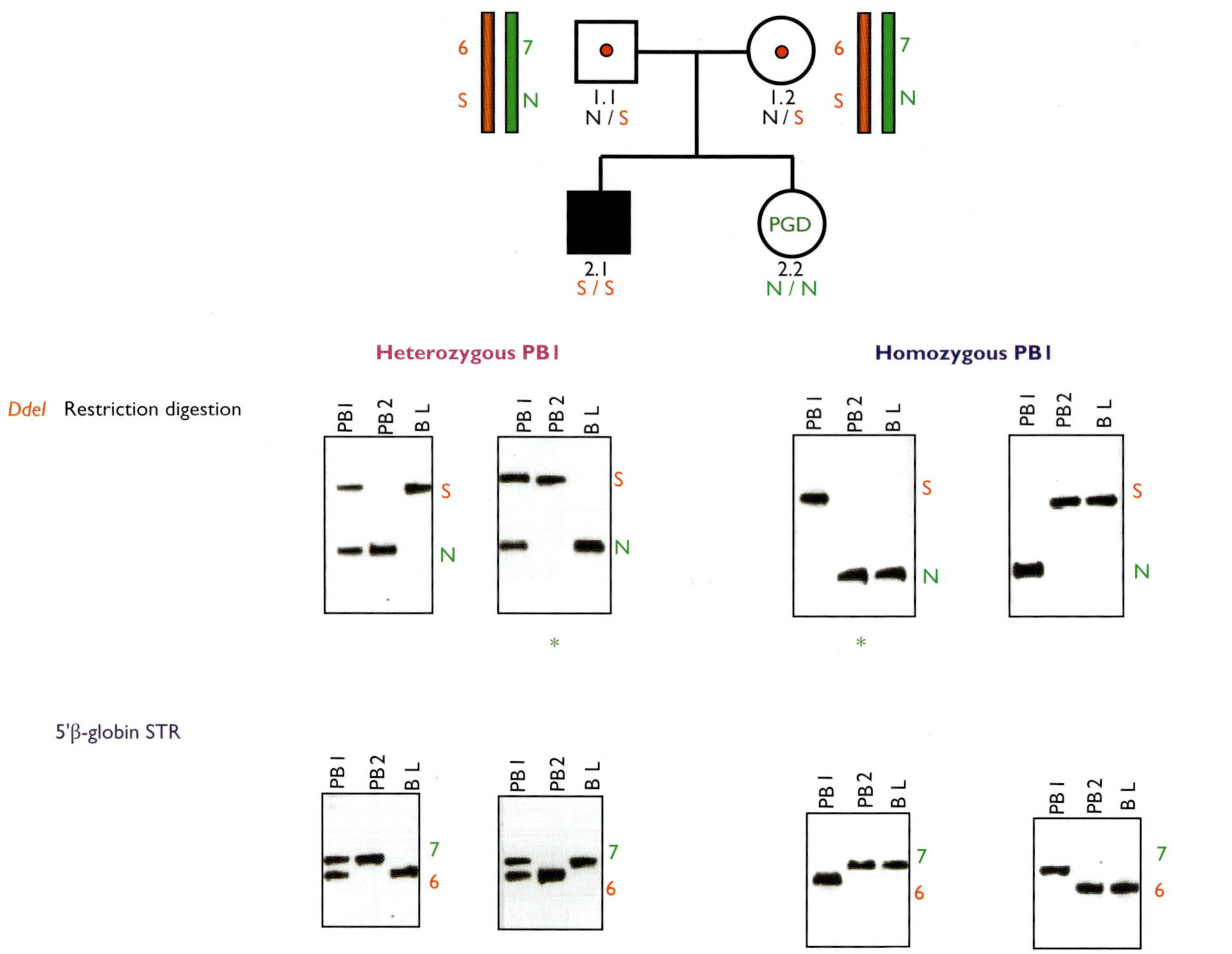

Figure 6.3 Principles of preselection of mutation-free oocytes using linked polymorphism: PGD for sickle cell disease. (Top): Haplotype prediction based on family pedigree genotypes (1.1, 1.2, and 2.1). PGD was performed for carriers (1.1 and 1.2) of sickle cell anemia missense A/T mutation, resulting in the birth of a healthy female child (2.2). Haplotype analysis shows that the girl inherited both normal alleles linked to the seven repeats from her parents. (Middle): *DdeI* restriction digestion of PCR products from first and second polar bodies (PB1 and PB2) and blastomeres (BL) to assay the sickle cell mutation. Examples of PGD based on the heterozygous status of the PB1 and hemizygous normal or abnormal status of the PB2 are shown on the left, demonstrating the prediction of normal unaffected status of the oocyte (*) based on the presence of a heterozygous PB1 and a mutant PB2. This is confirmed by blastomere analysis. An example of preselection of a mutation-free oocyte based on a homozygous mutant PB1 and normal PB2 (*) is shown on the right, also confirmed by blastomere analysis. (Bottom): 5'β-globin STR polymorphism analysis of the same oocytes (six-repeat polymorphism linked to mutant, seven-repeat polymorphism linked to normal allele) is in accordance with (top), confirming the correctness of preselection of normal oocytes (*) for transfer both on left and right. S, sickle cell allele; SS, homozygous for sickle cell mutation; SN, heterozygous sickle cell/unaffected; NN, homozygous unaffected.

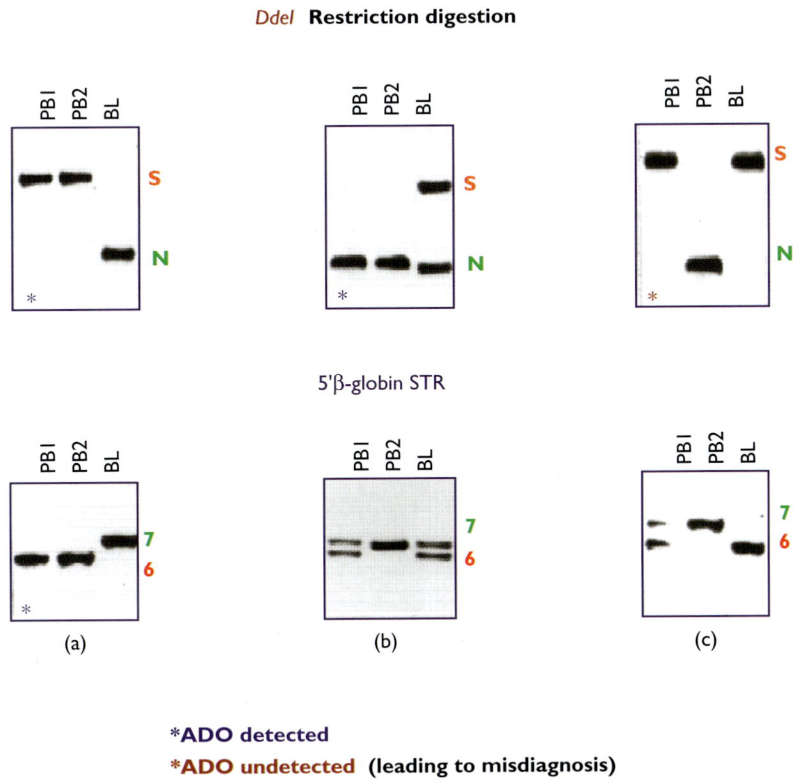

Figure 6.4 Examples of detected and undetected allele dropout (ADO) in the first polar body (PB1). (Top) *DdeI* restriction digestion of PCR products to assay sickle cell mutation. Three different cases, (a), (b), and (c), are assessed. The sickle cell allele (S) gives rise to a larger product than the normal allele (N). In case (a), both the PB1 and second polar body (PB2) are mutant, suggesting ADO of the normal allele in the PB1 (*), and thus implying a normal genotype of the corresponding oocyte. This was confirmed by blastomere (BL) analysis. The opposite situation is seen in case (b), with both the PB1 and PB2 apparently normal, suggesting ADO of the mutant allele in the PB1. The predicted mutant genotype of this oocyte is also in agreement with blastomere analysis showing the presence of both alleles. No accurate genotype prediction is possible for the oocyte in case (c), without linked marker analysis performed simultaneously with the gene (see below). (Bottom) 5'β-globin STR polymorphism (six-repeat polymorphism linked to the mutant allele, and seven-repeat polymorphism linked to the normal allele). In case (a), as is expected from the mutation analysis, both the PB1 and PB2 contain the six-repeat marker, evidencing ADO of the seven-repeat marker in the PB1 (*) and thus suggesting a normal genotype of the corresponding oocyte, as shown by the seven-repeat genotype in blastomere analysis. Marker analysis also confirms ADO of the mutant allele in the PB1 in case (b) (*), based on a PB1 heterozygous for six- and seven-repeat allele. Finally, marker analysis is of particular value in case (c), as it detects ADO of the normal allele in the PB1 (red*), which would have led to misdiagnosis and transfer of the affected embryo had linked polymorphic markers not been used.

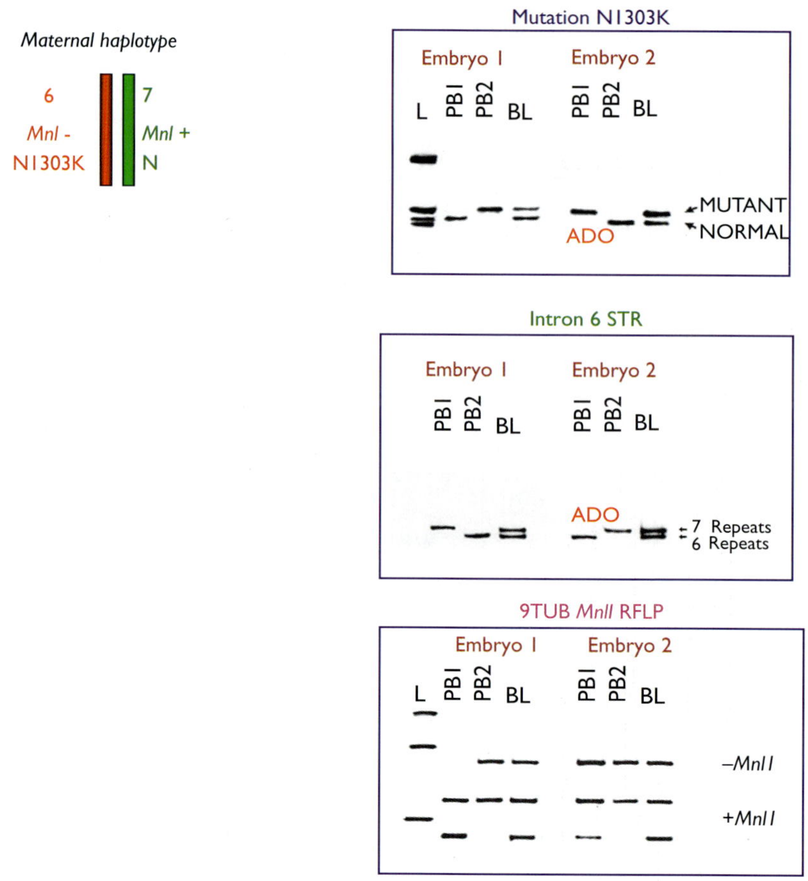

Figure 6.5 Allele dropout (ADO) detection by simultaneous application of two linked markers in PGD for CFTR N1303K mutation. (Upper left) Maternal haplotypes showing the linkage of normal allele to the seven repeats and *Mnl+*, and the mutant to six repeats and *Mnl–*. (Top right) *BstNI* restriction digestion of PCR product to assay N1303K mutation in *CFTR* gene indicates a homozygous normal first polar body (PB1) and affected second polar body (PB2), suggesting the presence of the mutant gene in the corresponding oocyte (embryo 1). This is in agreement with follow-up analysis of blastomeres from the resulting embryo, containing both mutant and normal alleles (left) (confirmation of diagnosis by linked markers is shown below). Mutation analysis of oocyte 2 from the same patient (right) revealed an opposite situation (homozygous mutant PB1/normal PB2), suggesting that the oocyte was normal. However, as shown by marker analysis below, oocyte 2 is actually mutant, due to ADO of the normal allele in the corresponding PB1. (Middle) Testing for intron 6 polymorphism in the PB1, PB2, and blastomeres (six repeats linked to the mutant and seven repeats linked to the normal allele) confirmed the results of mutation analysis, including ADO of the seven-repeat allele in agreement with ADO of the normal allele in the top right assay. (Bottom) Testing the same oocytes for *MnlI* RFLP. The normal allele contains a restriction site for *MnlI* (+) and the mutant allele lacks the site (–). RLFP analysis confirms the results of mutation and intron 6 polymorphism analysis in embryo 1, but contradicts that of embryo 2. In contrast to the initial diagnosis of oocyte 2 as normal by mutation and intron 6 polymorphism analysis (Top and Middle), this oocyte appears to contain a mutant gene, as evidenced by ADO of the normal allele in the corresponding heterozygous PB1, which was diagnosed as homozygous mutant by mutation and intron 6 polymorphism analysis. BL, blastomere; L, size marker ladder.

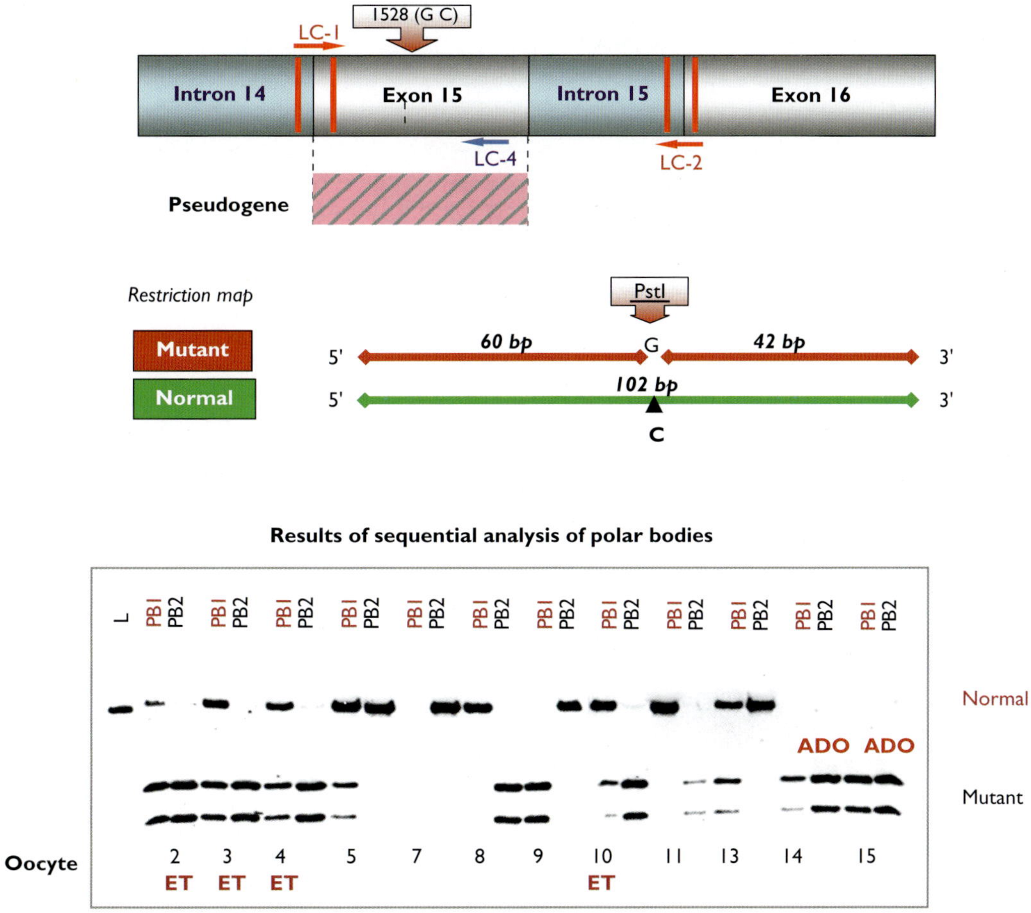

Figure 6.6 Design for PGD for long-chain 3-hydroxyacyl-CoA dehydrogenase deficiency (LCHAD) to overcome misdiagnosis due to pseudogene. (Top) Schematic diagram of heminested PCR for G1528C mutation in *LCHAD* gene on chromosome 2p24.1, showing positions of mutation site and primers involved in PGD. The syntenic pseudogene is shown as a shaded bar directly below exon 15. Outer primers lie outside of the pseudogene. First-round primers LC-1 and LC-2 are designed to span intron 14/exon 15 and intron 15/exon 16 boundaries, eliminating false priming to the pseudogene. Restriction maps of first- and second-round PCR products show band lengths and nucleotide substitution. The G1528C mutation causes formation of *PstI* restriction site in exon 15. Restriction digestion of second-round PCR product from the mutant allele produces two fragments of 60 and 42 bp, while the normal allele results in a single fragment of 102 bp. (Bottom) Polyacrylamide gel electrophoresis of *PstI*-digested PCR product of first (PB1) and second (PB2) polar bodies from 12 oocytes detects four normal oocytes (2, 3, 4, and 10) evidenced by heterozygous PB1 and abnormal PB2. Contradictory results of PB1 (mutant) and PB2 (also mutant) from oocytes 14 and 15 suggest allele dropout (ADO) of the normal allele in the corresponding PB1 (noted by ADO in red). ET, embryo transfer; L, size marker ladder.

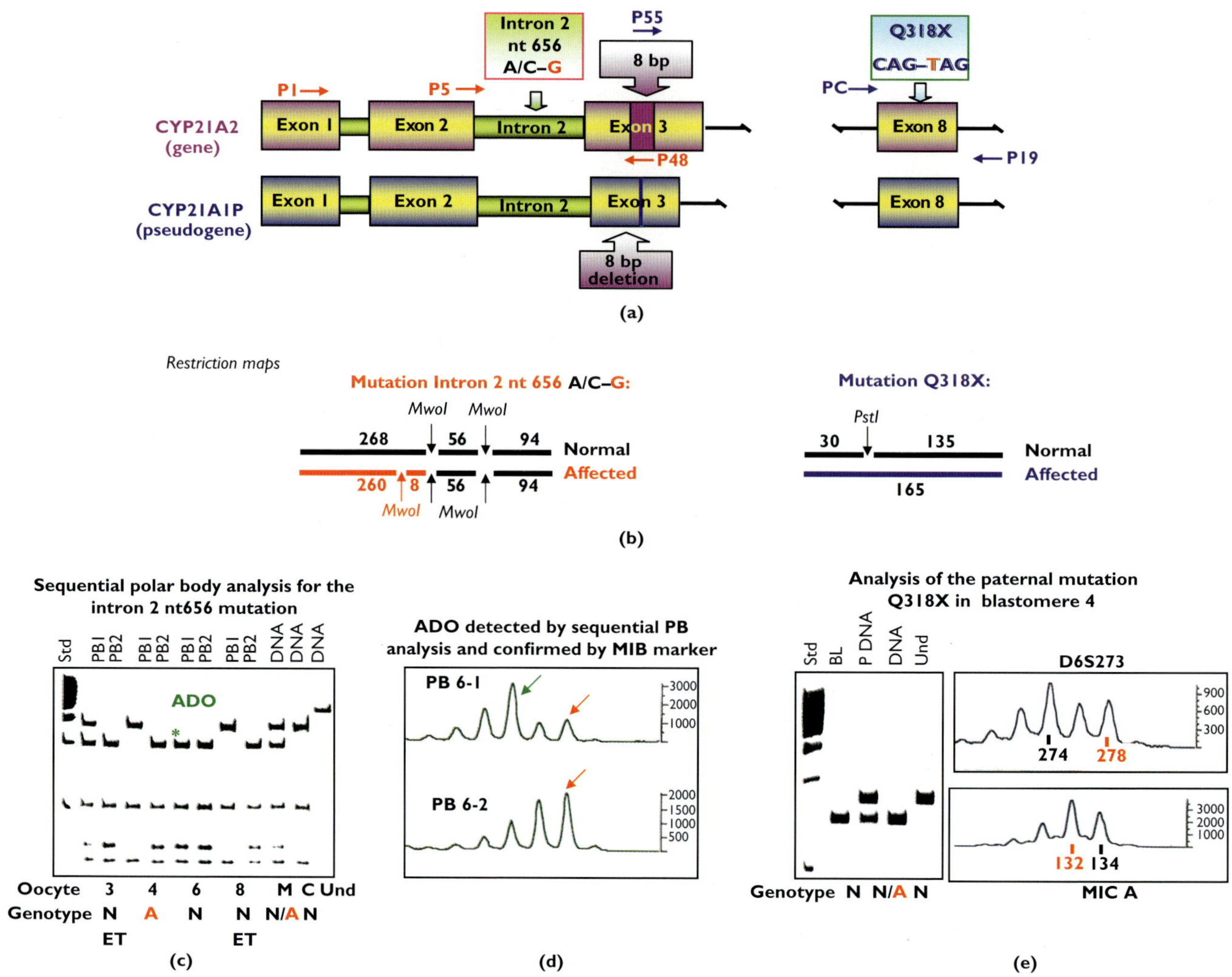

Figure 6.7 Principles of mutation testing in the presence of a pseudogene: PGD for congenital adrenal hyperplasia (CAH). (a) Schematic diagram of heminested PCR for the mutation nt656 located in intron 2 and mutation Q318X positioned in exon 8. The syntenic *CYP21A2* gene (purple) and CYP21A1P pseudogene (blue) share almost 99% of sequences. The major difference between them is an 8-bp deletion in exon 3 of the pseudogene (blue line). Specific primers have 3′ ends complementary to the 8-bp sequence present only in the gene, eliminating any chance of false priming to the pseudogene. Forward primer P55 is used to study mutations located after exon 3. Reverse primer P48 is designed to analyze mutations in exon/intron 1–2. To detect the nt656 mutation, the primer sets P1 and P48 are used in the first-round PCR. Second-round heminested PCR is performed with the primers P5 and P48. To study the Q318X mutation, the primer sets P55 and P19 are added to the first round of PCR. Second-round heminested PCR is performed with the primers PC and P19. (b) Restriction maps of the second-round PCR products showing restriction enzymes for the detection of normal and altered sequences and bended lengths. Mutation nt656 creates a second *MwoI* restriction site. Mutation Q318X eliminates the *PstI* restriction site. (c) Multiplex heminested PCR performed on the polar bodies (PB) to study the maternal mutation and informative linked polymorphic markers (see pedigree in Figure 6.45). Oocytes 3, 6, and 8 were predicted to be normal by mutation and linkage study. The identical affected status of both the first (PB1) and second (PB2) polar bodies from oocyte 6 provides evidence of allele dropout (ADO) of the normal allele (*) in the PB1. This is in agreement with the presence of two MIB markers in this PB1 (d). Oocyte 4 was predicted to be abnormal based on the mutation and linkage analysis. The blastomere from embryo 4 was removed and amplified to study the paternal mutation and polymorphic markers informative for both parents. A normal paternal allele was found, and a carrier status of the maternal mutation was confirmed (e). Std, size standard; N, normal; A, affected; Und, undigested PCR product; M, maternal amplified DNA; C, normal control amplified DNA; green arrow, marker linked to normal allele; red arrow, marker linked to maternal affected allele; PB6-1, the first polar body from oocyte 6; PB6-2, the second polar body from oocyte 6; BL, blastomere; ET, embryo transfer.

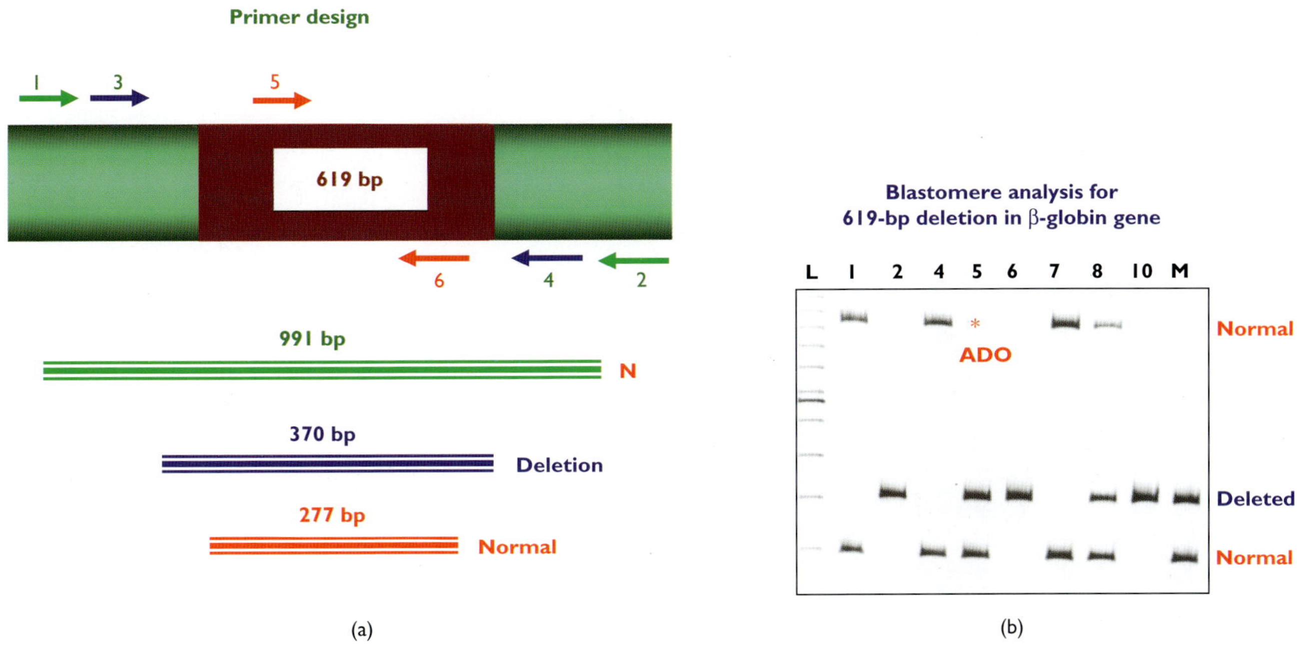

Figure 6.8 A fully nested PCR design for PGD of beta-thalassemia deletion mutation. (a) Primer design strategy for the detection of the 619-bp deletion in the β-globin gene. Fully nested primers positioned outside the mutation break point for simultaneous detection of the deleted and normal sequences in the β-globin gene. The first round of PCR was performed with a set of outside primers 1 and 2 (green arrows). Two separate second-round reactions were run. One tube contained nested primers 3 and 4 (blue arrows) surrounding the deletion, and the other had nested primers 5 and 6 (red arrows), which were specific for the sequence from the deleted area. Second-round PCR generated different-length fragments providing the information about the presence/absence of the deleted sequence and predicting normal, mutant, or heterozygous genotypes. The normal sequence is detected by the presence of either 991-bp and 277-bp PCR products, or the latter alone. The mutant sequence is predicted by the presence of the 370-bp fragment. (b) Blastomere analysis for the detection of the 619-bp deletion mutation in the β-globin gene, with both parents being carriers of the same mutation. Embryos 2, 6, and 10 are predicted to be affected based on the presence of the 370-bp band corresponding to the deleted sequence. Embryos 1, 4, and 7 are predicted to be normal based on the presence of both the 991-bp and 277-bp bands. Embryos 5 and 8 demonstrate a heterozygous genotype evidenced by the presence of two (370 and 277 bp) or three bands (991, 370, and 277 bp). The application of the second set of primers (5 and 6), which generate a much smaller (277-bp) normal band, allowed detection of allele dropout (ADO) of the 991-bp normal band in embryo 8. This approach greatly improves the ADO detection rate and the accuracy of the analysis. L, size standard; M, homozygous mutant genomic DNA (positive control).

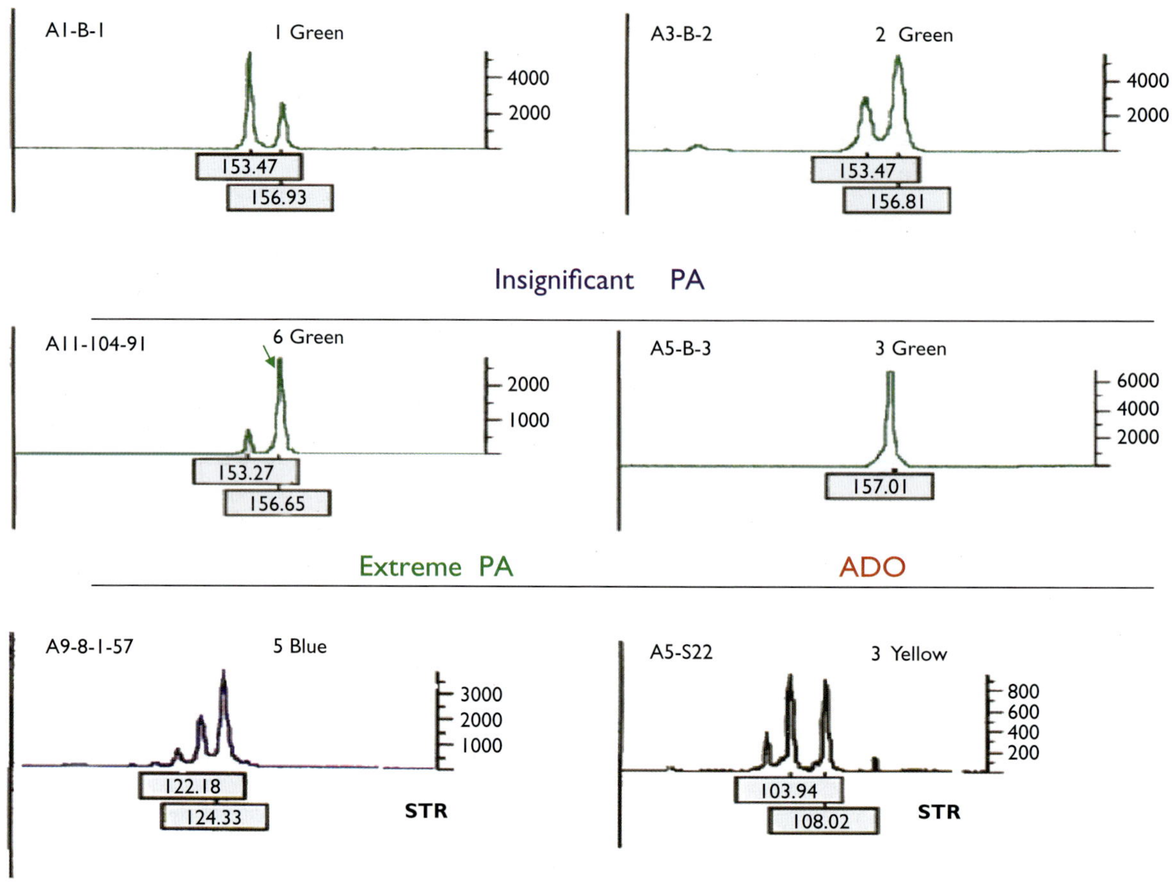

Figure 6.9 Examples of preferential amplification (PA) in single human fibroblasts heterozygous for ΔF508 mutation in the *CFTR* gene (capillary electrophoresis of fluorescent PCR product). (Top) Examples of PA with no significant difference in amplification of normal or mutant alleles (PA of mutant 153-bp allele (left) and PA of normal 156-bp allele (right)). (Middle) Examples of extreme differences in amplification of normal and affected alleles (left), and allele dropout (ADO) of the affected allele (completely missing 153-bp peak) (right). (Bottom) Insignificant PA of a 124-bp dinucleotide repeat in intron 8 (left), compared to equal amplification of intron 6 short tandem repeat (STR) (right).

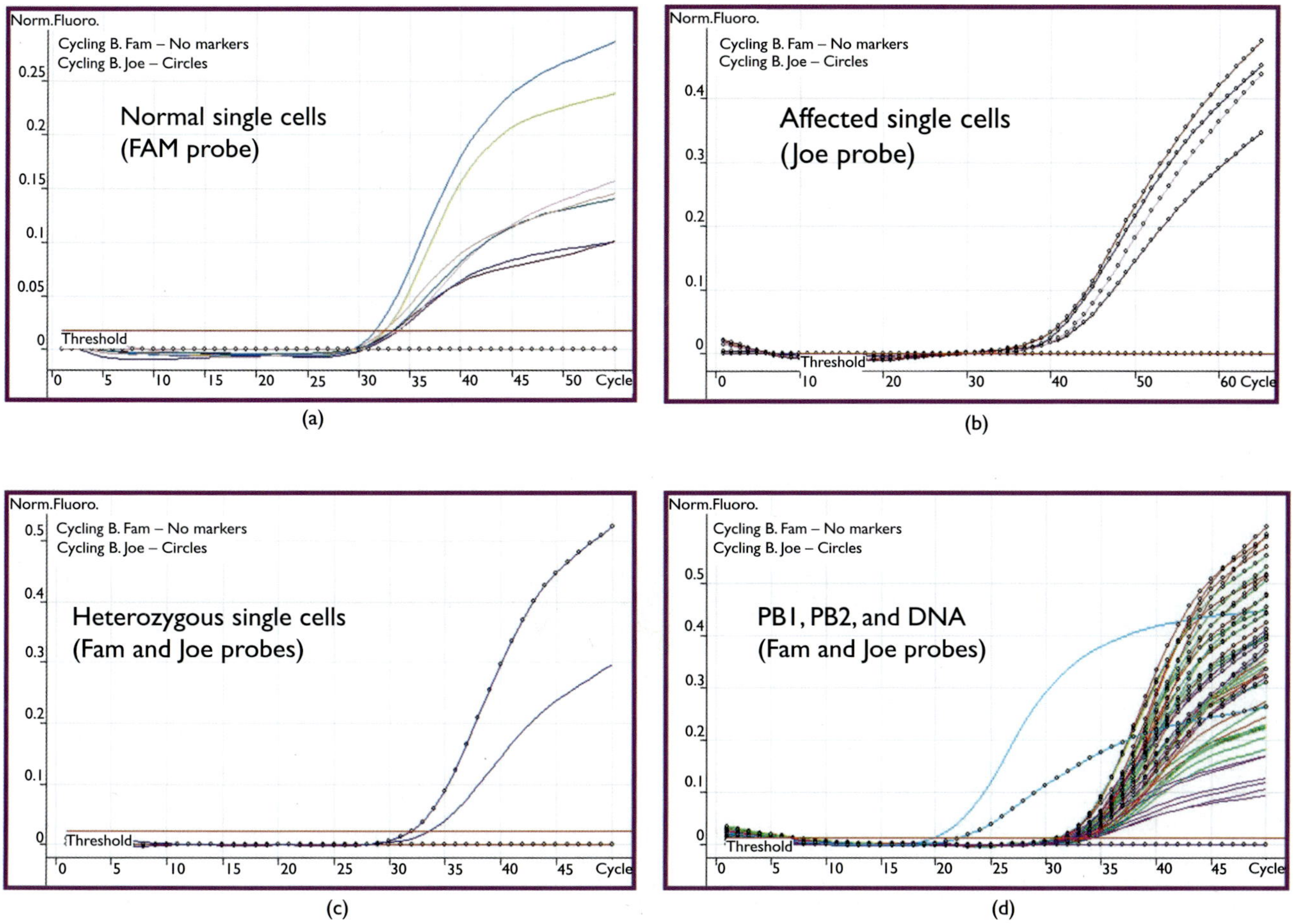

Figure 6.14 Dual-probe real-time PCR of single cells heterozygous for ΔF508. Forty-five cycles of first-round PCR were performed in the presence of both normal and mutant ΔF508 TaqMan probes. The solid lines correspond to the normal sequence generated as a result of normal probe displacement, cleavage, and the release of Fam reporter dye attached to this probe. The solid lines with circles correspond to the mutant sequence generated as a result of ΔF508 probe displacement, cleavage, and the release of Joe reporter dye attached to this probe. (a) Real-time amplification pattern obtained from seven single fibroblasts homozygous for the normal allele. The selective reaction with only the normal probe demonstrates the normal genotype of the cells. (b) Real-time amplification pattern obtained from four single fibroblasts homozygous for the affected allele. The selective reaction with only the mutant probe demonstrates the affected genotype of the cells. (c) Real-time amplification pattern from one fibroblast heterozygous for ΔF508 mutation in *CFTR* gene. The reaction with both probes confirms the heterozygous status of the cell. (d) Real-time amplification pattern obtained from first polar body (PB1), second polar body (PB2), and maternal genomic DNA during PGD for ΔF508 mutation in *CFTR* gene. Evaluation of the genomic DNA samples was possible after 25 cycles of PCR, while single-cell results were detectable only after 35 cycles. Single-cell amplification requires at least ten more cycles to generate detectable real-time PCR results.

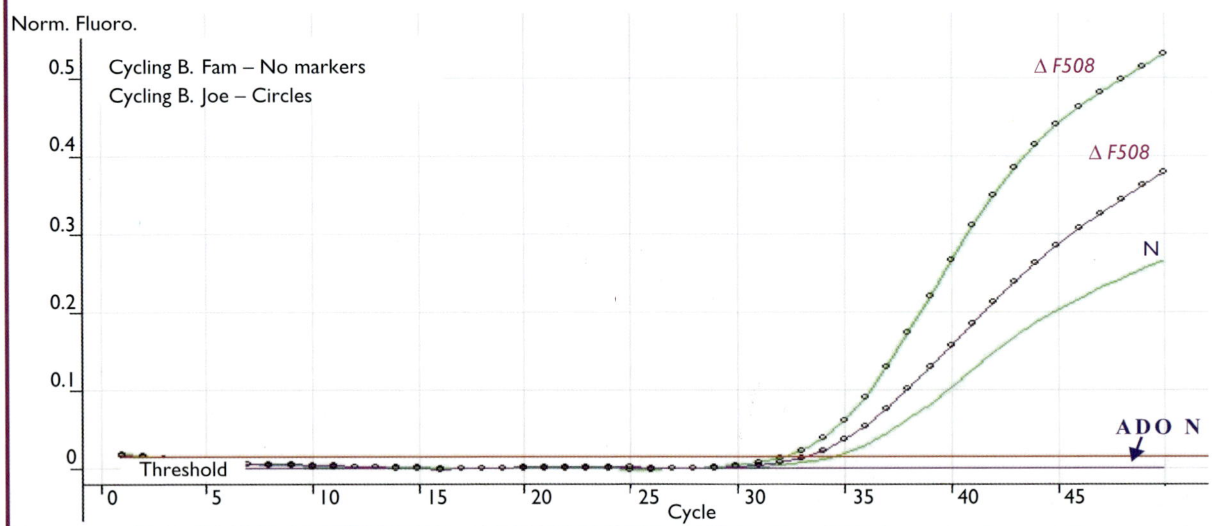

No.	Color	Name	Genotype	Cycling B.Fam	Cycling B.Joe
1		SC-1	Heterozygous	Reaction	Reaction
2		SC-2	**Normal**	No reaction	Reaction

Figure 6.15 Allele dropout (ADO) pattern generated by real-time PCR with TaqMan probe from single fibroblast heterozygous for ΔF508 mutation in *CFTR* gene. Forty-five cycles of first-round PCR were performed in the presence of both normal and ΔF508 mutant for cystic fibrosis TaqMan probes. Single cell 1 is indicated in green and single cell 2 in purple. Two green lines were generated from single cell 1, one solid green line corresponding to the normal allele and the other with circles corresponding to the mutant sequence, indicating the heterozygous status of the studied fibroblast. The presence of only the affected allele (purple solid line with circles) was detected in single cell 2, suggesting ADO of the normal allele, which occurred during the first round of PCR. This demonstrates the occurrence of ADO even in real-time PCR of single cells, indicative of an extremely sensitive detection system, which also cannot completely prevent misdiagnosis.

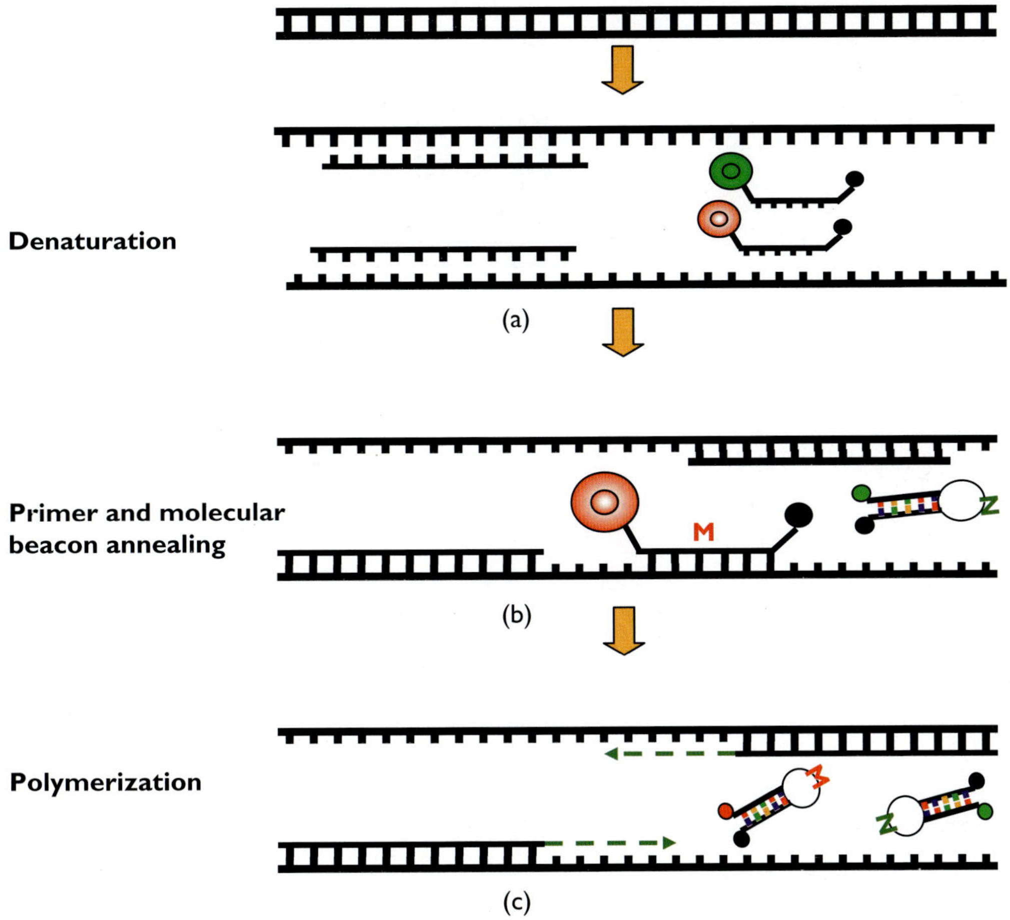

Figure 6.16 Dynamics of real-time PCR based on molecular beacons (MBs). (a) MBs are designed to be complementary to a sequence in the middle of the expected amplicon. During the denaturation step, the MB is uncoiled and fluorescence occurs. (b) In the presence of a target, a sequence-specific MB binds to the amplicons and generates fluorescence. (c) During the extension step, the MB dissociates from the targets, and fluorescence is again quenched. A new hybridization takes place in the annealing step of every cycle, and the intensity of the resulting fluorescence indicates the amount of accumulated PCR product at the end of the previous cycle. M, mutant; N, normal.

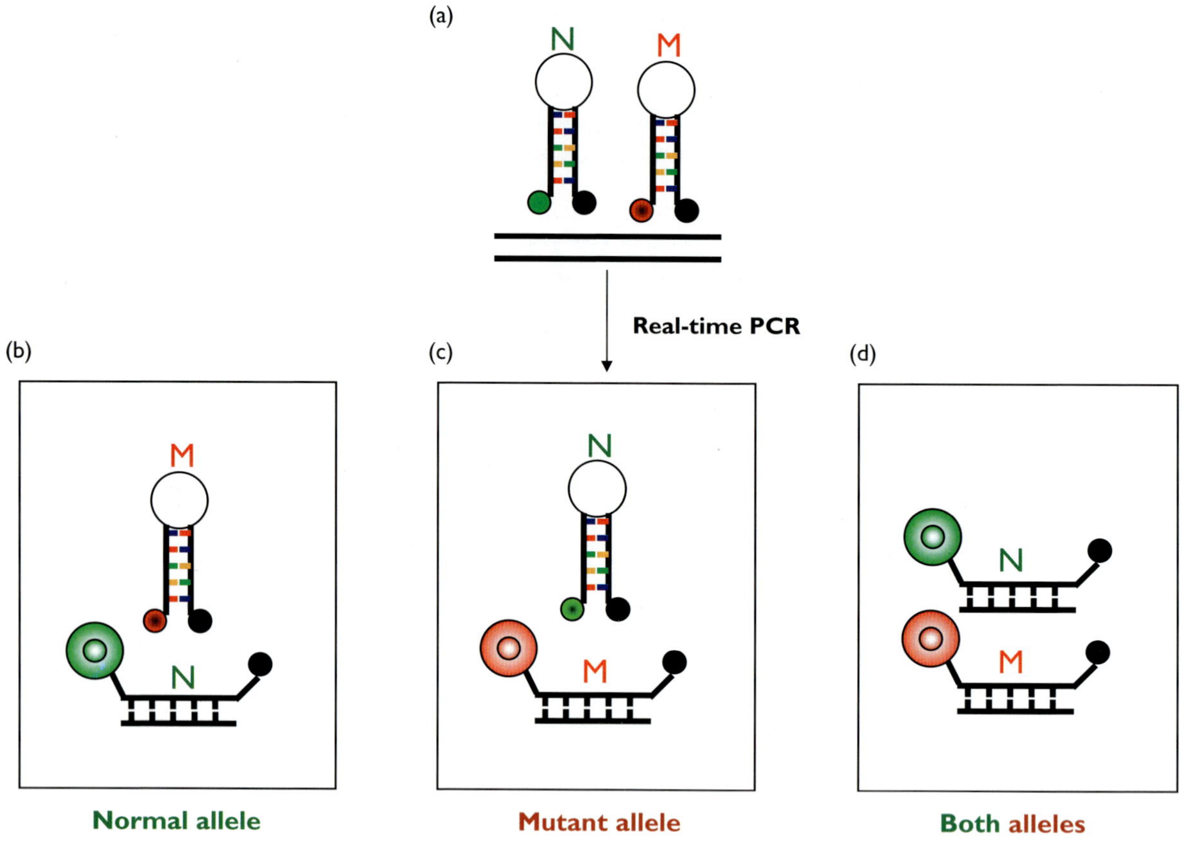

Figure 6.17 Genotyping of real-time PCR product using molecular beacon (MB) probes. (a) Two allele-specific MBs are added to the PCR tube. The green circle probe has a normal sequence (N), and the red circle probe has a mutant sequence (M). (b) The green signal indicates the presence of only a normal allele in the tube. (c) The red signal indicates the presence of only a mutant allele in the tube. (d) The presence of both the red and green signals indicates the amplification of both the mutant and normal alleles.

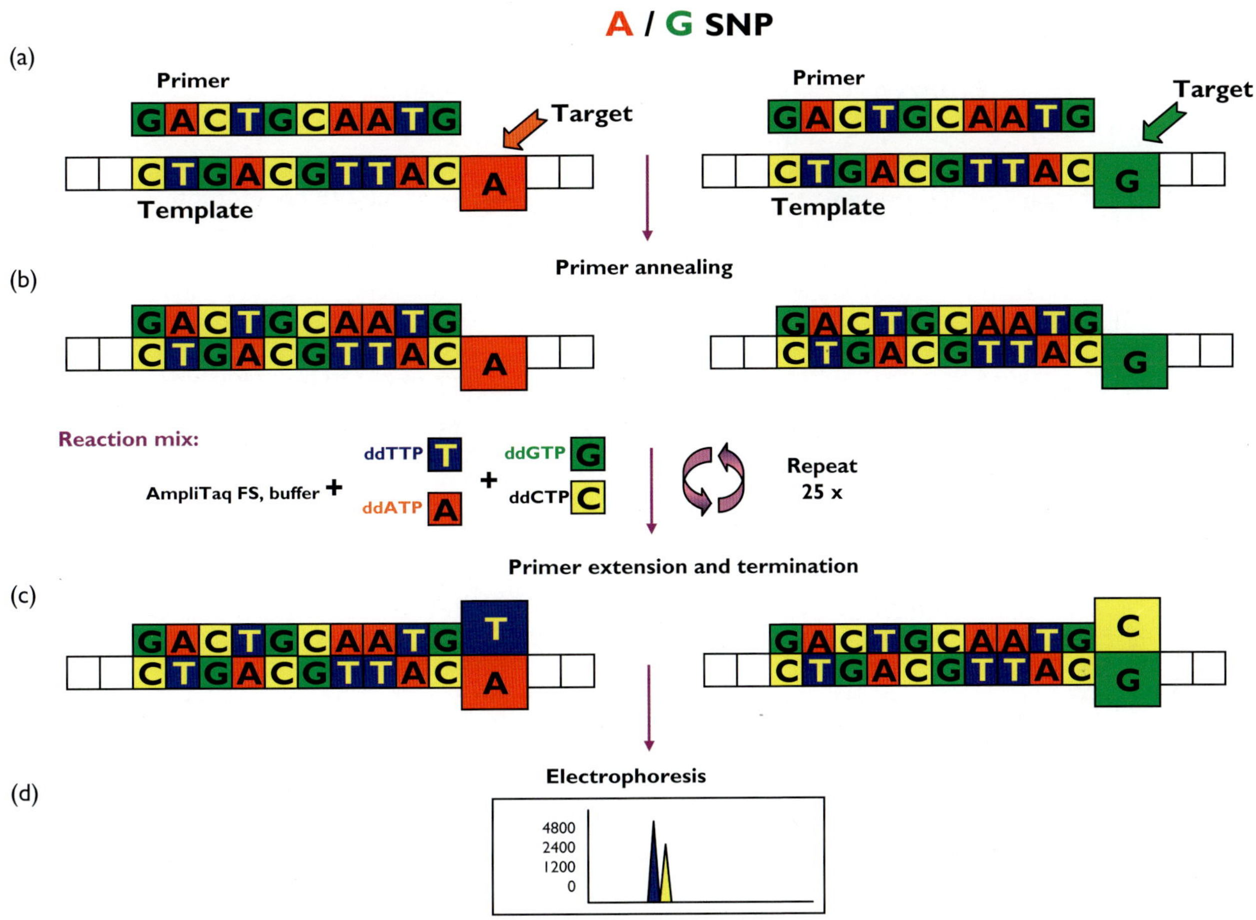

Figure 6.18 Single base-pair A/G polymorphism detection by minisequencing. Minisequencing is designed for the detection of single-nucleotide polymorphisms (SNPs). The distinction between SNP genotypes is based on the high accuracy of nucleotide incorporation by the Taq polymerase. Minisequencing technology involves the extension of a specific primer that hybridizes to the template with its 3' end immediately adjacent to the polymorphic or mutant site (a) and (b). Primer extension reactions contain four fluorescently labeled dideoxynucleotides (ddNTPs). Incorporation of the differently labeled ddNTPs depends upon the genotype. In the absence of ddNTPs the reaction is terminated after the incorporation of a single sequence-specific ddNTP (c). In this particular instance, the reaction was terminated by the incorporation of blue ddTTP (left) and yellow ddCTP (right). Primer annealing, extension, and termination are repeated during 25 cycles of PCR to generate fluorescently labeled fragments recognizable by capillary electrophoresis on a DNA sequencer (d).

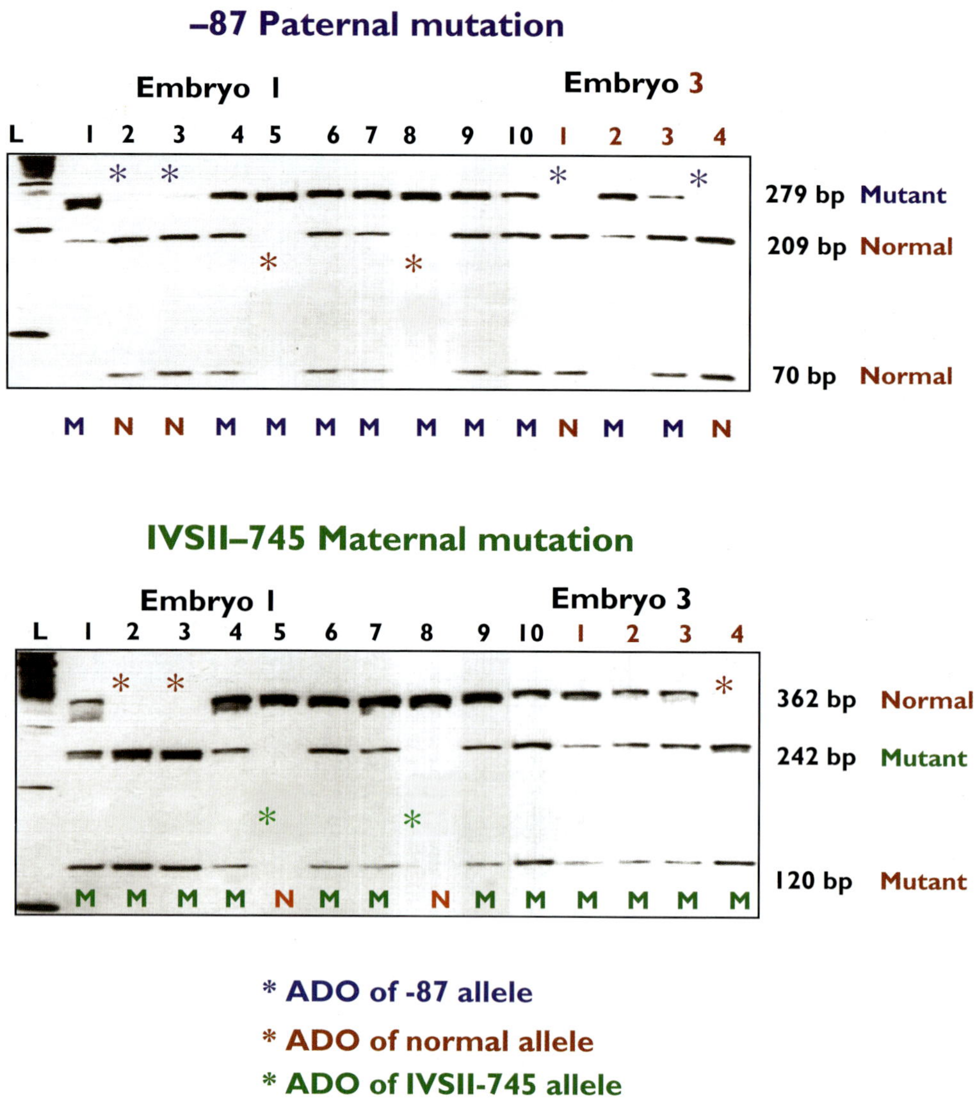

Figure 6.19 Allele dropout (ADO) as a possible cause of misdiagnosis in compound heterozygous blastomeres. (Top) Polyacrylamide gel analysis of -87 (paternal) mutation in the β-globin gene in dissociated single blastomeres from two compound heterozygous embryos (embryo 1, blastomeres 1–10; and embryo 3, blastomeres 1–4). PCR products were digested with restriction enzyme AvrII, giving rise to a 279-bp undigested fragment (mutant allele), a 209-bp restriction fragment (normal allele), and a 70-bp restriction fragment (normal allele). Blastomeres 2 and 3 from embryo 1, and 1 and 4 from embryo 3, demonstrate ADO of the mutant allele, while blastomeres 5 and 8 from embryo 1 failed to amplify a normal allele. ADO of the mutant allele in blastomeres of both embryos (blue asterisk) will potentially lead to misdiagnosis if not detected by marker analysis. (Bottom) Polyacrylamide gel analysis of IVSII-745 (maternal) mutation in the β-globin gene in dissociated single blastomeres from the same heterozygous embryos as above. PCR products were digested with restriction enzyme *RsaI*, giving rise to a 362-bp undigested fragment (normal allele), a 242-bp restriction fragment (mutant allele), and a 120-bp restriction fragment (mutant allele). Blastomeres 2 and 3 from embryo 1, as well as blastomere 4 from embryo 3, demonstrate ADO of the normal allele, while blastomeres 5 and 8 from embryo 1 failed to amplify a mutant allele. The latter will potentially lead to misdiagnosis in the absence of simultaneous amplification of linked markers. The results show that even simultaneous analysis of both paternal and maternal mutations does not eliminate the risk of misdiagnosis, since ADO cannot be detected for both paternal and maternal mutations in the same blastomeres (blastomeres 2, 3, 5, and 8 from embryo 1, and blastomere 4 from embryo 3). L, size marker ladder; M, mutant allele; N, normal allele.

(a)

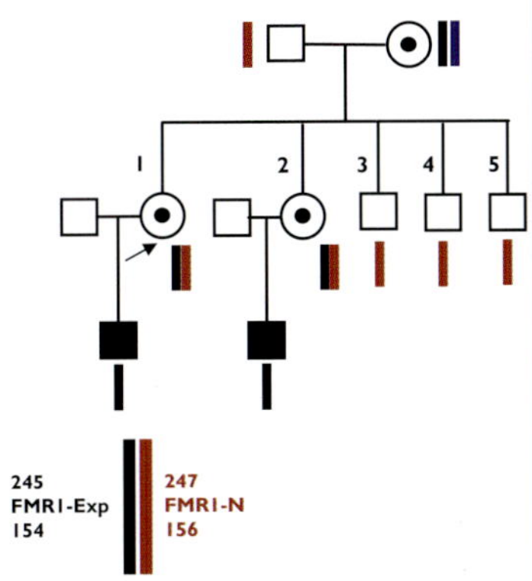

(b)

Oocyte	Cell type	DXs1193	DXs548	Predicted genotype
1	PB1	154 / 156	245 / 247	AFFECTED
	PB2	156	247	
3	PB1	154 / 156	245 / 247	AFFECTED
	PB2	156	247	
5	PB1	154 / 156	245 / 247	NORMAL
	PB2	154	245	
6	PB1	154 / 156	245 / 247	NORMAL
	PB2	154	247	
9	PB1	154*	245*	NORMAL*
	PB2	156	247	
10	PB1	154 / 156	245 / 247	AFFECTED
	PB2	156	247	
Cord blood		154	245	AFFECTED

Figure 6.20 Misdiagnosis in PGD for fragile-X syndrome: table (b) and pedigree (a) with PGD results of haplotype analysis for CGG expansion in *FMR1* gene using two linked markers. On the right of (a) haplotypes of the mother carrying an expanded allele shown linked to 154 and 245 markers (in black). The haplotype of two sisters with the same expanded allele inherited from their mother is shown in black. One of the sisters who presented for PGD is shown by the arrow. The other sister has an affected son, who carries only the expanded allele (linked to 154 and 245 markers). On the left of the pedigree, an affected child carrying only an expanded allele (linked to 154 and 245 markers) was born following PGD, due to the predicted 5% risk of misdiagnosis resulting from undetected allele dropout (ADO) of the normal allele in the first polar body (PB1) of the corresponding oocyte (* in the table (b)), from which the transferred embryo derived. As can be seen from the table, misdiagnosis originates from undetected ADO of both markers linked to the expanded allele in the PB1 of oocyte 9, which was erroneously considered to be homozygous mutant, while it was actually heterozygous; following the extrusion of the second polar body (PB2) with a normal allele, the maternal contribution to the resulting oocytes should have been considered mutant.

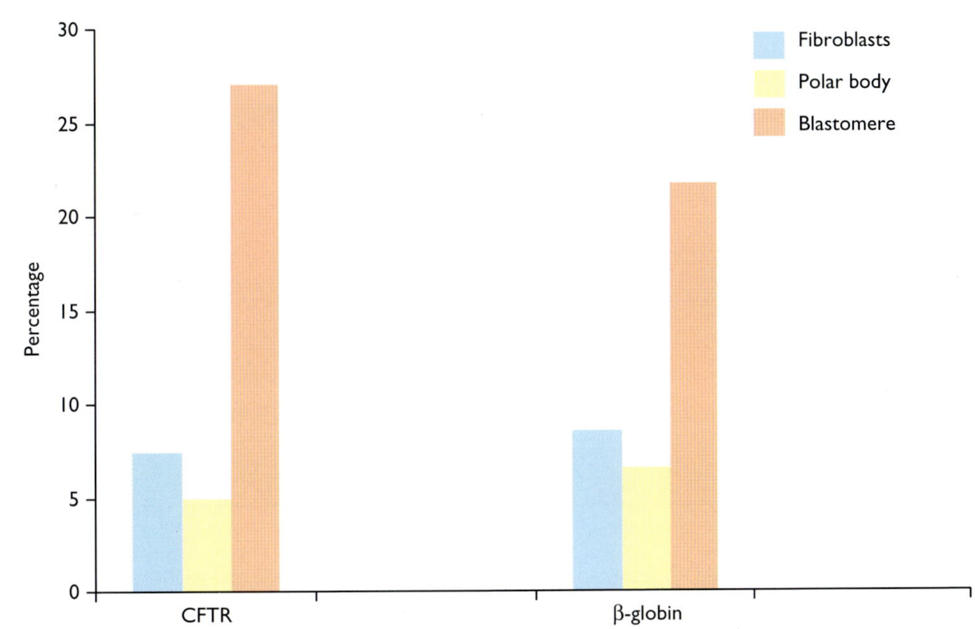

Figure 6.21 Allele dropout (ADO) rate in different types of single cells. In the case of the *CFTR* gene, a significantly higher ADO rate is seen in blastomeres (red bar: 27.1%) heterozygous for ΔF508 mutation than in single human fibroblasts (blue bar: 7.4%) and first polar bodies (PB1) (yellow bar: 5%). Similarly, a significantly higher ADO rate is seen in blastomeres (red bar: 27.1%) heterozygous for sickle cell anemia mutation in the β-globin gene compared to single human fibroblasts (blue bar: 8.6%) and PB1 (yellow bar: 6.6%).

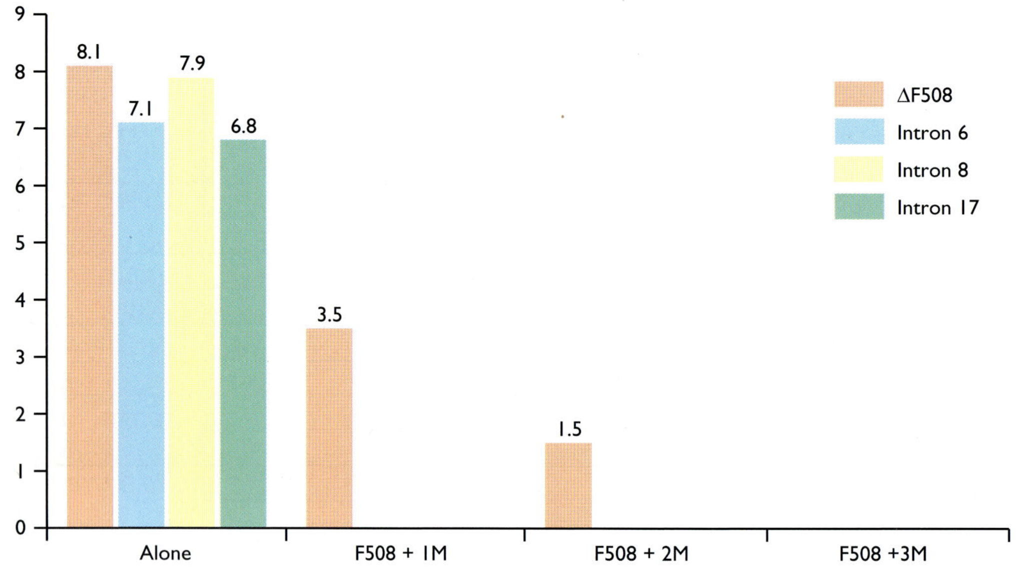

Figure 6.22 Allele dropout (ADO) detection with application of additional linked markers. ADO rates are shown for single and multiplex PCR reaction with single human fibroblasts heterozygous for ΔF508 mutation in the *CFTR* gene. Comparable ADO rates are seen in separate single PCR reactions for each of four loci, including ΔF508 mutation (red bar: 8.1%), linked intron 6 STR (blue bar: 7.1%), linked intron 8 dinucleotide repeat (yellow bar: 7.9%), and intron 17 dinucleotide repeat (green bar: 6.8%). However, simultaneous analysis of two linked loci (ΔF508 mutation and intron 6 STR) reduces ADO rates by more than half (second red bar: 3.5%). Simultaneous analysis of three loci (ΔF508 intron 6 STR and intron 8 dinucleotide repeat) further reduces the ADO rate. ADO is eliminated with multiplex PCR involving three markers in combination with ΔF508 mutation analysis. M, linked marker.

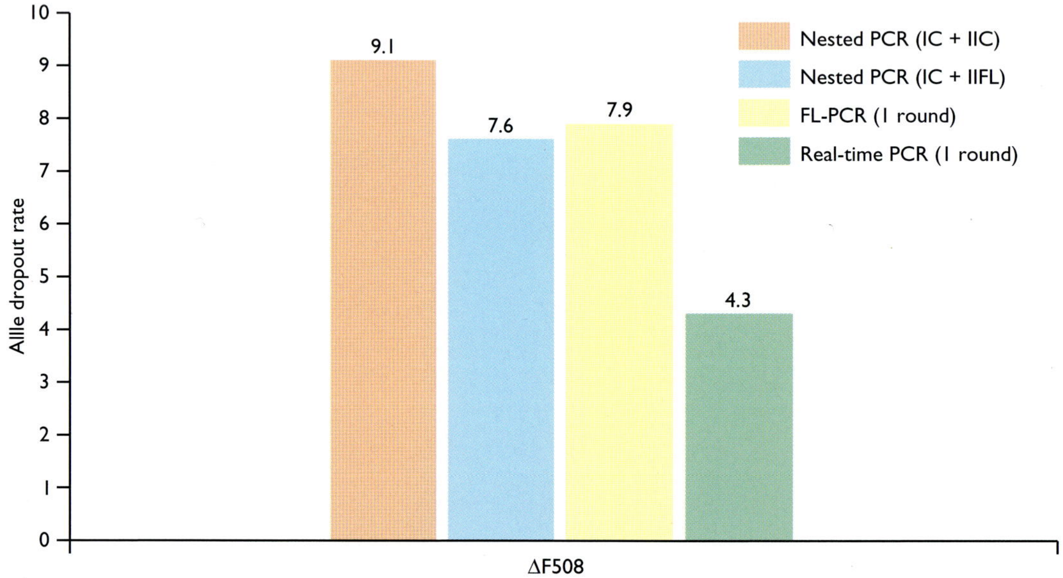

Figure 6.23 Comparison of allele dropout (ADO) rates following fluorescent, conventional, and real-time PCR. ADO rates are shown for nested conventional PCR (red bar), nested combined PCR (first-round conventional, second-round fluorescent: blue bar), one round of fluorescent PCR (yellow bar), and one round of real-time PCR (green bar) with single human fibroblasts heterozygous for ΔF508 mutation in the *CFTR* gene. Comparable ADO rates are seen in the first three types of PCR. The application of one round of real-time PCR reduces ADO in single fibroblasts by almost half. This demonstrates that real-time PCR is the most sensitive method for detection of ADO, although it cannot completely prevent misdiagnosis. IC, first round conventional PCR; IIC, second-round conventional PCR; IIFL, second-round fluorescent PCR.

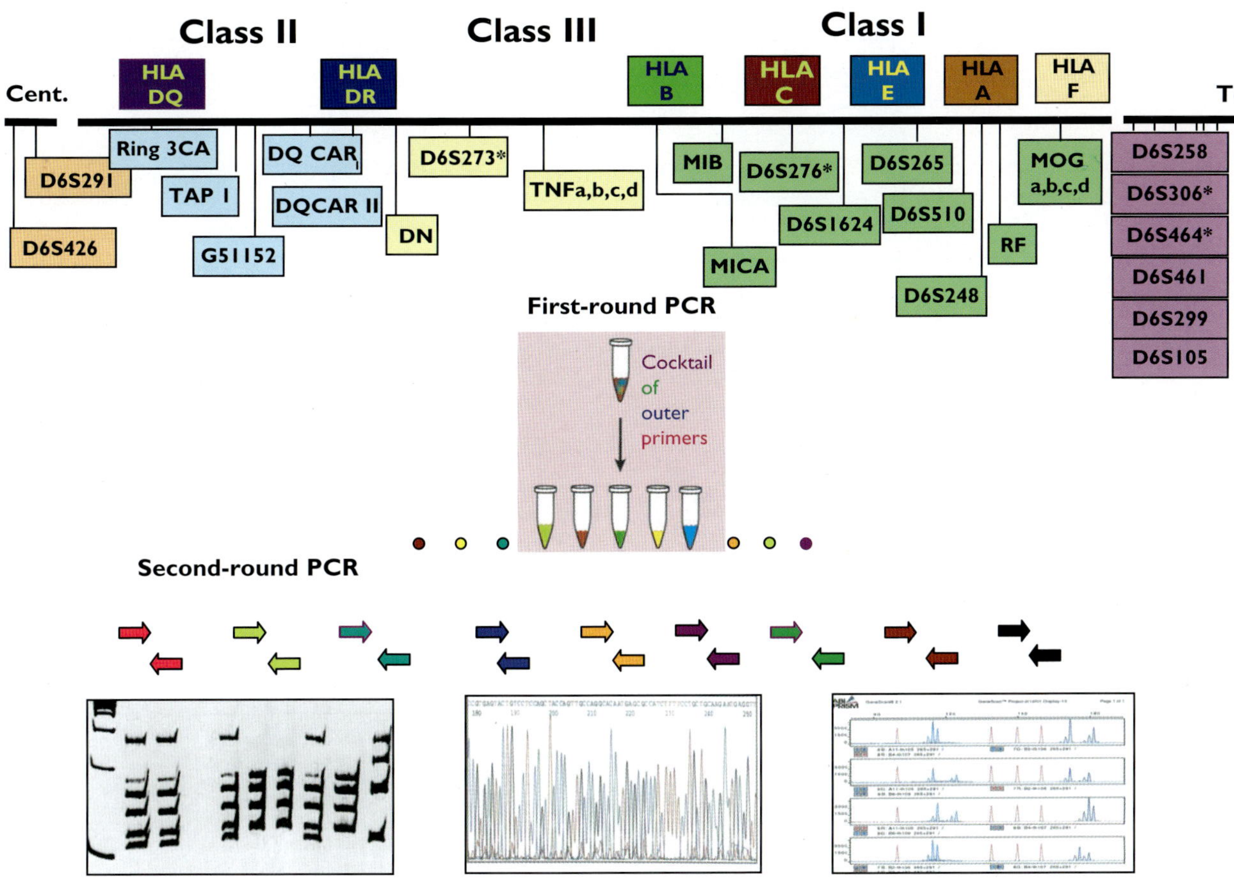

Figure 6.24 Flow chart for multiplex nested PCR applied for preimplantation HLA typing. (Top) Schematic representation of short tandem repeat (STR) and human leukocyte antigen (HLA) genes in HLA classes I, II, and III located on chromosome 6p21.3. All STR markers are dinucleotide repeats (AC)n, except for DQCARII, which is (CTG)n; TNF b, c, d, which are (CT)n; 62, which is (TC-CA)n; Mic A, which is (GCT)n; D6S510, which is (CA-GA)n; and MOG d, which is (CTC)n. Cent., centromere; Tel., telomere. (Middle) Scheme showing first-round PCR, with the addition of all sets of outside primers informative for the particular family, followed by transfer of the PCR product into separate second-round PCR tubes containing inside primers specific for each locus. (Bottom) Different approaches to PCR product detection and analysis. Amplification of HLA A, HLA B, and HLA C alleles with sequence-specific primers (left), fluorescent DNA sequence of HLA B allele from a single-cell nested PCR sequencing reaction (center), and fluorescent fragment-size analysis of D6S291 and D6D265 dinucleotide polymorphic markers (right).

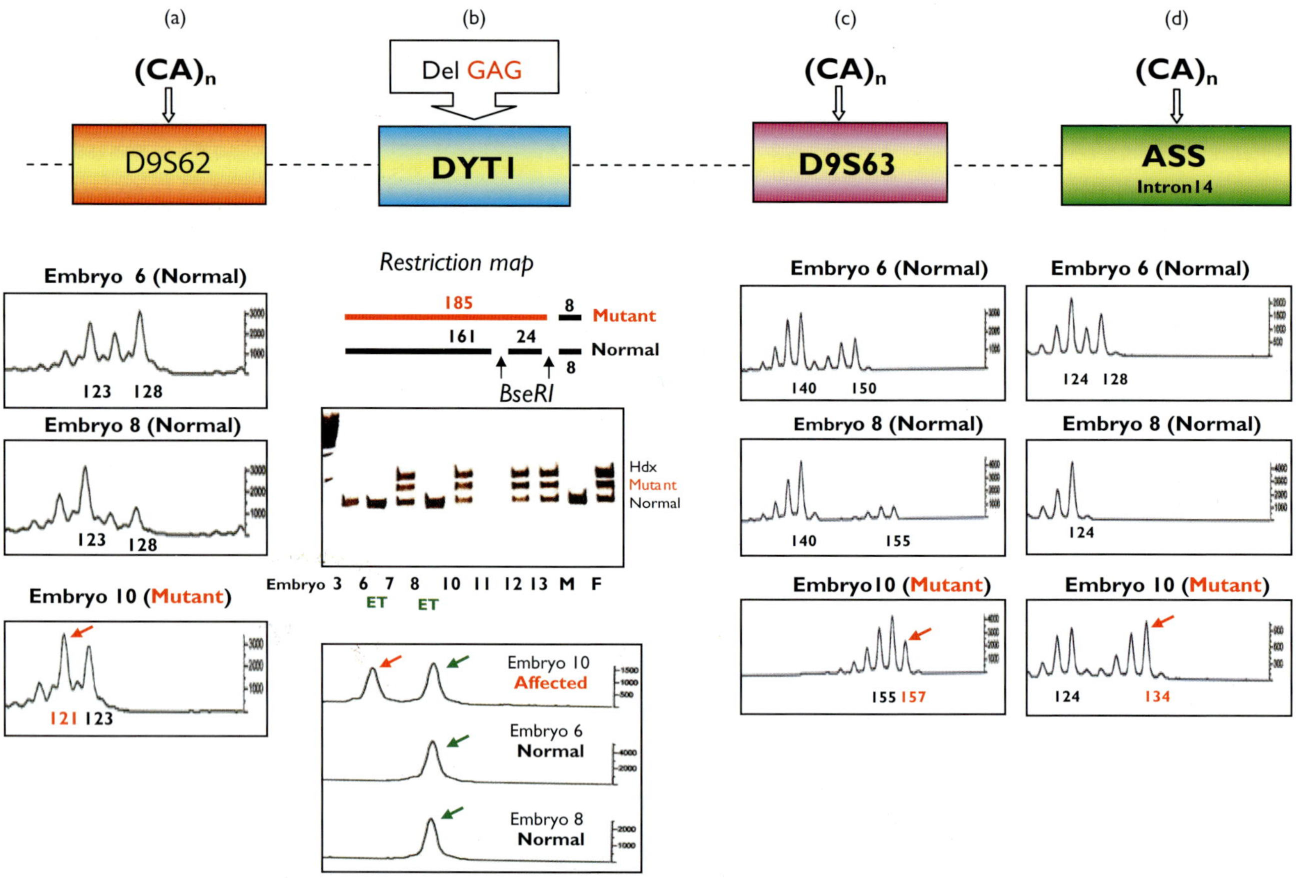

Figure 6.25 Preimplantation diagnosis for GAG deletion of *DYT1* gene, resulting in an ongoing mutation-free pregnancy. Panels (a), (c), and (d) capillary electrophoregrams of fluorescently labeled PCR products of linked markers D9S62 (a), D9S63 (c), and ASS (d), scored by Genotyper®. The data obtained by the genotyping of only three embryos are shown as examples, including two transferred normal (embryos 6 and 8), and one mutant (embryo 10) embryos. Paternally derived 128-, 140-, and 124-dinucleotides indicative of the *DYT1* mutation are evident in the blastomeres of embryos 6 and 8, together with the presence of maternal normal alleles. (b) The location (top) of the mutation in *DYT1*, restriction map for *DseRI* digestion (second from the top), creating three fragments of 161, 24, and 8 bp in the normal allele, in contrast to only two fragments of 185 and 8 bp in the mutant allele. However, because this required a long incubation period and a large amount of enzyme, fluorescent genotyping was also performed (see bottom of (b)). The middle section of (b) shows the polyacrylamide-gel electrophoregram of the *BseRI*-digested PCR products of eight blastomeres from one of the cycles of PGD, paternal DNA (F) from sperm, and maternal (normal) DNA. Hdx, an extra fragment in the heterozygous mutant embryos as a result of heteroduplex formation. The bottom section of (b) shows capillary electrophoregrams of fluorescently labeled PCR products of some of the above blastomeres, including two normal (embryos 6 and 8) and one mutant (embryo 10) embryos. The paternally derived GAG deletion shown by the red arrow is evident in embryo 10, but absent in embryos 6 and 8, in agreement with the linked marker analysis (see (a), (c), and (d)). These embryos inherited the paternal normal chromosome, but may be distinguished from each other by the inheritance of different maternal chromosomes, allowing the origin of the resulting mutation-free baby to be identified. ET, embryo transfer.

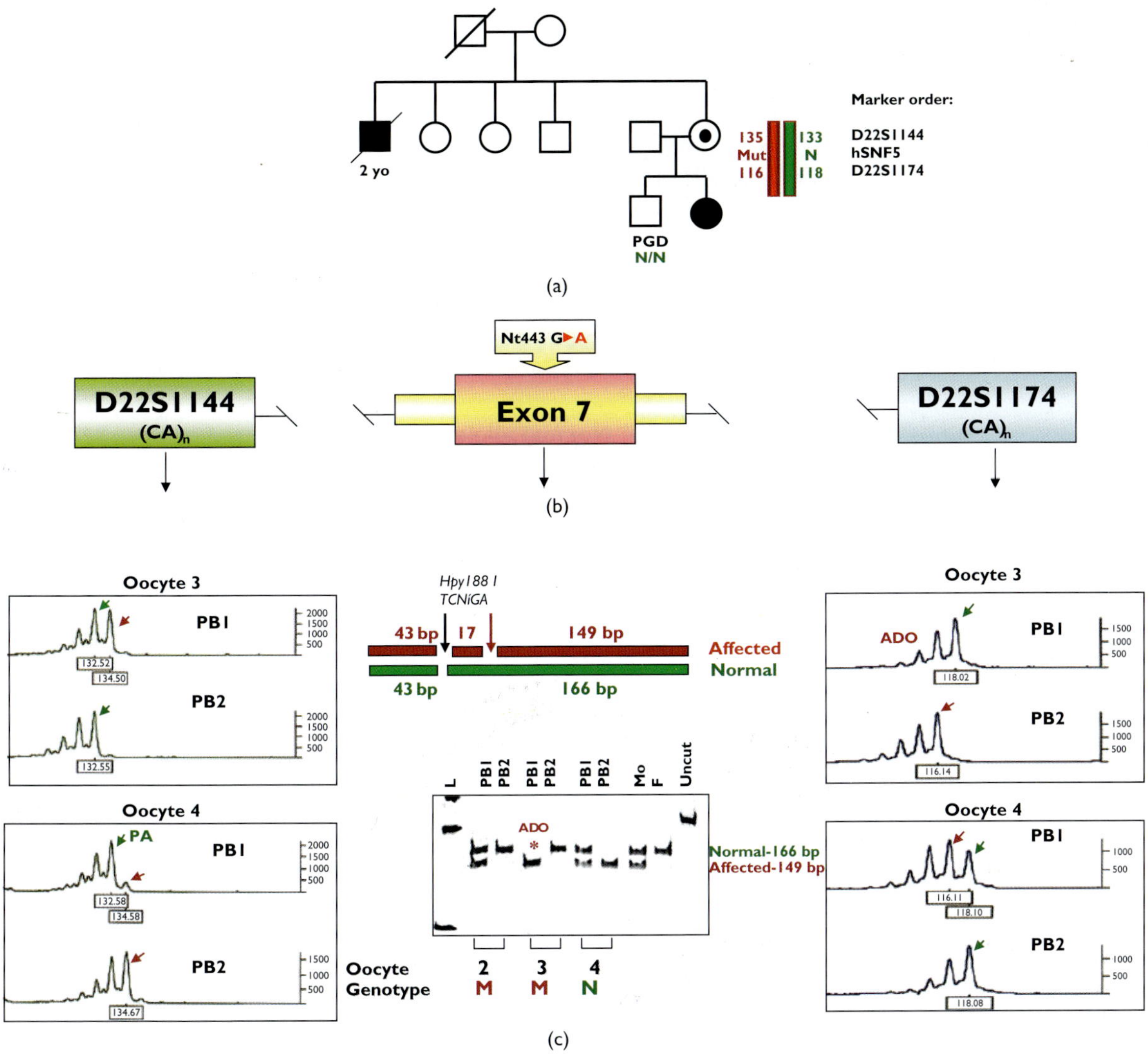

Figure 6.26 PGD for Nt443 G–A mutation in exon 7 of the *hSNF5* gene. (a) Family pedigree with posterior fossa tumors in two generations: an unaffected carrier haplotype was determined by sequential first and second polar body (PB1 and PB2) analysis. (b) Position of the Nt443 G–A mutation in exon 7 of the *hSNF5* gene and tightly linked dinucleotide polymorphic markers D22S1144 and D22S1174. (c) On the left, the fluorescent PCR results of the sequential PB1 and PB2 analysis are displayed. One of the second-round PCR primers was labeled with Hex fluorescent dye. Oocyte 3 is predicted to be affected based on the heterozygous (132/134) PB1 and the 132-bp PCR product linked to the normal maternal allele in the PB2. Preferential amplification (PA) of the 132-bp allele was detected in the PB1 from oocyte 4 in agreement with the mutation analysis and the second D22S1174 marker, suggesting that oocyte 4 can be predicted to be normal. (c) In the center, there is a restriction map and polyacrylamide gel analysis of Hpy188 I restriction digestion of PCR product from the PB1 and PB2. Based on this analysis, oocyte 2 is normal as evidenced by the heterozygous PB1 and mutant PB2. Allele dropout (ADO) was detected in the PB1 from oocyte 3 by polymorphic markers D22S1144 and D22S1174. Without these markers, oocyte 3 genotype would have been predicted to be normal based on the homozygous mutant PB1 and the hemizygous normal PB2, which might have led to misdiagnosis. Oocyte 4 is predicted to be normal based on the heterozygous PB1 and the mutant PB2, in agreement with marker analysis as mentioned. N, normal; M, mutant; F, paternal DNA; Mo, maternal DNA; Uncut, uncut PCR product; Nt, nucleotide; L, size marker ladder. (c) On the right, the results of fluorescent PCR (FL-PCR) of sequential PB1 and PB2 analysis are shown. One of the second-round PCR primers was labeled with Fam fluorescent dye. ADO of the 116-bp allele was detected in the PB1 from oocyte 3 by mutation analysis and D22s1144 marker study. The heterozygous PB1 from oocyte 4 confirmed PA suspected during the D22s1144 analysis.

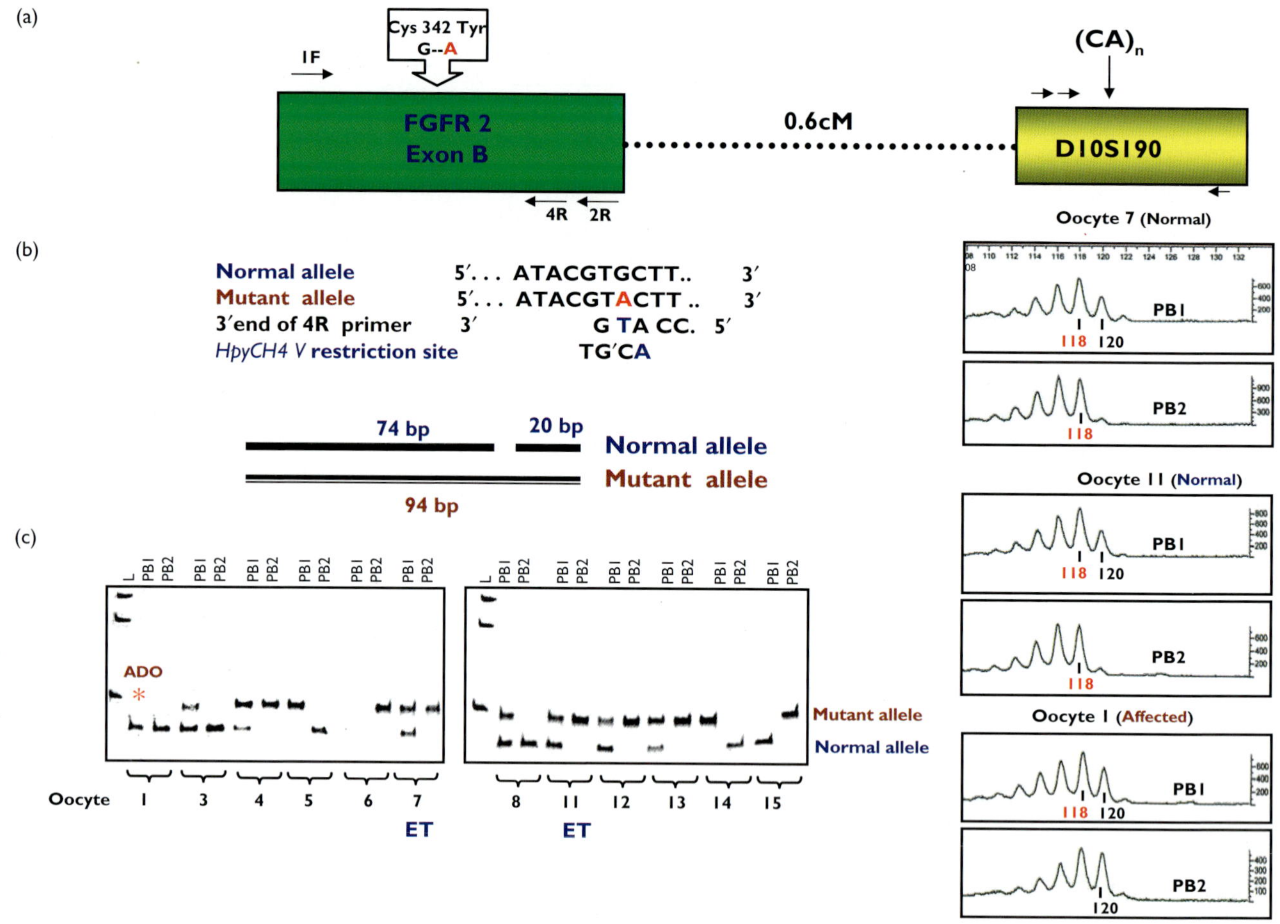

Figure 6.27 PGD for mutation in *FGFR2* gene causing Crouzon syndrome. (a) Map of human *FGFR2* gene, showing the sites and the location of C342Y mutation and the position of linked D10S190 dinucleotide STR. Horizontal arrows show primer sets for heminested PCR. (b) Primer design and (c) restriction map for normal and mutant alleles. (d) Mutation analysis of 12 oocytes by sequential first (PB1) and second (PB2) polar bodies. Allele dropout (ADO) of the mutant allele (*) was detected by both sequential PB1 and PB2 analysis (both having an identical genotype) and linked marker analysis (presence of 118-bp and 120-bp bands). STR profile for the PB1 and PB2 from oocytes 1, 7, and 11 confirmed the results of mutation analysis (e), suggesting that the latter two are normal and can be transferred. L, size standard; bp, base pair; ET, embryo transfer.

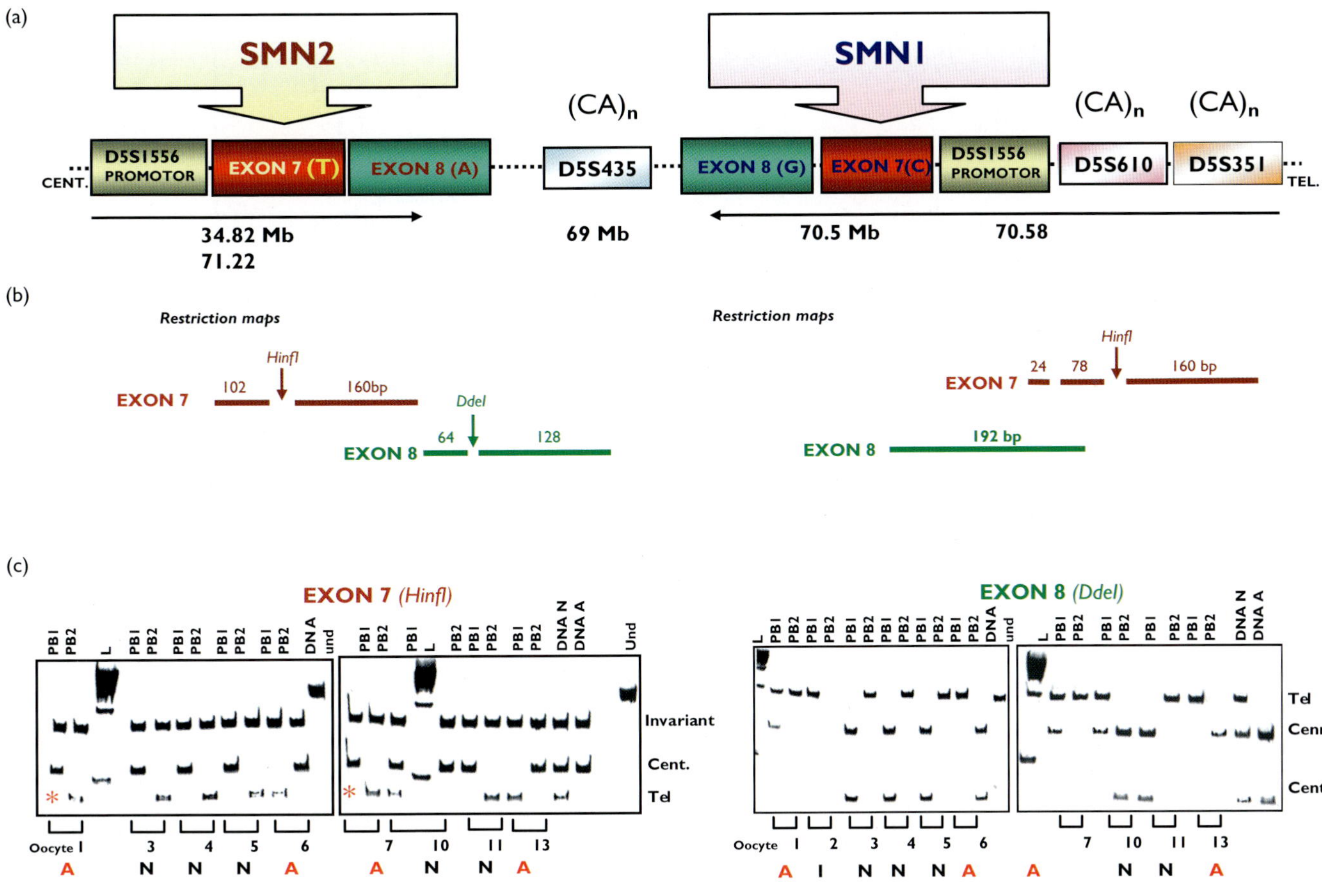

Figure 6.28 Genomic organization of the *SMN1* and *SMN2* genes and deletion detection system designed for PGD of spinal muscular atrophy (SMA). (a) Schematic representation of telomeric (SMN1) and centromeric (SMN2) copies of the *SMN* gene (5q13) and closely located polymorphic markers. Two SMA genes are highly homologous. Deletion of the *SMN1* gene is involved in 95% of spinal muscular atrophy (SMA) cases. The differences between exon 7 (C/T) and 8 (G/A) are used to distinguish SMN1 and SMN2 in the diagnosis of SMA. Mb, megabase; TEL, telomeric; CENT, centromeric. (b) Restriction maps for *HinfI* and *DdeI* enzymes. To distinguish between SMN1 and SMN2 copies, a mismatched second-round primer was designed to introduce an artificial second restriction to the *HinfI* site to exon 7 of the *SMN1* gene. The detection of a 78-bp band (red bar under the SMN1) confirms the presence of at least one copy of the *SMN1* gene. A centromeric SMN2 copy is detected by the presence of the 102-bp fragment (red bar under the SMN2). The presence of the 'C' variant in exon 8 sequence of the centromeric copy (SMN2) creates a natural *DdeI* restriction site. The centromeric copy of the gene (SMN2) can be detected by the presence of 128-bp and 64-bp bands. The undigested 192-bp fragment originated from the amplification of the *SMN1* gene. (c) Polyacrylamide gel analysis of the *HinfI* restriction digestion of exon 7 PCR product from the first and second polar bodies (PB1 and PB2) (left). Polyacrylamide gel analysis of the *DdeI* restriction digestion of exon 8 PCR product from the PB1 and PB2 (right). Allele dropout (*) was detected in the PB1 from oocytes 1 and 7 by simultaneous amplification of exons 7 and 8. L, size standard; A, affected (deleted SMN1) allele; N, normal (SMN1 present) allele; Und, undigested PCR product.

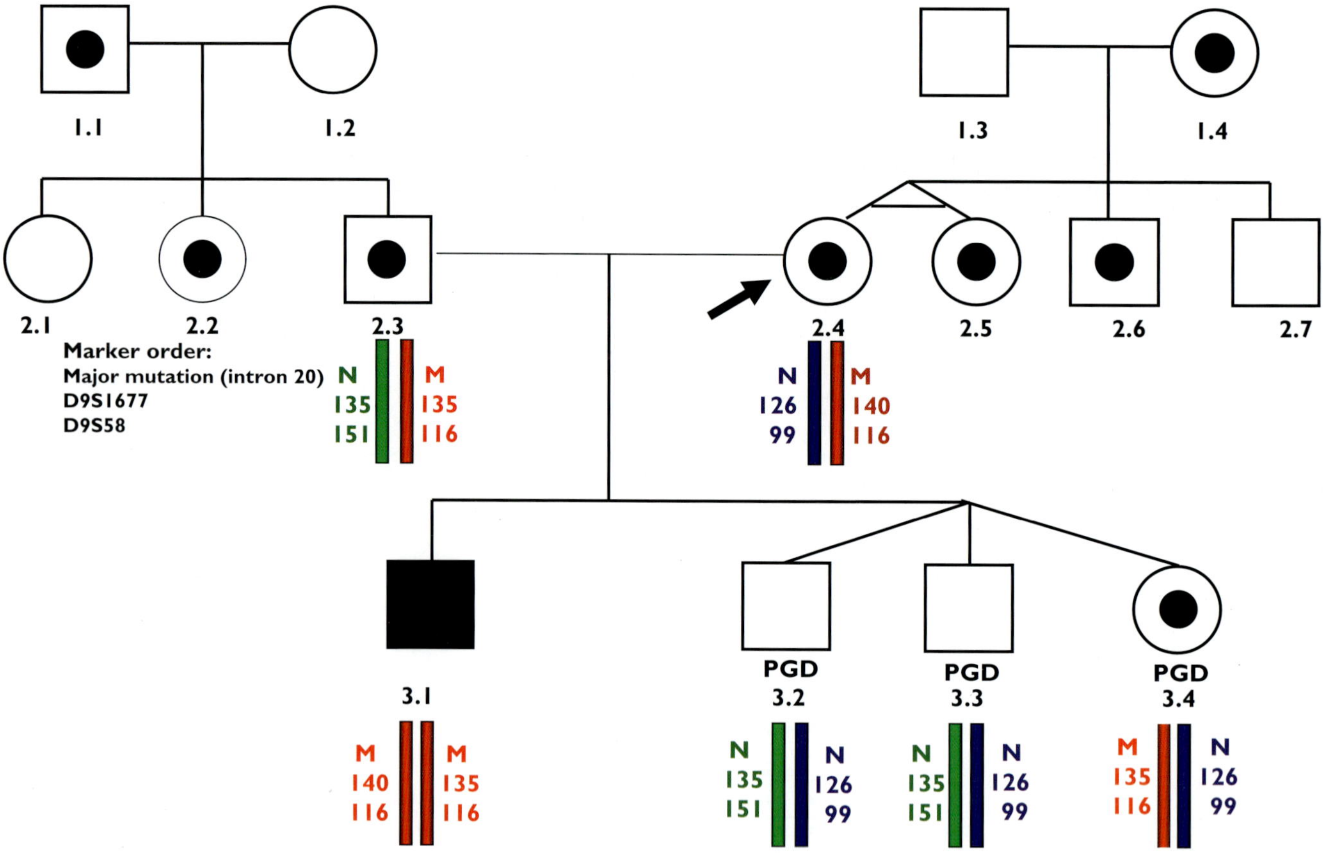

Figure 6.29 Family pedigree of a couple undergoing PGD for familial dysautonomia (FD). The father (2.3) is a carrier of the mutation of the donor splice site of intron 20 of the *IKBKAP* gene, which is linked to a 135-bp repeat of D9S1677 and a 116-bp repeat of D9S58, while the normal allele is linked to a 135-bp and a 151-bp repeat of the same polymorphic markers, respectively. The mother (2.4) is also a carrier of the same mutation, linked to a 140-bp and a 116-bp repeat, the normal gene being linked to a 126- and a 99-bp repeat, respectively. As seen from this panel, the paternal sister (2.2) and maternal sister (2.5) and brother (2.6) are also carriers of the mutation inherited from the paternal father (1.1) and the maternal mother (1.4). Reproductive outcomes of this couple, including one previous affected child with FD (3.1) and unaffected triplets born following PGD (3.2, 3.3, 3.4), are shown at the bottom.

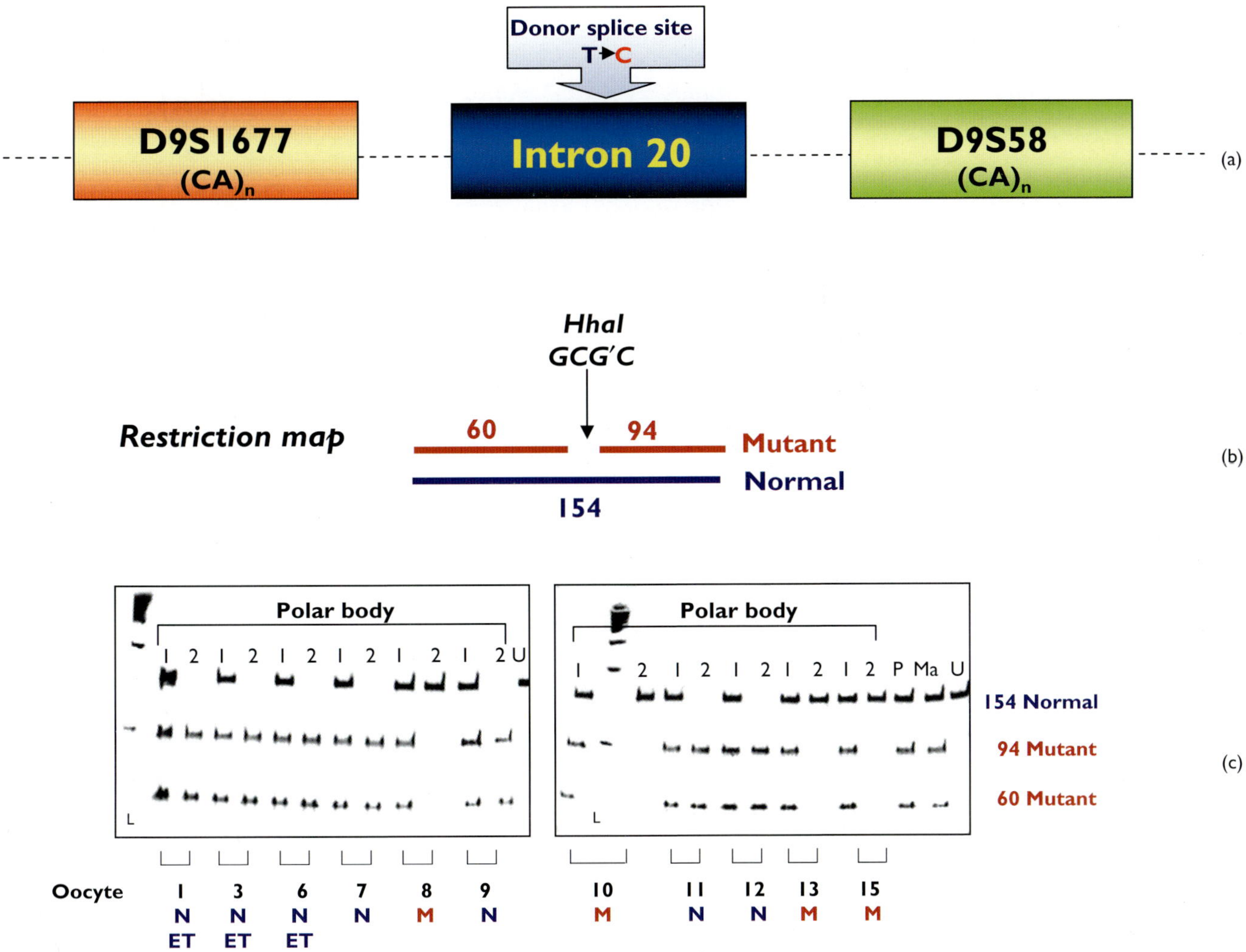

Figure 6.30 Preimplantation genetic diagnosis for major mutation in the *IKBKAP* gene, causing familial dysautonomia. (a) The position of a major splice donor mutation T–C in the *IKBKAP* gene and linked markers. (b) Restriction map showing the major mutation creating a restriction site for the *HhaI* enzyme. (c) Polar body (PB) analysis of normal and mutant sequences of the *IKBKAP* gene. Of 11 oocytes tested, seven were mutation-free based on heterozygous PB1 and affected PB2, of which oocytes 1, 3, and 6 were transferred, resulting in unaffected triplets. L, 100-bp ladder; N, normal; M, mutant; ET, embryo transfer; U, undigested PCR product; Ma, maternal genotype; P, paternal genotype.

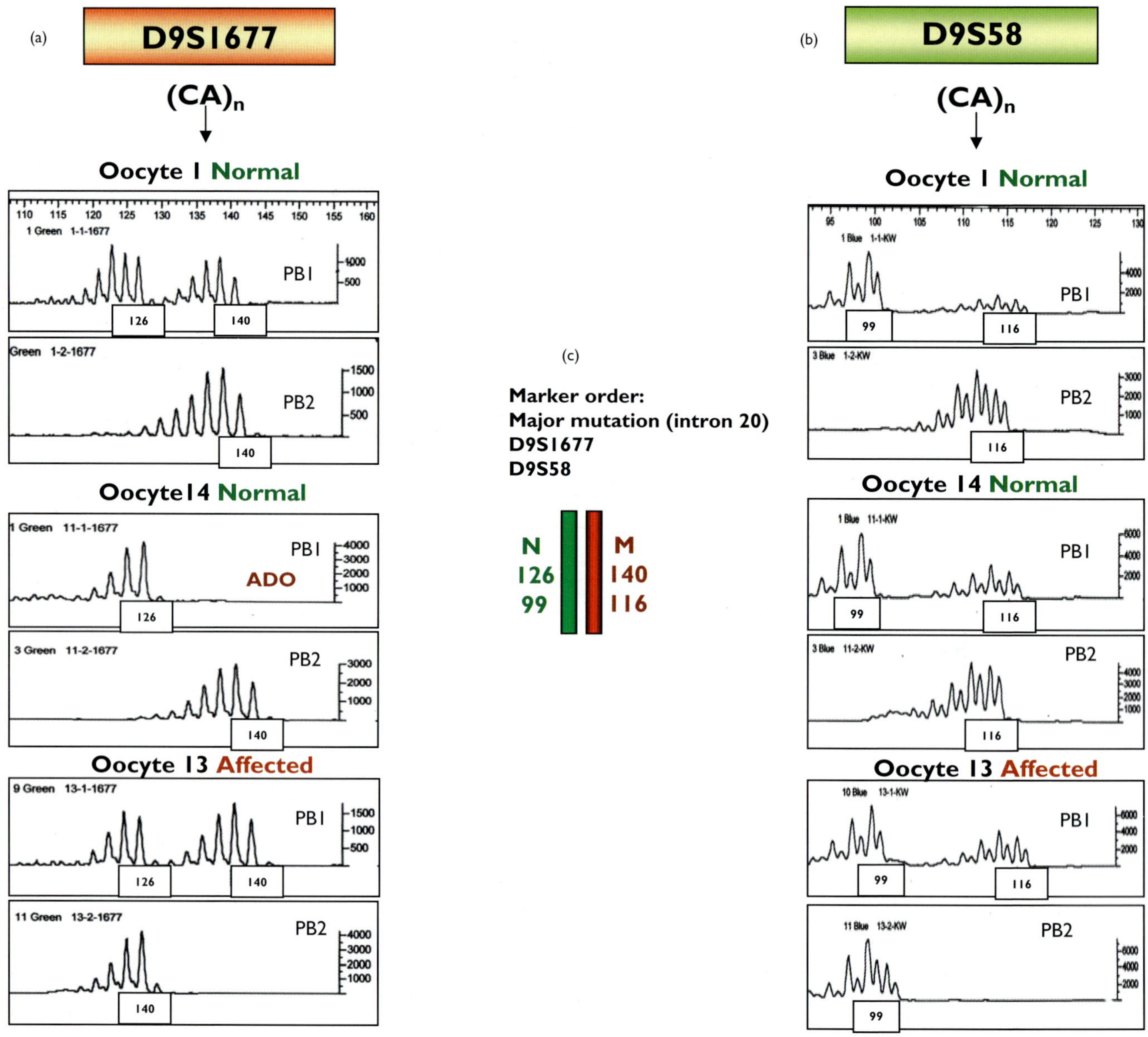

Figure 6.31 Capillary electrophoregrams of fluorescently labeled PCR products of tightly linked markers D9S1677 (a) and D9S58 (b) scored by Genotyper. (c) Maternal haplotype. (Top) Confirmation of the mutation-free status of oocyte 1, based on the presence of both polymorphic markers linked to normal and mutant genes in the first polar body (PB1) and marker linked only to the mutant gene in second polar body (PB2). (Middle) Confirmation of the mutation-free status of oocyte 14, based on the presence of one of the polymorphic markers linked to normal and mutant genes in the PB1 and the marker linked to the mutant gene in the PB2 (b). Allele dropout (ADO) of the marker linked to the mutant gene is seen in the PB1 (a). (Bottom) Confirmation of the mutant status of oocyte 13 based on the presence of both polymorphic markers linked to normal and mutant genes in the PB1 and the marker linked to the normal gene in the PB2.

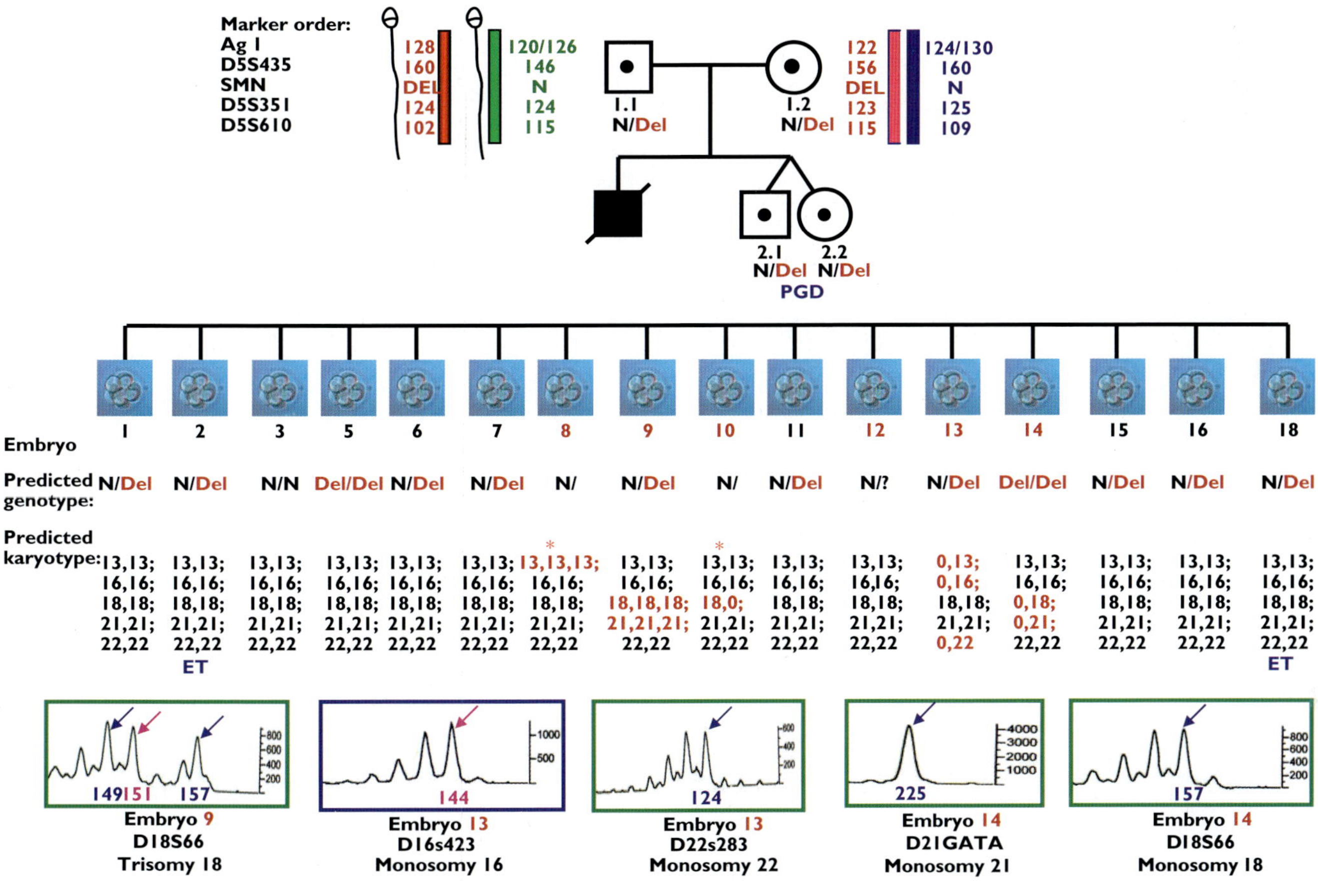

Figure 6.32 Combined PGD for spinal muscular atrophy (SMA) and aneuploidy by multiplex heminested PCR. (Top) Pedigree of a family undergoing PGD for SMA. Both parents (1.1 and 1.2) are carriers of the deletion in the *SMN1* gene. The paternal haplotype was predicted by multiplex heminested single-sperm PCR analysis. Maternal haplotype was established by sequential first and second polar body (PB1 and PB2) analysis. As a result of the IVF–PGD cycle, healthy twins were born (2.1 and 2.2). The positions of polymorphic markers linked to the *SMN1* gene and applied to improve the accuracy of the mutation analysis are shown next to paternal haplotypes. (Middle) Oocytes 3, 8, and 11 were predicted to be normal by polar body analysis. The embryos resulting from these oocytes were subjected to aneuploidy testing using five chromosome-specific probes. Trisomy for chromosome 13 was detected in embryo 8 and monosomy 18 in embryo 10. Blastomeres from the remaining 13 embryos were subjected to multiplex heminested PCR to perform simultaneous mutation, linked polymorphic marker, and aneuploidy analysis for chromosomes 13, 16, 18, 21, and 22. Of these, embryos 5 and 14 were affected, while embryos 1, 2, 6, 7, 9, 11, 13, 15, 16, and 18 were predicted to be heterozygous for the deletion in the *SMN1* gene. At least three STRs were amplified on each chromosome for aneuploidy testing, which revealed monosomies 13, 16, and 22 in embryo 13, monosomy 18 and 21 in embryo 14, and trisomy 18 and 21 in embryo 9. Chromosomal abnormalities predicted by PCR were confirmed by whole embryo fixation and fluorescent *in situ* hybridization (FISH) analysis. Embryos 2 and 18 were transferred, and healthy twins (2.1 and 2.2) were born. All unaffected and chromosomally normal blastocysts were frozen for a future cycle. (Bottom) Examples of chromosomal abnormalities (monosomy and trisomy) detected by PCR of different STRs. N, normal allele; Del, deletion; ET, embryo transfer; blue arrow, paternal allele; red arrow, maternal allele.

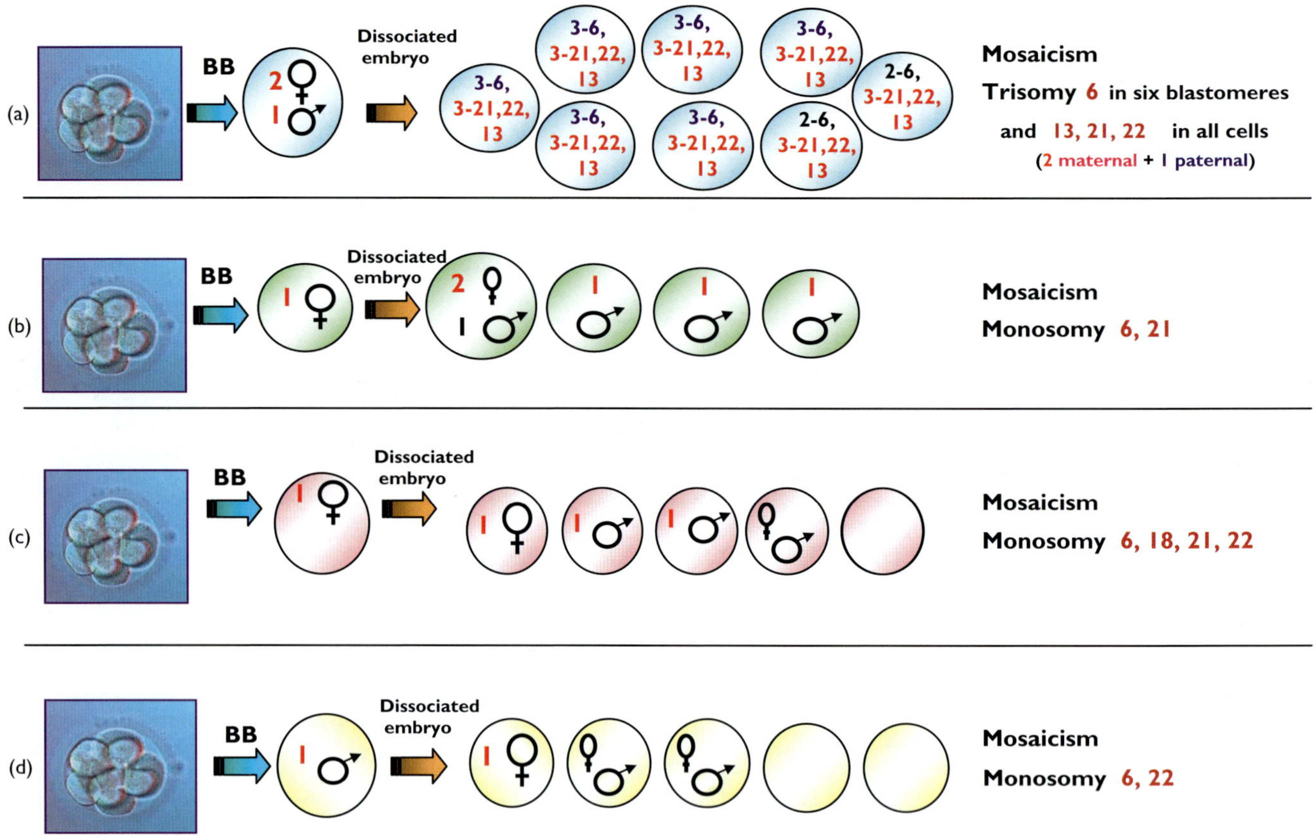

Figure 6.33 Preimplantation HLA genotyping combined with STR-based aneuploidy testing. Preimplantation HLA-matching based on multiplex heminested PCR of blastomeres by a set of informative polymorphic markers covering the complete HLA area and testing the number and origin of the paternal and maternal chromosomes 6. The multiplex system also makes it possible to test for aneuploidy of chromosomes 13, 16, 18, 21, and 22, which is required in patients with advanced reproductive age. (a) PCR-based detection of trisomy 6, 13, 21, and 22 in the blastomeres, confirmed by follow-up analysis of dissociated embryos. (b) Monosomy 6 and 21, as evidenced by the presence of only maternal markers in the blastomere, which appeared to have mosaicism in the follow-up study (one blastomere was trisomic, and three monosomic, with only paternal chromosomes 6 and 21 present). (c) Embryos with mosaicism for chromosomes 6, 18, 21, and 22. (d) Embryo with mosaicism for chromosomes 6 and 22. BB, blastomere biopsy; ♀ and ♂, show origin of chromosome 6 (numbers show the number of maternally and paternally originating chromosomes).

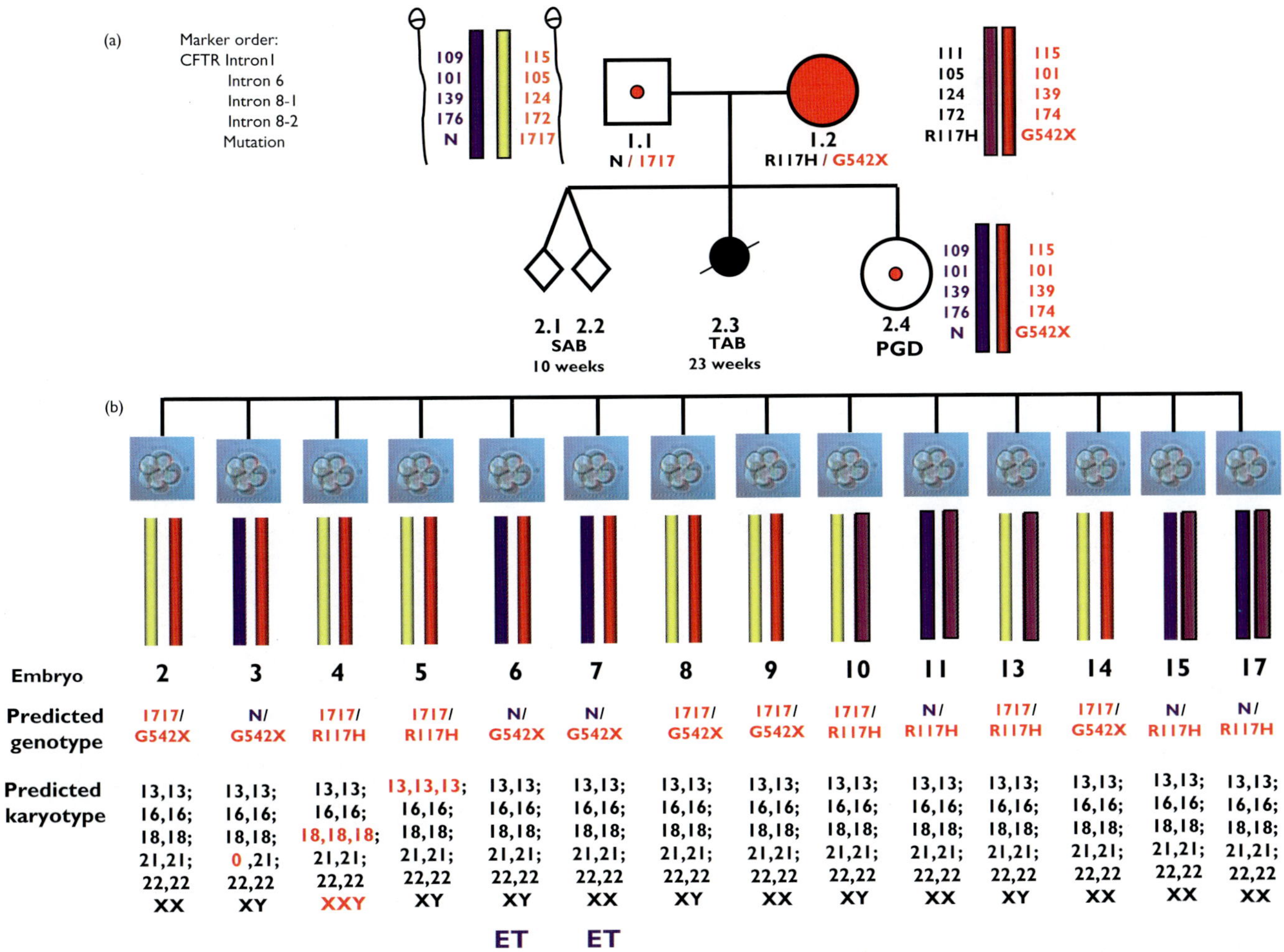

Figure 6.34 PGD in a couple with the affected female partner being double heterozygous with two different cystic fibrosis mutations. (a) Family pedigree of a couple with three different mutations in *CFTR* gene. The mother is affected with cystic fibrosis and has two different mutations (R117H and G542X). The father is a carrier of 1717 mutation in *CFTR* gene. The paternal haplotype was established by multiplex heminested single-sperm PCR. Maternal linkage was based on DNA amplification of the polar bodies. Marker order of the mutations and polymorphic markers in *CFTR* gene are shown (top left). The first pregnancy with twins (2.1, 2.2) resulted in a spontaneous abortion (SAB), the second pregnancy in an affected fetus (2.3) that was terminated (TAB); PGD was performed for three different mutations in the *CFTR* gene, resulting in an unaffected pregnancy and the birth of a healthy girl predicted and confirmed to be the carrier of the maternal mutation G542X (2.4). (b) The outcome of the PGD cycle for three mutations in the *CFTR* gene combined with age-related aneuploidy testing. Multiplex heminested PCR performed on blastomeres from 14 embryos allowing simultaneous detection of the paternal and maternal *CFTR* haplotypes and non-syntenic short tandem repeats (STRs) located on chromosomes 13, 16, 18, 21, 22, X, and Y. Six embryos (3, 6, 7, 11, 15, and 17) were predicted to be carriers based on the presence of the maternal mutation and normal paternal *CFTR* gene. Monosomy 21 was found in the blastomere from embryo 3, which was excluded from the transfer and freezing. Trisomy 18 and XXY were observed in the blastomere from embryo 4, and trisomy 13 was detected in the blastomere from embryo 5. Embryos 6 and 7 were transferred, resulting in pregnancy and the birth of a healthy girl. DNA analysis of the newborn baby revealed the genetic profile identical to that of embryo 7, evidencing the usefulness and accuracy of the combined mutations analysis, linkage, and aneuploidy testing in PGD for single-gene disorders in patients of advanced reproductive age.

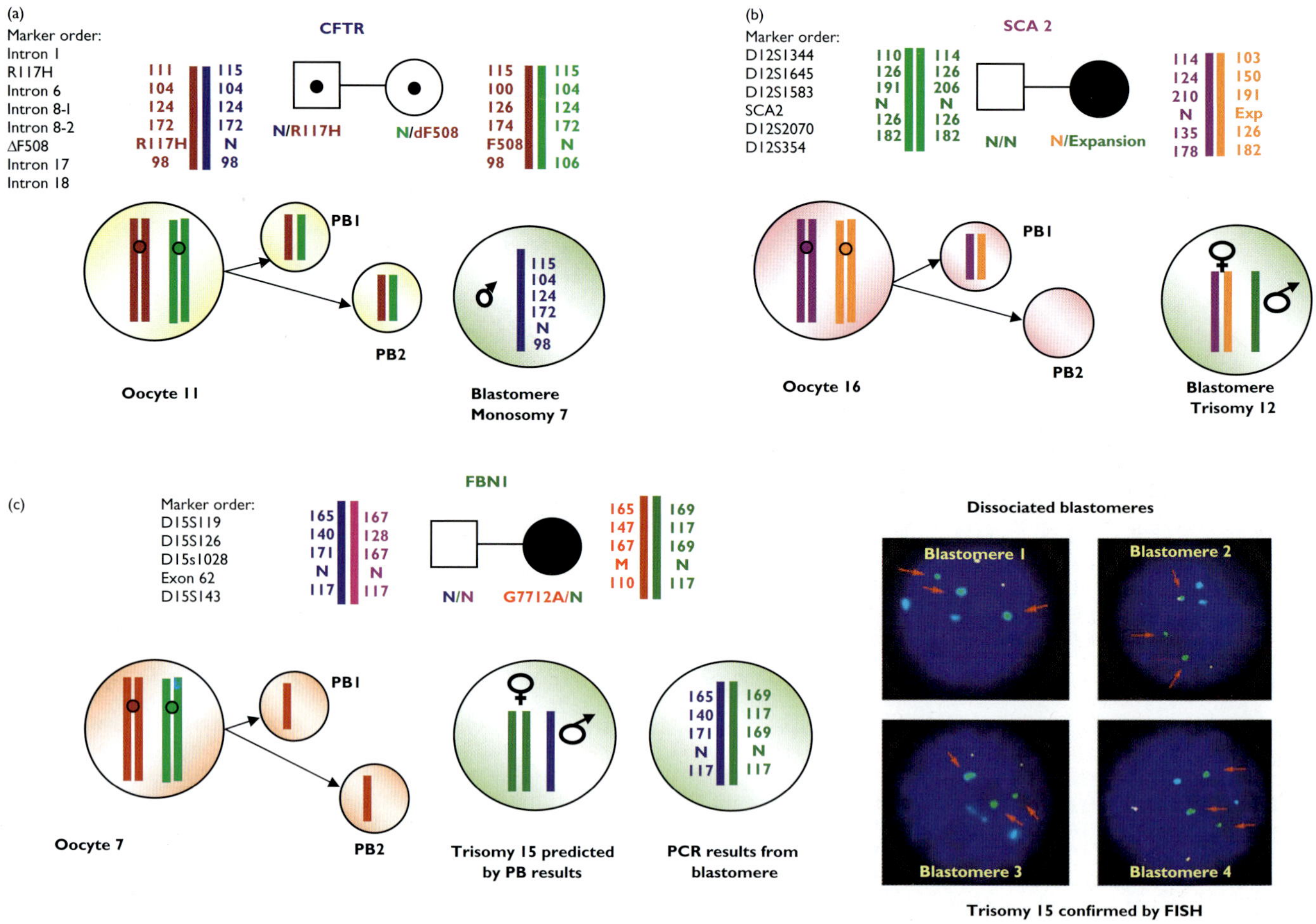

Figure 6.35 PCR-based detection of meiosis I and meiosis II errors affecting PGD results. (a) Monosomy 7 detected by a set of linked polymorphic markers in PGD for cystic fibrosis (CFTR). (Top) Paternal haplotype established by multiplex-nested PCR of single sperms, and maternal haplotype detected by first and second polar body (PB1 and PB2) multiplex DNA amplification. (Bottom) Heterozygous status of both the PB1 and PB2 confirmed by mutation analysis and five linked markers, providing the basis for the prediction of the lack of maternal chromosome 7 in the resulting embryo, which is confirmed by the presence of only the paternal chromosome 7 markers in the embryo. (b) Trisomy 12 predicted by a set of linked polymorphic markers for chromosome 12 in PGD for spinal cerebella ataxia type 2 (SCA2). (Top) Maternal haplotype revealed on the basis of PB1 and PB2 multiplex-heminested amplification. (Bottom) The heterozygous PB1 and lack of chromosome 12 polymorphic markers in the corresponding PB2 allowed the prediction of the extra chromosome 12 contribution of maternal origin in the resulting embryo. This was confirmed by blastomere analysis of the embryo, which appeared to contain both maternal chromosomes 12, in addition to paternal chromosome 12, evidencing trisomy 12 of maternal meiosis II origin, rather than ADO of all chromosome 12 alleles tested in the PB2, which could be the other possible interpretation of the PB2 results. (c) Trisomy 15 predicted in PGD for Marfan syndrome. (Top) Maternal haplotype detected by sequential PB1 and PB2 multiplex heminested PCR. (Bottom) Identical homozygous affected haplotype of both the PB1 and PB2 providing evidence for either ADO of an allele of one of the chromosomes 15 in the PB1, or prediction of an extra chromosome 15 of maternal origin in the embryo resulting from this oocyte. Embryo biopsy shows the presence of both maternal and paternal (normal) alleles, as well as corresponding linked polymorphic markers, which, however, could not detect the extra maternal chromosome 15, because both of these chromosomes are not distinguishable by linked markers, being originated from sestrid chromatids as a result of a meiosis I error. This was confirmed by fluorescent *in situ* hybridization (FISH) analysis in the corresponding embryos, which revealed trisomy 15. Without the polar body results the embryonic genotype might have been described as normal, and the error might have led to the transfer of the chromosomally abnormal embryo.

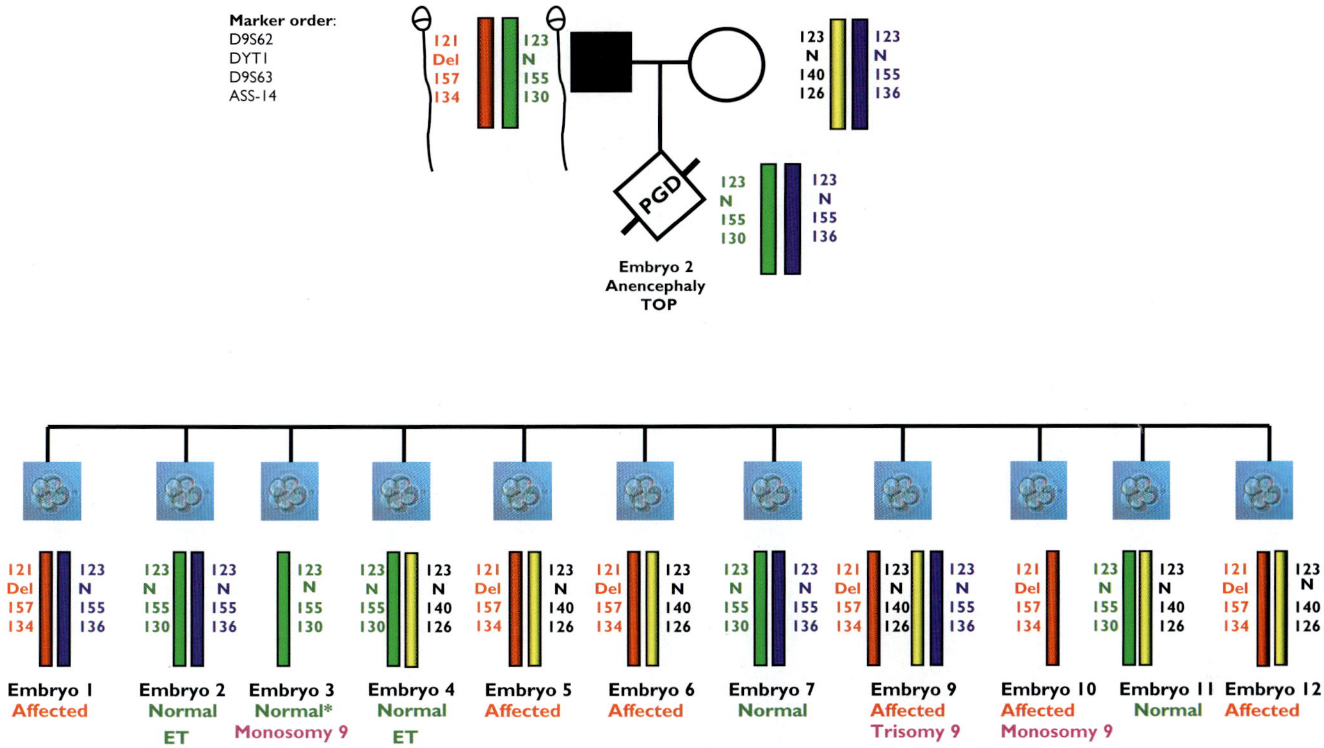

Figure 6.36 PGD for GAG deletion of the *DYT1* gene causing early-onset torsion dystonia together with aneuploidy testing for the chromosome in which the causative gene is located. (Top) Paternal haplotype (left) based on single-sperm DNA amplification. The red bar represents the chromosome with the affected allele, and the green bar corresponds to the normal allele and linked markers. The maternal haplotype (right) is based on blastomere results. The couple is informative for three polymorphic markers tightly linked to the *DYT1* gene. (Bottom) Multiplex heminested PCR performed for the detection of the mutant and normal sequences of the *DYT1* gene from 11 embryos. The presence or absence of the paternal affected allele in the embryo is confirmed by link marker analysis, which also provides information about the number of chromosomes 9, in which the *DYT1* gene is localized. Embryos 1, 5, 6, 9, 10, and 12 had an affected paternal allele (red bar) and were not suitable for transfer. Embryos 3 (green bar) and 10 (red bar) were missing the maternal chromosome 9 (monosomy 9), while embryo 9 (red, yellow, and blue bars) contained an extra maternal chromosome (trisomy 9), evident from the set of markers tested. The remaining embryos (2, 4, 7, and 11) were predicted to be normal, of which two (2 and 4) were transferred, resulting in a mutation-free pregnancy (terminated due to anencephaly). ET, embryo transfer; TOP, termination of pregnancy.

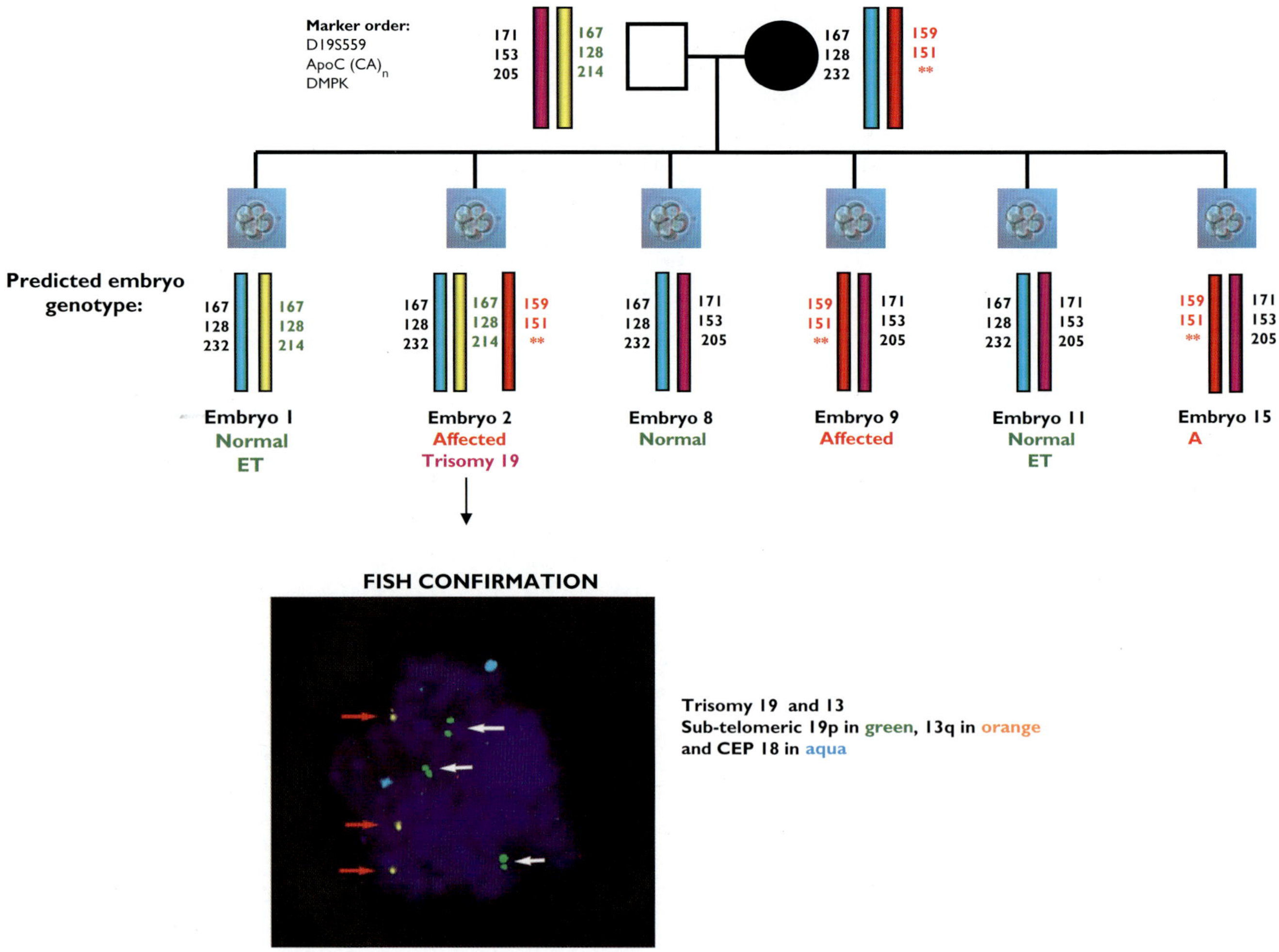

Figure 6.37 PGD for myotonic dystrophy combined with chromosome 19 aneuploidy testing. (Top) Maternal haplotype based on first and second polar body (PB1 and PB2) multiplex DNA amplification of the normal allele of the *DMPK* gene (19q13.2–13.3) and linked markers (right). The paternal haplotype is based on blastomere analysis (yellow and purple bars). As the expansion of (CTG)n repeats in the *DMPK* gene is not detectable at single-cell level (red bar in maternal haplotype corresponds to the affected allele **), linked polymorphic markers are used for diagnosis; blue bar represents the normal allele and tightly linked markers. (Bottom) Six embryos tested for the presence of the normal number of (CTG)n repeats in the *DMPK* gene and polymorphic marker pattern. Embryos 1, 8, and 11 were predicted to be normal based on the presence of the normal maternal chromosome (haplotype) (blue bar) and one paternal chromosome 19. Embryos 2, 9, and 15 were affected as evidenced by the presence of the maternal affected haplotype (red bar). Embryo 2 contains two sets of maternal and one set of paternal polymorphic markers (blue, red, and yellow bars), evidencing trisomy 19 of maternal origin. Therefore, amplification of only the (CTG)n repeat in the *DMPK* gene would have revealed a normal status based on the presence of only normal maternal and paternal alleles, which would have led to misdiagnosis. As seen from the whole embryo follow-up analysis by fluorescent *in situ* hybridization (FISH) (shown below embryo 2 and noted by arrows) the embryo was confirmed to have trisomy 19, as predicted, and also to have incidental trisomy 13. DMPK, dystrophia myotonica protein kinase; ET, embryo transfer.

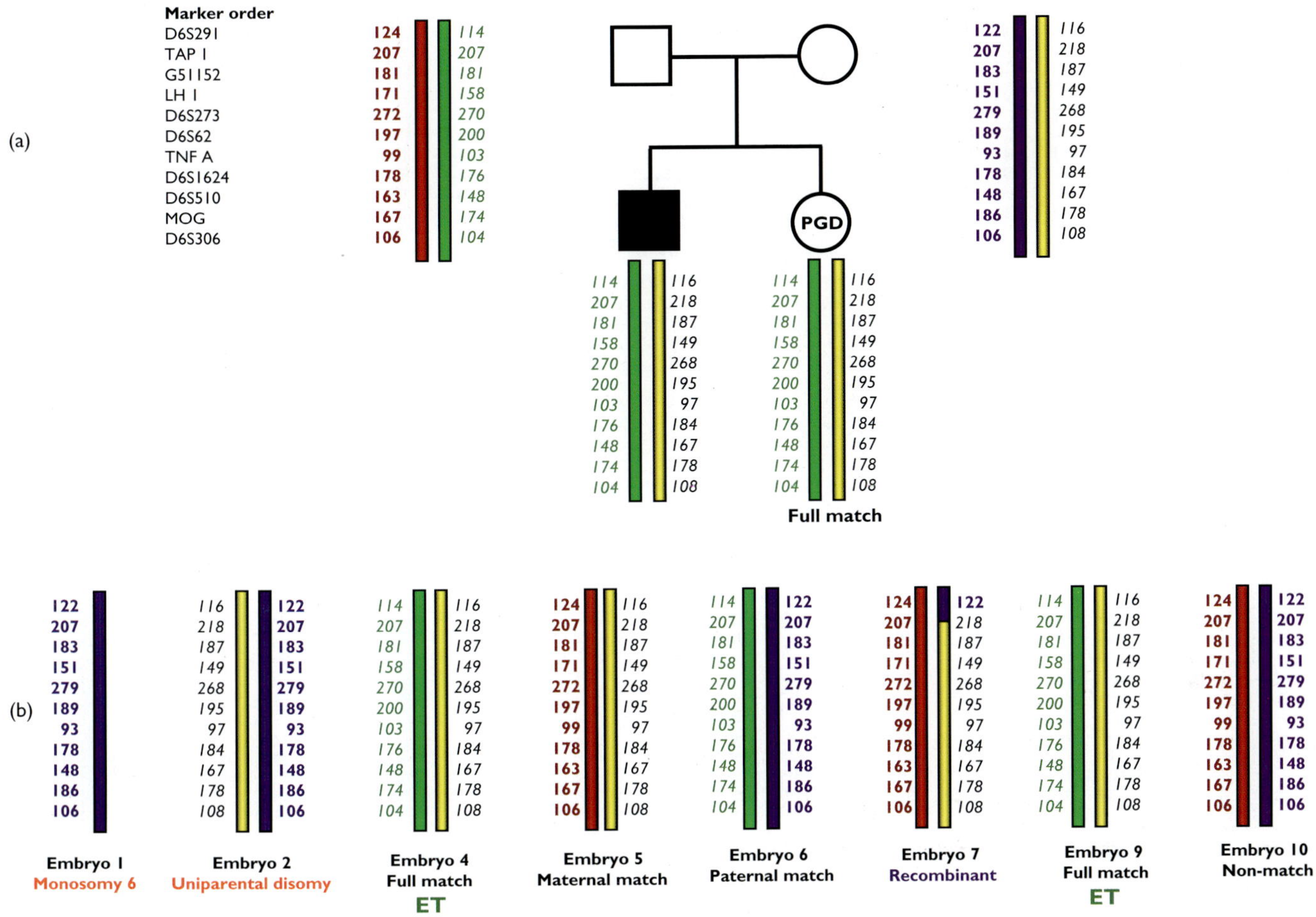

Figure 6.38 Preimplantation HLA typing for acute lymphoid leukemia (ALL), resulting in the birth of an HLA-matched baby. (a) Marker order and haplotypes of mother, father, and the affected child. (b) Results of HLA typing of biopsied blastomeres from eight embryos. Embryos 4 and 9 are an HLA match to the affected sibling (see (a)). Embryo 1 is a maternal non-match with no paternal chromosome present (monosomy 6). Embryo 2 is also a non-match due to only maternal chromosomes being present (uniparental disomy). Embryo 7 is both a paternal and a maternal non-match, the latter being due to maternal recombination after the D65291 marker. The other two embryos are non-matched, embryo 6 being a paternal non-match and embryo 10 being both a maternal and a paternal non-match. ET, embryo transfer.

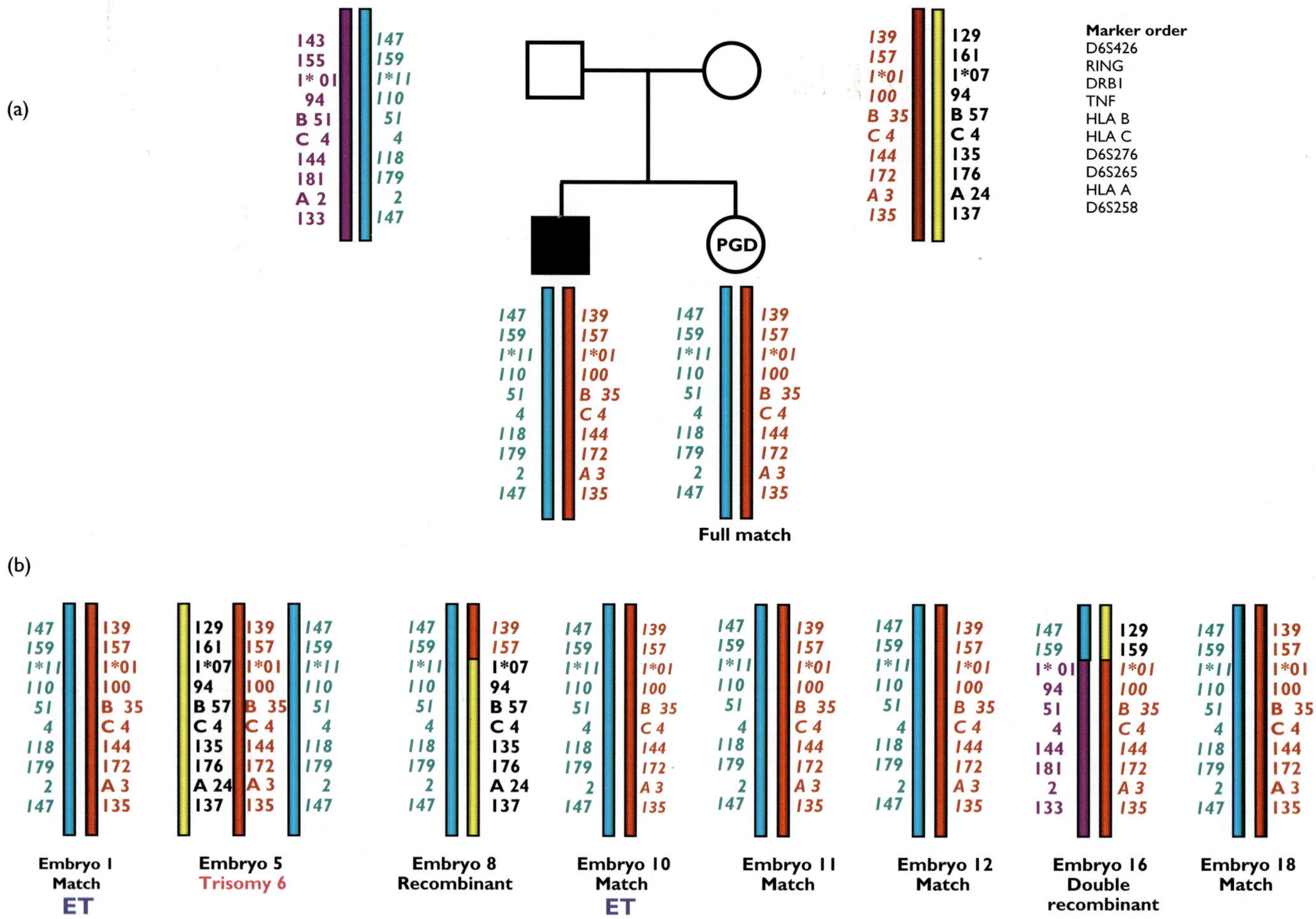

Figure 6.39 Preimplantation HLA typing for Diamond–Blackfan anemia, resulting in the birth of an HLA-matched child. (a) Marker order and haplotypes of mother, father, and the affected child. (b) Results of HLA typing of biopsied blastomeres from eight embryos (another eight embryos that were also tested are not shown). Embryos 1, 10, 11, 12, and 18 are HLA matched to the affected sibling (see (a)). Embryo 8 is a maternal non-match due to maternal recombination after Ring allele, as well as embryo 16, which is both a paternal and a maternal non-match, due to double recombination in the paternal and maternal Ring alleles. Embryo 5 is also a non-match due to an extra maternal chromosome, suggesting trisomy 6. ET, embryo transfer.

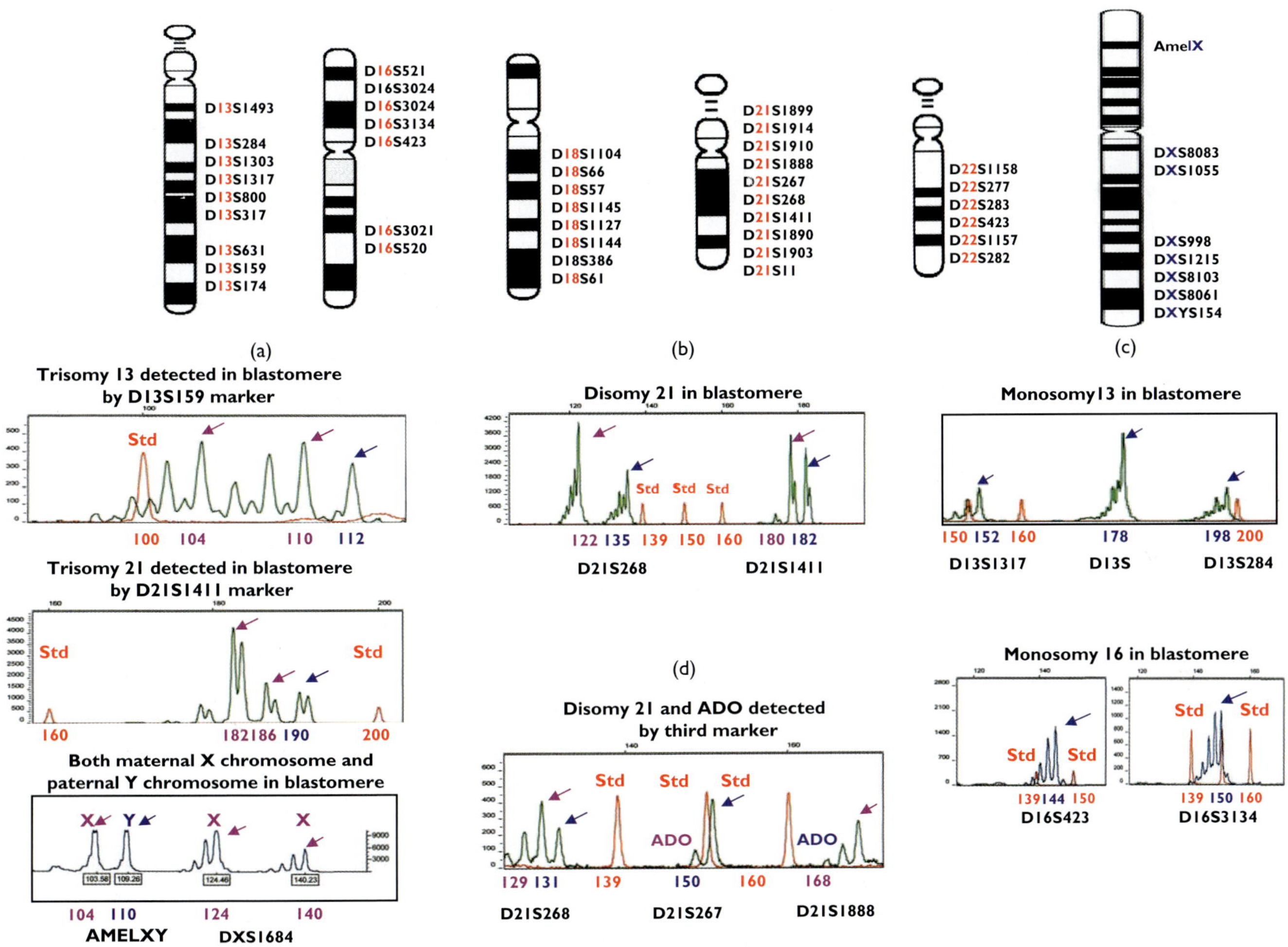

Figure 6.40 PCR-based aneuploidy testing performed simultaneously with PGD for causative genes. (Top) Positions of polymorphic markers applied for PCR-based aneuploidy testing. To distinguish between allele dropout (ADO) and the absence of the whole chromosome (monosomy), at least three informative polymorphic markers for each chromosome are tested. (Bottom) Examples of single-blastomere PCR results with trisomy 13, 21, and XXY (a); normal for chromosome 21 (b); monosomy 13 and 16 (c); and ADO, distinguished from monosomy 21 by the use of three linked markers (d). Std, ROX size standard; purple arrows, maternal bands; blue arrows, paternal bands.

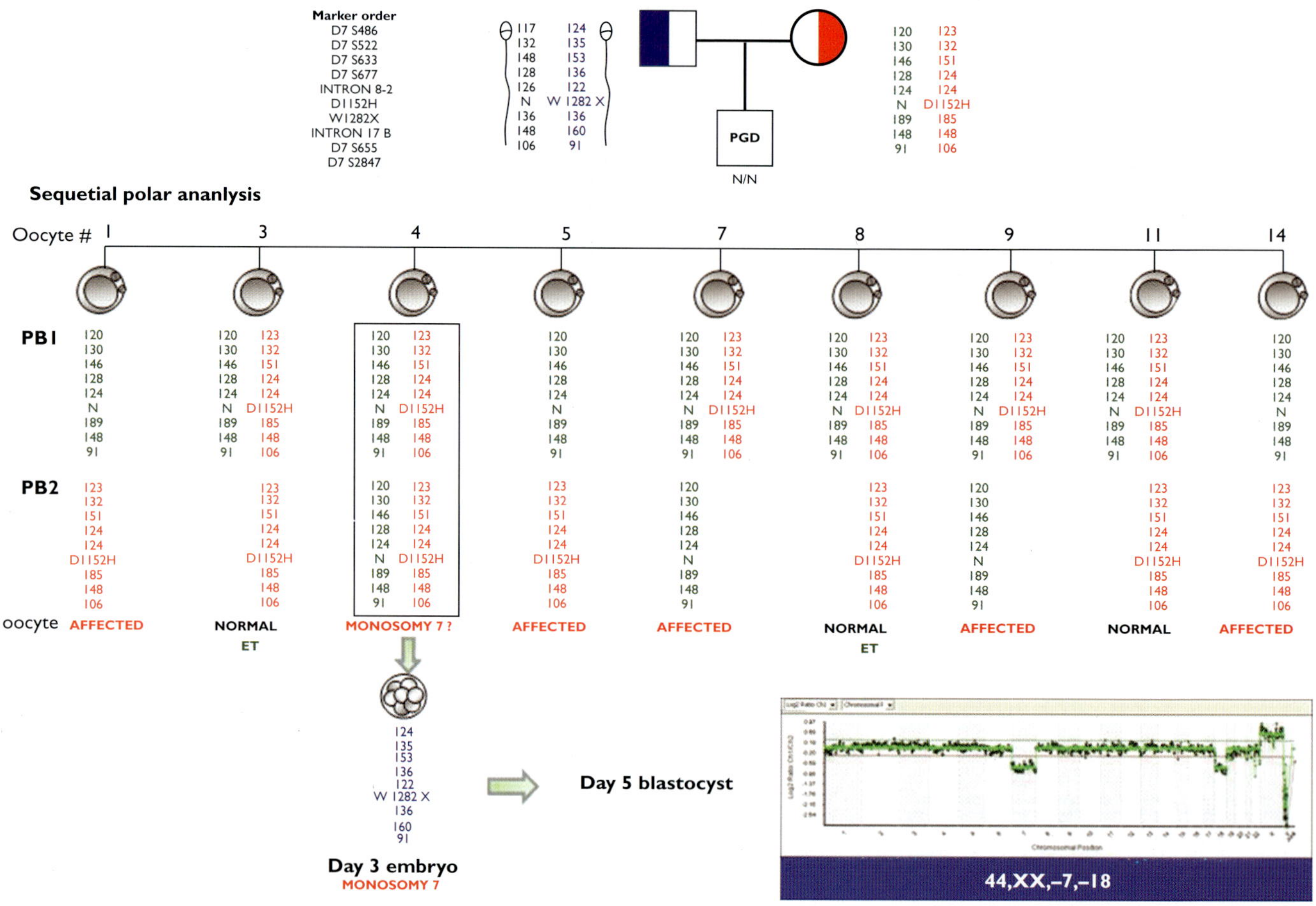

Figure 6.41 PGD for two different CFTR mutations by sequential polar body analysis combined by aCGH for 24-chromosome aneuploidy testing. (Upper panel) Pedigree, showing that the parents are carriers of different CFTR mutations: the mother is a carrier of D1152H mutation, and the father V1282X. (Middle panel) Sequential PB1 and PB2 analysis of nine oocytes, of which three were predicted to be free of maternal mutation, five affected, and one (oocyte 4) with both maternal copies of the *CFTR* gene extruded with PB2, predicting monosomy 7 in the resulting embryos. Embryos resulting from oocytes 3 and 8 were transferred, resulting in birth of unaffected baby boy (see PGD on the upper panel). (Lower panel) 24-chromosome testing of the embryo resulting from oocyte 4 on a trophectoderm biopsy, confirming monosomy 7 (also monosomy 18).

Figure 6.42 *(opposite)* Strategies for combined mutation, aneuploidy, and HLA testing. (a) First and second polar body (PB1 and PB2) testing for a maternally derived dominant mutation when aneuploidy testing is needed because of advanced maternal age. Embryos predicted to be free from maternal mutation are further tested for aneuploidies using fluorescent *in situ* hybridization (FISH) analysis or array-CGH 24-chromosome aneuploidy, while those with inconclusive results for the mutation are subjected to multiplex nested or heminested PCR for simultaneously testing the mutation site, linked to its polymorphic markers and STRs on chromosomes 13, 16, 18, 21, 22, X, and Y, for aneuploidies. Alternatively, whole genome amplification (WGA) of biopsied blastomeres or trophectoderm cells is performed, as for array-CGH, for 24-chromsomsome aneuploidy testing, using WGA product also for mutation and linkage analysis. (b) In case of a paternally derived dominant mutation and advanced maternal age, PB1 and PB2 testing for aneuploidy is performed first, followed by blastomere analysis of aneuploidy-free embryos for paternal mutations and polymorphic markers. Alternatively, whole genome amplification (WGA) of biopsied blastomeres or trophectoderm cells is performed, as for array-CGH, for 24-chromsomsome aneuploidy testing, using WGA product also for mutation and polymorphic markers. (c) In case of an autosomal recessive disorder and advanced reproductive age, PB1 and PB2 aneuploidy testing is done first, followed by blastomere analysis of aneuploidy-free embryos for mutations and polymorphic markers. Maternal mutation is also assessed by PB1 and PB2 analysis once the parents are known to have different mutations, so that the maternal mutation-free embryos can be further tested for the paternal mutation together with the linked markers. As above, all embryos derived from oocytes with inconclusive results in PB1 and PB2 analysis are subjected to multiplex nested or heminested PCR for simultaneous study of the mutation site, linked to its polymorphic markers and STRs on chromosomes 13, 16, 18, 21, 22, X, and Y for aneuploidies, or subjected to WGA and array-CGH for 24-chromsome aneuploidy testing, using WGA product also for mutation and linkage analysis. (d) The strategy is similar to the one applied for recessive disorders and aneuploidy, except HLA typing is performed on all blastomeres in combination with mutation analysis or aneuploidy STR, or array-CGH typing for the same embryos. (e) HLA typing combined with PCR aneuploidy testing is done either by PB FISH analysis followed by HLA typing on blastomeres, or a combined HLA and 24-chromosome aneuploidy testing in WGA product obtained in the first step of the array-CGH procedure.

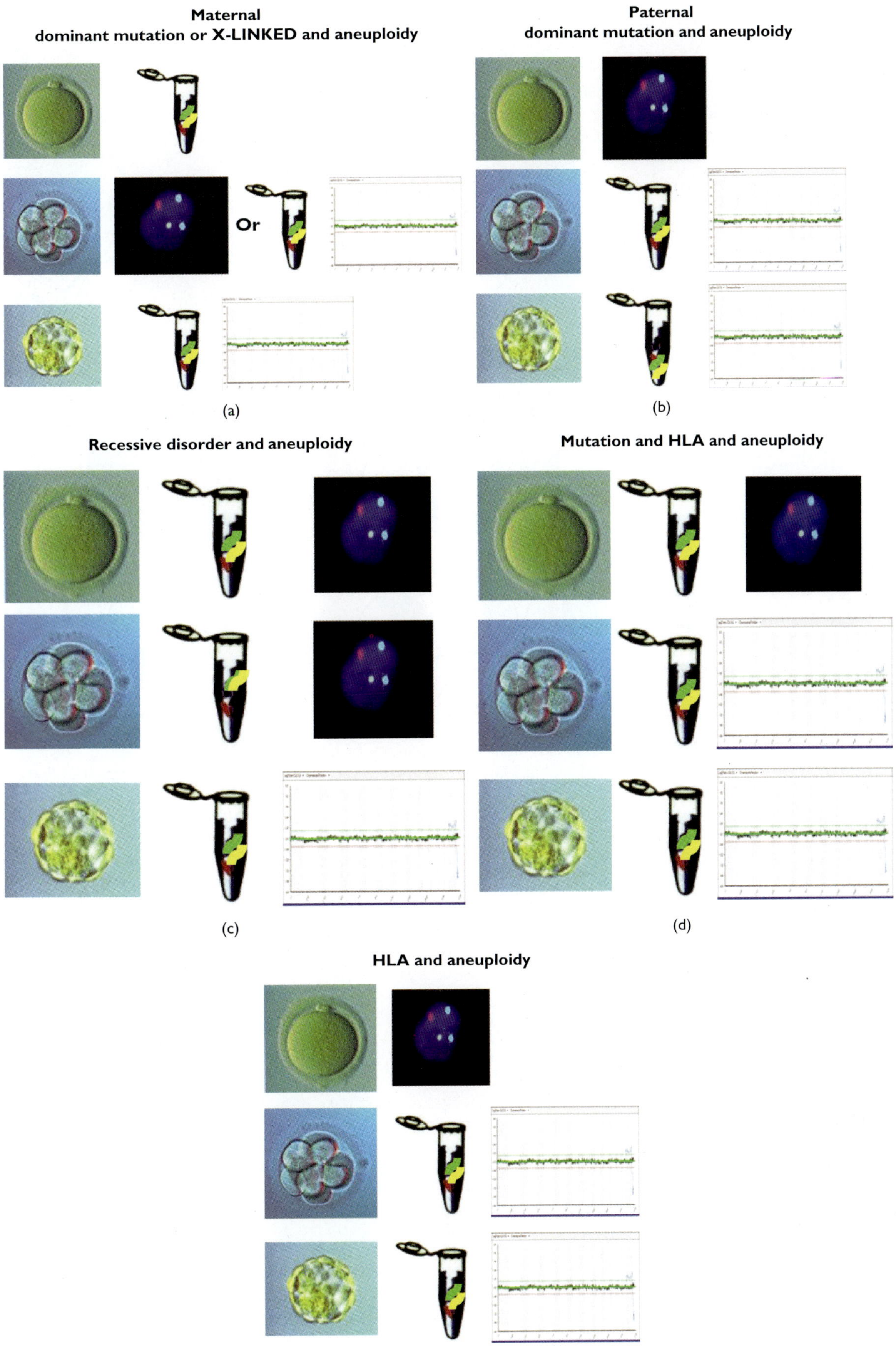
Maternal
dominant mutation or X-LINKED and aneuploidy
Or
(a)
Paternal
dominant mutation and aneuploidy
(b)
Recessive disorder and aneuploidy
(c)
Mutation and HLA and aneuploidy
(d)
HLA and aneuploidy
(e)

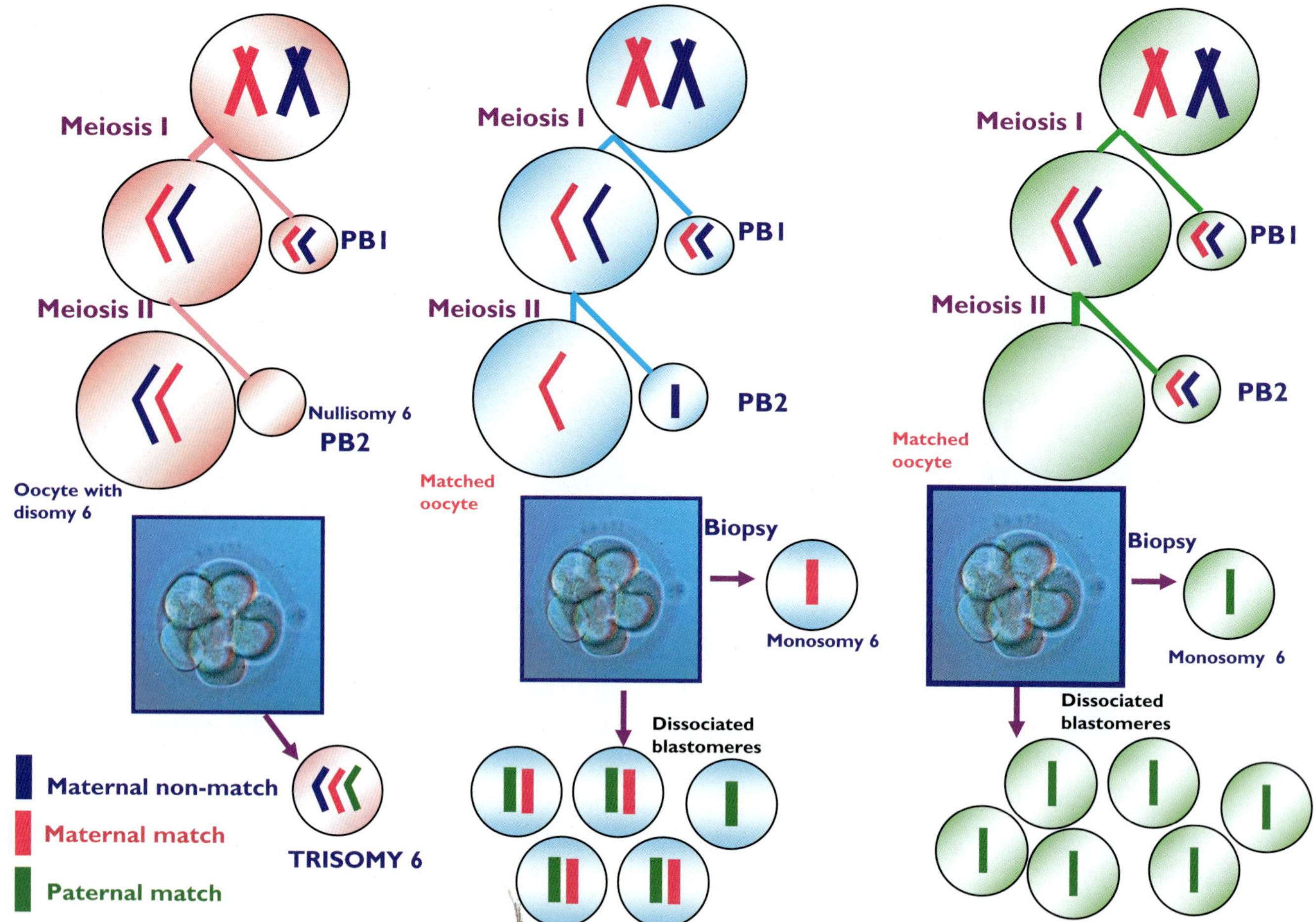

Figure 6.43 The value of chromosome 6 aneuploidy testing for accuracy of preimplantation HLA typing. (a) Matched maternal chromosome 6 is shown in pink, and non-matched in blue. Maternal disomy 6 was predicted based on the heterozygous first polar body (PB1) and "empty" (absence of DNA material) second polar body (PB2). Blastomere biopsy confirms the presence of two maternal and one paternal set of markers, evidencing trisomy 6 in the resulting embryo. (b) Sequential PB1 and PB2 analysis, suggesting maternal chromosome 6 matching, while the lack of the paternal markers in the blastomere indicates a potential monosomy 6. The follow-up analysis of the dissociated single blastomeres from this embryo revealed monosomy 6 in one of the blastomeres with the presence of the paternal matching chromosome 6. The rest of the blastomeres had both maternal and paternal matching chromosomes 6. (c) Monosomy 6 of maternal origin is inferred from the heterozygous PB1 and PB2, in agreement with the finding of only a paternal matching chromosome in the blastomere biopsy. This is further evidenced by the follow-up study of the dissociated blastomeres of this embryo, showing monosomy 6 in all the cells.

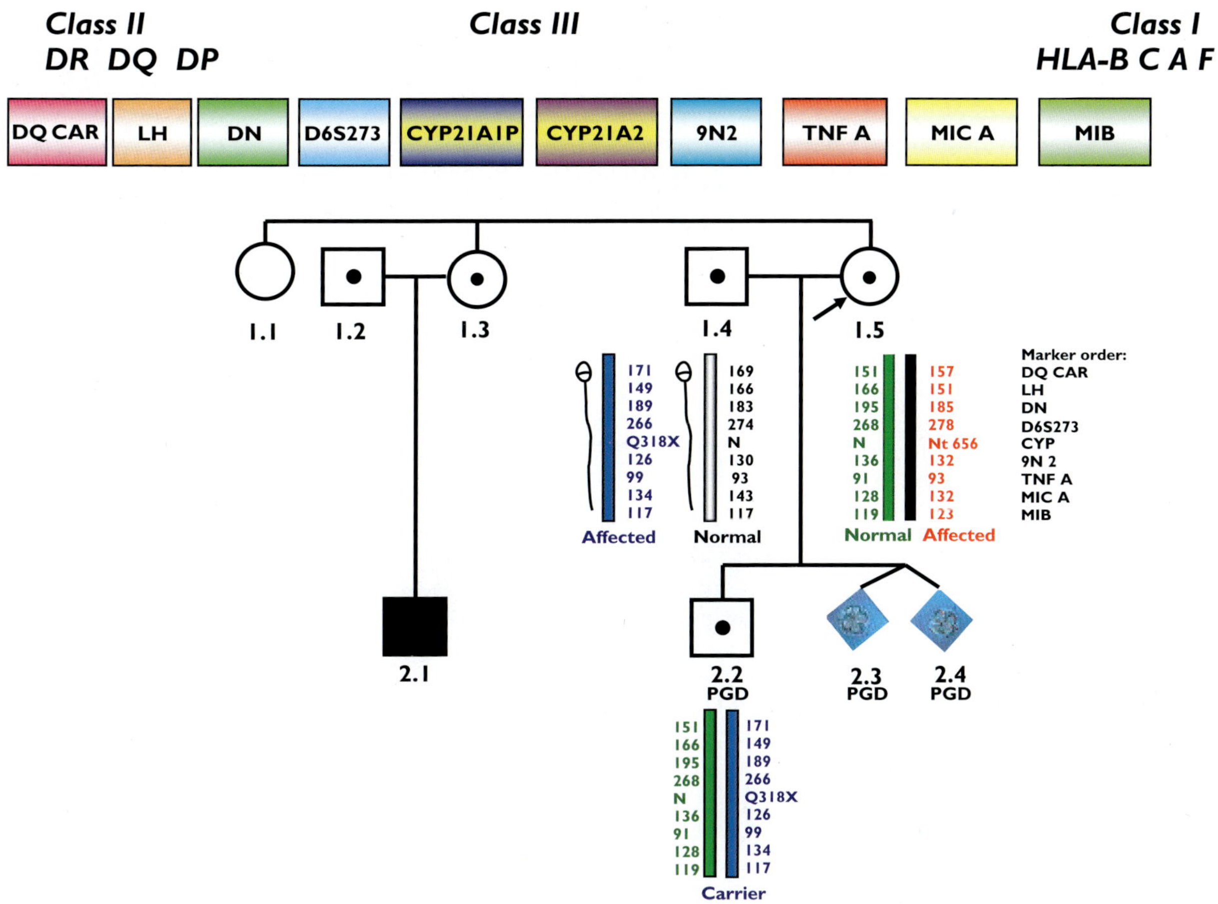

Figure 6.44 PGD for congenital adrenal hyperplasia (CAH). (Top) Location of the *CYP21A2* gene, *CYP21A1P* pseudogene, and tightly linked polymorphic markers on chromosome 6p21.3. (Bottom) Pedigree of a family undergoing PGD for CAH: husband (1.4) and wife (1.5) are carriers of two different mutations in the *CYP21A2* gene (the maternal nephew (2.1) is affected with CAH). As per the strategy of the mutation detection described on Figure 6.7, the paternal haplotype was established by multiplex single-sperm analysis, showing seven informative polymorphic markers wrapping the mutation site, with the maternal haplotype detected based on sequential analysis of the first and second polar bodies (PB1 and PB2). The mother was informative for eight markers. High similarity between the gene and pseudogene makes the application of polymorphic markers extremely important for testing accuracy. Following two PGD cycles, a healthy boy (2.2) was born after the first, and an ongoing twin pregnancy (2.3 and 2.4) has resulted after the second.

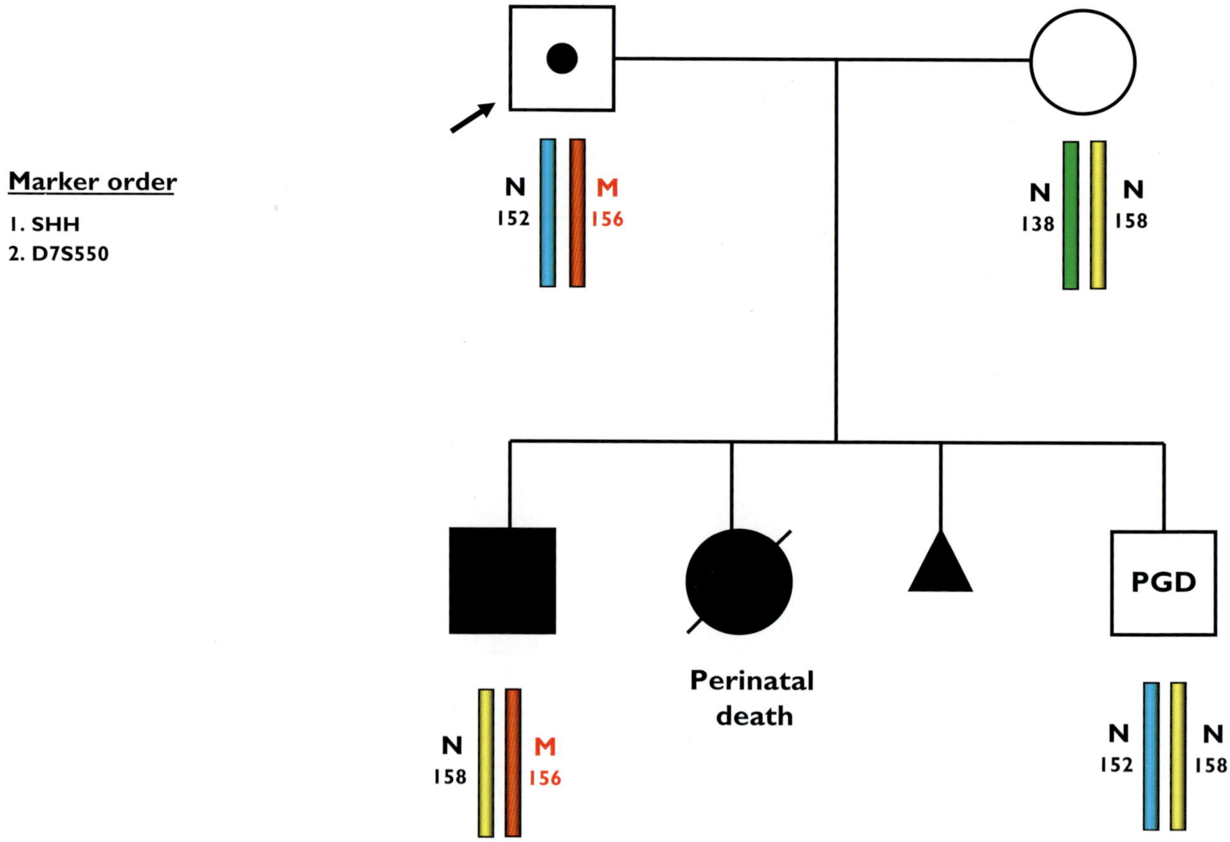

Figure 6.45 Family pedigree of a couple undergoing PGD for sonic hedgehog (*SHH*) mutation. (Top) The father has a gonadal mosaicism for the SHH mutation, which is linked to a 156-bp dinucleotide CA repeat allele of D7S550 polymorphic marker, while the mother is normal, with one normal allele linked to a 158-bp repeat and the other to a 138-bp repeat allele. (Bottom) Reproductive outcomes of this couple, including three previous pregnancies, one resulting in the birth of an affected child with holoprosencephaly, carrying the mutant gene (lower left), one in perinatal death, also carrying the mutant gene (lower center (circle)), and one in a spontaneously aborted fetus with Turner syndrome, free from SHH mutation (lower center (triangle)). The lower right (PGD) shows the outcome of preimplantation diagnosis, resulting in an unaffected clinical pregnancy and the birth of a healthy child, following confirmation of the mutation-free status by amniocentesis.

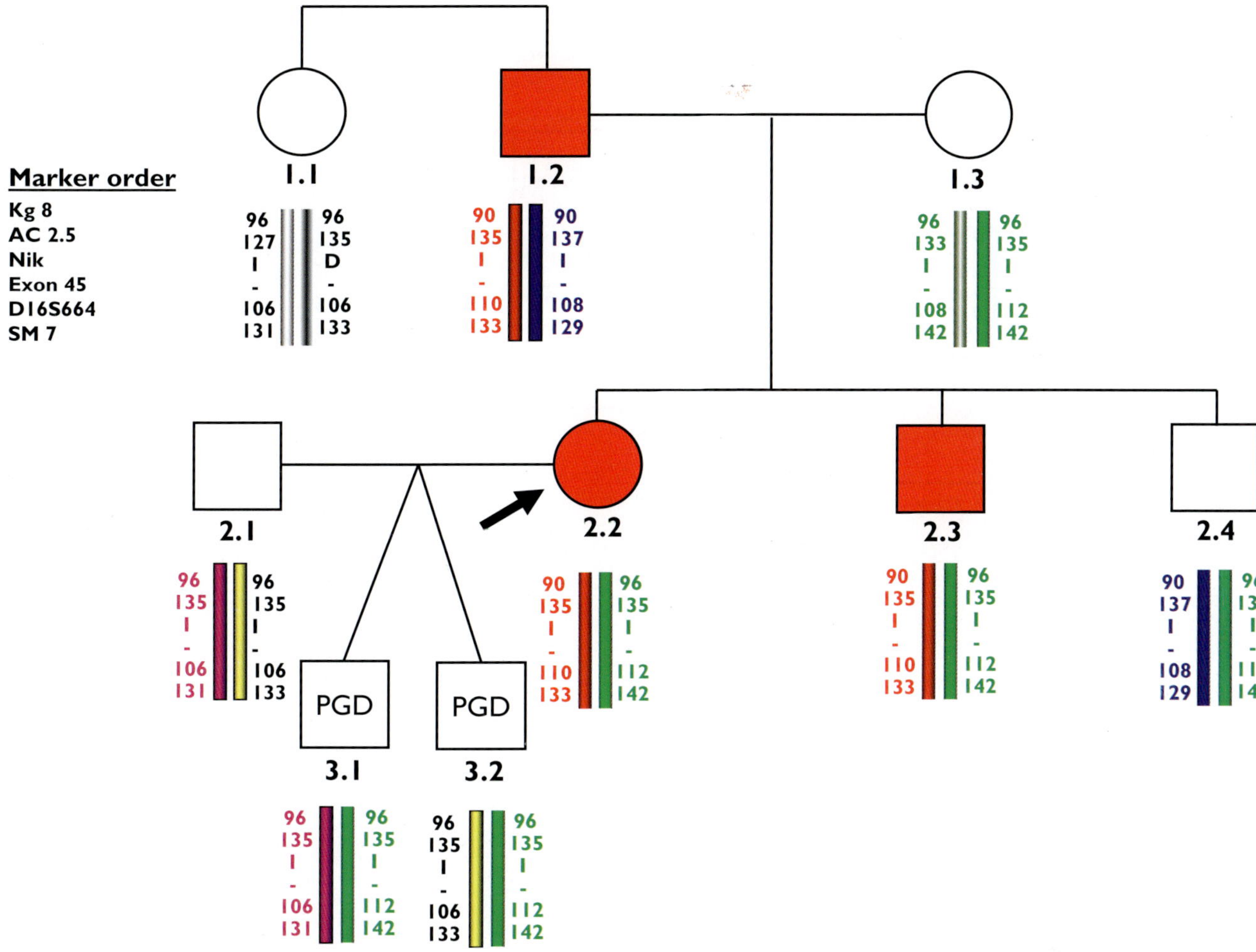

Figure 6.46 Preimplantation linked marker analysis for polycystic kidney disease (PKD)-1 resulting in the birth of unaffected twins. (Top) ADPKD mutation (mutant chromosome 16 is shown in red) originating from the affected maternal father (1.2), from whom the patient (2.2) inherited a possibly mutant chromosome 16 (red); mutation-free chromosomes of maternal mother (1.3) are shown in green. (Middle) The affected patient (2.2) had one affected brother (2.3), who also inherited the mutant chromosome from his father, and the same normal chromosome 16 from his mother. Her unaffected husband's (2.1) normal chromosomes 16 differ by one of the markers (131 bp vs. 133 bp), which makes it possible to identify the twins, resulting from PGD (3.1 and 3.2) (Bottom).

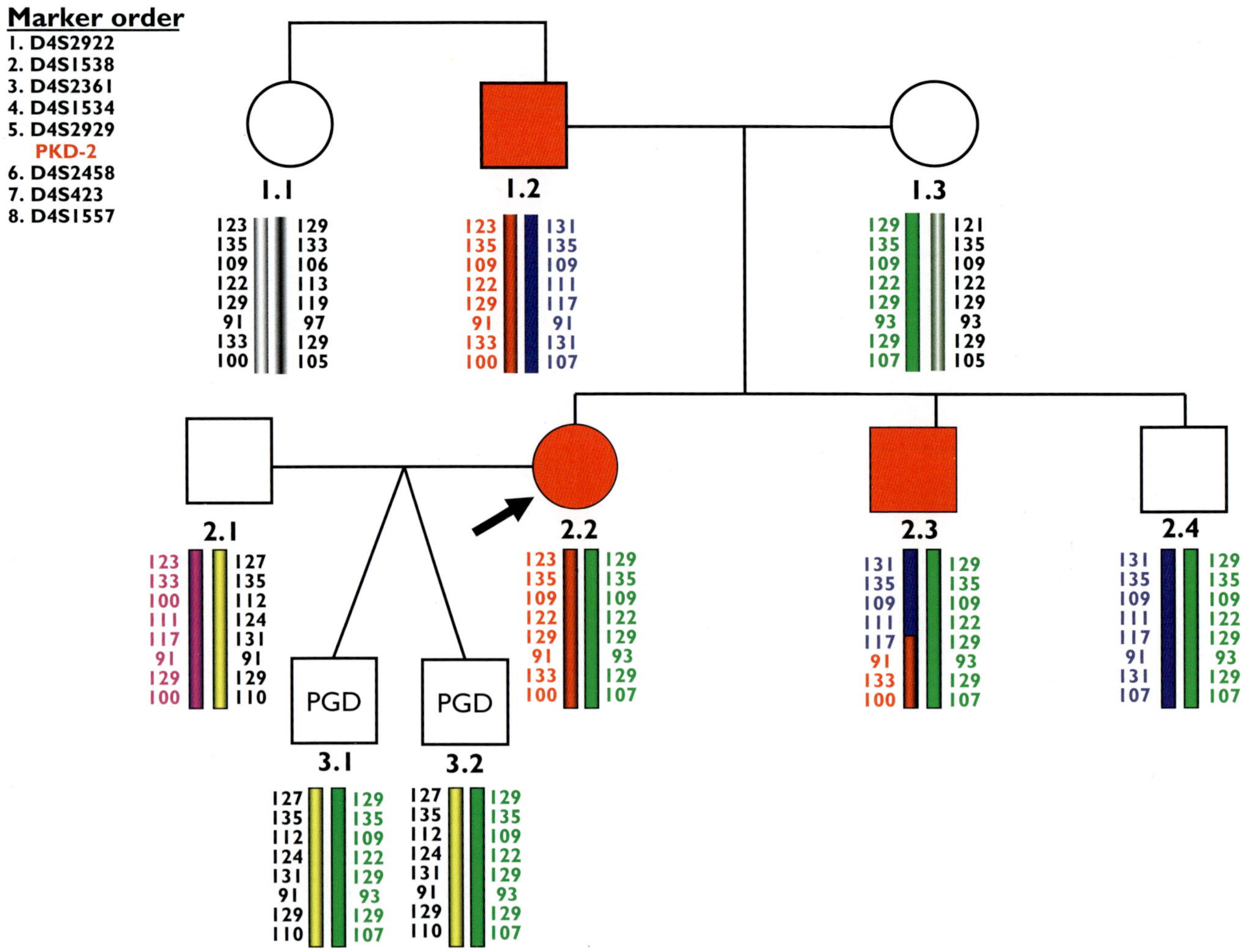

Figure 6.47 Preimplantation linked marker analysis for polycystic kidney disease (PKD)-2 resulting in the birth of unaffected twins (same pedigree). (Top) An ADPKD mutation (mutant chromosome 4 is shown in green) originating from the affected maternal father (1.2), from whom the patient (2.2) inherited a possibly mutant chromosome 4 (green); mutation-free chromosomes of maternal mother (1.3) are shown in red and black. (Middle) The affected patient (2.2) had one affected brother (2.3), who also inherited the mutant chromosome from his father, but following recombination between D4S2929 and D4S2458, which resulted in a recombinant chromosome 4 (blue and green), and the same normal chromosome 4 from the mother. Her unaffected husband's (2.1) normal chromosomes 4 cannot be distinguished as a consequence of sharing the same markers, so the fact that the resulting PGD twins are dizygotic cannot be demonstrated (3.1 and 3.2) (Bottom).

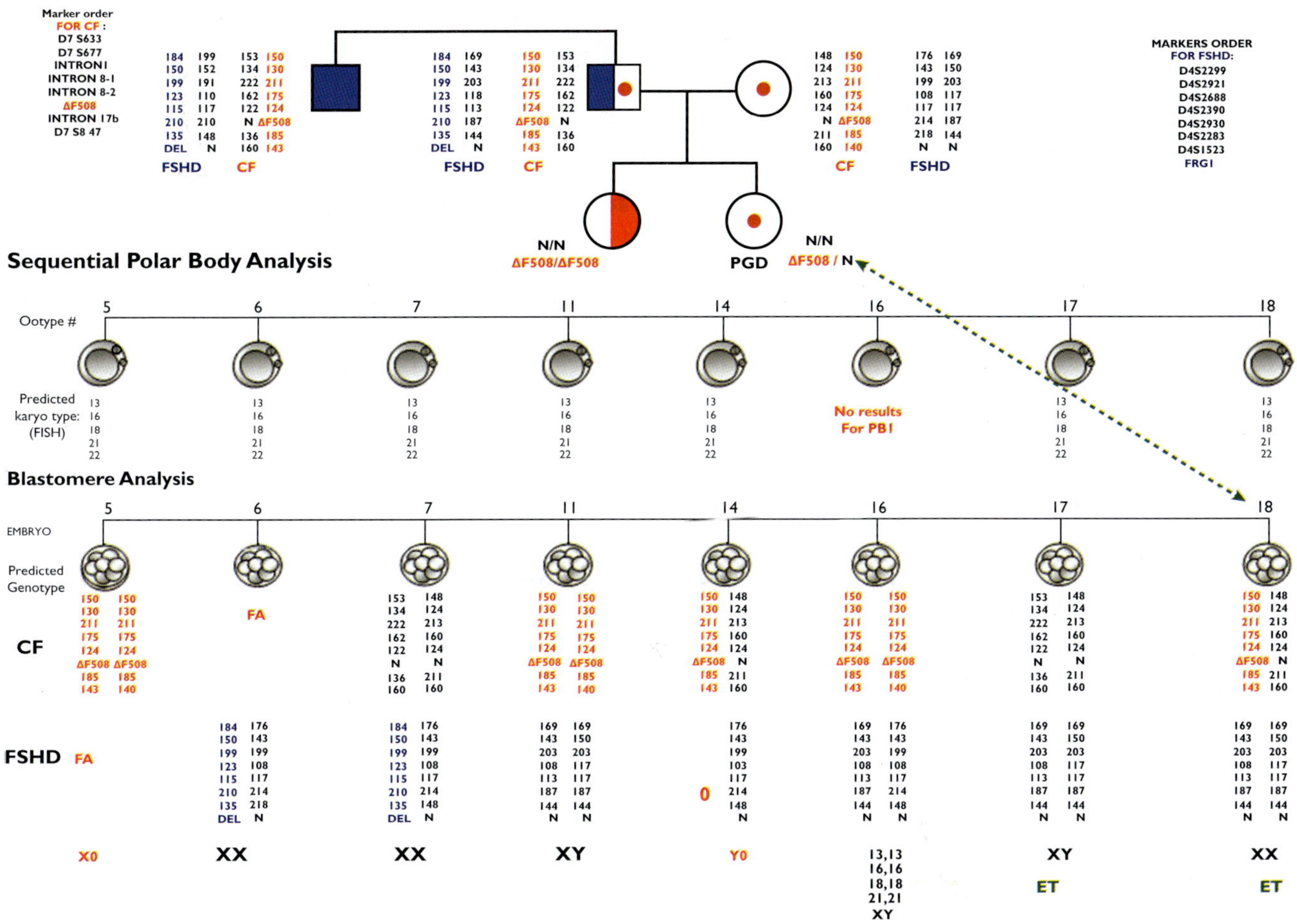

Figure 6.48 PGD for CF combined with testing for autosomal dominant disease and aneuploidy testing. (Upper panel) Pedigree, showing that both maternal and paternal partners are heterozygous carriers of ΔF508 mutation, while the latter is also a carrier of facioscapulohumeral muscular dystrophy 1A (FSHMD1A), (FRG1) (FSHD) mutation. Marker order used for testing CFTR mutation shown on the left as well as markers for testing *FRG1* gene deletion. (Middle panel) Sequential PB1 and PB2 aneuploidy testing of eight oocytes by FISH, showing normal results for all but one (oocyte 16). (Lower panel) Blastomere analysis of all eight resulting embryos for both ΔF508 and FRG1 mutations showed results for seven of them for CF (amplification failed in embryo 6) and for seven for FSHD (amplification failed in embryo 5). Embryos 5, 11, and 16 were homozygous affected for CF, embryos 14 and 18 were heterozygous carriers of ΔF508 mutation, and embryos 7 and 9 were free of ΔF508 mutation. Only embryos 6 and 7 were with FSHD mutation, and one (embryo 14) was aneuploid, missing the X-chromosome, while the remaining four embryos were unaffected for FSHD. Embryos 17 and 18 were unaffected for both mutations and so were transferred, resulting in a singleton pregnancy and birth of a healthy baby girl free of both diseases. As seen from marker analysis this baby originated from the transfer of embryo 18.

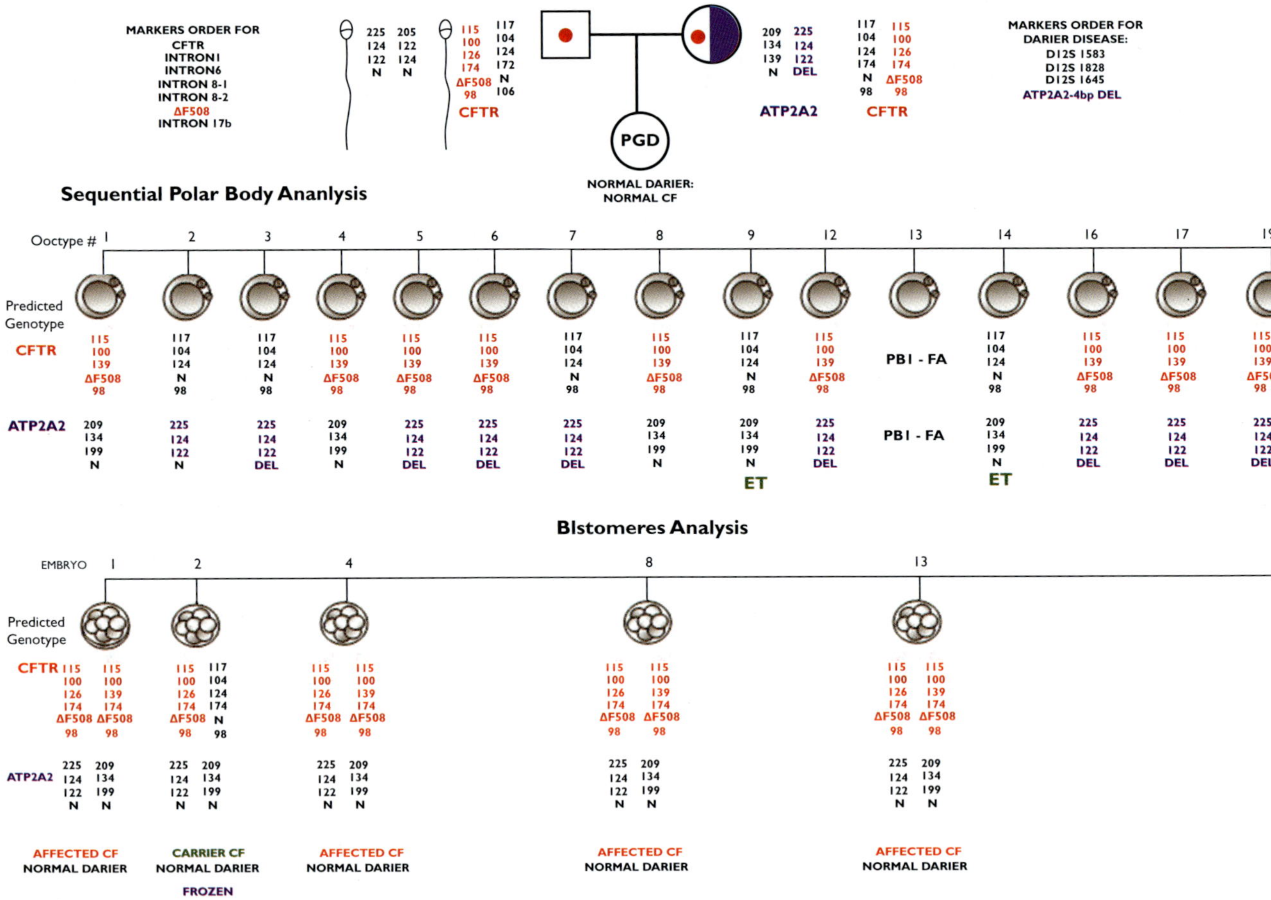

Figure 6.49 Combined PGD for *CFTR* gene and Darier disease *de novo* maternal mutation in ATP2A2. (Upper panel) Pedigree, showing that the both paternal and maternal partners are heterozygous carriers of ΔF508 mutation, while the latter also appeared to have a *de novo* mutation in *ATP2A2* gene. (Middle panel) Sequential PB1 and PB2 testing for both mutations. Of 15 oocytes tested by sequential PB1 and PB2, only two (oocytes 9 and 14) appeared to be free of both mutations, so the embryos resulting from these oocytes were transferred, resulting in a singleton pregnancy and birth of a healthy baby girl, free of both diseases. (Lower Panel) A sequential blastomere analysis of the four embryos resulting from the oocytes with DF508 mutation and without ATP2A2 deletion (one of the tested embryos was without PB results) allowed preselection of one embryo (embryo 2), a carrier of ΔF508 mutation, frozen for future use by the couple.

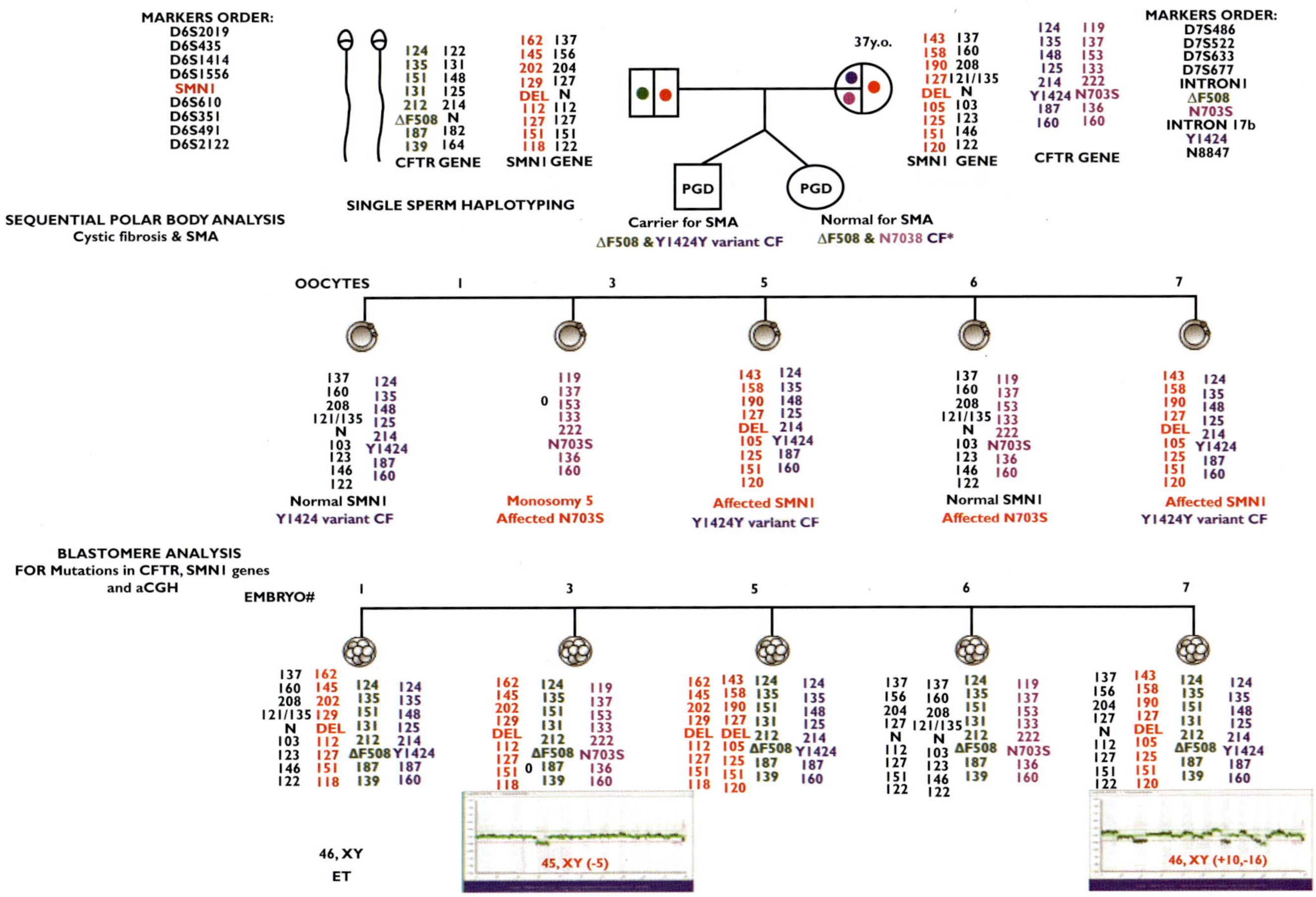

Figure 6.50 Combined PGD for CF and SMA with 24-chromosome aneuploidy testing. (Upper panel) Pedigree showing that both partners are carriers of *SMN1* gene, while father is also a carrier of DF508 and mother also a carrier of N703S CFTR mutation. (Middle panel) Sequential PB1 and PB2 testing in five oocytes, showing that only one (oocyte 1) appeared to be free of both SMN1 and N703S mutations, while others were with either the CFTR or SMN1 mutation, with further testing of the resulting embryos for 24-chromosome aneuploidy. (Lower panel) Testing of the resulting embryos, confirming unaffected status of the embryo resulting from oocyte 1, which was also aneuploidy free in array-CGH analysis for 24 chromosomes. The embryos resulting from the oocytes 2 and 7, although unaffected carriers of CFTR and SMA mutations, appeared to be with monosomy 5 (embryo 2) and trisomy 10 and monosomy 16 (embryo 7). The embryo resulting from oocyte 5 was affected for SMA and carrier of DF508 mutation in CFTR. Finally, the embryos resulting from oocyte 6 appeared to be an unaffected carrier of DF508 mutation and free of aneuploidy. Therefore, two embryos (embryos 1 and 6) were transferred, resulting in a twin pregnancy and birth of two unaffected carriers of SMA and CFTR.

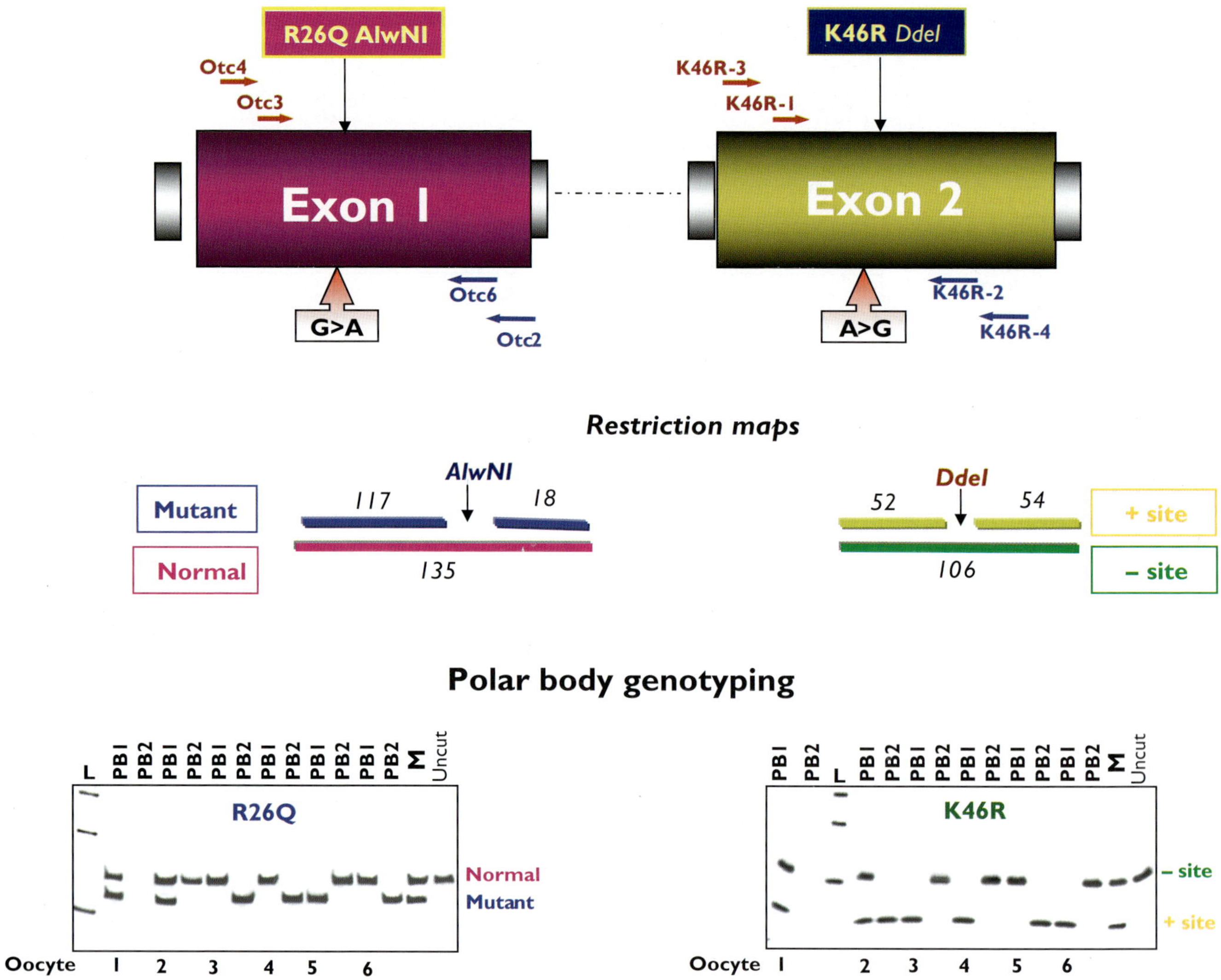

Figure 6.51 PGD for R26Q mutation in ornithine transcarbamylase (*OTC*) gene. (Top) Diagram of *OTC* gene exons 1 and 2, primers, and single nucleotide substitution mutation. Horizontal arrows show primer sets for nested PCR; vertical arrows show restriction sites for various enzymes. (Middle) Restriction map for mutation (R26Q) analysis and linked polymorphism. (Bottom) Mutation analysis of six oocytes by first (PB1) and second (PB2) polar bodies, suggesting mutant status of oocytes 2 (heterozygous PB1/normal PB2), 3, 4, and 6 (normal PB1/mutant PB2), and normal oocyte 5 (mutant PB1/normal PB2) (left). This is confirmed by linked marker analysis (right), in which the mutant allele lacks a *DdeI* site (– site) and the normal allele contains the site (+ site). The genotype of oocyte 1 cannot be predicted owing to the absence of information about the PB2. Uncut, undigested PCR product control; L, size marker ladder; M, maternal DNA.

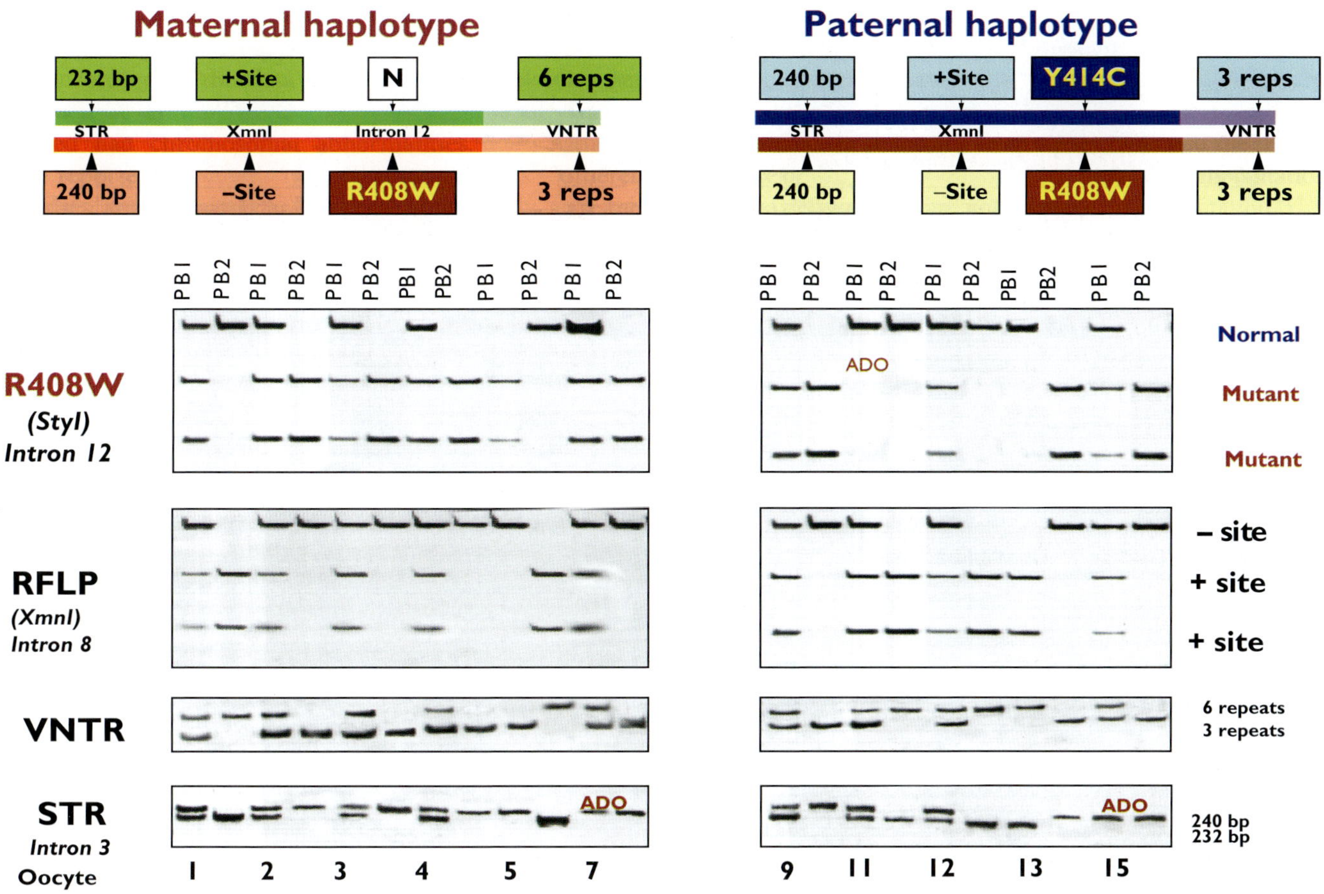

Figure 6.52 PGD for R408W mutation in phenylalanine hydroxylase (*PAH*) gene in a couple with the male partner being homozygous affected. (Top) Schematic representation of maternal (left) and paternal (right) haplotypes. The heterozygous mother has an R408W mutation linked to short tandem repeats (STR) in intron 3, a variable number of tandem repeats (VNTR) close to the 3′ end of the gene (3 reps), and restriction fragment length polymorphism (RFLP) in intron 8 (– site). The homozygous affected father has two different mutations, one the same as the maternal (R408W) mutation, and the other (Y414C mutation) with its own linkage pattern. (Bottom) Genotyping of oocytes by sequential analysis of first (PB1) and second (PB2) polar bodies for R408W mutation and informative linked markers (RFLP, VNTR, and STR). All series include the PB1 followed by the PB2 in the column immediately to its right, corresponding to 11 oocytes studied (oocytes are numbered at the bottom). As the R408W mutation creates a restriction site for the *StyI* enzyme, oocytes 2, 3, 4, 7, 9, and 15 were predicted to be normal based on heterozygous PB1 and a homozygous mutant PB2. Oocyte 5 was also predicted to be normal, but this was based on a homozygous mutant PB1 and a normal PB2 (which was in agreement with marker analysis), excluding the possibility for allele dropout (ADO) in the corresponding PB1. ADO of the mutant allele is evident from the identical genotype of the PB1 and PB2 in oocyte 11 (confirmed by all three markers), suggesting affected status of this oocyte. Three other oocytes were predicted to be affected based on a heterozygous PB1 and a normal PB2 (oocytes 1 and 12), and a homozygous normal PB1 and mutant PB2 (oocyte 13). ADO was also detected in intron 3 STR in oocytes 7 and 15 (identical genotype of PB1 and PB2). These data are not in conflict with the unaffected genotype of the resulting embryos, which were transferred together with two other unaffected embryos (2 and 4). This resulted in twin pregnancy and the birth of two healthy children, following confirmation of PGD by prenatal diagnosis.

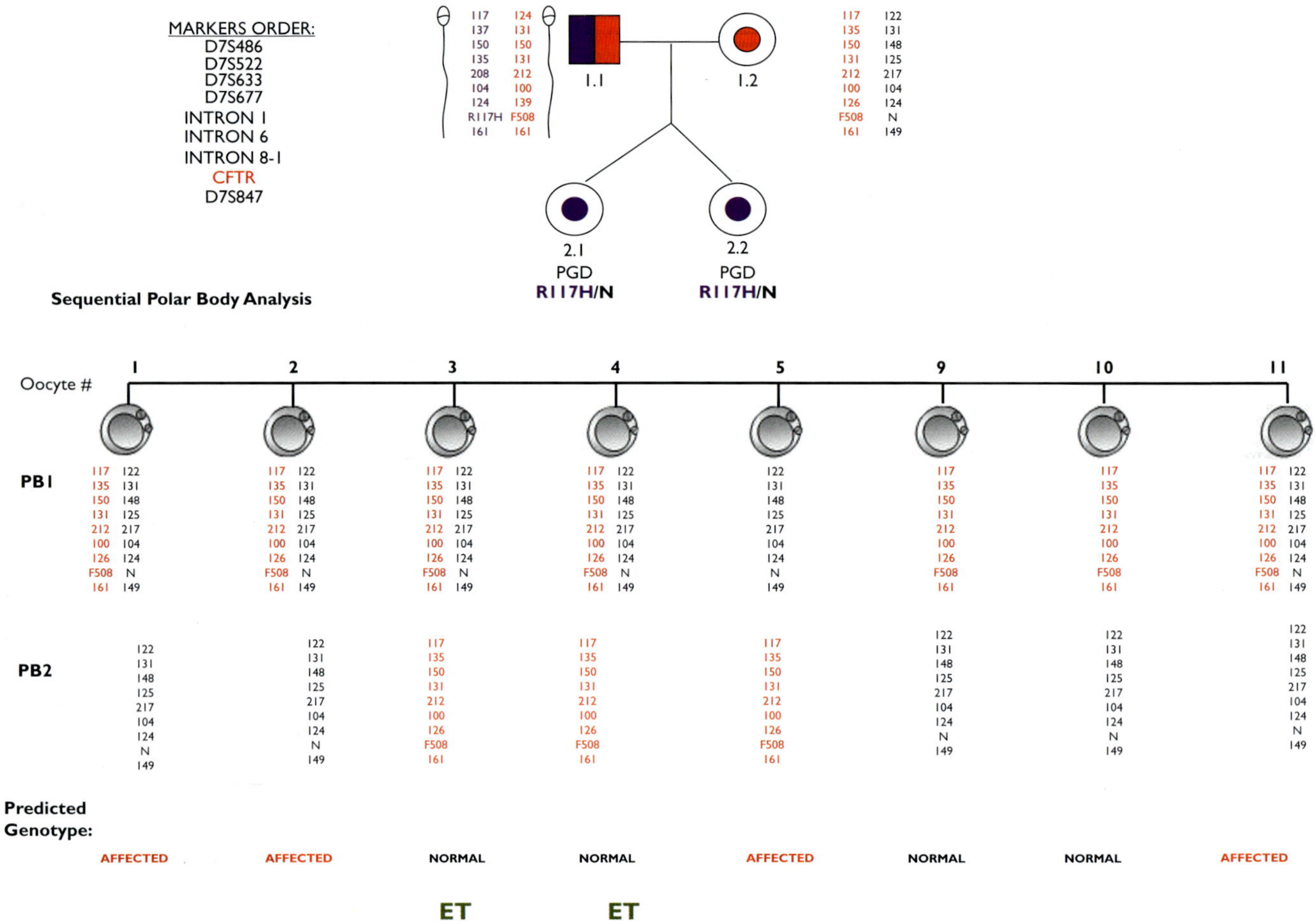

Figure 6.53 PGD for double heterozygous CF male patient by sequential polar body analysis. (Upper panel) Pedigree, showing that the paternal partner is a double heterozygous affected CF patient, with two different CFTR mutations, ΔF508 and R117H, while the maternal partner is a carrier of the ΔF508 mutation. (Lower panel) Sequential PB1 and PB2 analysis of eight oocytes, of which four were predicted to be free of maternal mutation, one of which (oocyte 4) had heterozygous PB1 and mutant PB2, with no risk for misdiagnosis due to ADO. Two embryos resulting from oocytes 3 and 4 were transferred, resulting in an unaffected twin pregnancy and birth of two healthy baby girls carrying the paternal R117H mutation.

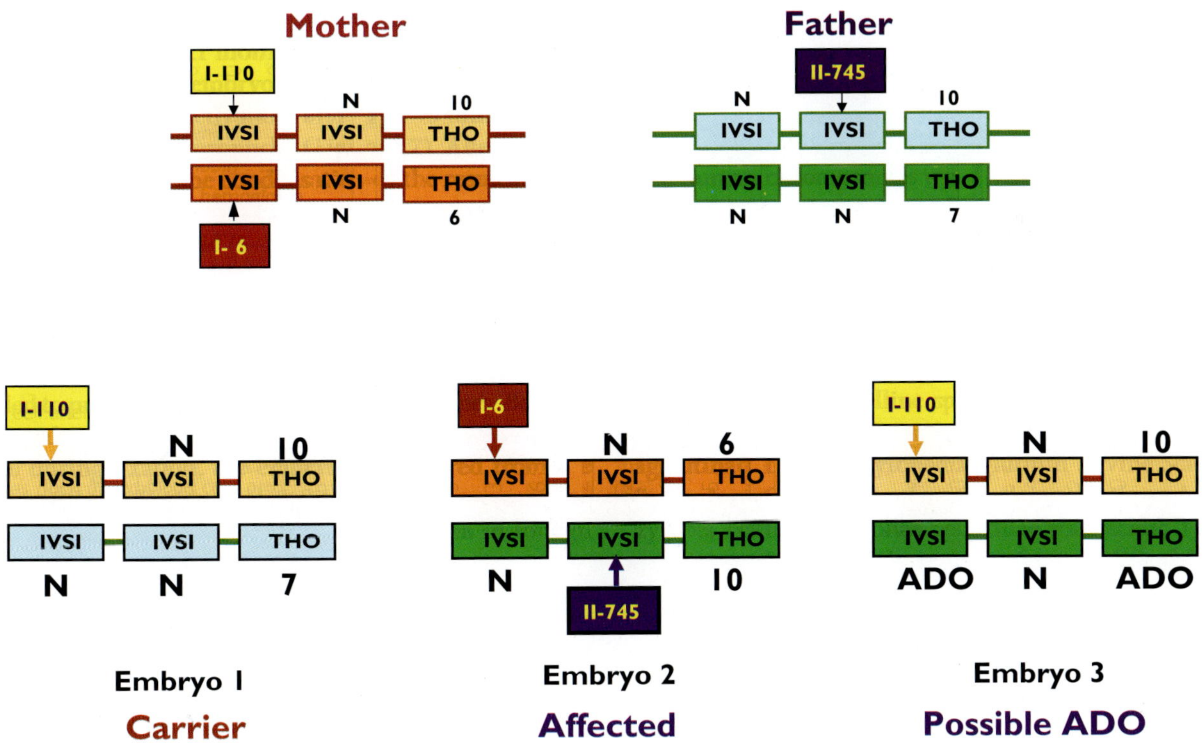

Figure 6.54 PGD in a couple with three different β-globin gene mutations. (Top) Schematic representation of maternal and paternal haplotypes, showing linkage of maternally derived mutations IVSI-110 and IVSI-6 to ten and six repeats, respectively, and linkage of paternally derived mutation IVSII-745 to ten repeats in the THO (thyrosin hydroxylase) polymorphic site. The normal paternal allele is linked to seven THO repeats, as detected by sperm haplotyping analysis. (Bottom) Genotyping three embryos for both paternal (IVSII-745) and maternal (IVSI-110, IVSI-6) mutations simultaneously with linked markers in the THO site. Only one mutation (IVSI-110) is detected in embryo 1, along with the paternally derived normal allele, as evidenced by the presence of seven repeats in the THO site, suggesting carrier status of embryo 1 (suitable for transfer). Embryo 2 is predicted to be affected based on the presence of maternal mutation IVSI-6 and paternal mutation IVSII-745. This was confirmed by linked marker analysis (presence of six and ten repeats in the THO site). No decision can be made regarding the transfer of embryo 3, owing to possible dual allele dropout (ADO) of the paternal allele and the linked marker. N, normal allele.

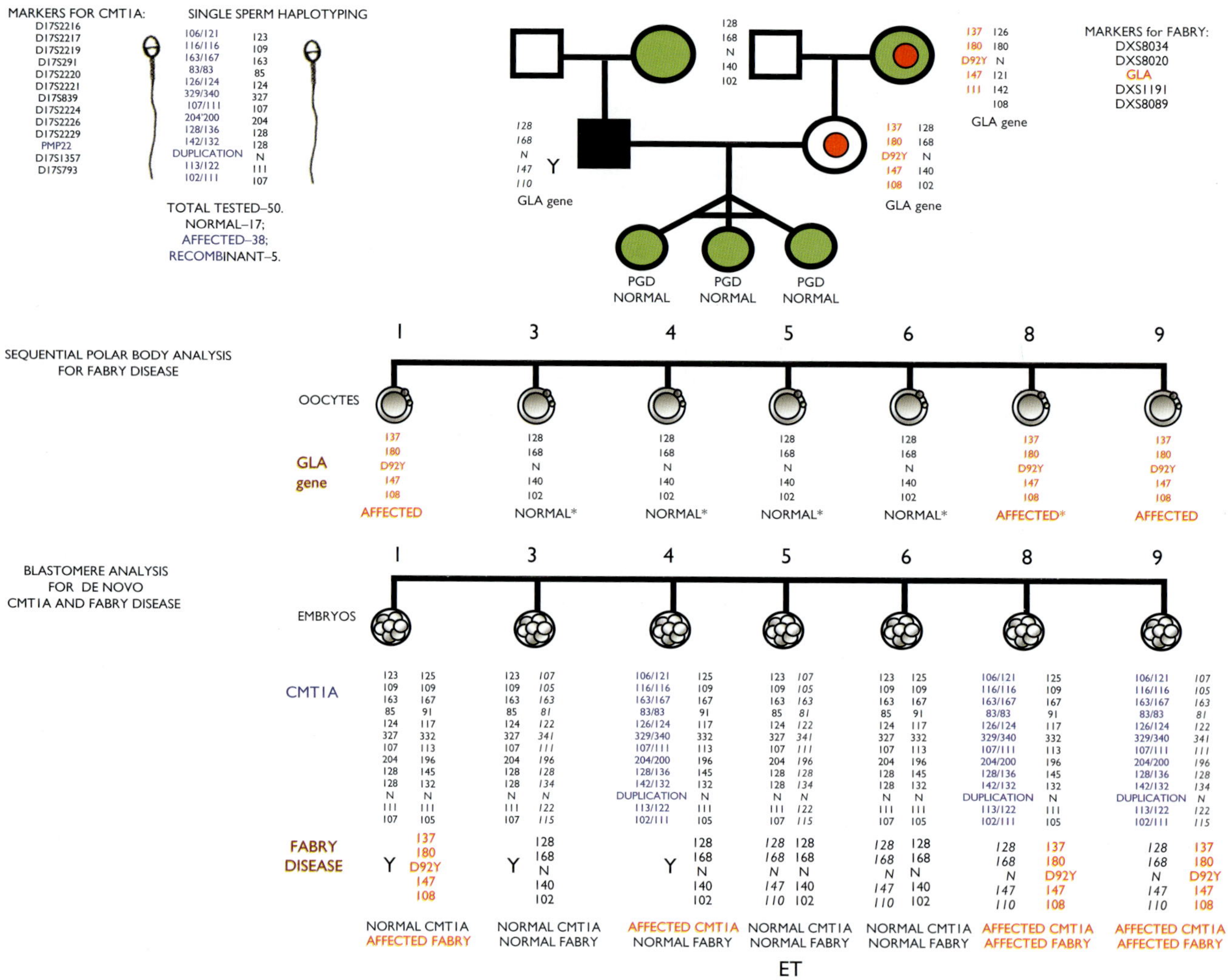

Figure 6.55 Combined PGD for paternal *de novo* duplication in *PMP22* gene (Charcot–Marie–Tooth disease, CMT1a) and Fabry disease. (Upper panel) Pedigree, showing the origin of both mutations in maternal and paternal partners: paternal partner is unaffected, but duplication of *PMP22* gene was detected in single sperm typing (the mutant sperm haplotype is shown on the left, as well as marker orders). Maternal partner is a carrier of *GLA* gene originating from her mother (maternal mutant and normal haplotypes are shown on the right, as well as marker order). (Middle panel) Sequential PB1 and PB2 analysis of oocytes for Fabry disease, showing that oocytes 1, 8, and 9 are affected (shown in red), while the remaining four oocytes (oocytes 3, 4, 5, and 6) are free of mutation. (Lower panel) Blastomere analysis for CMT1A, Fabry disease, and aneuploidy testing, showing that the embryos originating from oocytes 3, 8, and 9 are affected by CMT1A, while embryos 1 and 9 were confirmed affected by Fabry disease. Taking into account the finding on both mutations, three embryos were unaffected by both conditions and euploid (embryos 3, 5, and 6), one of which was transferred (embryo 5), resulting in the triplet pregnancy and birth of monozygotic triplets free of both CMT1A and Fabry diseases (shown in green on the bottom of pedigree).

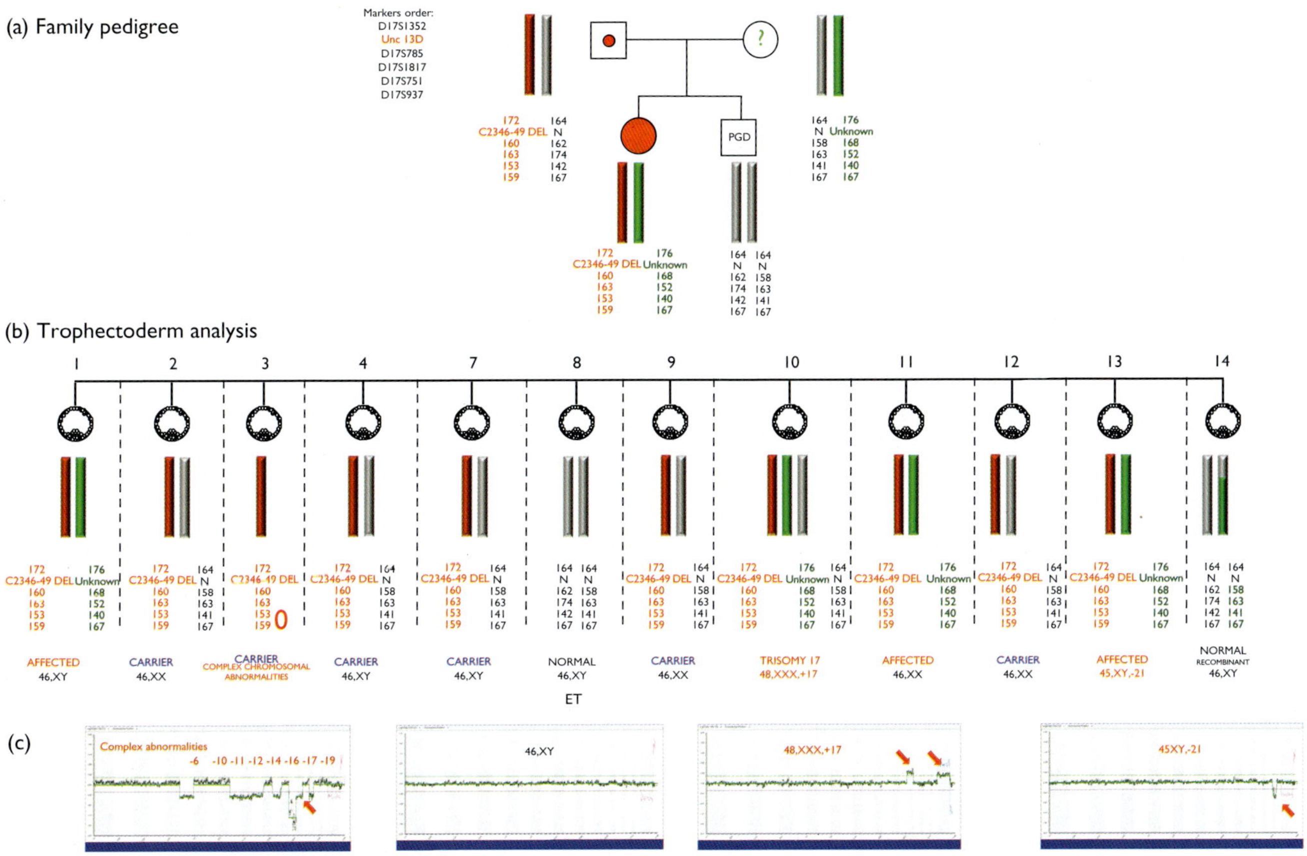

Figure 6.56 PGD for familial hemophagocytic lymphohistiocytosis, a *de novo* recessive mutation in the *Unc13D* gene, combined with aneuploidy testing by array-CGH. (a) Family pedigree showing that the unaffected paternal partner is a carrier of C246-49 Del in the *Unc13D* gene. No mutation was identified in the unaffected maternal partner, but she could have had gonadal mosaicism for unknown *Unc13D* mutation, not identified also in her affected daughter, shown in red. The PGD was based on tracing against both haplotypes of the affected child (shown in red and green). Marker order for *Unc13D* gene testing is shown on the left. (b) Trophectoderm analysis in 12 embryos detected three affected embryos (embryos 1, 11, and 13), six carriers (embryos 2, 3, 4, 7, 9, and 12), and two normal (embryos 8 and 14), the latter however being recombinant and thus ruled out for transfer. (c) Results of aCHG for 24-chromosome aneuploidy testing, showing complex aneuploidy in embryo 3, double trisomy X and 17 in embryo 10, and trisomy 21 in embryo 13. Embryo 8, which was free of both mutant haplotypes, was also euploid, based on array-CGH analysis for 24 chromosomes. This embryo was transferred, resulting in a singleton pregnancy and birth of an unaffected baby boy (PGD, shown on the bottom of the pedigree in panel (a)).

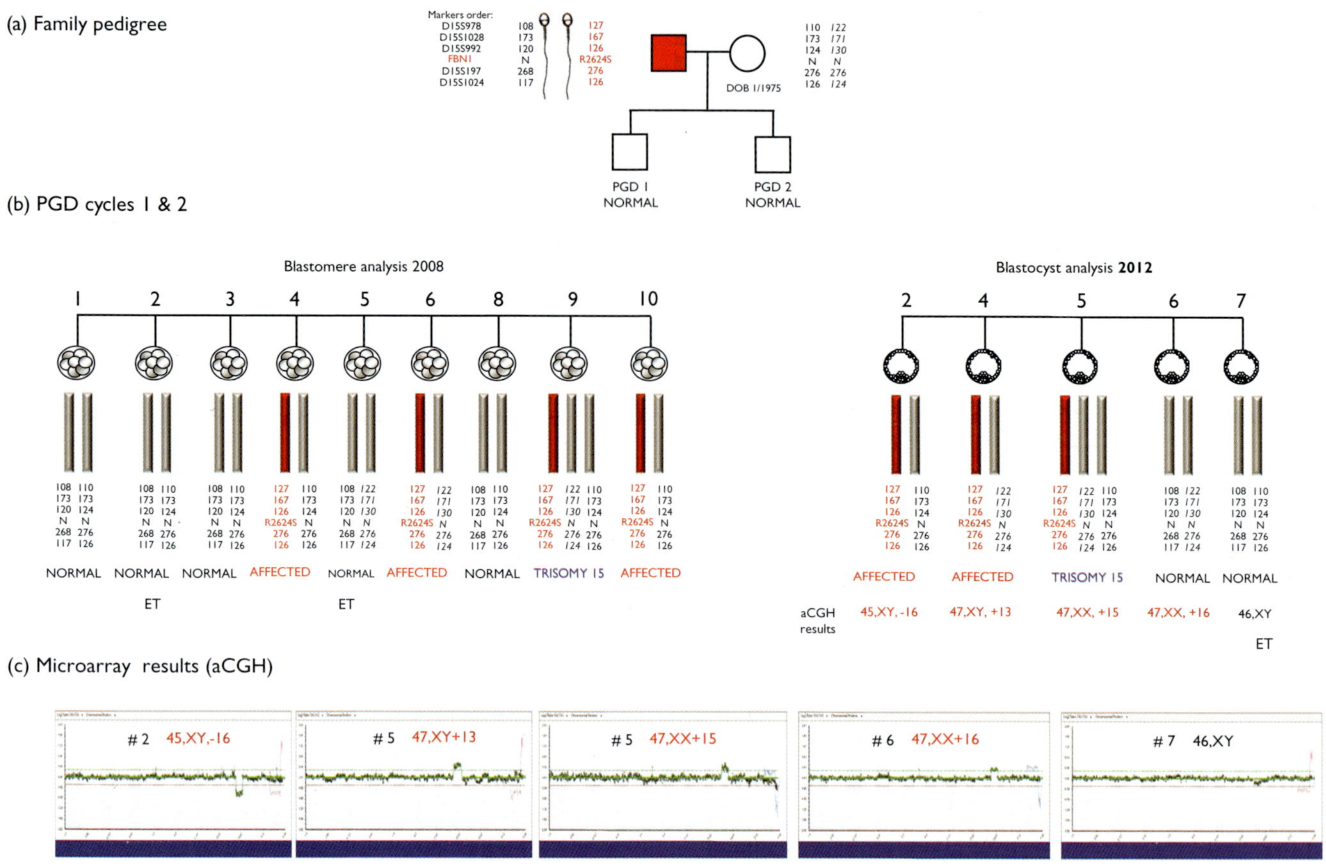

Figure 6.57 PGD for *de novo* paternal mutation in *FBN1* gene causing Marfan syndrome. (a) Family pedigree, showing also the results of single sperm typing from the affected paternal partner, who is a carrier of *FBN1* mutation, but has no family history of the disease in any of his family members. Marker order for the mutation testing is shown on the left. (b) Results of PGD in two cycles performed in 2008 (left portion of Panel (b)) and 2012 (right portion of Panel (b)). The first PGD cycle in 2008 was performed by blastomere analysis, which detected three affected embryos from the nine embryos tested (embryos 4, 6, and 10), one trisomy 15 (embryo 9), and the remaining five embryos free of FBN1 mutation (embryos 1, 2, 3, 5, and 8), two of which (embryos 2 and 5) were transferred, resulting in a singleton pregnancy and birth of an unaffected baby boy (shown as PGD1 in the bottom of pedigree). The second PGD cycle in 2012 (right portion of Panel (b)) was performed by trophectoderm analysis, combined with array-CGH testing for 24-chromosome aneuploidy, which detected only one of five embryos (embryo 7) being mutation free and euploid. (c) The array-CGH 24-chromosome aneuploidy testing of five embryos in 2012 PGD cycle, showing aneuploidy for different chromosomes in all but one embryo (embryo 7), which was also free of mutant gene (see above in Panel (b)) and transferred, resulting in an unaffected singleton pregnancy and birth of a healthy baby boy (see PGD2 in the bottom of pedigree).

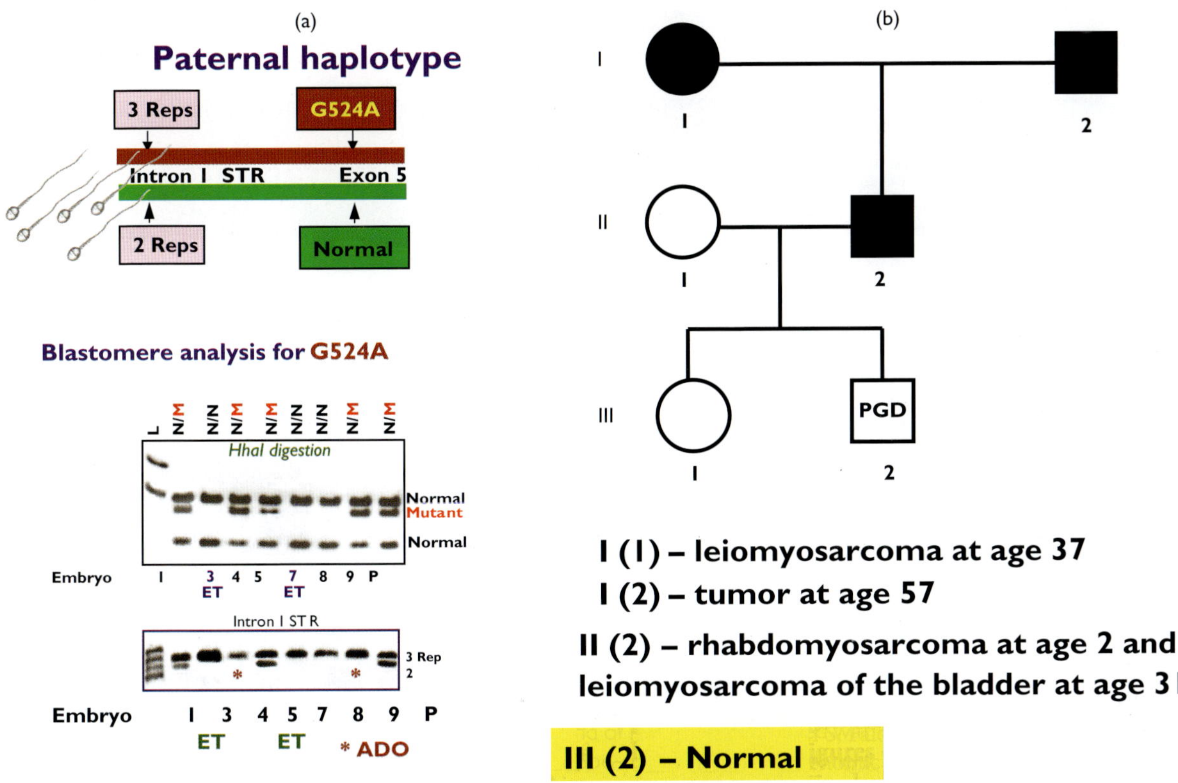

Figure 6.58 PGD for *p53* tumor suppressor gene mutations. (a) PGD for paternally derived G524A mutation in *p53* tumor suppressor gene. The paternal haplotype based on single-sperm analysis shows linkage of the affected allele to three repeats and the normal allele to two repeats in intron 1 STR (top). Duplex blastomere analysis for G524A mutation in exon 5 and linked STR in intron 1 (bottom), showing that embryos 1, 4, 5, and 9 are affected, while embryos 3, 7, and 8 are mutation free and suitable for transfer. Allele dropout (ADO) of three repeats in intron 1 STR was detected in the blastomeres from embryos 4 and 9. (b) Family pedigree for three generations.

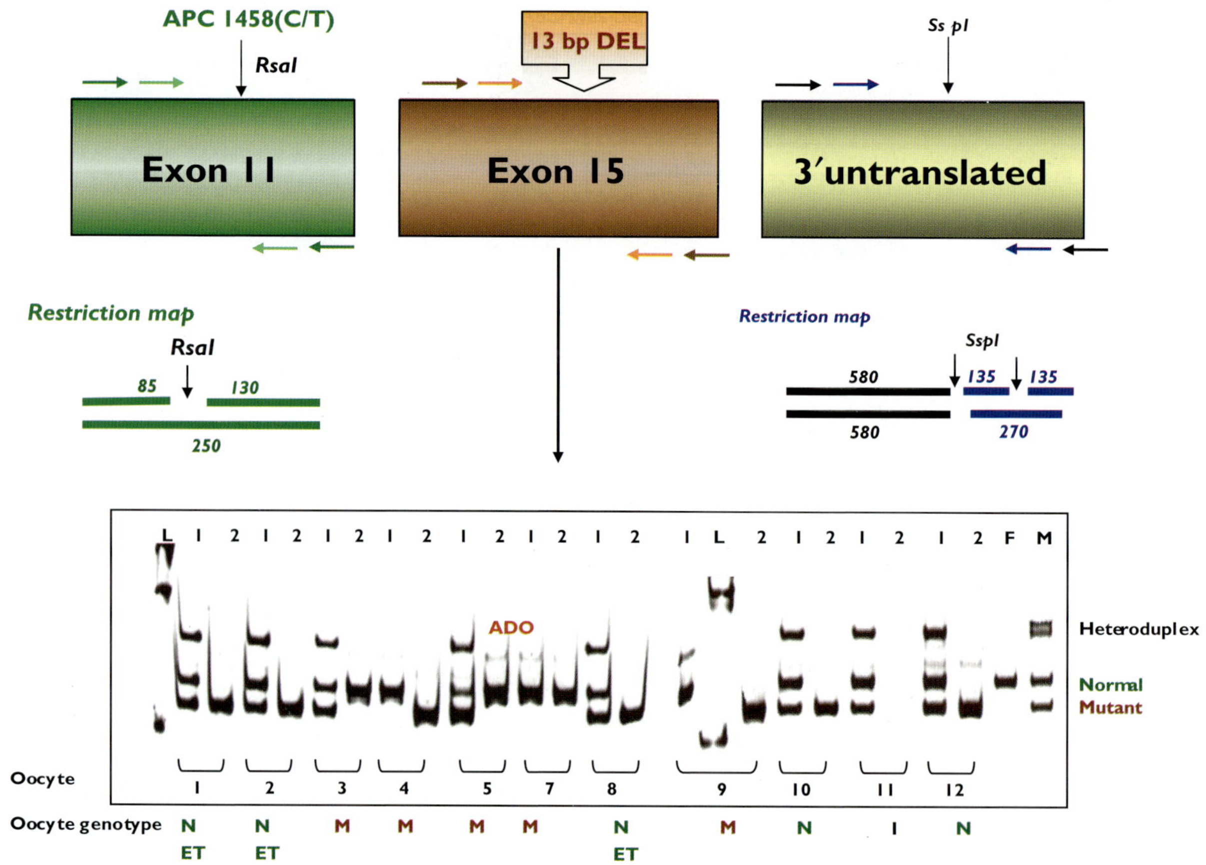

Figure 6.59 PGD for 13-bp deletion in adenomatous polyposis coli (*APC*) gene. (Top) Schematic diagram of the mutation and linked markers on chromosome 5q21. (Bottom) Polyacrylamide gel electrophoresis of the PCR products of the first (PB1) and second (PB2) polar bodies from 11 oocytes in one of the cycles of PGD for familial adenomatous polyposis coli (FAP), showing mutation-free oocytes 1, 2, 8, 10, and 12, evidenced by normal (N) and mutant (M) fragments in the PB1 and a mutant fragment in the PB2, in agreement with linked marker analysis (results not shown). ET, embryo transfer.

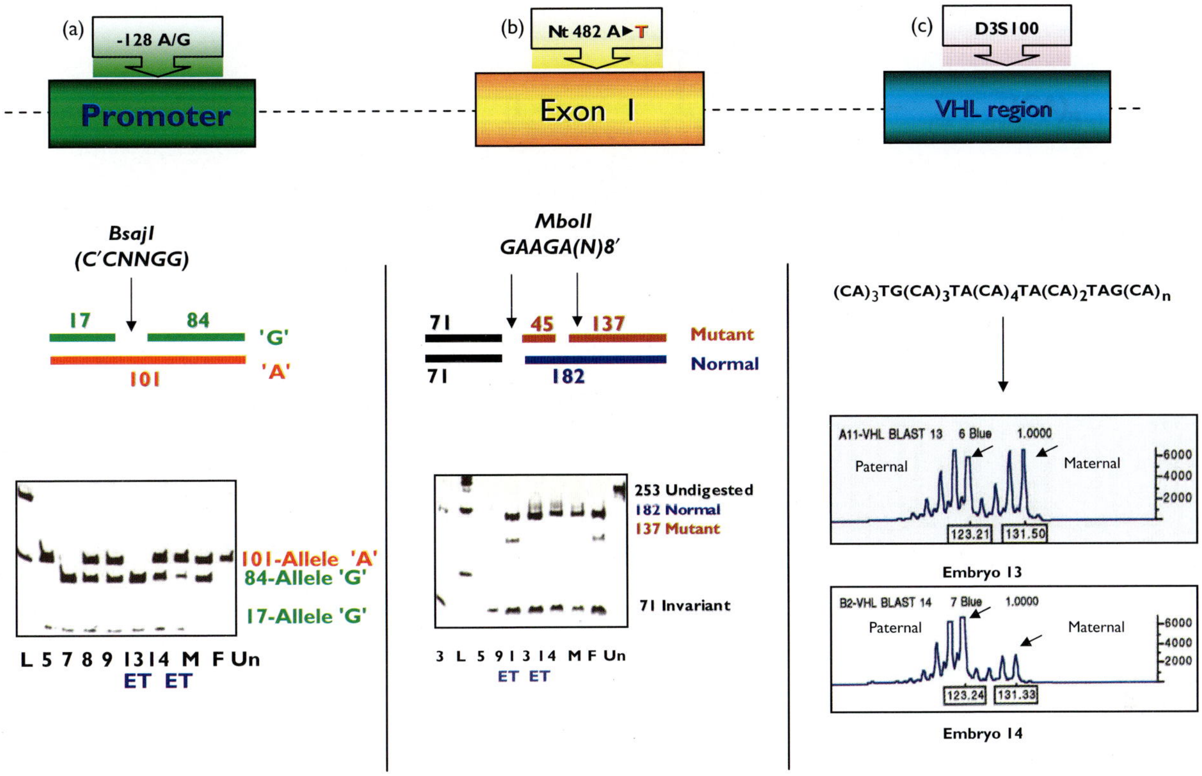

Figure 6.60 PGD for Nt 482 A–T mutation in exon 1 of von Hippel–Lindau (*VHL*) gene. (Top) Schematic diagram of the mutation and linked markers. (a) Position of G/A single-nucleotide polymorphism (SNP) in the promoter area of the gene and restriction map. Restriction digestion with *BsaJI* enzyme distinguished 'A' and 'G' sequences. (b) Position of Nt 482 A–T mutation in exon 1 of *VHL* gene and the restriction map. Amplified sequence has an invariant restriction fragment (71 bp). The enzyme *MboII* digests the mutant sequence into two fragments of 45 bp and 137 bp, with the size of the normal allele being 182 bp. Polyacrylamide gel electrophoresis of the *MboII* restriction-digested PCR products of blastomeres detected mutation-free embryos 13 and 14, evidenced by the presence of a 182-bp undigested fragment, as compared to the presence of a digested 137-bp fragment in the affected embryos. ET, embryos transferred; Un, undigested; M, maternal DNA; F, paternal DNA containing the mutation; L, 100-bp standard. (c) Position and sequence of D3S100 dinucleotide repeat in *VHL* region. Capillary electrophoregrams of fluorescently labeled dinucleotide repeat PCR products scored by Genotyper®. The presence of the 123-bp paternal allele in embryos 13 and 14 confirmed the normal status of these embryos as predicted by mutation analysis.

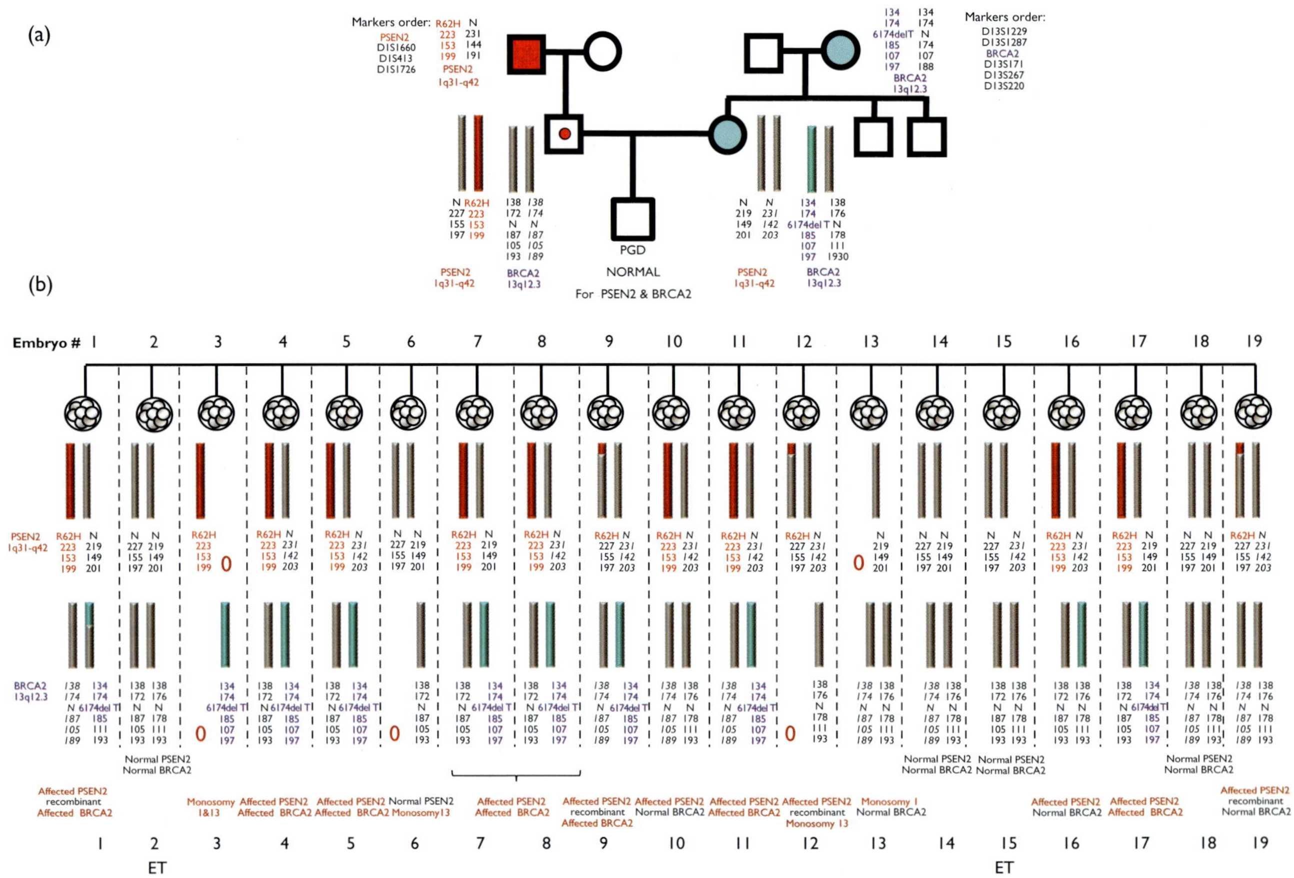

Figure 6.61 PGD for breast cancer (6174del T mutation in *BRCA2* gene) and early Alzheimer disease (R62H mutation in *PSEN2* gene). (a) Pedigree, showing that the maternal partner and her mother are carriers of *BRCA2* mutation (6174del T shown in blue). Linked markers are listed on the right. The paternal partner is a carrier of R62H mutation in the *PSEN2* gene, inherited from his father (shown in red). Linked markers are listed on the left. (b) Nineteen embryos were tested by blastomere analysis, simultaneously for both mutations, which detected only two embryos (embryos 2 and 15) that were free of both mutations, the remaining 15 being either with PSEN2 mutation (shown in red) (upper level of Panel (b)) or with BRCA2 mutation (shown in blue) (lower level of Panel (b)). Some of these embryos were also with monosomy of the chromosome in which the genes are located: monosomy chromosome 1 (embryos 3 and 13), and monosomy 13 (embryos 3, 6, and 12). There were also three recombinant embryos for the *PSEN* gene (embryos 9, 12, and 19) and one for the *BRCA2* gene. Both unaffected embryos (embryos 2 and 15) were transferred, resulting in a singleton unaffected pregnancy (see the bottom of pedigree).

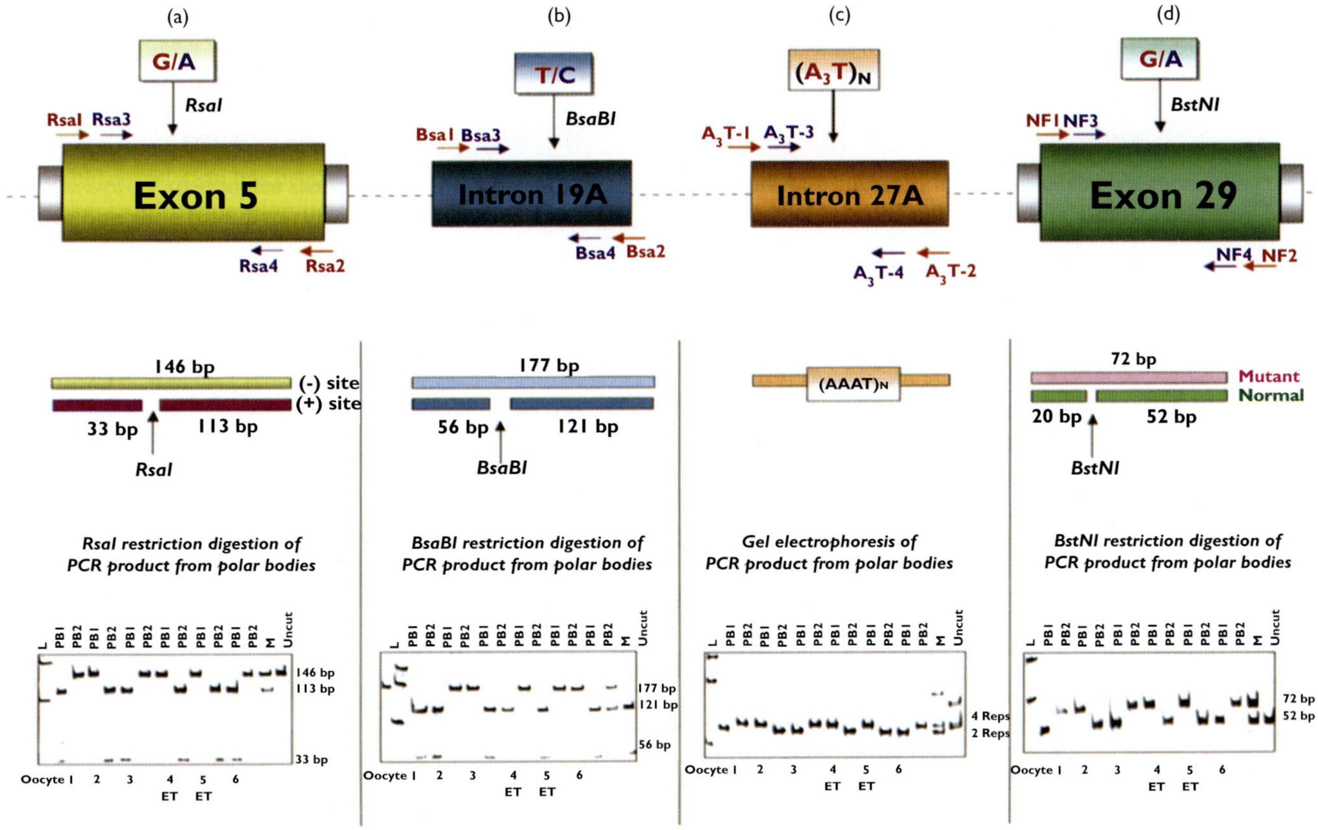

Figure 6.62 PGD for neurofibromatosis (NF1) nonsense mutation Trp→Ter (TGG→TGA) in exon 29. (Top) Schematic diagram of the mutation (d), and linked markers (a), (b), and (c) on chromosome 17q11.2. (Middle) Restriction maps for *BstNI* (d), *RsaI* (a), and *BsaBI* (b) restriction fragment length polymorphisms, and short tandem repeat in intron 27A (c). (Bottom) Polyacrylamide gel electrophoresis of the restriction-digested PCR products of the first (PB1) and second (PB2) polar bodies from six oocytes in the PGD cycle for NF1, showing mutation-free oocytes 2, 4, and 5, evidenced by a 72-bp undigested fragment in PB1 and a 52-bp digested fragment in the PB2 (d), in agreement with all three marker analyses (a), (b), and (c) (for linkages to mutant and normal alleles). L, standard size; M, maternal DNA; P, paternal DNA; ET, embryo transfer.

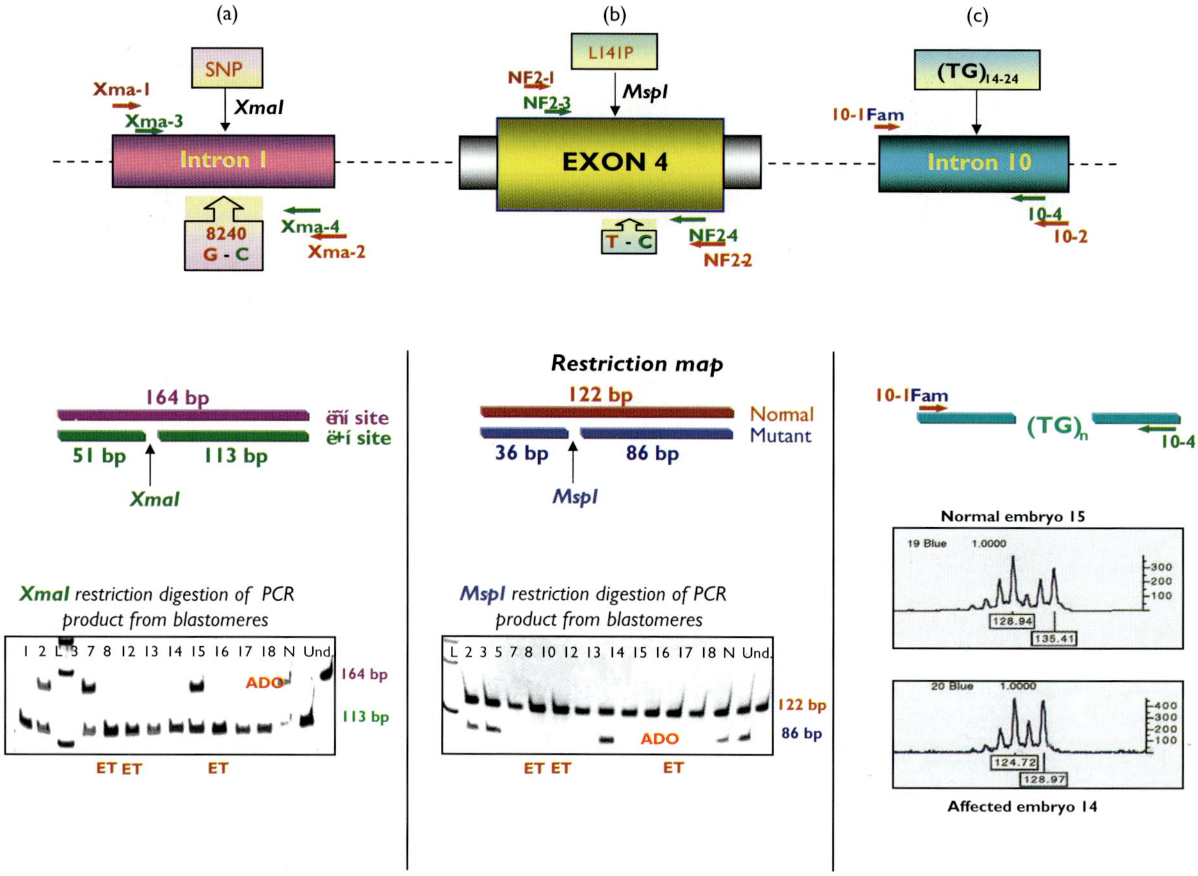

Figure 6.63 PGD for L141P mutation in exon 4 of neurofibromatosis 2 (*NF2*) gene. (Top) Schematic diagram of the mutation (b), and linked markers (a) and (c) on chromosome 22q12.2. (Middle) Restriction maps for *MspI* (b) and *XmaI* (a) restriction digestion in exon 4 and intron 1 of the *NF2* gene, and design for the dinucleotide TG repeat testing in intron 10 (c). (Bottom) Polyacrylamide gel electrophoresis of the restriction-digested PCR products of blastomeres, showing seven mutation-free embryos (5, 7, 8, 10, 13, 15, and 16), evidenced by the presence of a 122-bp undigested fragment, as compared to the presence of a digested 86-bp fragment in addition to a 122-bp fragment in the remaining embryos (b), in agreement with *XmaI* restriction length polymorphism in intron 1 (a), and dinucleotide TG repeats in intron 10 (the latter being detected by fluorescent capillary electrophoresis (c)) shown for normal embryo 14, as an example (for the linkages to normal and mutant genes, see Figure 6.62). ET, embryo transfer; ADO, allele dropout.

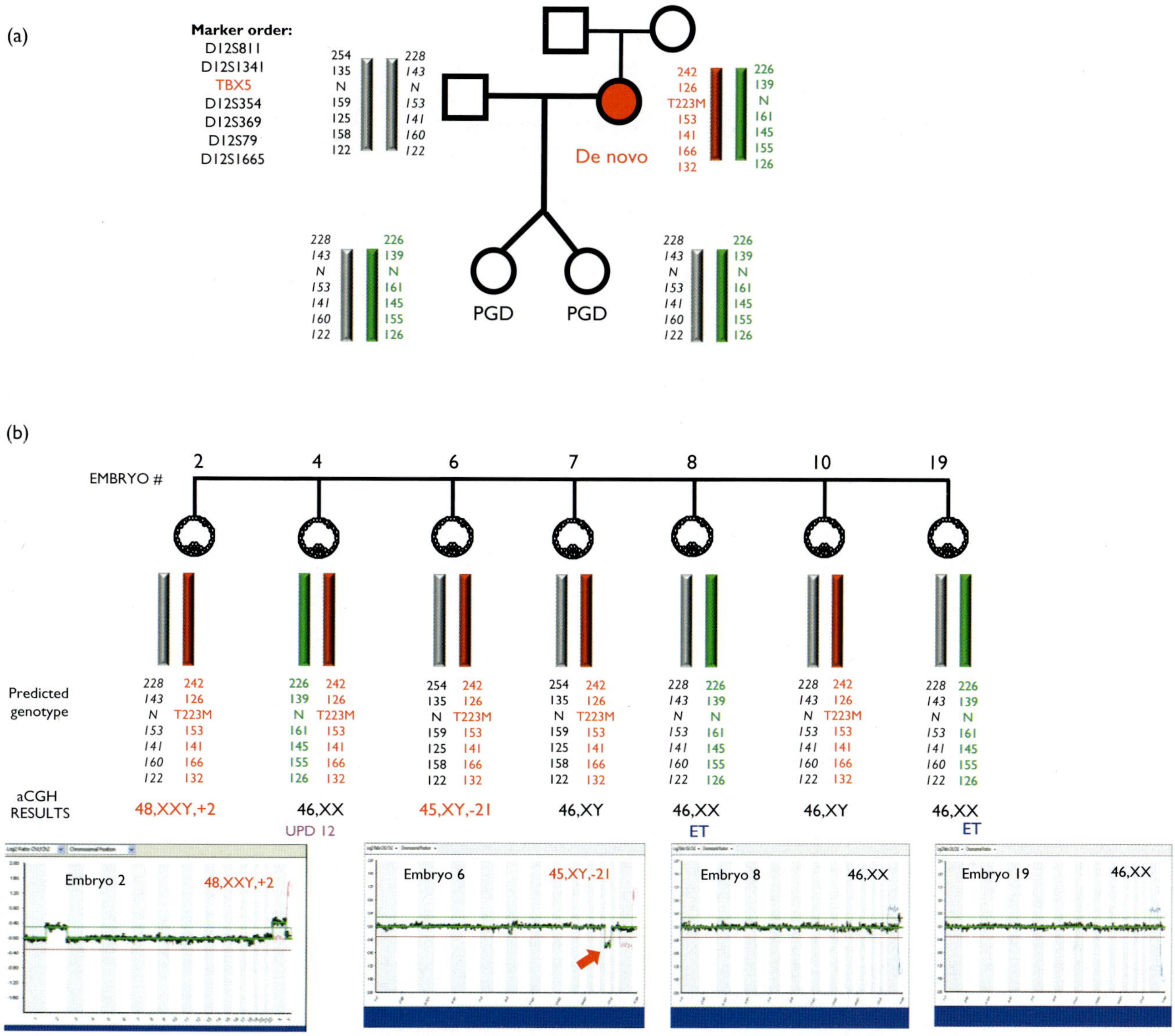

Figure 6.64 PGD for Holt–Oram syndrome, determined by missense mutation (T223M) in *TBX5* gene, combined with 24-chromosome aneuploidy testing by array-CGH. (a) Family pedigree, showing that female partner has a *de novo* mutation (marker order is presented on the left). (b) Trophectoderm analysis of seven embryos detected only two mutation-free embryos (embryos 8 and 10), the remaining five embryos containing the T223M mutation. As seen on the bottom of Panel (a), embryo 2 also has a trisomy 2, and embryo 6 also has monosomy 21. Mutation-free embryos (embryos 8 and 19) were also euploid, so were transferred, resulting in a twin pregnancy and birth of unaffected twins free of T223M mutation.

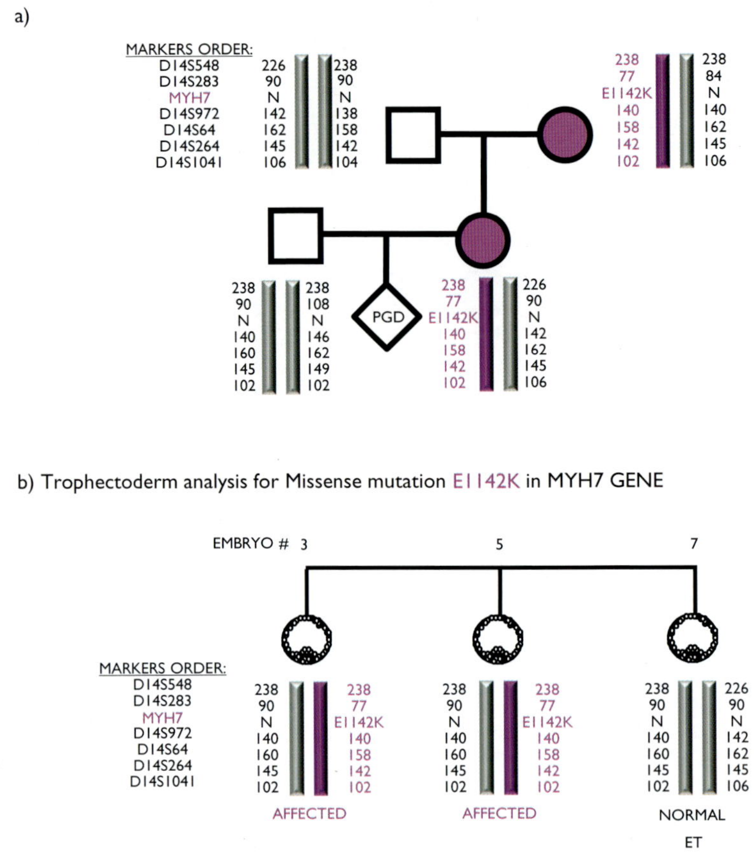

Figure 6.65 PGD for familial hypertrophic cardiomyopathy (CMH1), determined by dominant missense mutation E1142K in *MYH7* gene located in chromosome 14 (14q12). (a) Family pedigree of a couple with affected female partner carrying mutation E1142K in the *MYH7* gene. Maternally linked polymorphic markers are shown on the right, and paternal on the left, and the order of the maternal markers and mutation in the *MYH7* gene are shown on the upper left. Despite only a possible few symptoms, related to the heart function, the patient was at risk for cardiac failure and sudden death provoked by excessive exercise. The gene was inherited from her mother, who has no clinical symptoms. (b) Blastocyst biopsy and trophectoderm analysis for missense mutation in *MYH7* gene, showing that only one embryo is free of mutation, with the other two embryos containing the mutant gene. This single normal embryo (embryo 7) was transferred, resulting in an ongoing unaffected pregnancy.

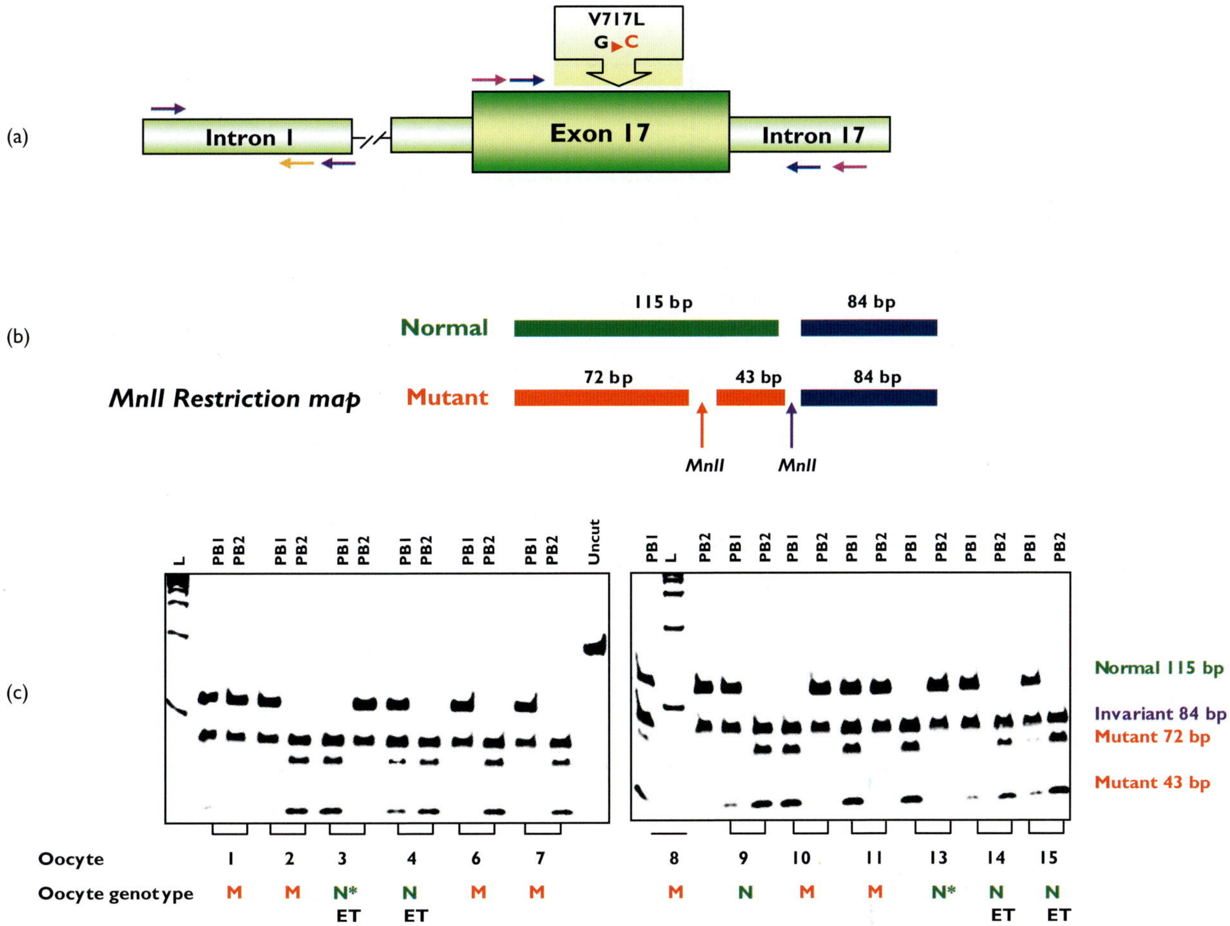

Figure 6.66 PGD for V717L mutation in the amyloid precursor protein (*APP*) gene, causing early onset of Alzheimer disease. (a) Map of the human *APP* gene, showing sites and location of V17L G–C mutation and polymorphic markers. (b) Restriction map for normal and abnormal alleles. (c) Polyacrylamide gel analysis of *MnlI* restriction digestion, showing six unaffected (N) oocytes (3, 4, 9, 13, 14, and 15), and seven mutant (M) oocytes (1, 2, 6, 7, 8, 10, and 11). Four of six embryos resulting from unaffected oocytes (3, 4, 14, and 15) were transferred back to the patient, resulting in an unaffected pregnancy. Three of these oocytes had a heterozygous first polar body (PB1) and mutant second polar body (PB2) (noted as N), and only one oocyte (3) had a homozygous mutant PB1 and normal PB2, leaving a 5% probability for misdiagnosis, noted as N*. ET, embryo transfer; L, ladder (size standard); Uncut, the undigested PCR product. Arrows indicate fully nested primer sets.

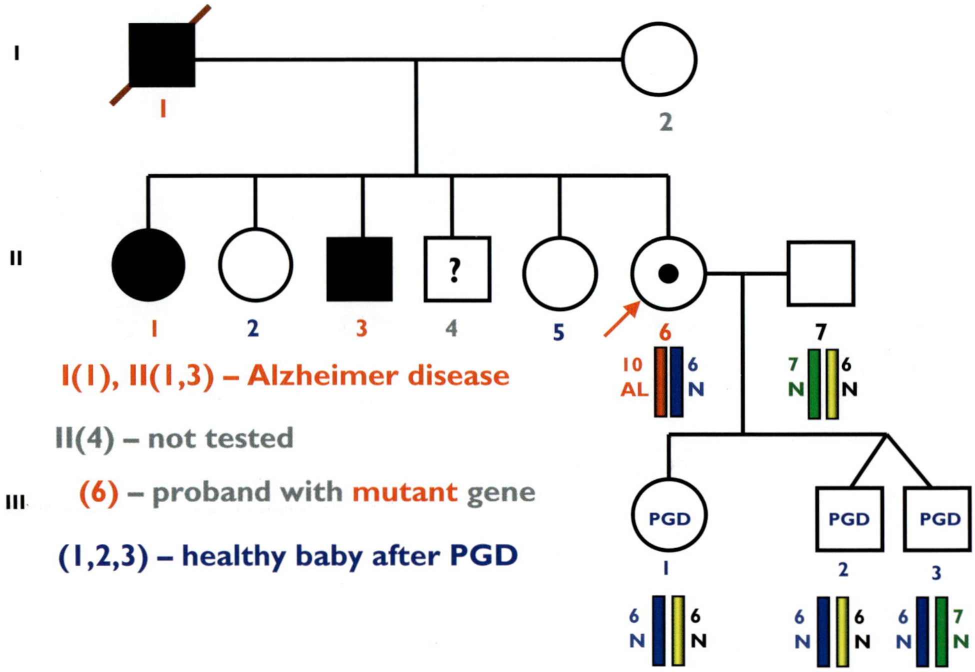

Figure 6.67 Pedigree of a family with early-onset Alzheimer disease (AD). Two PGD cycles for an asymptomatic carrier of the mutant gene (II,6) both resulted in the birth of an unaffected child (III). The haplotype analysis shows that these children inherited the normal maternal allele linked to the six repeats. Her sister (II,1) and brother (II,3) were affected by early-onset AD, as well as her father (I). N, normal.

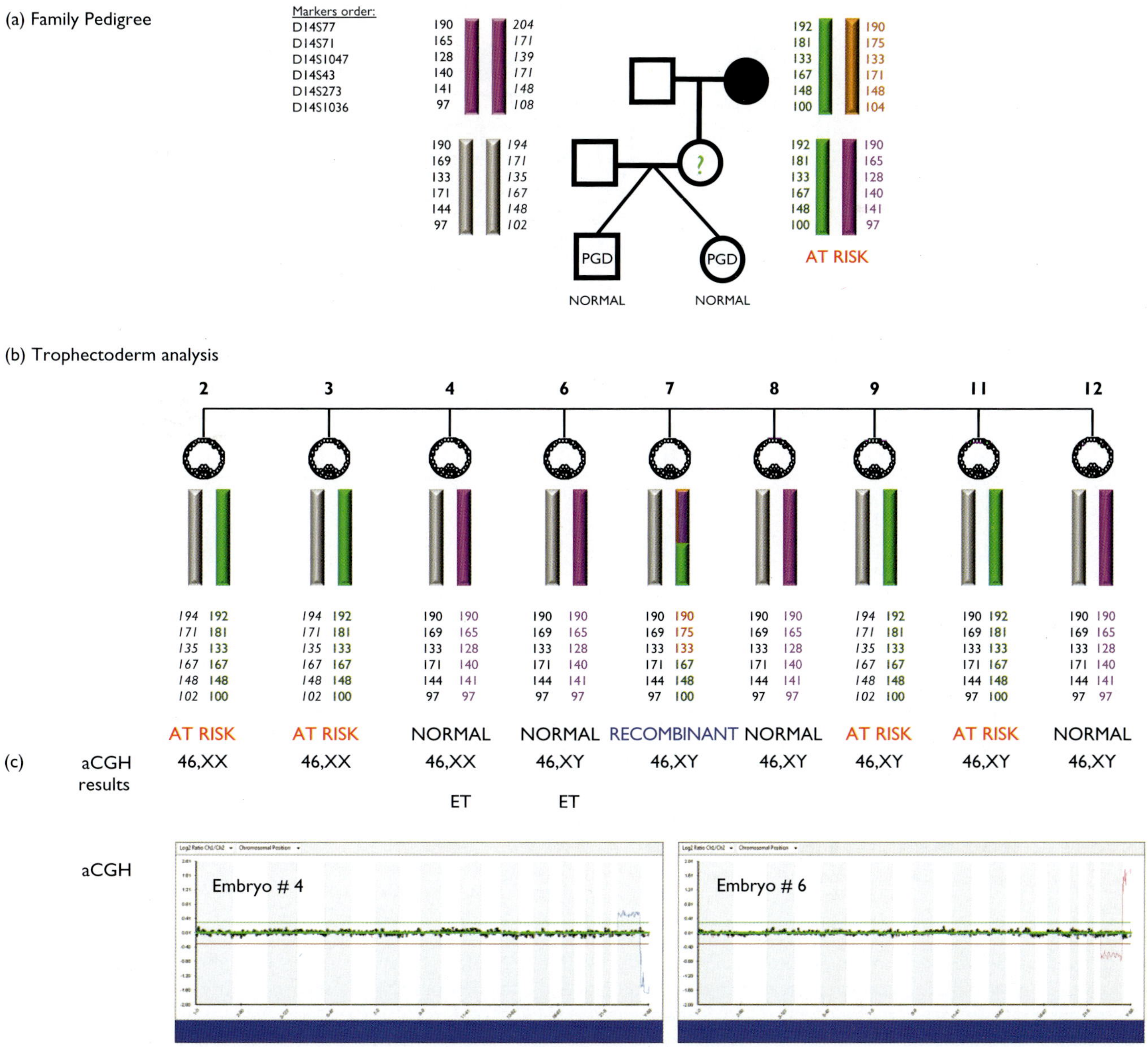

Figure 6.68 Indirect non-disclosure PGD for early Alzheimer disease (*PSEN1* gene) combined with aneuploidy testing by array-CGH. (a) Pedigree of a family with early-onset Alzheimer disease (AD) detected in the mother (the mutant haplotype is shown in green) of the female partner, who does not want to know her carrier status, but requested that her embryos be tested to avoid the inheritance of early onset AD gene (*PSEN1*) by her progeny. Marker order for tracing this gene is shown on the left. (b) Trophectoderm analysis of nine embryos revealed four embryos at risk (embryos 2, 3, 9, and 11) and one recombinant (embryo 7). Four embryos (embryos 4, 6, 8, and 12) were free of the gene predisposing to early AD. These embryos were also aneuploidy free, based on 24-chromosome testing by array-CGH analysis (results of array-CGH for embryos 3 and 4 are shown on the bottom panel). The latter two embryos were transferred, resulting in the birth of twins free from *PSEN1* gene, so with no risk of development of early onset AD (see the bottom line of pedigree).

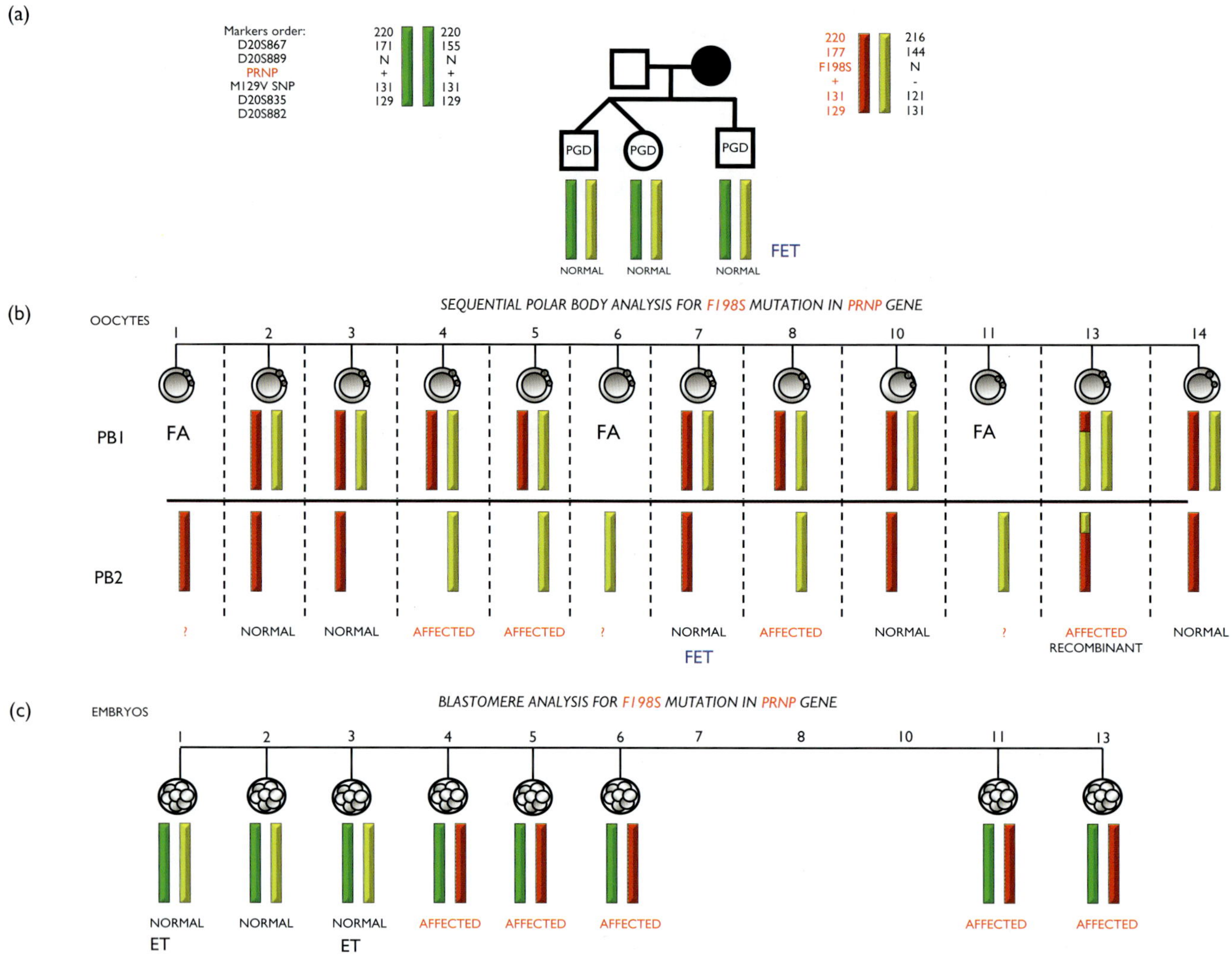

Figure 6.69 PGD for Gerstmann–Sträussler–Scheinker syndrome, a familial fatal neurodegenerative disorder determined by an autosomal dominant mutation in the prion protein gene (*PRNP*) with extremely high penetrance. (a) Pedigree, showing that maternal partner is a 28-year-old asymptomatic woman with a F198S mutation identified by predictive testing in a family with a known history of Gerstmann–Sträussler–Scheinker syndrome (GSS) due to a mutation in *PRNP* gene, causing phenylalanine to serine substitution at codon 198 (F198S) in the *PRNP* gene. Marker order in relation to the gene is shown on the left. (b) Sequential PB1 and PB2 mutation analysis of 12 oocytes, with the results available for nine oocytes, four of which were with the mutation, including one recombinant oocyte (oocyte 13). The remaining five oocytes with DNA results were free of F198S mutation (oocytes 2, 3, 7, 10, and 14), three of which were from oocytes with heterozygous PB1 and hemizygous mutant PB2 (oocytes 7, 10, and 14). (c) Blastomere analysis of eight embryos deriving either from the oocytes with failed amplification of PB1, or with ADO of linked markers, or from affected oocytes for confirmation. This analysis allowed detection of one additional mutation-free embryo for transfer (embryo 2), deriving from a mutation-free oocyte and confirmed normal. Two embryos (1 and 3) were transferred, resulting in the birth of healthy twins free of F198S mutation, thus with no predisposition to this familial fatal prion-related neurodegenerative disorder. The third mutation free baby was born following frozen transfer of embryo deriving from mutation free oocyte 7.

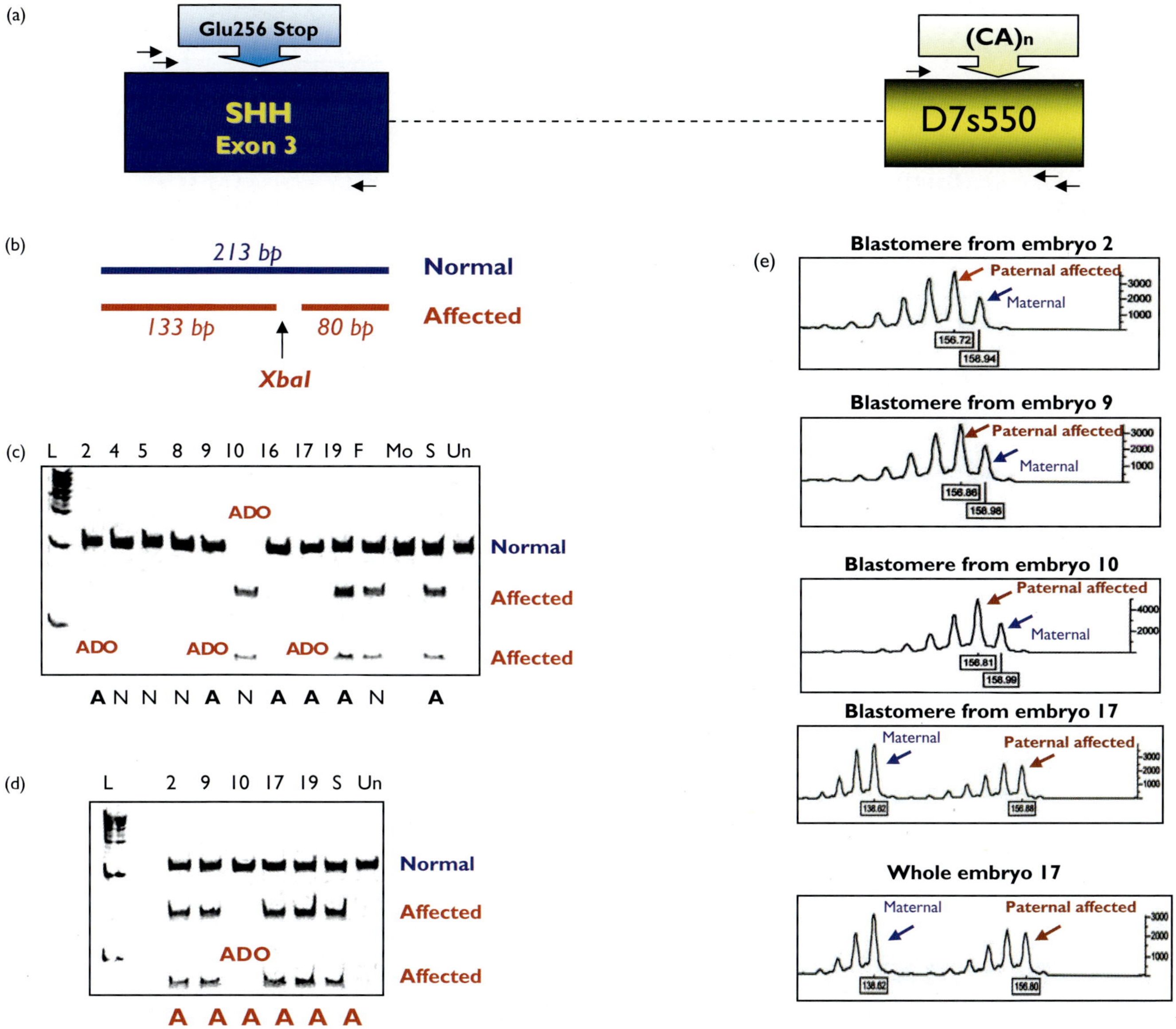

Figure 6.70 Preimplantation diagnosis for nonsense mutation Glu256 stop in exon 3 of sonic hedgehog (*SHH*) gene, causing holoprosencephaly. (a) Schematic diagram of the mutation and D7S550 linked marker on chromosome 7. The black arrows demonstrate the positions of heminested primers. (b) Restriction map for *XbaI* digestion, showing the gain of *XbaI* site by the mutant allele (lower line). (c) Polyacrylamide gel electrophoresis of the *XbaI*-digested PCR products of nine blastomeres from PGD cycle. L, 100-bp standard; ADO, allele dropout; F, paternal DNA amplified from sperm; Mo, maternal normal amplified DNA; S, amplified DNA from affected baby; Un, undigested PCR product; A, affected blastomere; N, normal blastomere. (d) Follow-up DNA analysis of genomic DNA from five embryos predicted to be affected by blastomere testing. (e) Capillary electrophoregrams of the fluorescently labeled PCR product of tightly linked marker D7S550. The paternally derived 156-bp dinucleotide C–A repeats linked to the *SHH* mutation are shown by arrows (noted as "Paternal affected") in the blastomeres of embryos 2, 9, 10, and 17 and the genomic DNA of the whole embryo 10, in which ADO of the mutant gene was seen in the follow-up study (see (d), embryo 10). Maternally derived 158-bp dinucleotide C–A repeats of D7S550 polymorphic marker are shown by arrows (noted as "Maternal") in the blastomeres of embryos 2, 9, and 10, while the other maternally derived 138-bp repeats of D7S550 are shown in the blastomere of embryo 17.

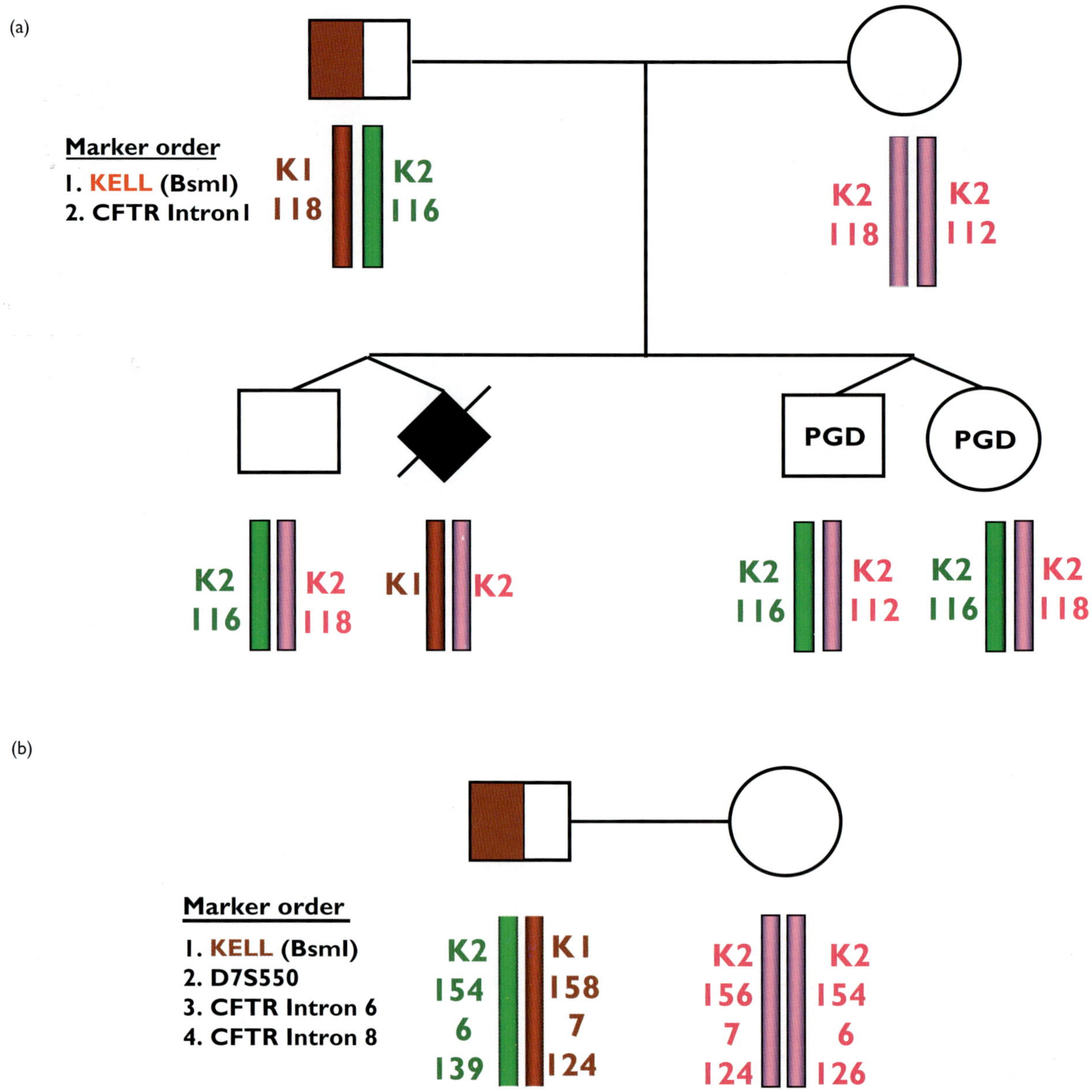

Figure 6.71 Pedigree of couples at risk for producing children with Kell disease presented for PGD. (a) Pedigree of the first family. (Top) The father (upper left) has K1/K2 genotype, K1 allele linked to 118-bp repeats and K2 allele to 116-bp repeats of intron 1 of the CFTR polymorphic marker, while the mother (upper right) has the K2/K2 genotype, one allele linked to 118-bp repeats and the other to 112-bp repeats of intron 1 of CFTR polymorphic marker. (Bottom) Reproductive outcomes of this couple, including previous twin pregnancy resulting in the neonatal death of one of the twins due to hemolytic disease of the newborn (HDN) (lower left). Two healthy twins with K2/K2 genotype resulting from PGD are shown on lower right, as also seen from the information on linked polymorphic markers. (b) Haplotypes of the second couple. The father (upper left) has the K1/K2 genotype, with linkage shown for K1 and K2 alleles, while the mother (upper right) has the K2/K2 genotype, with linkage shown for both normal alleles.

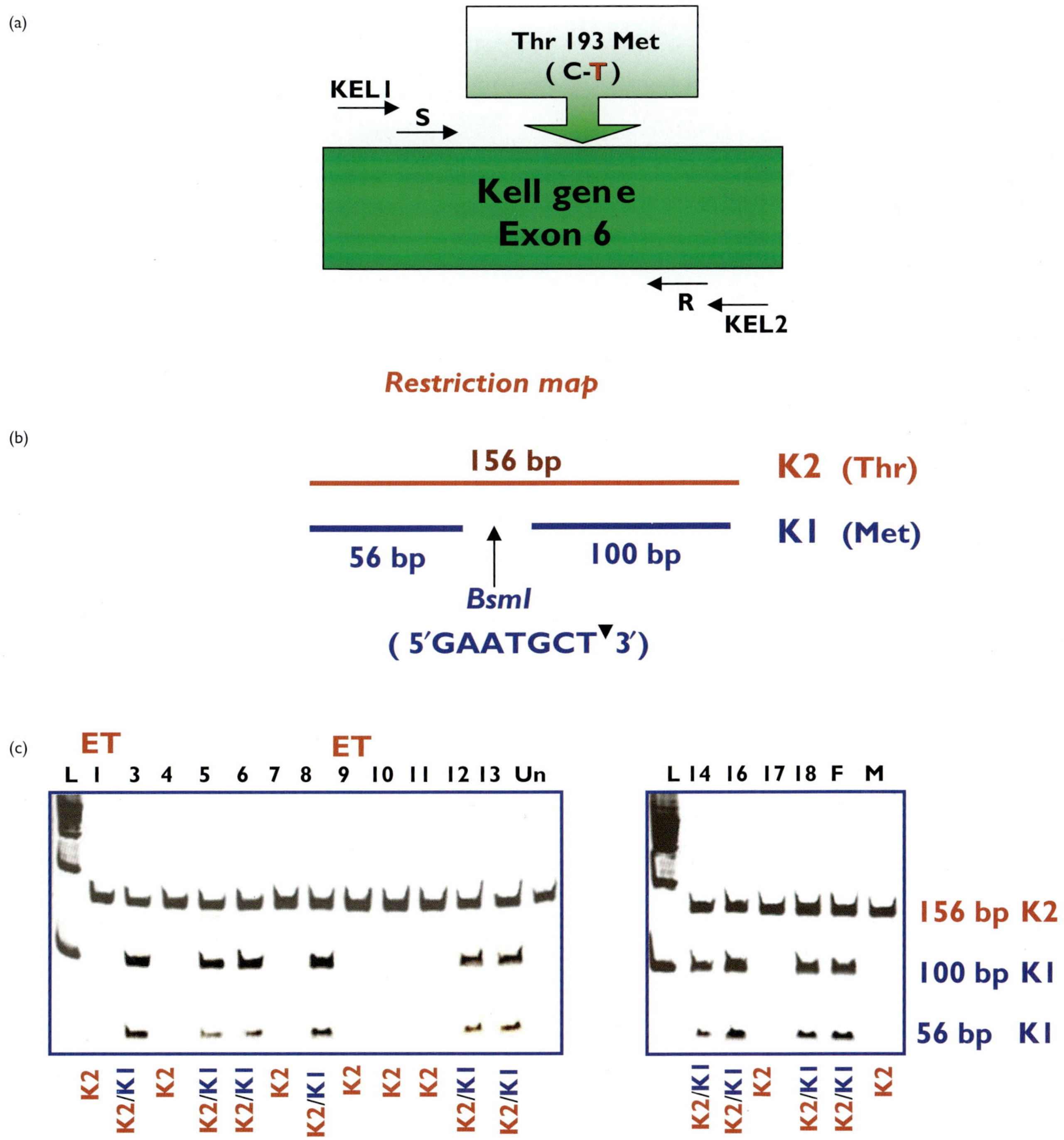

Figure 6.72 Preimplantation genetic diagnosis for Kell genotype. (a) Schematic diagram showing C>T substitution in exon 6 of *KEL* gene on chromosome 7. Black arrows demonstrate the positions of nested primers. (b) Restriction map for *BsmI* digestion, showing the gain of *BsmI* site by the K1 allele (lower line). (c) Polyacrylamide gel electrophoresis of the *BsmI*-digested PCR products of 16 blastomeres from the first PGD couple (shown in Figure 6.71a), demonstrating K1-allele-free genotype in embryos 1, 4, 7, 9, 10, 11, and 17, from which embryos 1 and 9 were transferred, resulting in a twin pregnancy and birth of healthy K1-allele-free children. The remaining nine embryos had the K1/K2 genotype. L, standard; F, paternal DNA amplified from sperm; M, maternal normal amplified DNA; Un, undigested PCR product; K1/K2, affected blastomere; K2/K2, normal blastomere.

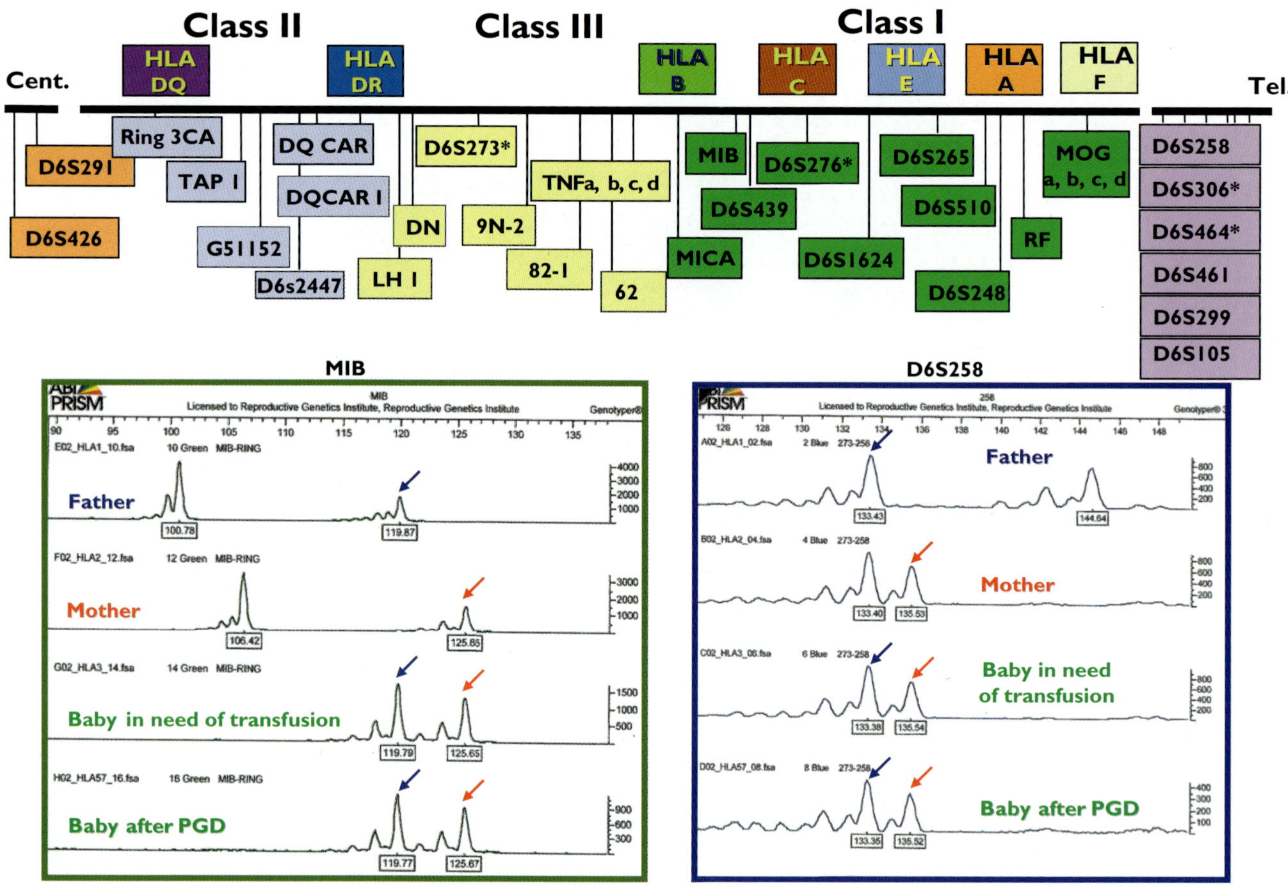

Figure 6.73 A set of polymorphic short tandem repeat (STR) markers in the HLA region used for preimplantation HLA typing. (Top) Schematic representation of STRs in HLA classes I, II, and III on chromosome 6. All STR markers are dinucleotide repeats (AC)n, except for DQCAR II, which is a (CTG)n; TNF b, c, d, which are (CT)n; 62 which is a (TC-CA)n; Mic A, which is a (GCT)n; D6S510, which is a (CA-GA)n; MOG d, which is (CTC)n. Cent., centromere, Tel., telomere. (Bottom) Examples of capillary electrophoregrams of fluorescently labeled PCR products of MIB marker (left) and D6S258 marker (right). Blue arrow, paternal matching marker; red arrow, maternal matching marker.

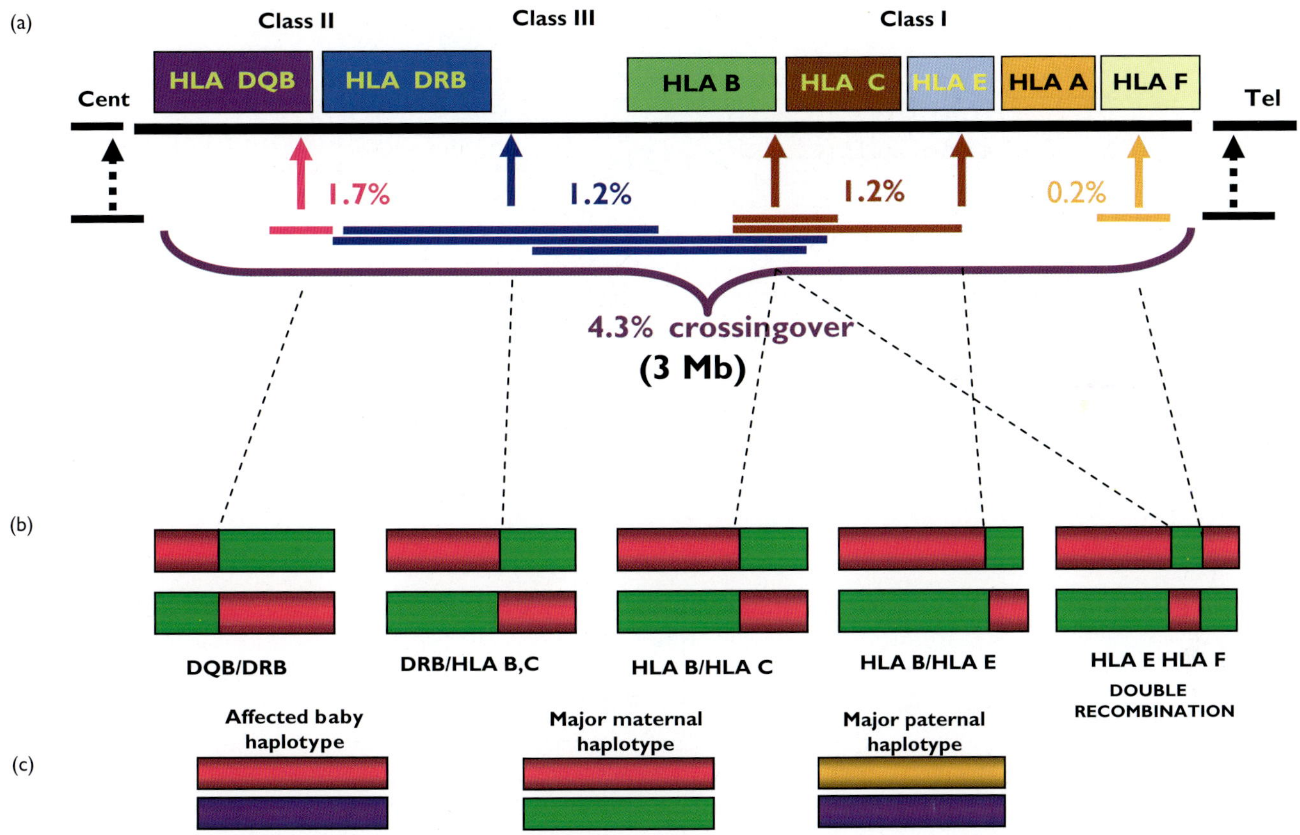

Figure 6.74 Recombination in HLA region observed in preimplantation HLA typing of 330 embryos (frequency and position). (a) Position of HLA genes of class II, III, and I. Pink line and arrow show recombination observed between *DQB* and *DRB* genes. Blue lines and arrow correspond to the recombination detected between class II and III HLA genes. Brown lines and arrows indicate recombination detected between HLA B and HLA C genes and between HLA B and HLA E genes from class I. Yellow line and arrow show recombination occurring between HLA A and HLA F genes from class I. The size of the HLA area is approximately three megabases (Mb). Overall, the observed recombination rate was 4.3%. (b) Maternal haplotype disruption as a result of meiotic recombination between the different HLA genes (based on short tandem repeat (STR) analysis of the HLA area). (c) Schematic representation of the paternal, maternal, and affected child haplotypes. Successful cord blood stem cell transfusion depends upon the number of HLA alleles in the sample matching that of the affected child. Recombination of maternal and paternal (not shown) alleles during meiosis leads to the haplotype changes, affecting the chances for identification of matching alleles. Application of a set of polymorphic markers throughout the HLA area improves the accuracy of preimplantation HLA matching. Cent, centromeric area; Tel, telomeric area.

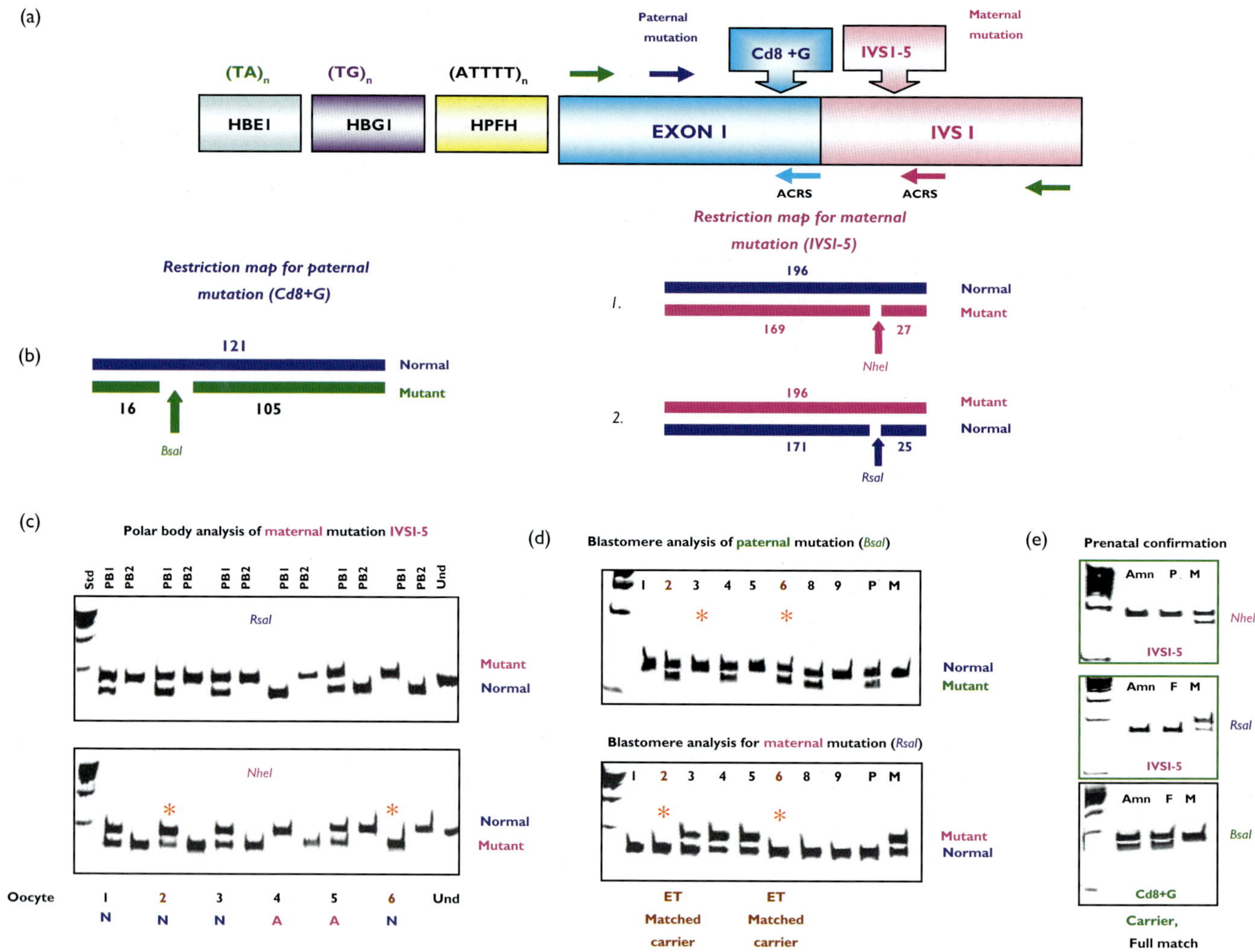

Figure 6.75 Preimplantation HLA typing combined with PGD for β-globin mutation, resulting in the birth of an unaffected HLA-matched healthy child. (a) Position of two different mutations and informative linked polymorphic markers used in PGD. Colored arrows represent heminested primers designed for the mutation analysis. Application of outside primers for testing both maternal and paternal mutation improves the allele dropout (ADO) detection rate. Two different artificially created restriction site (ACRS) primers were used in the second round of heminested PCR to detect the maternal and paternal mutations. (b) Restriction maps for the paternal (left) and maternal (right) mutation. The previously mentioned ACRS primers introduce the *BsaI* restriction site to the mutant paternal sequence. Two different ACRS primers were designed to detect the maternal mutation: one introduced the *NheI* restriction site to the mutant sequence, and the other introduced the *RsaI* restriction site to the normal β-globin sequence, with both increasing the reliability of the mutation analysis to overcome potential problems due to incomplete digestion of the PCR product. (c) First (PB1) and second (PB2) polar body analysis for the maternal mutation IVSI-5. Polyacrylamide gel electrophoresis of PCR product digested with *RsaI* (upper panel) and *NheI* (lower panel) restriction enzymes. Based on this analysis, the oocytes 4 and 5 are predicted to contain the affected allele, and the remaining oocytes (1, 2, 3, and 6) are mutation free. (d) Blastomere analysis of paternal and maternal mutations. Polyacrylamide gel electrophoresis of the PCR product from blastomere amplification digested with *BsaI* restriction enzyme for the paternal (cd 8+G) mutation (top) and *RsaI* (bottom) confirming the presence of the maternal mutation (IVSI–5). (Haplotypes are shown in Figure 6.77 below). Two embryos (2 and 6) that were predicted to be carriers of the paternal mutation and to represent a full HLA match to the affected baby were transferred, resulting in a clinical pregnancy and the birth of a healthy child. (e) Prenatal confirmation of PGD results. Gel electrophoresis of digested PCR product from amniocytes and genomic DNA, confirming the unaffected status of the fetus carrying paternal mutant allele. Std, size standard; A, affected; N, normal; M, maternal genomic DNA; P, paternal genomic DNA; Und, undigested PCR product; * transferred embryos; ET, embryo transfer; Amn, amniocentesis.

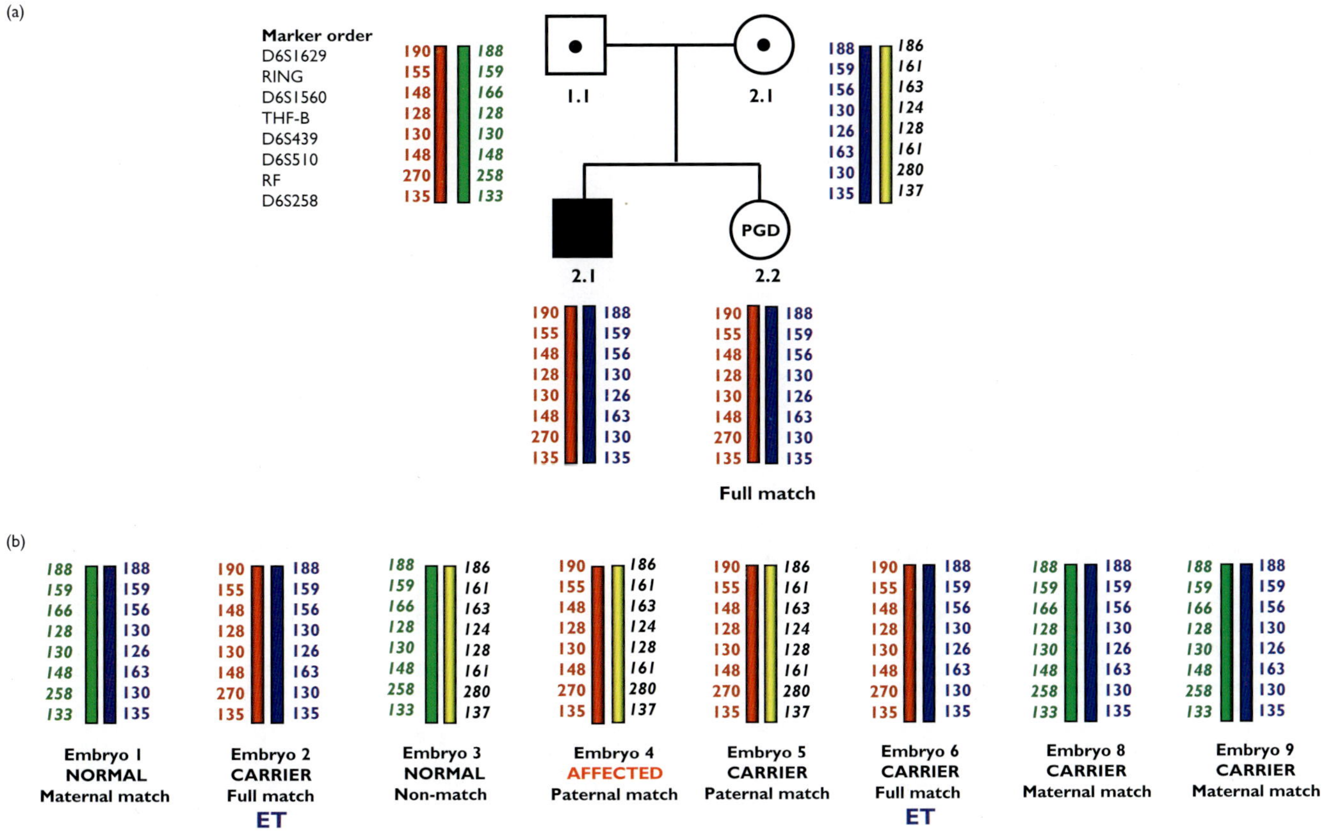

Figure 6.76 Preimplantation HLA matching combined with PGD for thalassemia (continued). (a) A family pedigree with HLA haplotype analysis based on parental (1.1 and 1.2) and affected child's (2.1) genomic DNA testing. HLA marker order is presented at the upper left. Red bar, matching paternal HLA haplotype; green bar, non-matching haplotype; blue bar, maternal matching haplotype; yellow bar, non-matching haplotype. (b) HLA typing by short tandem repeats (STRs) along with mutation analysis was performed on blastomeres from eight embryos, two of which (2 and 6) were predicted to be an HLA match to that of the affected sibling (2.1), although they carried the paternal mutation (also see Figures 6.75 and 6.77). Prenatal testing confirmed these results, and a healthy baby girl with an HLA type matching that of the sick sibling was born. Cord blood stem cells were collected during delivery and frozen for future use.

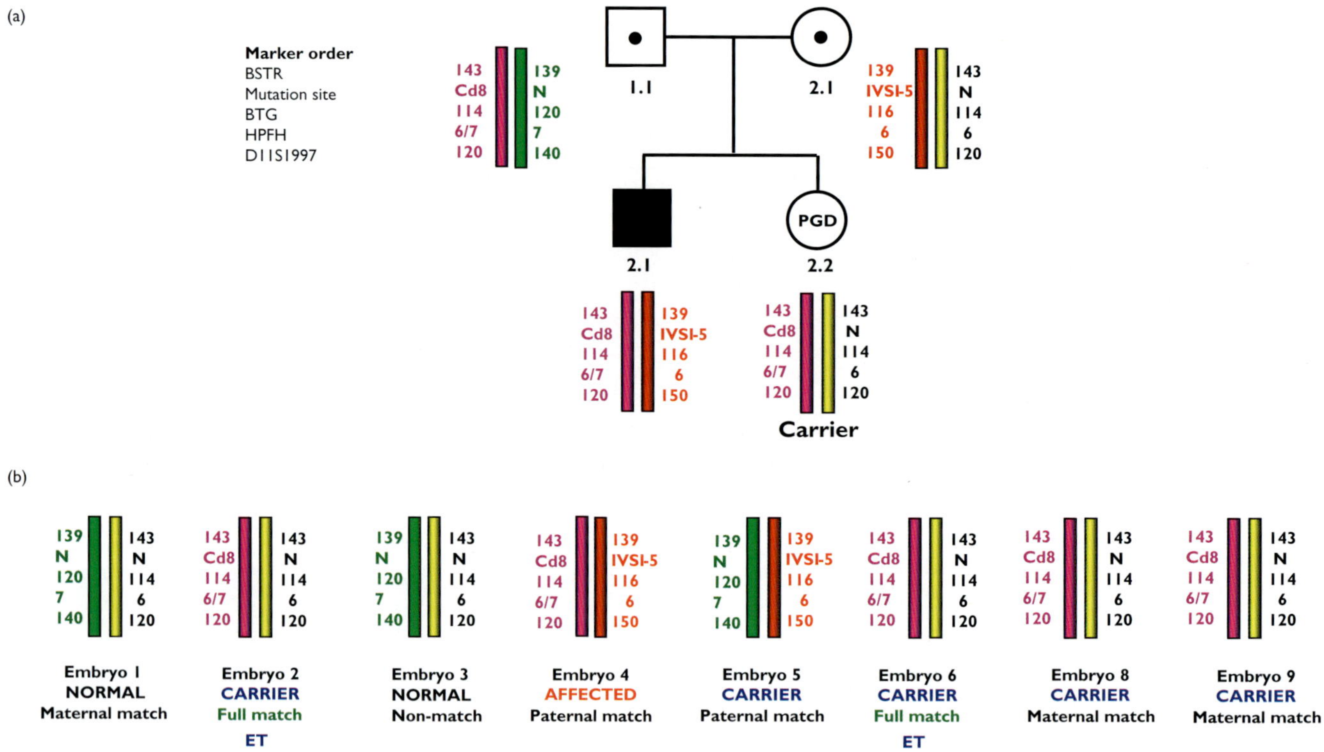

Figure 6.77 Preimplantation HLA matching and PGD for thalassemia (continued). (a) A family pedigree with β-globin haplotype analysis based on parental (1.1 and 1.2) and affected child's (2.1) genomic DNA testing. β-globin mutation and marker order are shown at the upper left. Red bar, maternal mutant haplotype; yellow bar, maternal normal haplotype; purple bar, paternal affected haplotype; green bar, normal paternal sequence and markers. (b) Maternal mutation and linked polymorphic markers were first assessed by sequential multiplex polar body analysis (see Figure 6.75). Two oocytes (4 and 5) had an affected allele, while the remaining six (oocytes 1, 2, 3, 6, 8, and 9) were normal. Based on blastomere results, one embryo was affected (number 4), two were homozygous normal (1 and 3), and five were carriers of paternal (2, 6, 8, and 9) or maternal (5) mutations. Embryos 2 and 6 are fully HLA-matched to the sick sibling (2.1) (see also Figure 6.74). Prenatal testing confirmed these results, and a healthy HLA-matching sibling baby girl was born.

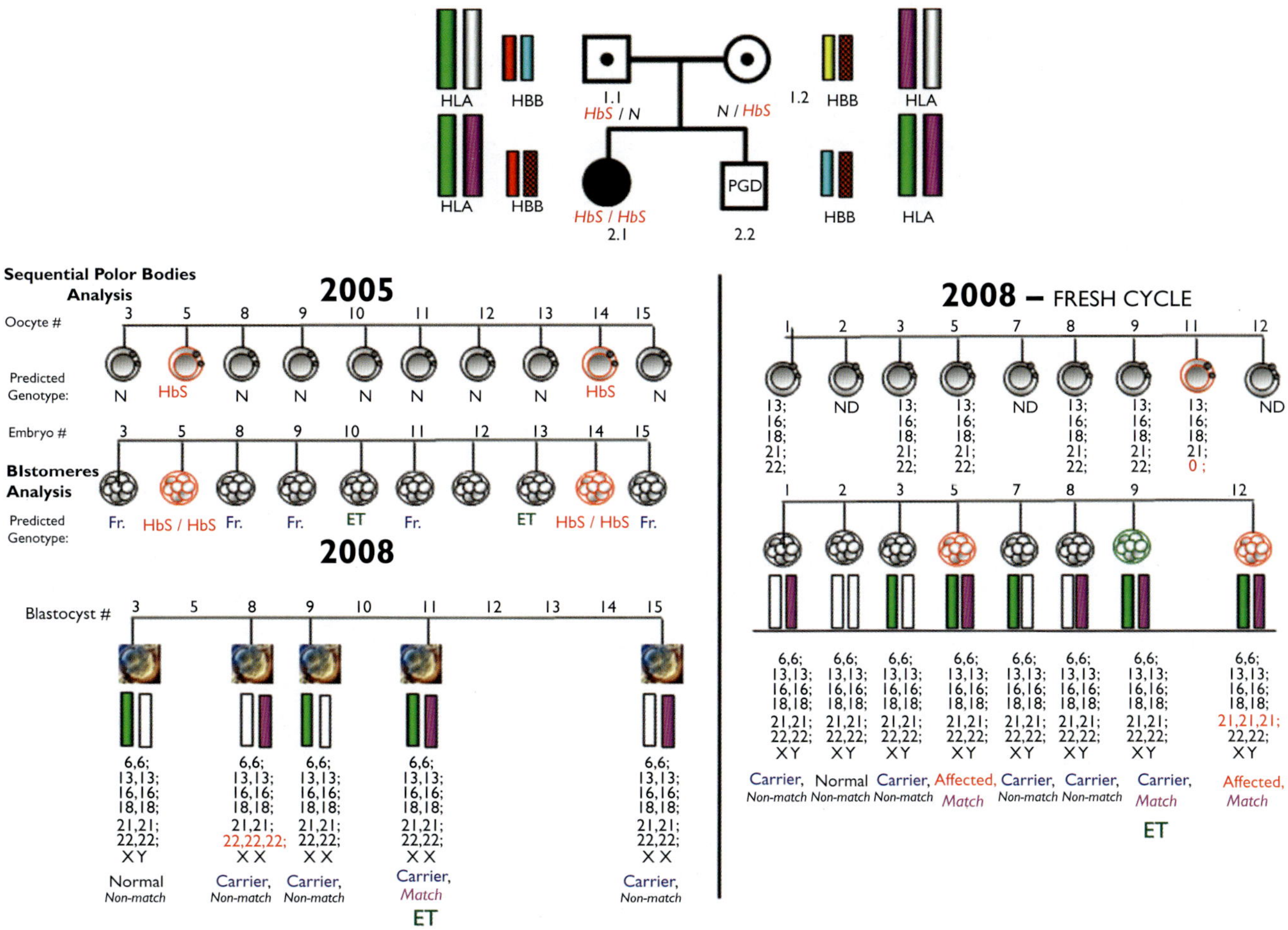

Figure 6.78 PGD for sickle cell anemia with HLA and aneuploidy testing. (Upper panel) Family pedigree showing maternal (1.1) and paternal (1.2) matching HLA haplotypes (violet for maternal and green for paternal). Both parents are carriers of *HbS* gene (shown in red). Affected sibling (shown in black) has sickle cell disease (HbS/HbS) requiring HLA matched stem cell transplantation. (Middle left panel) Results of PGD cycle in 2005, without HLA typing, involving mutation testing by polar body analysis of ten oocytes, two of which (oocytes 5 and 14) were predicted to be affected, also confirmed by blastomere analysis, shown under each oocyte. Only one of the unaffected embryos (embryo 10) was transferred, while others were frozen and reanalyzed in 2008 for HLA typing and aneuploidy. (Bottom left panel) This resulted in finding one HLA-matched embryo (embryo 11). This embryo was transferred together with another matched unaffected embryo, detected in the fresh PGD cycle shown in the right panel. (Middle right panel) Results of PGD cycle for HbS in 2008, with aneuploidy testing by polar body analysis of nine oocytes, followed by mutation testing and HLA typing in each resulting embryo (shown under each oocyte). Only one unaffected heterozygous embryo (embryo 9) appeared to be HLA-matched and was transferred together with another unaffected HLA-matched embryo from the frozen cycle mentioned (see above), resulting in a singleton pregnancy and birth of an unaffected HLA-matched baby boy (shown as 2.2 in the upper panel), as a donor of stem cell transplantation for the affected sibling (2.1 in the upper panel).

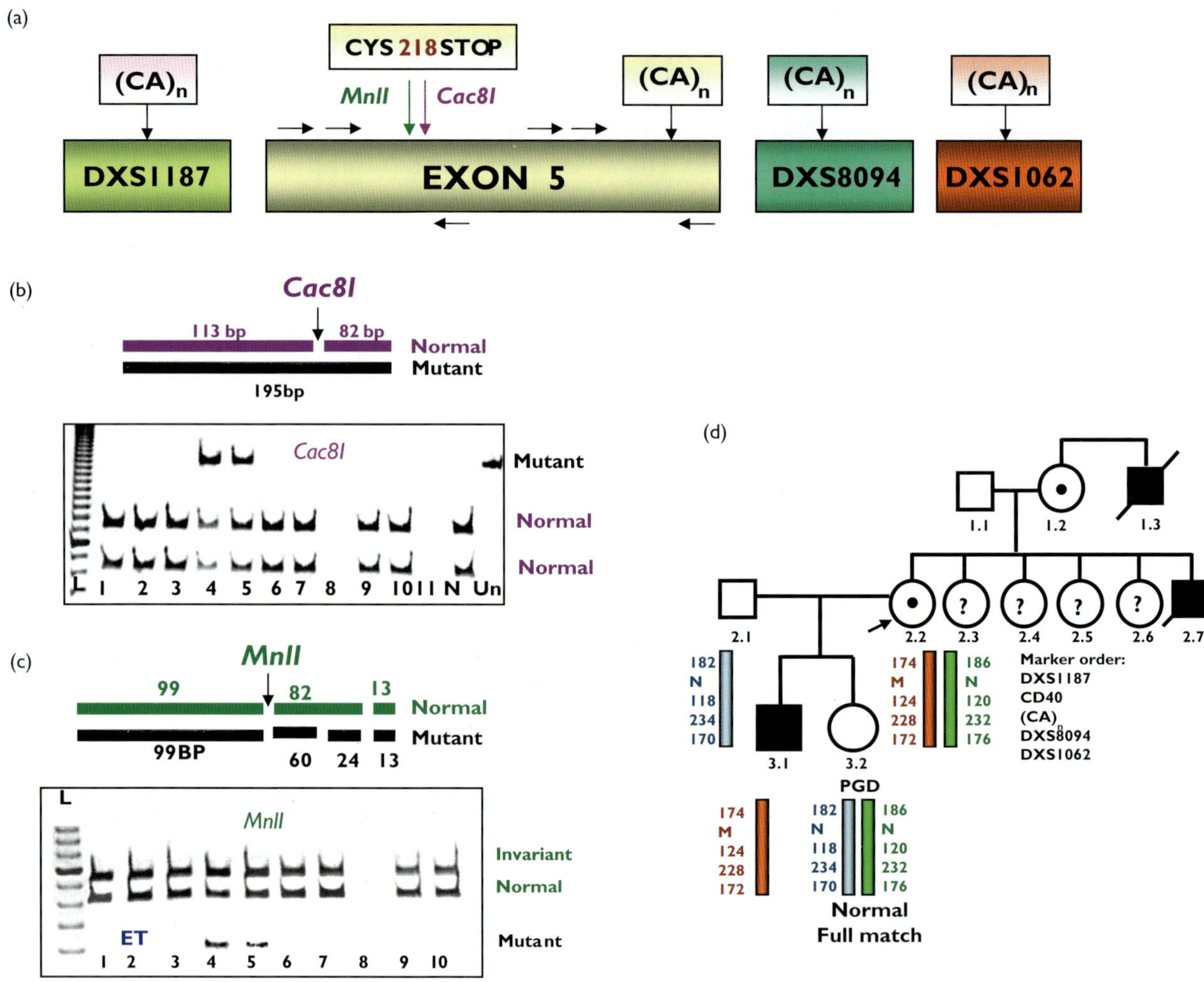

Figure 6.79 Preimplantation HLA typing combined with PGD for X-linked hyper-IgM syndrome. (a) The position of the C218X mutation in exon 5 of CD40 ligand gene (Xq26.3) and tightly linked dinucleotide polymorphic markers inside the gene (exon 5) and outside the gene (DXS1187, DXS8094, DXS1062). Horizontal arrows represent primer positions. Vertical arrows indicate the location of the *MnlI* and *Cac8I* restriction sites and the positions of the dinucleotide polymorphic markers. (b) Restriction map of the *CacI* restriction digestion and polyacrylamide gel analysis of PCR product from 11 blastomeres digested with Cac8I restriction enzyme. All but two embryos (4 and 5) were predicted to be normal based on the presence of two bands of 113 bp and 82 bp. Mutant 195-bp fragment was detected in blastomeres 4 and 5. L, size standard; bp, base pairs; N, normal control DNA; Un, undigested PCR product. (c) Restriction map for the *MnlI* digestion and polyacrylamide gel analysis of PCR product from ten blastomeres digested with *MnlI* restriction enzyme. Embryos 1, 2, 3, 6, 7, 9, and 10 were predicted to be normal based on the presence of 82-bp bands. A mutant 60-bp fragment was detected along with the normal 82-bp band in embryos 4 and 5. By the presence of both normal and affected sequences and polymorphic markers DXS1187, DXS8094, and DXS1062, these embryos were predicted to be carriers. HLA typing was performed simultaneously with mutation analysis on all blastomeres. Embryo 2 was predicted to be a normal female and to have the same HLA profile as the affected sibling (3.1). The transfer of this embryo resulted in pregnancy and the birth of a healthy unaffected HLA-matched baby girl (3.2). Cord blood stem cells were collected at birth and stored for the future transfusion. (d) The family pedigree of this family with hyper-IgM syndrome in three generations. Marker order is located next to maternal haplotypes. Paternal (2.1), maternal (2.2), and the affected sibling (3.1) CD40 gene haplotype assignment is based on genomic DNA testing.

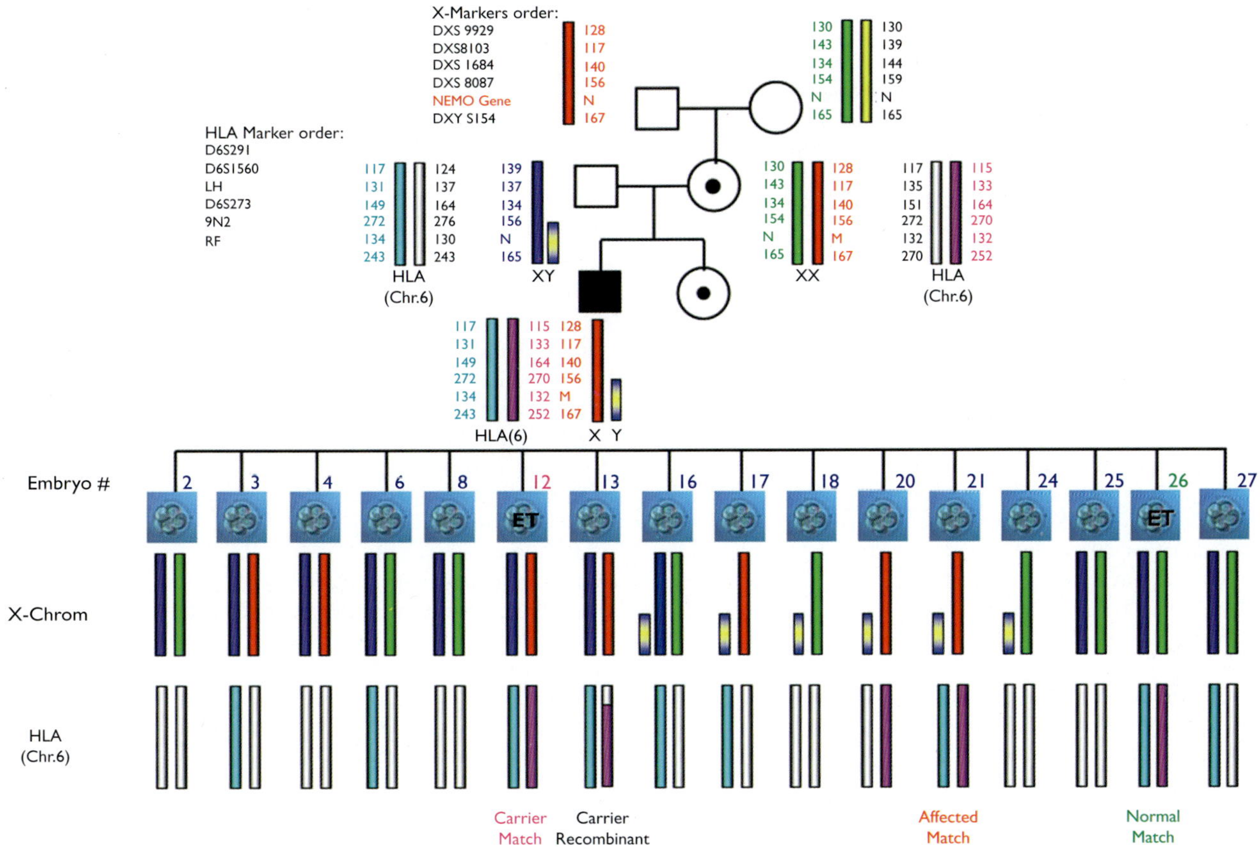

Figure 6.80 PGD for X-linked hypohidrotic ectodermal dysplasia (*NEMO-IKBKG* gene) with immune deficiency and HLA typing. (Upper panel) Family pedigree showing maternal and paternal matching HLA haplotypes (red for maternal and green for paternal). Marker order for testing *NEMO* gene is located next to maternal haplotypes (red). Paternal, maternal, and the affected sibling's (shown in black) *NEMO* gene haplotype assignment is based on genomic DNA testing. As seen from the pedigree, the mutant haplotype originated from the grandfather, who has no mutant gene in his blood cells, but seems to harbor *de novo* mutation of the *NEMO* gene in his gonads, inherited by affected sibling's mother. (Middle panel) Results of blastomere DNA analysis from 16 embryos showing that three embryos were affected (embryos 17, 20, and 21), one with extra X chromosome, suggesting the XXY genotype (embryo 16), with the remaining being either carriers or unaffected. (Lower panel) HLA typing was performed simultaneously with mutation analysis of all blastomeres, showing that two of the unaffected embryos (embryos 12 and 26) were also HLA matched to the affected sibling (one embryo, embryo 13, was recombinant). In addition one embryo, embryo 21, was also HLA matched but affected. Embryos 12 and 26 were transferred, resulting in a pregnancy and birth of a healthy unaffected HLA-matched baby girl, shown in the upper panel. Cord blood stem cells from this child were collected at birth and transplanted to the affected child, resulting in a total cure.

Index